SKIN DEEP

SKIN DEEP

An A–Z of Skin Disorders,
Treatments and Health

Updated Edition

Carol A. Turkington
and
Jeffrey S. Dover, M.D.

Medical Illustrations by
Birck Cox

☑® Facts On File, Inc.

Skin Deep: An A–Z of Skin Disorders, Treatments and Health, Updated Edition

Facts On File, Inc.
11 Penn Plaza
New York, NY 10001

Library of Congress Cataloging-in-Publication Data
Turkington, Carol.
Skin deep : an A–Z of skin disorders, treatments and health /
Carol A. Turkington and Jeffrey S. Dover ; medical illustrations by
Birck Cox.—Updated ed.
p.   cm.
Includes bibliographical references and index.
ISBN 0-8160-3826-0 (pbk.)
1. Dermatology—Encyclopedias.   2. Skin—Diseases—Encyclopedias.
3. Skin—Encyclopedias.   I. Dover, Jeffrey S.   II. Title.
RL41.T87   1998
616.5'003—dc21   98-11760

Facts On File books are available at special discounts when purchased in bulk
quantities for businesses, associations, institutions or sales promotions. Please
call our Special Sales Department in New York at 212/967-8800 or 800/322-8755.

You can find Facts On File on the World Wide Web at
http://www.factsonfile.com

Cover design by Cathy Rincon
Illustrations by Birck Cox

Printed in the United States of America

RRD VC 10 9 8 7 6 5 4 3 2 1

This book is printed on acid-free paper.

To Dottie Kennedy,
for her unfailing support

CONTENTS

ACKNOWLEDGMENTS

Thanks to Birck Cox for providing terrific drawings; to my editor Michelle Fellner for patient editing; and, as always, to my agent Bert Holtje for his tireless efforts.

Thanks also to the staffs of the American Academy of Dermatology, the American Dermatological Association, the American College of Allergy and Immunology, Jeff Bender at the American Academy of Allergy and Immunology, the American Hair Loss Council, Susan Kastner at the American Leprosy Missions, the American Society for Dermatologic Surgery, the American Society of Plastic and Reconstructive Surgeons, the Dystrophic Epidermolysis Bullosa Research Association of America, the Foundation for Ichthyosis and Related Skin Types, the National Tuberous Sclerosis Association, the National Institutes of Health, Maggie Bartlett and Donna at the National Cancer Institute, the National Institute of Arthritis, Musculoskeletal and Skin Diseases, Dr. Amy Paller at the Society for Pediatric Dermatology, the Psoriasis Research Institute, the National Vitiligo Foundation, the Skin Cancer Foundation, Suzanne Corr at the National Rosacea Society.

Thanks also to the librarians of Hershey Medical Center medical library, the National Library of Medicine, the Reading Public Library, the Reading Hospital Medical Library, the Chester County Library and the Pennsylvania State Library/Berks Campus.

Finally, thanks to Kara and Michael for unfailing support.

SKIN DEEP

Updated Edition

A

abdominoplasty A surgical technique used to tighten up a sagging abdominal wall that has become flaccid due to pregnancy or weight loss. The most common of these techniques involves a long incision in the lower abdomen or directly above the pubic hairline. The skin and subcutaneous tissues of the abdominal wall are lifted off the muscle, where they are redraped and the excess skin removed. After the wounds are closed, a new opening is made for the belly button and it is sutured into place.

This operation is considered major surgery and requires general anesthesia and post-surgical recovery of up to a week in a hospital and several weeks more rest at home.

Risks Scars, numbness in the lower abdominal wall and blood clots in the veins of the lower legs.

abrasion A graze, a superficial loss of EPITHELIUM, the tissue that covers the external surface of the body (usually due to friction), that results in oozing and crusting. No treatment is necessary.

abscess An inflammatory nodule containing a collection of pus, usually caused by a bacterial infection. The pus is made up of dead and live microorganisms and destroyed tissue from white blood cells carried to the area to fight the infection. An abscess may either grow larger or smaller depending on whether the white blood cells or the bacteria win the fight.

Abscesses may be found in the soft tissues beneath the skin, such as the armpit and the groin—two areas with a large number of lymph glands responsible for fighting infections.

Cause Bacteria (such as staphylococci) are the most common cause of abscesses. The bacillus responsible for tuberculosis used to be an abscess-forming type, but is now very rare. Fungal infections sometimes cause abscesses as well.

Symptoms Most larger abscesses cause systemic symptoms such as fever and chills because they are a source of infection within the body. Abscesses close to the skin usually cause inflammation with redness, increased skin temperature and tenderness.

Diagnosis Abscesses can usually be diagnosed visually, although an imaging technique (CAT scan, MRI or radionuclide scans) may also be used to confirm the extent of the abscess.

Treatment Antibiotics are usually prescribed to treat a bacterial infection, and antifungal agents treat fungi. However, the lining of the abscess cavity tends to cut down on the amount of drug that can get into the source of the infection from the blood. Therefore, the cavity itself needs to be drained via a cut in the lining, allowing the pus to escape either through a drainage tube or by leaving the cavity open to the skin. Many abscesses heal after drainage alone; others require both drainage and drug treatment.

acantholysis Disruption of intercellular connections between keratin-producing cells in the outer skin layer. It is caused by the dissolution of the cementing substance between cells and is associated with a form of blisters in disease like PEMPHIGUS.

acanthosis Increased thickness of the EPIDERMIS that is found in a wide variety of skin disorders. See ACANTHOSIS NIGRICANS.

1

acanthosis nigricans A rare untreatable condition characterized by thick velvety dark gray or brown patches of skin on the groin, armpits, neck and other skin folds. It can either be an inherited genetic disorder appearing during youth, the result of an endocrine or metabolic disorder (such as CUSHING'S SYNDROME) or a symptom in those with malignant tumors of the lung or other organs. In addition, at least one drug (nicotinic acid) may cause *acanthosis nigricans.*

When caused by obesity or heredity, the condition progresses very slowly; *acanthosis nigricans* associated with cancer appears and develops more rapidly. With treatment of the malignancy, the condition improves.

Pseudoacanthosis nigricans is a far more common condition that is found in overweight patients with dark complexions. Skin in the fold areas (groin, armpits or neck) is both thicker and darker than the surrounding skin. There is also usually excessive sweating in this area.

Treatment Therapy for patients with *acanthosis nigricans* is aimed at recognizing and treating the underlying disorder.

acarophobia See DELUSIONS OF PARASITOSIS.

Accutane See ISOTRETINOIN.

acid mantle A fluid of fresh sebum (oily substance), sweat and dissolved cells that bathes the top layer of the skin and protects against skin infection. Care of this acidic fluid mantle is very important, especially in those with oily skin prone to acne lesions and infection.

acne A very common inflammatory reaction in oil-producing follicles. While most common in adolescence, the problem may affect people of any age, including infants and the middle-aged. Acne is the most common skin disease in the United States, and accounts for 25 percent of all visits to dermatologists. Because it most commonly affects the face and can lead to permanent scarring, acne can have profound and long-lasting psychological effects.

In males, acne usually begins in early adolescence; it tends to be more severe than in females and resolves in the early to mid-twenties. In females, acne usually begins slightly later (mid-teens), and is less severe. In some individuals acne can last into the 30s. Patients with severe acne often have a family history of severe acne.

Cause Normally, oil is produced in the oil glands in the skin; the oil travels up to the hair follicles and flows out onto the surface of the skin. When oil glands within the hair follicles are stimulated and begin to enlarge (usually as a result of the hormonal change at puberty), they produce more oil. Acne bacteria inside the follicles multiply and produce fatty acids, which irritate the lining of the pores. Simultaneously, there is an increased number of thicker cells in the lining of the pores, which tend to clump together, narrowing and clogging the pore openings with a backup of oil, skin cells and debris inside the pores.

As the pressure builds within these clogged pores, the constant production of oil together with irritation from bacterial action ruptures the pore walls. When the oil pathway gets blocked and the plug pushes up to the surface, it causes a blackhead (or open comedo). When the opening is very tightly closed, the material behind it causes a whitehead (or closed comedo).

While there are many factors behind the inflammatory changes in acne, one of the most important is the different levels of microflora (mainly bacteria) found on the skin. While acne is *not* a bacterial infection, it is believed that inflammation results from the byproducts released by the bacterium *Propionibacterium acnes,* found deep in the sebaceous follicle.

Emotional stress, cosmetics and certain drugs (such as the birth control pills that have higher amounts of progesterone and lower amounts of estrogen) may worsen the condition. Estrogen, however, will improve acne; women who use an estrogen-dominant birth control pill usually notice their acne improves.

Acne is hereditary, and the tendency to develop it runs in families. If both parents have acne, then three out of four of their children also will have acne.

Oil in cosmetics can also contribute to acne. Cosmetic products that contain lanolin, sodium lauryl sulfate, isopropyl myristate, laureth-4 and D&C red dyes should be avoided, since all of these ingredients can promote acne. Makeup should be washed off each night with a mild soap, being sure to rinse six or seven times with fresh water.

(To find out how oily your cosmetics are, rub a thick blob of your makeup on a piece of typing paper; within 24 hours, the oil will make a ring on the paper; the bigger the ring, the more oil in the makeup.)

Acne is *not* caused by diet, dirt or surface oil. Oily foods have nothing to do with the oil on your skin; oil on the skin is manufactured locally in the oil glands, no matter *what* you eat.

Treatment There are excellent types of therapy for all kinds of acne, including topical treatment, systemic antibiotics and hormonal manipulation. A properly structured regimen is required for all those with acne, but most people benefit from a regimen that combines peeling of the skin, destroying bacteria and applying comedolytic agents.

First, wash with soap and water every night, and make sure you eat well and exercise regularly. For milder cases of acne, try medications containing BENZOYL PEROXIDE (start with a 5 percent solution) or those containing SULFUR, a combination of sulfur and RESORCINOL or SALICYLIC ACID.

Since oil accumulation attracts bacteria and the bacteria's enzymes produce fatty acids that irritate the skin and cause inflammation, one of the best ways to fight acne is to kill the bacteria. Those products that are effective in treating acne actually cut down the oil production of the glands slightly, and destroy (or decrease) bacteria in the follicles. The most popular antibiotics in the treatment of acne are tetracycline, minocycline and erythromycin.

For mild cases of acne, antibiotics are used topically. For more advanced disease, they are taken by mouth.

RETIN-A, a drug made with TRETINOIN (an acid related to vitamin A) is an effective treatment for comedones, inflammatory papules and pustules. It is often used in combination with benzoyl peroxide or antibiotics. Those with the most severe types of acne may be given a stronger vitamin-A related drug called Accutane (ISOTRETINOIN). This drug has more serious side effects, including birth defects, and requires strict medical supervision. *No one should became pregnant when taking Accutane.* It is not safe to become pregnant until two months after the course of medication is finished. (See also ACNE, TREATMENT FOR)

It's possible that some cases of acne can be controlled by regulating the androgen/estrogen hormone balance in those women who have an increased activity of the enzyme that converts testosterone (a male androgen) into a more potent form that affects the oil glands. And since androgen has been implicated in the increased secretion of sebum that starts an acne blemish, androgen blockers that reduce the size of oil glands may help women whose acne is associated with other changes, such as excessive hair growth or balding. These drugs could be in the form of high-estrogen birth control pills.

Steroids (cortisone) are very effective for inflammatory or cystic acne when injected into a lesion; it can heal the cyst in about 24 hours. The injection is relatively painless, clears the skin rapidly and prevents scarring. See also ACNE, ADULT; ACNE, COSMETIC; ACNE, CYSTIC; ACNE DETERGENS; ACNE, DRUG-IN-

DUCED; ACNE FULMINANS; ACNE KELOIDALIS; ACNE, INFANT; ACNE MECHANICA; ACNE MYTHS; ACNE, OIL; ACNE VULGARIS.

TYPES OF ACNE

Acne conglobata Severe hereditary acne that generally causes scarring on face and back

Acne detergens Acne caused by overuse of abrasive cleansers

Acne excoriee A psychosomatic disease involving neurotic picking of the face

Acne mallorca Acne caused by sunbathing

Acne mechanica Acne caused by mechanical irritation (such as under the chin straps in football players)

Acne medicamentosa Acne caused by medications

Acne neonatorum Infant acne caused by hormones from the mother to the newborn that usually disappears without treatment

Chloracne Acne induced by constant exposure to hydrocarbons in motor oil or insecticides

Imaginary acne Imagining acne where none exists

Pitch acne Lesions caused by coal tars or dandruff tar shampoos

Premenstrual acne Acne breakouts induced by hormonal change that flare each month prior to starting a period

Steroid acne An inflammation of hair follicles caused by internal steroids or from topical corticosteroids on the face

Tropical acne Acne first described in World War II by soldiers in the tropics who developed severe acne with terrible scars

Extra Y chromosomes People with XYY chromosomes may have quite severe acne

---

acne, adult Pimples, pustules and papules may be the bane of the teenage years, but they can also crop up in adulthood—even in people who were never troubled with breakouts during their adolescence. In fact, some estimates suggest that acne affects 70 to 80 percent of all individuals in their 20s and 30s.

Why these skin blemishes suddenly occur in older patients is a mystery. The hormonal upheaval that triggers acne in teenagers is not usually a factor in adult acne, and while stress, dirt and pollution are prime suspects, there is no direct evidence that either is the cause. In 30- to 40-year-old women the cause is clearly related to hormones.

Treatment See ACNE, TREATMENT OF. See also ACNE; ACNE, COSMETIC; ACNE, CYSTIC; ACNE DETERGENS; ACNE, DRUG-INDUCED; ACNE FULMINANS; ACNE KELOIDALIS; ACNE, INFANT; ACNE MECHANICA; ACNE MYTHS; ACNE, OIL; ACNE VULGARIS.

acne, cosmetic True cosmetic ACNE is probably quite rare, according to acne experts. While it is commonly believed that much of the acne seen in adult women is related to their use of cosmetics containing comedogenic material, this is probably inaccurate. See also ACNE, ADULT; ACNE, CYSTIC; ACNE DETERGENS; ACNE, DRUG-INDUCED; ACNE FULMINANS; ACNE, INFANT; ACNE KELOIDALIS; ACNE MECHANICA; ACNE MYTHS; ACNE, OIL; ACNE VULGARIS.

acne, cystic A type of severe ACNE in which the sebum (together with dead cells and bacterial products) ruptures through the follicle wall, causing an inflammatory reaction that may end in scarring. See also ACNE, ADULT; ACNE, COSMETIC; ACNE, DETERGENS; ACNE, DRUG-INDUCED; ACNE FULMINANS;ACNE, INFANT; ACNE KELOIDALIS; ACNE MECHANICA; ACNE MYTHS; ACNE, OIL; ACNE VULGARIS.

acne detergens This form of ACNE occurs in some patients who are compulsive face washers. However, there is some evidence that this may be a variety of ACNE MECHANICA. See also ACNE, ADULT; ACNE, COSMETIC; ACNE, CYSTIC; ACNE, DRUG-INDUCED; ACNE FULMINANS; ACNE, INFANT; ACNE KELOIDALIS; ACNE MECHANICA; ACNE MYTHS; ACNE, OIL; ACNE VULGARIS.

acne, drug-induced Many drugs can cause ACNE when administered systemically. The most common are phenytoin (Dilantin), isoniazid, lithium, bromides, iodides, androgens and corticosteroids. Of these, topical and systemic corticosteroids are the most common acne inducers. In drug-induced acne there may not be any blackheads; instead, there are uniform papules and pustules.

Lithium worsens *acne vulgaris,* and can cause a severe case of acne in patients who never before had a skin problem. Oral contraceptives containing agents such as norgestrel or norethindrone can induce or worsen *acne vulgaris;* this may improve when pill prescriptions are switched. Medications containing potassium iodide, bromide (especially cold remedies) and chlorine (chloral hydrate) may cause acne with very small pustules.

Steroids may cause acne several days to weeks into treatment with either oral or topical steroids. Steroid-induced acne is distinctive, with tiny red papules and pustules limited to the area where the steroid was applied, or on the chest, back and shoulders in people on systemic therapy. Steroids thin the outer skin layer, making follicles more susceptible to rupture. Because inflammation is controlled by steroids, the lesions are usually small or they may appear after the drug is stopped. Acne fades after medicine is stopped, but it may take some time to completely clear.

Other drugs associated with acne are actinomycin D, cod liver oil, halothane, thiouracil, thiourea, trimethadione and vitamin B_{12}. See also ACNE, ADULT; ACNE, COSMETIC; ACNE, CYSTIC; ACNE DETERGENS; ACNE FULMINANS; ACNE, INFANT; ACNE KELOIDALIS; ACNE MECHANICA; ACNE MYTHS; ACNE, OIL.

acne excoriée One of a group of disorders in which a patient, because of an exaggerated sense of abnormal conditions, causes a skin rash by constantly picking or squeezing facial blemishes. In these cases, one or a few small blemishes so concern the person that he or she constantly picks or washes them, actually making the lesions worse. People with this problem may refuse to believe they are making the lesions worse by constant irritation, and may seek plastic surgery to correct the problem. However, in these cases they are quite often dissatisfied with the results. Severely distraught patients may even attempt suicide. See also ACNE, ADULT; ACNE, COSMETIC; ACNE, CYSTIC; ACNE DETERGENS; ACNE, DRUG-INDUCED; ACNE, INFANT; ACNE KELOIDALIS; ACNE MECHANICA; ACNE MYTHS; ACNE, OIL; ACNE VULGARIS.

acne fulminans This is an acute, severe necrotic variety of acne that is accompanied by systemic symptoms and signs, including fever and joint pain. This rare form of acne usually requires treatment with systemic corticosteroids. See also ACNE, ADULT; ACNE, COSMETIC; ACNE, CYSTIC; ACNE DETERGENS; ACNE, DRUG-INDUCED; ACNE, INFANT; ACNE KELOIDALIS; ACNE MECHANICA; ACNE MYTHS; ACNE, OIL; ACNE VULGARIS.

acne, infant Acne is not unusual among newborns; it is brought on by hormones passed from the mother to the child before birth. The hormones cause the SEBACEOUS GLANDS in the skin to produce oil; if these glands become blocked and inflamed, whiteheads and pimples may develop on the baby's face. Newborn acne usually clears up on its own in three or four months. If it's troublesome or persistent, a pediatrician may prescribe a topical medication. Contrary to popular belief, infant acne is not associated with the development of acne in adolescence or later in life. However, an uncommon problem is infantile acne that becomes severe and persists for months to a few years. This is associated with a family history of acne, usually in the father, and often is followed by severe acne at adolescence. See also ACNE, ADULT; ACNE, COSMETIC; ACNE, CYSTIC; ACNE DETERGENS; ACNE, DRUG-INDUCED; ACNE FULMINANS; ACNE, KELOIDALIS; ACNE MECHANICA; ACNE MYTHS; ACNE, OIL; ACNE VULGARIS.

acne keloidalis Also called *dermatitis papillaris capillitii,* this disorder affects hair follicles in people of African descent, creating firm papules and pustules on the nape of the neck. In severe cases, large lesions can result in significant scarring and permanent hair loss. Complications may include infection, scarring resulting in limited range of neck movement; squamous cell cancer may rarely develop.

Treatment While no single treatment is effective for all patients, therapies include corticosteroid injections and topical corticosteroid preparations, which may limit the formation of scars. A variety of surgical techniques may also be attempted, including removal of individual papules with scissors, a scalpel or lasers. In more severe cases, the entire affected area is cut out and the wound is stitched closed. See also ACNE, ADULT; ACNE, COSMETIC; ACNE, CYSTIC; ACNE DETERGENS; ACNE, DRUG-INDUCED; ACNE FULMINANS; ACNE, INFANT; ACNE MECHANICA; ACNE MYTHS; ACNE, OIL; ACNE VULGARIS.

acne mechanica Acne that occurs from physical trauma such as rubbing, found most often underneath chin straps of helmets worn by athletes. Heat and sweat also contribute to this condition. See also ACNE, ADULT; ACNE, COSMETIC; ACNE, CYSTIC; ACNE DETERGENS; ACNE, DRUG-INDUCED; ACNE FULMINANS; ACNE, INFANT; ACNE, KELOIDALIS; ACNE MYTHS; ACNE, OIL; ACNE VULGARIS.

acne medicamentosa See ACNE, DRUG-INDUCED.

acne myths A wide range of ACNE taboos have recently been proven to be groundless, such as the idea that acne is worsened by chocolate, nuts, fatty foods and shellfish.

In one study, 65 people ate chocolate bars every day for a month, but although the bars contained 10 times the normal amount of chocolate, the subjects experienced no worsening of blemishes. Other research also found that nuts, shellfish and fatty foods did not affect blemishes, either. See also ACNE, ADULT; ACNE, COSMETIC; ACNE, CYSTIC; ACNE DETERGENS; ACNE, DRUG-INDUCED; ACNE FULMINANS; ACNE, INFANT; ACNE, KELOIDALIS; ACNE MECHANICA; ACNE, OIL; ACNE VULGARIS.

acne neonatorum See ACNE, INFANT.

acne, oil A form of ACNE caused by heavy petroleum lubricating oils and greases that irritate the follicles, resulting in plugging of comedones or pustular folliculitis. The lesions usually occur on the hands and forearms, but they may be severe on covered areas of the body if clothing is saturated with oil. The appearance of lesions outside the typical acne distribution (bridge of nose, chin, forehead, back and chest), plus a history of exposure to oils, is a good way to distinguish oil acne from ACNE VULGARIS or bacterial FOLLICULITIS. See also ACNE, ADULT; ACNE, COSMETIC; ACNE, CYSTIC; ACNE DETERGENS; ACNE, DRUG-INDUCED; ACNE FULMINANS; ACNE, INFANT; ACNE, KELOIDALIS; ACNE MECHANICA; ACNE MYTHS.

Treatment This condition responds immediately when the exposure to the irritating oil is stopped. Eliminating skin and clothing contact with the offending oil and grease is the best way to avoid oil acne, and BENZOYL PEROXIDE may also help.

acne, pomade A type of ACNE that occurs primarily in black patients who use pomades or thick oils daily on their hair to eliminate the curl. The pomade gets transferred to the skin from the fingers and hair, and blocks the skin's oil glands, causing acne-like lesions. In this condition, which was first described in 1970, many closed comedones and sometimes inflamed lesions are packed close together on the head and temples near the hairline. (See also BLACK SKIN.)

Treatment Wash hands after applying the oil, keep hands away from the face and avoid hairstyles where the hair constantly touches the skin of the face.

acne products, over-the-counter There are a number of ingredients found in non-prescription products that are considered safe and effective in the treatment of ACNE by the U.S. Food and Drug Administration. They include BENZOYL PEROXIDE 2.5 to 10 percent, RESORCINOL 2 percent (in certain combinations), resorcinol monacetate 3 percent (in certain combinations), SALICYLIC ACID 0.5 to 2 percent and SULFUR 3 to 10 percent (in certain combinations).

All of these products dry, exfoliate and peel the skin to some degree. Used together they may increase the dryness and cause irritation.

Acne Research Institute An organization of research scientists, physicians and ACNE sufferers that provides technical assistance to federal, local, professional and industrial groups engaged in acne treatment. The institute, founded in 1974, supports basic research into the cause and treatment of acne and hopes eventually to find a cure for acne. The group plans to establish a center for multidisciplinary research where dermatologists, biochemists, bacteriologists and endocrinologists can cooperate on various projects, including basic studies, experimental clinical studies to improve acne treatment, workshops and conferences, standardization of testing for new drugs, and effective public education for the cause of acne.

The institute publishes a quarterly, *Update*, and two books, *Let's Talk Cosmetics* and *Acne: A Treatable Disease.*

acne rosacea See ROSACEA.

acne, treatment for There are a range of therapies for all kinds of acne, including topical treatment, systemic antibiotics, hormonal manipulation or ISOTRETINOIN (Accutane), a synthetic derivative of vitamin A.

For milder cases, some people find relief with over-the-counter medications containing BENZOYL PEROXIDE or SULFUR, a combination of sulfur and RESORCINOL, or SALICYLIC ACID. These medications are sold as liquids, gels, lotions or creams; the water-based gels are least likely to irritate the skin.

Probably the most popular of these over-the-counter products is benzoyl peroxide, an extremely effective topical antibacterial agent. When applied to the skin, it markedly suppresses the bacterium *Propionibacterium acnes.* The benzoyl in the product draws the peroxide into the pore where it releases oxygen, killing the bacteria that can aggravate acne. Benzoyl peroxide also suppresses fatty acid cells that irritate pores, and it helps to open up blackheads and whiteheads. Benzoyl peroxide it is most effective for patients with inflammatory acne; by inhibiting bacteria growth, it decreases the inflammatory components in the skin.

Benzoyl peroxide is sold in strengths ranging between 2.5 percent to 10 percent, but dermatologists usually advise patients to start with a 2.5 or 5 percent product, since the lower concentration is usually just as effective and less likely to cause irritation. Most over-the-counter products contain benzoyl peroxide in a lotion base or in treated pads; the prescription items contain the chemical in a gel base. Some irritation, redness and swelling may follow use of benzoyl peroxide, and allergic sensitization has occasionally occurred.

For more severe cases, dermatologists may prescribe RETIN-A, a drug made with TRETINOIN (an acid related to vitamin A), or topical or oral antibiotics. Tretinoin is the principal drug for topical use in acne with comedones (open whiteheads), and is available as a gel, cream or lotion. (The lotion is potentially more irritating and the creams are less irritating.) Less irritation develops if tretinoin is applied at least 30 minutes *after* washing. Tretinoin, like benzoyl peroxide, should be started in the lowest concentration available and be applied only every other day. Patients should protect their skin from exposure to the sun, since tretinoin increases the skin's sensitivity to ultraviolet radiation.

While tretinoin is best used for acne with open whiteheads, it may also help patients with inflammatory acne since it helps to prevent inflammation.

Topical antibiotics (including TETRACYCLINE, ERYTHROMYCIN, CLINDAMYCIN and MECLOCYCLINE) have been used topically as an antibacterial approach to treating acne. Experts believe antibiotics are not as effective as benzoyl peroxide except in mild inflammatory acne. A fairly new preparation combining 3 percent erythromycin with 5 percent benzoyl peroxide in a gel base may be more effective than either component by itself.

Systemic therapy About 10 percent of all tetracycline sold in the United States is used to treat acne, although the condition is not a bacterial disease. The effectiveness of systemic antibiotics is probably related to the fact that the drugs interfere with inflammatory byproducts of some types of bacteria, which prevents the development of new inflammatory lesions. It does take some time, however, before the systemic antibiotic approach works. Erythromycin and minocycline are probably as effective as tetracycline, but minocycline is much more expensive.

Preparations that interfere with the production of sebum (an oily substance produced by sebaceous glands) may also be effective, including corticosteroids and estrogens. (Estrogens should only be used for women whose acne has not responded to other types of treatment). In addition, a medication called cyproterone acetate has been used in Europe to successfully treat acne.

Those with the most severe types of acne may be given an even stronger vitamin-A related drug called Accutane (ISOTRETINOIN). Accutane is very effective against the most stubborn cases of acne, and has produced remarkable clearing in those with severe cystic acne. The drug has also resulted in remissions that have persisted for years in most patients. When treated with the correct dosage, 9 out of 10 patients with severe cystic acne do not require any subsequent therapy.

Unfortunately, Accutane has serious side effects and requires strict medical supervision. Side effects include those found in excess levels of vitamin A (dry mouth, itching, small red spots on the skin and eye irritation). Its most serious side effect is that it can cause serious birth defects. Treatment *may not* be given during pregnancy.

Acne medications may cause reactions if the skin is exposed to the sun; experts recommend staying away from sunlight, infrared heat lamps and sunscreens until you're sure how the product works on your skin.

Physical therapy Acne surgery removes open and closed comedones and sometimes very small pustules; removal of the closed comedones is important, since they can lead to inflammatory lesions. Open comedones are removed only for cosmetic reasons, since they don't usually become inflamed.

The direct injection of corticosteroids into the lesion can reduce inflammation in larger cysts in order to avoid a depressed scar. This technique is not used for papules and pustules.

Prevention Acne sufferers should try to avoid excess stress if prone to breaking out. Patients taking birth control pills (especially Ovral, Loestrin, Norlestrin and Norinyl) may be able to switch to a different pill or use an alternative birth control method.

Application The directions on most topical acne medications say to "apply to the affected area" after washing. This does *not* mean apply to pimples only, since these medications don't really fight pimples that already exist. However, there is the possibility that benzoyl peroxide applied to a pimple may cause it to go away a bit faster.

It's not a good idea to mix acne medications. If you are using a nonprescription acne product, you should stop using it if you are given a prescription product.

What NOT to do Picking or squeezing blemishes can inhibit healing and lead to scarring. For this reason, you should never squeeze pimples or whiteheads. Because regular pimples are the result of inflamation, squeezing can simply worsen the inflammation and cause an infection. However, pimples with a little yellow pus head in the middle *can* be gently squeezed, which will pop the pimple and allow it to heal more quickly. Unfortunately, nothing you can do to a pimple will make it go away faster—the life of a pimple lasts between one and four weeks.

Whiteheads, which do not involve inflammation, should never be squeezed. If you squeeze a whitehead, the wall of the plugged pore can break and the contents can leak out into the skin, causing a pimple. (A pimple forms from the rupture of a whitehead pore.)

Blackheads may be squeezed, since they won't result in a pimple. Blackheads are simply open comedones or open whiteheads. The black color is from melanin and from oxidation of the pore contents.

acne vulgaris Another name for common ACNE.

acrochordon See SKIN TAG.

acrocyanosis A condition induced by abnormal cold sensitivity, which causes spasms in small blood vessels. These spasms result in a loss of oxygen in the blood, which makes hands and feet blue, cold and sweaty. The problem is usually worsened by cold weather, and young women are particularly susceptible. Acrocyanosis is distantly related to RAYNAUD'S DISEASE, a more serious circulatory disorder in which the skin of the fingers and toes may be damaged by chronically reduced blood flow.

Treatment Treatment is often unnecessary; prevention involves avoiding cold and tobacco use. Drugs to dilate the blood vessels are not usually prescribed.

acrodermatitis enteropathica A rare inherited disease in which the skin of the fingers, toes, mouth, anus, mouth and scalp of infants is reddened, ulcerated and covered with pustules. In rare instances, the disorder can lead to blood poisoning and death if unrecognized and untreated.

Symptoms Symptoms appear about 4 to 10 weeks after birth in bottle-fed babies, or after weaning in breastfed babies: failure to thrive, diarrhea, hair loss, nail problems, conjunctivitis and photophobia (hypersensitivity to light), emotional instability, decreased appetite, and skin problems. The disease usually improves during adolescence, but it may persist into adulthood when it begins to resemble PSORIASIS.

Cause The disease is caused by low levels of zinc in the skin as a result of problems in zinc metabolism. The problem occurs after weaning because human breast milk contains a substance (believed to be picolinic acid) that permits zinc absorption even when the intestinal factor normally controlling the absorption of zinc is deficient or absent. After weaning from breast milk, symptoms in affected babies occur in both males and fe-males.

Treatment Zinc dietary supplements reverse all symptoms. The supplements should not be taken with food (especially bread); nausea is a common side effect. While the disease is lifelong, proper treatment leads to remission and a normal life span.

acrodermatitis, papular See GIANOTTI-CROSTI SYNDROME.

acroparesthesia A medical term for the feeling of tingling in the fingers or toes. See also PINS AND NEEDLES SYNDROME.

actinic Pertaining to changes caused by the ultraviolet rays of the sun.

actinic conditions Conditions caused by overexposure to the sun. These include ac-tinic dermatitis (inflammation of the skin), ACTINIC KERATOSIS (a sun-induced premalig-nant condition characterized by redness and swelling), BASAL CELL CARCINOMA and SQUA-MOUS CELL CARCINOMA. All these conditions can be prevented by avoiding the sun and using sunscreens from an early age. See also DERMATITIS, ACTINIC.

actinic dermatitis See DERMATITIS, ACTINIC.

actinic keratosis Also known as solar kera-tosis, this lesion is a dry, scaly, rough pink-to-tan thickening of the skin caused by long-standing overexposure to the sun. The condi-tion is usually found in older patients; however, with increased exposure to the sun it is being seen in younger and younger pa-tients. This common skin lesion affects one out of six people; it is a precancerous condi-tion that can lead to malignant skin tumors (SQUAMOUS CELL CARCINOMA).

Untreated, this type of cancer can invade the surrounding tissues or internal organs. The presence of this skin lesion indicates that the sun has damaged the skin, and any type of skin cancer can develop.

Lesions occur most often on the face, back of the hands and forearms, neck and exposed scalp. The lesions develop slowly, eventually growing to the size of a quarter inch, some-times fading and reappearing. There are usu-ally several keratoses at one time on areas of the body exposed to sunlight.

The skin surrounding the lesion often shows evidence of chronic sun damage, in-cluding scaling, pigment variation, wrinkling and atrophy.

Actinic damage of the lips is called "ac-tinic cheilitis," if it proceeds to squamous cell carcinoma, about one-fifth of these lesions will spread.

Those at greatest risk for these lesions have fair skin, blonde or red hair, and blue, green or gray eyes because their skin has less protective pigment. But even those with dark skin can develop keratoses if they are ex-posed to the sun without protection, al-though those with black skin rarely have these lesions. Individuals with compromised immune systems as a result of chemotherapy, AIDS or organ transplants are at higher risk.

Actinic keratoses are more likely to appear in older people because of the cumulative ef-fects of the sun; one recent survey of individ-uals who had been exposed to large amounts of sunlight found keratoses in more than half of the men and a third of the women aged 65 to 74. Some experts believe that most people who live to be 80 or older have actinic kera-toses.

Since more than half a person's lifetime sun exposure occurs before age 20, keratoses *can* appear in a person's 20s if that person has not been sufficiently protected from sun damage.

Treatment While not all keratoses need to be removed, there are a number of treatments for those that do. The most common treat-ment is cryotherapy with LIQUID NITROGEN. With CRYOSURGERY, the physician freezes the lesions by applying liquid nitrogen with a special spray or a cotton-tipped applicator and removes the lesions. This method doesn't require anesthesia and produces no bleeding. White spots may sometimes appear afterward on the skin's surface, but if done properly this is relatively uncommon. By another method, CURETTAGE AND ELECTRODESICCATION, the physician scrapes the lesion and does a biopsy to test for malignancy. During the procedure, bleeding is controlled by electrocautery (heat produced by an electric needle).

Alternatively, a physician could shave the keratosis by a process called "shave removal" to obtain a specimen for testing; the base of the lesion is destroyed and the bleeding is stopped by cauterization (heat).

DERMABRASION removes the upper layers of the skin by sanding or using a fine wire brush; redness and pain usually disappear after a few days. Chemical peeling causes the top layers of the skin to slough off by applying glycolic acid, trichloroacetic acid or phenol while the patient is sedated; the skin is usually replaced within seven days by a new growth of skin.

LASER SURGERY may be used to treat actinic cheilitis by focusing a beam of light from a carbon dioxide laser onto the lips; the damaged skin can be vaporized.

Two medicated creams—5-FLUOROURACIL or MASOPROCOL are also effective in removing keratoses (especially when there are many lesions). A solution or cream of 1 to 5 percent fluorouracil is applied by the patient twice a day as infrequently as two days per week to as often as daily for four to nine weeks. Treatments cause the skin to become intensely red, causing some pain and skin breakdown. After treatment, the skin may be treated with a topical steroid (such as hydrocortisone 1 percent) to alleviate the inflammation.

Masoprocol cream (10 percent), the newest topical treatment, is applied for four weeks and is now available by prescription. Redness and flaking are common side effects.

actinic lentigo See LENTIGO SIMPLEX.

actinomycosis A deep bacterial infection of the skin caused by *Actinomyces israelii* or *Arachnia propionica,* normal bacteria always present in the mouth and tonsils that can cause infection when introduced into broken tissue. It's also possible to transmit this bacteria via a human bite.

Symptoms The most common form of the disease affects the mouth and jaw, causing a painful swelling. Small openings later develop on the skin of the face around the mouth, discharging pus and characteristic yellow granules. Poor oral hygiene may contribute to this form of the infection. A diagnosis is usually confirmed by presence of the granules.

Treatment Adequate surgical drainage is important, together with bed rest and good diet. Treatment with large doses of penicillin injections is usually successful, although medication may be needed for several months in severe infections.

acyclovir (Trade name: Zovirax) An antiviral drug introduced in 1982 used in treating the virus causing HERPES SIMPLEX INFECTION, SHINGLES and CHICKENPOX. Acyclovir is available in topical or oral form.

Oral acyclovir Acyclovir is effective in managing both the initial infection and recurrent infections of herpes (including ECZEMA HERPETICUM) and in the treatment of shingles. It is effective in preventing subsequent viral attacks if taken continuously soon after infection. In patients with recurrent genital herpes, acyclovir therapy reduces the duration of viral shedding, and makes the lesions heal quicker, providing symptom relief.

In addition, acyclovir has been helpful to patients receiving bone marrow transplants to prevent the subsequent development of herpes simplex infection.

Topical acyclovir The topical form does not prevent new lesions from forming during the course of the disease, nor does it prevent the development of latency. When applied to an existing blister, however, it may relieve symptoms, speed healing and shorten the duration of the infection and the contagious period.

Adverse effects Adverse effects are rare. The ointment may cause skin irritation or rash. Taken by mouth, the drug may cause headache, dizziness, nausea/vomiting. Rarely, acyclovir injections may cause kidney damage.

Addison's disease A rare disorder in which symptoms are caused by a deficiency of the hormones hydrocortisone and aldosterone. It was invariably fatal before hormone treatment became available in the 1950s.

Symptoms The disease, named for the English physician Thomas Addison (1793–1860) who first diagnosed the disorder, begins with feelings of malaise. One of its most specific symptoms is a darkening of the skin in the creases of the palms and pressure areas of the body, especially in the mouth. It is caused by excess production of the hormone that stimulates melanin production.

Treatment The pigmentation disappears slowly when the patient receives glucocorticosteroid replacement therapy. Still, most patients retain a slight tan color for the rest of their lives.

adenoma sebaceum Flesh- to reddish-colored papules on the face and nose that appear in the first 10 or 20 years of life. It is associated with TUBEROUS SCLEROSIS, a condition characterized by convulsions, retardation, and light-colored areas of skin. See also ANGIOFIBROMA.

adenosine monophosphate (AMP) A metabolism byproduct that may help ease the pain of SHINGLES. In one uncontrolled trial, 15 out of 17 shingles patients who took the drug reportedly felt no pain within two weeks, and were still pain-free two years later. The treatment has no side effects, and works best within the first few months of pain when the nerve endings have experienced minimal damage.

Otherwise, the pain following a shingles outbreak (postherpetic neuralgia) is treated with painkillers, Tylenol and codeine if necessary. In addition, ZOSTRIX (capsacin) has been shown in double blind studies to be effective.

adenovirus infection One of a group of viruses that cause infections of the upper respiratory tract, producing measles-like eruptions and symptoms of the common cold. Adenoviruses are often diagnosed in the winter and spring.

adipose nevi A rare type of connective tissue nevus (birthmark) characterized by grouped yellowish nodules that form plaques, usually appearing on the lower torso and upper thighs. The condition, also known as *nevus lipomatosus superficialis Hoffmann and Zurhelle*, does not require treatment.

adipose tissue A layer of fat beneath the skin and around internal organs. After puberty, the distribution of this superficial adipose tissue changes in males and females; women have a greater proportion of total body weight in adipose tissue accumulated on breasts, hips and thighs. In adult males, adipose tissue accumulates around the shoulders, waist and abdomen.

Adipose tissue is constructed from fat deposits left by excess food intake and serves as an energy store; too much adipose tissue causes obesity. The tissue is an insulator and keeps the body warm, especially in babies, and it also helps absorb shock in areas subject to sudden or frequent pressure (such as the buttocks and feet).

adnexa of skin The cutaneous structures that make up the hair, nails and sebaceous, eccrine and APOCRINE GLANDS. See also SEBACEOUS GLANDS.

age spots Blemishes that appear on the skin as a person ages. The most common of these spots are seborrheic keratoses—brown or yellow-brown raised spots that may occur anywhere on the body. Other common age spots in the elderly are liverspots (lentigenes), actinic keratoses and Campbell De Morgan's spots (cherry angiomas)—red, pinpoint blemishes.

Treatment is usually not necessary except for actinic keratoses, which may become malignant. Freezing the keratoses with liquid nitrogen and removing them is the usual treatment, although they may be removed surgically with a local anesthetic. While most age spots are harmless, any inexplicable blemish (or one that bleeds or grows rapidly) may represent skin cancer and should be examined by a physician. Brown spots that have irregularities of brown color or irregular borders also should be shown to a physician. See also KERATOSIS.

aging and skin Loss of elastic tissue and collagen causes the skin to sag and wrinkle; weakened blood capillaries cause skin to bruise more easily. This damage is accelerated by exposure to the sun or by smoking. In fact, there are really two types of skin aging—chronological aging and photoaging. Chronological aging is just what it sounds like—the inherited tendency to age. Photoaging (or solar-induced aging) is caused by damage from exposure to the sun, and this type of skin problem is more common today than skin problems due to chronological aging.

As we age, the skin produces fewer cells and repairs damaged cells more slowly, while cells in the horny layer of the skin become dryer and rougher. At the same time, the number of MELANOCYTES (melanin-producing cells) drops, leading to patchy skin color. Wound healing is also slowed down, and there is usually a decreased ability to clear foreign material and fluid. Increasing rigidity, inelasticity and a decrease of dermal COLLAGEN and elastin fibers mean the skin begins to wrinkle and sag.

Fat distribution in the skin also changes with age, being redistributed to the waist in men and the thighs in women. At the same time, the SUBCUTIS begins to thin in certain areas (such as the face, hands, feet and shins).

In addition, aging glands produce less oil and smaller amounts of perspiration, and so there is less oil to trap moisture on the skin's surface and less perspiration to moisturize skin. Environmental factors (heat, air conditioning and wind) can further dehydrate the skin.

Age also affects hair color, graying or whitening it because of a decrease in the number of melanin-producing cells. Most people also notice thinning and slower hair regrowth rate, while on the other hand, hair begins to appear in unwanted places (ears, nose and eyebrows in men and upper lip and chin in women).

Treatment Today there are literally hundreds of products on the market that claim to reverse the consequences of aging. Lotions containing ALPHA HYDROXY ACID and RETIN-A have been shown to reverse some features of skin aging; no other skin products have ever been shown to improve or slow the aging process.

Prevention Obviously, prevention offers the best chance to avoid excess age-related damage to the skin. Those who have stayed away from the sun's rays for most or all of their lives will have much healthier skin than the senior citizen who has been a sun-worshipper for decades.

Health habits also play a role—getting enough sleep, fresh air, exercise and good food. Cutting down or eliminating smoking will also improve the condition of the skin. In one study at Bowman Gray School of Medicine, researchers discovered that smokers (whether young or old, male or female, smiling or unsmiling) tended to look five or more years older than their actual age.

AIDS and skin disorders The skin symptoms of AIDS can range from a severe form of normally mild eruptions to unusual lesions such as the pink-purple spots of KAPOSI'S SARCOMA, and oral hairy LEUKOPLAKIA. In fact, skin symptoms may be the very first sign of a suppressed immune system.
Viral infections A wide range of viral infections may plague the patient with AIDS, including HERPES SIMPLEX (1 and 2), SHINGLES, MOLLUSCUM CONTAGIOSUM, WARTS and oral hairy leukoplakia. Herpes attacks are far more common in patients with AIDS than in the general population, and they are more likely to be deep, painful and slow to heal (especially in the perianal area). Occasionally, herpes simplex infections in patients with AIDS are resistant to ACYCLOVIR, the primary drug treatment for herpes simplex.

The appearance of shingles in an individual is highly suggestive of HIV infection, and the likelihood that the patient will go on to develop full-blown AIDS is high. In addition, recurrent shingles may also occur in patients with AIDS.

Both common WARTS and CONDYLOMATA ACUMINATA are common and can be very difficult to treat in this patient population. Warts in the anal area may become large and require surgical removal.

The lesions of oral hairy leukoplakia which are fairly specific to patients with AIDS, appear on the side of the tongue as white linear lesions.
Bacterial infections Treatment of SYPHILIS may be difficult in patients with AIDS, and one dose of penicillin may not cure the disease. Other bacterial infections that may be seen include CAT SCRATCH FEVER, mycobacte-

rial infections, ECTHYMA, CELLULITIS, ABSCESSES, IMPETIGO and FOLLICULITIS.
Fungal infections Oral CANDIDIASIS is very common. Dermatophyte (fungal) infections are frequent (including ATHLETE'S FOOT, JOCK ITCH and nail infection). CRYPTOCOCCIS (as either a single skin lesion or as herpes-like ulcers) or HISTOPLASMOSIS are also seen.
Parasitic infections AMEBIASIS or SCABIES may also occur among patients with AIDS.
Skin tumors In addition to Kaposi's sarcoma, patients with AIDS have a high incidence of lymphoma.
Miscellaneous skin lesions Patients with AIDS are much more likely than other patients to experience drug reactions. Explosive PSORIASIS may occur in these patients. Often, patients with AIDS develop seborrheic dermatitis of the scalp, face (especially center of the face), armpits, chest, groin and genitals.

In addition, these patients may experience itchy papular eruptions over the body, acquired ICHTHYOSIS and very dry skin. And an atopic-like DERMATITIS has developed in about half of all children with AIDS.
Hair problems As the disease progresses, patients report their hair becomes softer, lighter, thinner and silkier.
Nail problems Yellow colored nails have been reported; others notice bluish bands that occur during administration of zidovudine (AZT).

air travel and the skin Frequent airplane travel can have a negative effect on skin and hair, especially for those with dry skin. The low humidity and lack of fresh air on board can greatly increase flaky skin, dryness and irritation. Even those with oily skin complain that they develop dry patches of skin on cheeks and chin during plane travel, followed by a "rebound effect" of excess oiliness.

If possible, women should not wear makeup during air travel, but apply a moisturizer and eye cream the morning of the flight, reapplying it during any trip longer than two hours. For those who *must* wear makeup during air travel, use a water-based foundation and undermakeup primer or moisturizer.

Never drink alcohol or caffeinated beverages on a plane, since alcohol and caffeine are natural diuretics, minimizing the amount of moisture available to skin cells. Some travelers carry a mineral water spritzer to refresh and moisturize complexions. Always wear a lip balm or moisturized lip color on board, to prevent lips from drying and cracking. Reapply hand cream several times during the trip (especially if you wash your hands during the flight).

For irritated eyes (especially for those who wear contact lenses), apply cotton pads soaked in distilled water or milk to closed lids for several minutes. Contact lens wearers might consider abandoning the lenses altogether for the duration of the flight.

A few minutes before landing, cleanse your face and apply moisturizer; women can then apply water-based foundation, mascara, blusher and lip gloss.

albinism A rare congenital inherited condition characterized by a partial or total lack of the pigment MELANIN that gives color to skin, eyes and hair. Found in people of all races, albinos often suffer visual problems, skin inflammations, severe sunburn and a tendency toward SKIN CANCER.

The most common type of albinism is called oculocutaneous albinism, in which the hair, skin and eyes are all affected. In the more severe form, the skin and hair are snowy white throughout life. Less severely affected individuals may be born with white skin and hair, but both darken slightly with age and numerous freckles develop on sun-exposed parts of the body. In both forms, the eyes cannot tolerate bright lights and are often affected with nystagmus (abnormal flickering movements), strabismus (squinty

eyes) and myopia (nearsightedness). More rare types of albinism affect either only skin, hair or the eyes.

Oculocutaneous albinism has an autosomal recessive pattern of inheritance. Usually parents have normal skin coloring, but they carry the gene defect in a hidden form. If parents with normal pigmentation have an albino child, there is a one in four chance that future children will be affected.

Less than five per 100,000 people in the United States and Europe are affected, although the prevalence is much higher in some parts of the world (about 20 per 100,000 in southern Nigeria, for instance).

The most serious complication of the disease is the lack of melanin, which protects the skin against the harmful radiation in sunlight. Because the skin cannot tan, it ages prematurely and is prone to SKIN CANCERS. Visual problems common in albinos can also cause problems.

Albright's syndrome The popular term for polyostotic fibrous dysplasia, a condition characterized by a few large dark flat spots with very irregular borders (often compared to the coast of Maine). There may also be developmental abnormalities, such as bony lesions and endocrine problems, such as precocious sexual development.

The syndrome is not genetic, although it is more common in girls.

Other related symptoms include mental deficiency, epilepsy and headaches.

alcohol An organic compound with strong grease-cutting properties used in many cosmetics as an antiseptic astringent. Alcohol cools the skin as it evaporates. It is very drying, however, and people with dry skin should avoid products containing alcohol. Alcohol can be found in some soaps, deodorants, skin fresheners, colognes, acne products, mousses, gels and setting lotions.

alcohol and skin cancer New research suggests that alcohol use can contribute to malignant melanoma (the most deadly form of skin cancer), according to Australian researchers. Several studies appear to have uncovered a link between alcohol and melanoma; in the Australian study, women who drank two or more drinks per day had two and a half times the chance of developing melanoma. A Harvard University study found that drinking more than one beer, glass of wine or cocktail daily led to an 80 percent higher melanoma risk. See also MELANOMA, MALIGNANT.

alkaptonuria See OCHRONOSIS

allergens Antigens (foreign substances) that induce allergic reactions. Some common examples are insect bites, certain foods, dust, plants, etc.

allergies and the skin The skin is one of the first sites where the symptoms of allergy may appear. An allergic dermatitis (rash) occurs when the immune system tries to fight off a foreign substance (called an "allergen") that comes into contact with the skin. Some of the most common skin allergens include poison ivy (more than 50 percent of people are allergic to these plants), fragrances, preservatives, hair dyes, formaldehyde, nickel, cement, shoe leather and rubber.

Chromium/chromates This is the most common cause of contact dermatitis in men, usually occurring on the job. Chromium is commonly found in the environment and therefore is not easy to avoid. A primary source of chromium is in cement, often present in machining and building trades. In addition, shoes made from leather tanned with chromates can cause ECZEMA on the feet of sensitive people.

Collagen (injectable) About 3 percent of healthy people are allergic to injectable collagen, used to reverse facial wrinkles and creases; about half of them experience the allergy after the actual treatment has begun. Once an allergy develops, further treatments are not advisable.

Foods A range of common foods may bring on allergic reactions on the skin, including citrus fruits, eggs, fish, artificial coloring or milk. Acute hives usually result from an allergic reaction to foods such as shellfish, nuts, berries, tomatoes, eggs, citrus fruits, chicken and pork. Less commonly, individuals develop hives from contact of food with skin (chicken, fish and certain vegetables). Allergy prick or scratch skin testing to determine food allergies is often ineffective, sometimes producing a false positive (showing an allergy when no symptoms actually appear when the food is eaten) or a false negative (showing no reaction when tested on the skin but having strong reactions when the food is eaten).

Footwear It is possible to develop a contact allergy to footwear chemicals, especially rubber or rubber cements, leather-tanning products, or dyes. They cause itching, redness, swelling and small blisters. These symptoms appear most readily on the thin sensitive skin of the tops and sides of the feet. Avoiding such an allergy may mean buying special shoes and keeping the feet dry, since potential allergens can be leached out of footwear by sweat.

Fragrances A wide variety of products contain fragrances that may set off an allergic reaction in some people, including soaps, tissues, creams and deodorants. Since manufacturers closely guard the specific ingredients in scented products (the products usually simply list "fragrance" on their label), sensitive consumers may find the "fragrance free" products to be their best choice. Those marked "hypoallergenic" while good for sensitive people may still contain some scent that may cause a reaction in very sensitive individuals. "Unscented" products are not a good choice because they contain some fragrance traces that have been included to mask unpleasant odors naturally found in the product.

Allergic reactions to cosmetics are usually caused by fragrances such as cinnamic alcohol, cinnamic aldehyde, hydroxycitronnella, musk ambrette, isoeugenol and geraniol. Some eaux de cologne, which contain oil of bergamot (see BERGAMOT, OIL OF), can cause a berloque dermatitis (dark color when exposed to the sun on neck and cleavage of women) in the area of skin where the cologne is applied. Those sensitive to some types of perfume could try spraying the product on hair or clothing instead of skin.

Genital deodorants These products can produce a contact dermatitis, including swelling and itching.

Hair dye Permanent dyes contain *paraphenylenediamine,* which can cause an oozing red rash in allergic patients. This is the reason why patch tests are recommended before dying hair. For sensitive people, temporary or vegetable hair dyes are a good alternative.

Lanolin A type of animal fat derived from sheep oil glands, lanolin is commonly included in moisturizers. Many people with sensitive skin are allergic to lanolin.

Nail products Allergic reactions can occur from a wide variety of nail products, including nail polishes, nail hardeners and artificial nails. Most nail products contain *toluenesulfonamide formaldehyde resin,* which can set off an allergic response when it comes in contact with eyelids, the neck or other sensitive skin while nails are drying. If your nail products contain this chemical, be sure the nails have dried for an hour before touching skin.

Nickel This shiny stainless metal is often used in surface plating of metal objects such as buttons, costume jewelry and kitchen equipment. It is also an element in many alloys, and is widely used in dentistry. Allergy to nickel occurs 10 times more often in women then men, and is often triggered by

ear piercing. Having the ears pierced and using earrings with nickel posts causes subsequent rashes to appear in other areas of the body whenever the person touches objects containing nickel. In allergic individuals, necklaces, bracelets, belt buckles and other jewelry that have never before caused a problem may suddenly cause a rash after the ears are pierced. Those at high risk for developing an occupational nickel allergy include hairdressers, nurses, cashiers and metal industry employees.

If you have newly pierced ears, wear only steel posts until earlobes heal (about three weeks). Surgical steel is the best choice and is available most often in earrings specifically designed for sensitive skin. Avoid the heat when wearing this type of jewelry, and buy only high-quality jewelry that is at least 14-karat gold; the higher the karat, the lower the percentage of nickel. A few dermatologists warn highly sensitive patients to avoid foods containing traces of nickel, such as coffee, beer, tea, apricots, chocolate, and nuts.

Parabens A group of often-used preservatives, parabens can be found in a variety of products, especially cosmetics.

Plastics Plastics such as epoxy resin can affect workers; finished plastic products rarely cause sensitivity.

Preservatives A wide variety of cosmetics, shampoos, creams and lotions contain preservatives to extend their shelf life and prevent bacteria buildup. The most toxic of these are *quaternium 15, imidazolidinyl urea* and *dialozolidinyl urea.* (See also FORMALDEHYDE, SENSITIVITY TO.)

Rubber (latex) The stretchy material used in surgical gloves and condoms, bras, waistbands and sneakers cause two types of allergic reactions. Most common is a red, oozing, blistering eruption. Less common are hives. About a third of those who develop hives from contact with latex also develop other symptoms, including hay fever, asthma and even anaphylactic shock. This type of reaction is often seem among medical workers because of the extensive use of latex gloves. If you are sensitive to rubber, avoid clothes with exposed rubber, since rubber covered by cloth usually doesn't cause a problem. Women who are allergic to rubber condoms should have their partner wear a lambskin condom over a latex one (a lambskin condom alone won't protect against HIV). Males allergic to rubber should wear the lambskin condom *under* the latex condom.

Sun While most people think of the sun as the source of a so-called "healthy" tan, it can also cause allergies in some people, who develop bumps, blotches, hives or blisters. Some are allergic to the sun alone, others to a combination of cosmetics, soaps, detergents, perfumes or topical or systemic medications with the sun (See also SOLAR URTICARIA; POLYMORPHIC LIGHT ERUPTION.)

Topical agents Many people are sensitive to the active or inactive ingredients in topical drugs or cosmetics, including lanolin, bacitracin, neomycin, local anesthetics, formaldehyde and preservatives.

allergy tests See PATCH TESTS.

allograft A type of tissue (or organ) graft (also known as homograft) between two members of the same species.

aloe vera A wild succulent (*Aloe barbadensis* Miller) of the lily family used for centuries as a healing agent and beauty aid. Aloe vera juice (obtained from slicing the tip of leaf and squeezing out the gel) appears to be effective in relieving the pain and inflammation of sunburn. The aloe vera gel contains vitamins B_1, B_2 and B_6, calcium, potassium, chlorine, enzymes and other ingredients that have not yet been identified.

alopecia, androgenetic This is the most common type of hair loss. The condition includes hereditary hair loss and male pattern baldness. Normal genes and androgens (especially testosterone) cause progressive shrinking of certain scalp follicles over time. The shrinking follicle produces a smaller, finer hair with each growth cycle. In addition to a smaller follicle, androgenetic alopecia is characterized by a shortened growth phase, which results in shorter hair.

The balding process is a gradual conversion of active, large hair follicles to less active, smaller follicles, resulting in short, thin hairs that are barely visible and that eventually disappear completely. In men, hereditary baldness is characterized by a receding hairline above the forehead and loss of hair at the crown. If male pattern baldness progresses to its final stage, the person is left with hair only around the sides and back of the head.

In women, hereditary hair loss is a general or diffuse thinning of the hair over the top of the head; half of all women have a notable thinning by age 50, but rarely lose all their hair. The hairline in front is almost always maintained.

Treatment A topical solution of MINOXIDIL 2 percent applied twice daily to the scalp lessens falling hair and stimulates new hair growth; one third of patients using this product report moderate hair growth after one year. Beginning treatment with minoxidil is most effective if begun early; patients who have been balding for less than five years or who have smaller bald patches report the best results. It may take several months for hair growth to begin, and if the treatment is stopped, the newly regrown hair will fall out. Minoxidil is effective for both men and women. It was developed to treat high blood pressure, and it increases the diameter of blood vessels.

Alternatively, HAIR TRANSPLANTS or scalp reduction (removal of the bald area of the scalp) are effective treatments for men with male pattern baldness.

See also ALOPECIA AREATA; ALOPECIA, FRICTION; ALOPECIA, TRACTION; HAIR LOSS.

alopecia areata Alopecia areata is a common form of hair loss that usually begins with a small, round bare spot on the scalp; in extreme cases it progresses to total hair loss on the entire body. It can affect people of all ages, although it most often occurs in children and young adults.

In *alopecia totalis*, hair suddenly falls out in a generalized pattern, ending in complete baldness of the scalp but body hair is preserved. In *Alopecia areata universalis* all body hair is lost, including head, pubic, underarm, eyebrow and eyelid hair. The most common form of alopecia areata (localized alopecia) is characterized by a complete loss of hair on the head in one circular patch from 1 to 10 cm. in diameter; the nails may also be affected by pitting, ridging or splitting.

Cause The condition is generally believed to be an autoimmune disorder in which the body produces antibodies that cause hair follicles to stop hair production. It may run in families, especially those with a history of asthma, ECZEMA or autoimmune disorders such as rheumatoid arthritis or LUPUS ERYTHEMATOSUS.

Treatment While there is no cure, hair frequently regrows in the localized form without treatment. Otherwise, physicians may recommend cortisone injections, topical MINOXIDIL (Rogaine) or other medications that trigger the follicles to start producing hair again. Treatment must continue until the condition goes away, which may take months or years. See Appendix E; see also ALOPECIA, ANDROGENETIC; ALOPECIA, FRICTION; ALOPECIA, TRACTION; HAIR LOSS.

For more information, contact the National Alopecia Areata Foundation, PO Box 150760, San Rafael, CA 94915; (415) 456–4644.

alopecia, friction The loss of hair caused by constantly wearing snug-fitting wigs or hats. See also ALOPECIA, ANDROGENETIC; ALOPECIA AREATA; ALOPECIA, TRACTION; HAIR LOSS.

alopecia, traction Loss of hair caused by ponytails, braids or cornrows that are pulled too tight, pulling the hair out by its roots. See also ALOPECIA, ANDROGENETIC; ALOPECIA AREATA; ALOPECIA, FRICTION; HAIR LOSS.

alpha hydroxy acids (AHA) A generic term that refers to any one of several organic chemicals that serve as mild chemical peels, working to loosen and slough off dead skin cells to expose newer, fresher skin. In six to eight weeks, skin treated with alpha hydroxy acids appears softer and smoother; AGE SPOTS and FRECKLES also appear to fade.

Also called "fruit acids," these products are derived from sugar cane, apples, grapes and citrus. The popular GLYCOLIC ACID derived from sugar cane is one of the alpha hydroxy acids, all of which are applied as an ointment, cream or lotion directly to the skin.

Alpha hydroxy acids are available over the counter in mild strengths of 10 percent; in beauty shops in concentrations of up to 40 percent, and in dermatologist's office in concentrations of up to 70 percent.

Precisely how the acids interact with the skin is not entirely understood, but the products do improve the appearance of the skin by accelerating the natural process of shedding dead skin cells. Used properly, the acids work gently, producing only a slight tingling or stinging sensation in some users.

With repeated use, the acids can clear up acne-prone skin, soften tiny lines around the eyes and mouth, smooth dry skin, and fade dark spots caused by sun or hormonal changes (such as those caused by pregnancy). Fastest results occur in the physician's office, since dermatologists can prescribe the strongest products.

Legally, these acid products are considered COSMETICS, not drugs, and therefore are not regulated by the Food and Drug Administration. However, alpha hydroxy acids can be dangerous; the availability of "bootleg" formulations in high concentrations have caused irritations and even burns in some. Due to a rising number of lawsuits by injured parties, the FDA is reviewing the products to see whether strength thresholds should be established by law.

Over-the-counter products manufactured by reputable companies are safe and generally quite mild, containing less than 10 percent AHA. Responsible firms don't sell products with stronger concentrations over the counter because of the danger to consumers and the resulting liability threat. Because these acids have caused problems for people with sensitive skin (being acids, they can sting), the newest products are formulated to work effectively without irritating.

Some of these products contain only 4 percent glycolic acid. Many company experts state that many women can safely switch to the new 8 percent formula once their skin adjusts to this acid. Other companies have introduced a four-step program that gradually accustoms skin to increasing levels of AHAs. However, some experts believe these nonprescription products are not really strong enough to do anything more than soften the skin.

While the acids are less powerful than RE-TIN-A for wrinkle removal, AHA formulations, according to some dermatologists, may prove useful in preventing and treating fine wrinkles.

aluminum acetate See BUROW'S SOLUTION.

amebiasis Infection with the protozoa *Entamoeba histolytica*, which is found throughout the world (primarily in the tropical countries) and produces painful skin ulcers. Skin symptoms with this infection are not common.

The ameba is transmitted by contaminated food and beverages. Infections with *E. histo-lytica* are primarily in people who show no symptoms.

The skin also may be invaded by infection following surgical procedures, by direct extension of amebic liver abscess or by direct inoculation by the protozoa.

The skin ulcer is a painful lesion that can last from 10 days to two years. Rapid skin destruction occurs more often among children.

Treatment Combinations of medication may be required; in those with skin symptoms, metronidazole is probably the safest drug and is most effective when given in single daily doses.

American Academy of Allergy and Immunology A professional society of physicians specializing in allergy and allergic diseases that sponsors annual two-day postgraduate courses and three-day scientific sessions. The group conducts research and educational programs, maintains a speakers' bureau, bestows annual grants and research awards, operates a placement service and compiles statistics. The group was formed by the merger of the American Association for the Study of Allergy and the Association for the Study of Asthma and Allied Conditions. Founded in 1943, the academy has 4,900 members and publishes the annual journal *American Academy of Allergy and Immunology—Abstract Book*, the quarterly newsletter *News and Notes*, the quarterly newsletter *Practical Information and Health Tips from Your Allergist* and the monthly journal, *Journal of Allergy and Clinical Immunology*. See also AMERICAN ALLERGY ASSOCIATION.

American Academy of Cosmetic Surgery A professional group of licensed plastic surgeons that seeks to encourage high-quality cosmetic medical and dental care, provides continuing education for cosmetic surgeons, and promotes research. The academy also compiles statistics, operates the American Board of Cosmetic Surgery and maintains a speakers' bureau. Founded in 1985, the academy has 1,250 members and publishes a quarterly newsletter.

American Academy of Dermatology
A professional society of 8,800 physicians specializing in skin diseases. The academy conducts educational programs, provides placement services, bestows awards and compiles statistics. It also offers computerized services: DERM/INFONET, an online service containing 14 databases.

Established in 1938, the academy was formerly known as the American Academy of Dermatology and Syphilology.

Its publications include the bimonthly *Bulletin*, the biennial *Directory of the American Academy of Dermatology*, and the monthly *Journal of the American Academy of Dermatology*. It also issues *Dialogues in Dermatology* (audiotapes).

American Academy of Facial Plastic and Reconstructive Surgery
A professional association for physicians specializing in facial plastic surgery that promotes research and study in the field. It maintains a speakers' bureau, conducts education and charitable programs, and compiles statistics.

Founded in 1964, the academy has 2,900 members and publishes the quarterly *Facial Plastic Surgery Today*, the monthly *Facial Plastic Times* and brochures and directories. The group sponsors a semiannual meeting.

American Allergy Association
A support group for allergy patients and those interested in problems created by allergies that disseminates information on diet, environmental control and other allergy advice. Founded in 1978, the association publishes an annual handbook and holds an annual September meeting. For address, see Appendix D; see also AMERICAN ACADEMY OF ALLERGY AND IMMUNOLOGY.

American Association of Plastic Surgeons
A professional group of plastic surgeons founded in 1921, with 425 members. Formerly the American Association of Oral and Plastic Surgeons, the group sponsors an annual scientific program in April or May.

American Behcet's Association
A support group that gathers statistics on patients with BEHCET'S SYNDROME and educates the public and medical community about the disease. (Behcet's syndrome is characterized by skin lesions and mouth ulcers, among other symptoms.) The association conducts educational programs, maintains a speakers bureau and publishes a quarterly newsletter, brochures and pamphlets. Founded in 1986, the association holds a biennial conference. See Appendices D and E.

American Board of Dermatology
The examining and certifying body for United States dermatologists that seeks to assure competent care for patients with skin diseases by offering board certification to those who meet its requirements and pass its examination.

The board establishes requirements of postdoctoral training and creates and conducts an annual comprehensive examination to determine the competence of physicians who meet the requirements. It issues appropriate certificates to those who complete the exam satisfactorily. The board is also a member of the American Board of Medical Specialties.

Founded in 1932, the board has 14 directors and offers a *Booklet of Information*.

American Board of Plastic Surgery A group established in 1937 by representatives of various groups interested in encouraging well-rounded training in plastic surgery. Officially recognized in 1941 as the only specialty board responsible for certifying plastic surgeons, the board has 19 directors who meet twice a year to judge the education, training and knowledge of plastic surgeons. Certification by the board is not required to practice plastic surgery, but it is a status that plastic surgeons voluntarily obtain as an indication of competence.

Requirements for certification include graduation from an accredited medical school; at least three years of clinical training in general surgery, completion of an approved residency in orthopedic surgery, or certification by the American Board of Otolaryngology; at least two years of approved residency training in plastic surgery in the United States or Canada; and successful completion of the certification examination.
See also AMERICAN SOCIETY OF PLASTIC AND RECONSTRUCTIVE SURGEONS.

American Burn Association A professional organization for anyone interested in the care of burn injuries dedicated to improving the care and treatment of BURNS, including a program of preventing burn injuries. Founded in 1967, the association has 3,500 members and publishes an annual book of abstracts, a directory of burn care services in North America listing specialized burn care facilities in the United States and Canada, and a bimonthly *Journal of Burn Care and Rehabilitation*. The association sponsors an annual scientific meeting and regional seminars. For address, see Appendix E; see also BURNS UNITED SUPPORT GROUPS, INTERNATIONAL SOCIETY FOR BURN INJURIES, NATIONAL BURN VICTIM FOUNDATION, PHOENIX SOCIETY FOR BURN SURVIVORS, NATIONAL INSTITUTE FOR BURN MEDICINE.

American Dermatologic Society of Allergy and Immunology A professional group for physicians with practices in dermatology, allergy and immunology. Established in 1974, the society has 150 members and sponsors semiannual lectures on immunodermatology.

American Dermatological Association Founded in 1876, this professional society of physicians specializing in dermatology promotes teaching, practice and research in dermatology.

American Electrology Association A professional group for electrologists united for education, professional advancement and the protection of public welfare that promotes uniform legislative standards throughout the country. The association coordinates efforts of affiliated associations in dealing with problems, and sponsors the International Board of Electrologist Certification. The group also maintains referral, reference, advisory and consulting services.

Founded in 1958, the association has 2,000 members and publishes brochures and the quarterly newsletter *Electrolysis World* and the semiannual journal *Journal of the American Electrology Association* and the semiannual *Medical/Professional News*. The group also sponsors an annual conference, plus seminars and workshops. For address, see Appendix D; see also COUNCIL ON ELECTROLYSIS EDUCATION; INTERNATIONAL GUILD OF PROFESSIONAL ELECTROLOGISTS; NATIONAL COMMISSION FOR ELECTROLOGIST CERTIFICATION; SOCIETY OF CLINICAL AND MEDICAL ELECTROLOGISTS.

American Hair Loss Council A professional group for dermatologists, plastic surgeons, cosmetologists, barbers and interested lay members that provides non-biased information regarding treatments for hair loss in both men and women. The group facilitates communication and information exchange between specialists in different areas, maintains a library, conducts educational programs, offers children's services and a placement service, and compiles statistics. Founded in 1985, the council has 320 members and hosts an annual conference.

Its publications include the quarterly *Hair Loss Journal,* a newsletter reporting on hair loss and treatment ($30/year). For address, see Appendix D.

American Leprosy Foundation A health and research foundation concerned with microbiological research of LEPROSY (Hansen's disease), conducting research programs in the United States and the Philippines. The foundation supports clinical and basic lab research and epidemiological surveys and sponsors an exchange program. Formerly known as the Leonard Wood Memorial for the Eradication of Leprosy, the group was founded in 1928 and holds a semiannual scientific advisory board meeting. For address, see Appendix D. See also DAMIEN DUTTON SOCIETY FOR LEPROSY AID.

American Leprosy Missions An international medical Christian mission for those with Hansen's disease (LEPROSY) supporting more than 100 programs in approximately 30 countries with antileprosy drugs, surgical intervention for disabilities, training of health workers, research, public information, and physical and vocational rehabilitation assistance. Also known as ALM International, the group collaborates with member agencies of the International Federation of Anti-Leprosy Associations. As leprosy treatment becomes integrated with community health care, ALM includes those who are disabled from causes other than leprosy in its rehabilitation programs.

Founded in 1906 by Protestant missionaries, the group works closely with committees of the World Health Organization and with the U.S. Public Health Service Hospital in Carville, La. ALM also supports training and research centers in India, Ethiopia and Brazil. The group also publishes a quarterly newsletter *(Word & Deed),* pamphlets, reports and brochures. See Appendices D and E. See also DAMIEN DUTTON SOCIETY FOR LEPROSY AID; AMERICAN LEPROSY FOUNDATION.

American Lupus Society, The A support group for those interested in information on LUPUS ERYTHEMATOSUS, a noncontagious disease that may affect the skin, alone or in addition to other symptoms. The society helps lupus patients and their families cope with the daily problems associated with the disease. The group collects and distributes funds for research; chapters hold patient meetings and occasional medical seminars. Founded in 1973, the society publishes the quarterly newsletter *The American Lupus Society—Lupus Today,* plus booklets and pamphlets, and sponsors an annual conference. See Appendices D and E; see also LUPUS NETWORK; LUPUS FOUNDATION OF AMERICA; L.E. SUPPORT CLUB.

American Osteopathic College of Dermatology A professional association for osteopaths or those involved in dermatology that conducts specialized education programs. Founded in 1955, it has 130 members and hosts an annual convention in conjunction with the American Osteopathic Association.

Publications include the annual *Directory* and a quarterly *Newsletter.*

American Porphyria Foundation A support group for anyone interested in the treatment of PORPHYRIA, a class of seven rare (usually inherited) metabolic disorders that affect either the skin or the nervous system. The foundation provides financial support for research, offers educational programs and maintains a lending library of videotapes, papers and pamphlets. Founded in 1981, the group has 900 members and sponsors an annual meeting and physician lecture series. See Appendices D and E.

American Society for Dermatologic Surgery A professional organization for physicians specializing in dermatologic surgery that seeks to maintain the highest possible standards in medical education, clinical practice and patient care. The group endeavors to promote high standards in allied health professions and services as they relate to dermatology and maintains an audiovisual library.

Founded in 1970, the society has 2,157 members and hosts an annual conference. Its publications include the monthly *Journal of Dermatologic Surgery and Oncology* and an annual *Roster*. The group can provide consumers with a list of local physicians qualified to perform dermatologic laser surgery. For information, call (800) 441–2737.

American Society for Laser Medicine and Surgery A professional group for physicians, physicists and other scientists, nurses, dentists, podiatrists, veterinarians, paramedical personnel, technicians and commercial representatives concerned with the medical application of LASERS. The society exchanges information about lasers and publishes the bimonthly journal *Lasers in Surgery and Medicine*. Founded in 1980, the group has 1,902 members and holds an annual meeting.

American Society of Dermatological Retailers A professional group for board-certified dermatologists that promotes ethical and professional marketing standards for skin care products. The society conducts educational and research programs, sponsors competitoins, compiles statistics, maintains a library, speakers bureau, hall of fame and museum.

The group publishes *Epex Quarterly* (free) and *Health and Beauty*, plus the annual newsletter *Skin Saver* (free).

American Society of Dermatopathology A professional association that seeks to improve the quality of dermatopathology (the study of abnormal skin conditions, especially the structural and functional changes produced by disease). The group provides information, supports continuing education and research, conducts seminars and courses and bestows awards.

Founded in 1962, it has 880 members and hosts an annual scientific conference and an annual meeting in conjunction with the International Academy of Pathology.

Its publications include the bimonthly *Journal of Cutaneous Pathology* and its annual *Membership Directory*.

American Society of Plastic and Reconstructive Surgeons A professional organization founded in 1931 to promote optimal quality care for plastic surgery patients, to provide educational programs and to support the activities of its 2,900 members. To become a member, each plastic surgeon must be certified by the AMERICAN BOARD OF PLASTIC SURGERY.

In addition to its professional activities, the society maintains a patient referral service to help patients choose a plastic surgeon (call 800-635-0635) and a speakers' bureau. Material describing procedures and results are also available.

amino acids The basic building blocks of protein that make up the skin and hair. The process by which amino acids build skin is extremely complex, and slathering on products containing amino acids will not necessarily help the skin utilize these chemicals to produce new skin. However, shampoos and hair conditioners that contain amino acids do help fill in cracks in the hair shaft caused by harsh soaps and processing; these new proteins don't *rebuild* the hair shaft, but they do lend support.

ammoniated mercury A bleaching agent that reduces skin color by stopping the formation of MELANIN. It is not very effective and has several potentially harmful effects on the skin, including allergic reactions. Ammoniated mercury in cosmetics has been banned by the Food and Drug Administration.

amphotericin B An intravenous drug used to treat fungal infections of the skin. Fungus infections may mean anything from a minor problem such as ATHLETE'S FOOT or vaginal yeast infections to more serious problems if these infections invade the blood or internal organs when the immune system is not working well. Amphotericin B is only used for life-threatening systemic fungal infections.

Over the past 10 years, the incidence of serious fungus infections has risen dramatically in this country, mostly because profoundly ill patients are living longer than in the past. Those most susceptible to the serious fungal infections include cancer chemotherapy patients, AIDS and burn patients, and transplant recipients.

Adverse effects Vomiting, fever, headache or seizures are among the drug's adverse effects. Amphotericin B is administered in a hospital setting because side effects may be severe. See also KETOCONAZOLE; FLUCYTOSINE; ANTIFUNGAL AGENTS; FUNGAL INFECTIONS.

amyloidosis The general term for a group of fairly uncommon conditions in which amyloid (which contains protein and starch) builds up in tissues and organs.

Primary amyloidosis is often characterized by deposits of amyloid in the skin, causing raised, waxy spots clustered around the armpits, groin, face and neck. Male Caucasians between age 50 and 60 are most commonly affected; skin manifestations occur in 40 percent of patients. The most common sign is a "pinch purpura" (development of a purple lesion after pinching or stroking the skin). Lesions may appear to be translucent, waxy or amber-colored papules or nodules; less often the skin may look yellow, red or with heightened pigment. There may be a thickening of the palms and enlargement of ears, lips and eyelids, and the scalp may develop deep folds; there may be hair loss and some patients develop blisters. The nails may be brittle, crumbling or streaked, and on some fingers there may be no nails. About 40 percent of deaths related to this condition occur because of heart problems; 30 percent of deaths may result from kidney failure caused by deposits of amyloid. Diagnosis depends on microscopic examination of a biopsy of tissue from the affected organ.

Secondary amyloidosis (or reactive systemic amyloidosis) often occurs as a result of an infectious process such as tuberculosis or osteomyelitis, or a chronic noninfectious inflammatory disease such as rheumatoid arthritis. It also may occur in association with certain nonlymphoid tumors and some lymphomas (the two most common are renal cell carcinoma and Hodgkin's disease).

There are no skin symptoms in secondary amyloidosis.

Treatment Primary amyloidosis can be treated with anti-cancer drugs; secondary amyloidosis may be stopped or even reversed when the underlying disorder is treated.

anaphylaxis A severe, life-threatening, allergic reaction that occurs rarely in those who have an extreme sensitivity to a particular substance (allergen).

Cause The reaction, which often includes an itchy red rash or HIVES, is most common after an insect sting or as a reaction to an injected or ingested drug, such as penicillin or tetanus serum. As the allergen enters the bloodstream, it provokes the release of massive amounts of histamine and other chemicals that affect the body by widening blood vessels and lowering blood pressure.

Treatment A person who experiences such a reaction following a sting or injection should lie down with legs raised to improve blood flow to the heart and brain. An injection of epinephrine can save the victim's life and must be given as soon as possible.

Ancobon   See FLUCYTOSINE.

anergy Inability to react to common skin test ALLERGENS (foreign substances that produce allergic reactions), which represents a deficit in the cellular arms of the immune system.

angioedema An allergic reaction characterized by HIVES of large, well-defined swellings that appear suddenly in the skin and larynx. The swellings may last several hours (or days, if untreated). Angioedema is primarily found in young people in their 20s and those who tend to have allergies.

Cause The most common cause of angioedema is a sudden allergic response to food (especially strawberries, eggs or seafood). Less often, it occurs in response to drug injections or ingestion (especially penicillin), insect stings, snake bite, infection, emotional stress, exposure to animals, molds, pollens or cold.

Symptoms Angioedema may cause sudden breathing problems, difficulty swallowing, and obvious swelling of the lips, face and neck. The swelling it produces in the throat may lead to suffocation by blocking the victim's airway.

Treatment Severe cases respond to injections of epinephrine, but use of a breathing tube or even tracheostomy may be necessary to prevent suffocation. In less severe cases, antihistamine drugs often relieve symptoms.

angioedema, hereditary Hereditary forms of acquired ANGIOEDEMA (an allergic reaction characterized by itching and swelling). Attacks, which are characterized by diffuse nonitching swelling, are not usually accompanied by hives.

Cause Hereditary forms of angioedema are transmitted in an autosomal dominant manner. Attacks may be set off by trauma or may appear to occur spontaneously.

Symptoms In addition to the swelling of the skin, symptoms may include swelling of the gastrointestinal tract that may cause abdominal pain severe enough to suggest the need for surgery. Swelling of the upper respiratory tract may cause marked swelling of the uvula and larynx, leading to suffocation. Acute laryngeal swelling is the most serious manifestation of this disorder and can be fatal (due to asphyxiation) in nearly 20 percent of patients. Attacks usually fade within three to to four days, but during this time the individual must be observed careful for signs of laryngeal obstruction.

Treatment Epinephrine, antihistamines and corticosteroids are usually used in treatment, but the success of these agents is limited. If the larynx becomes obstructed, tracheostomy (a surgical hole in the trachea to relieve obstruction) may be needed.

angiofibroma Several different types of benign lesions may be included under the term "angiofibroma" (also called ADENOMA SEBACEUM). The angiofibroma may appear as a solitary lesion or in groups (and may be an important skin symptom of TUBEROUS SCLEROSIS).

The condition may include fibrous papule of the nose—a single lesion on the nose that sometimes looks like a red or flesh-colored mole that is not related to tuberous sclerosis. Lesions on the face that show a great deal of fibrous tissue around hair follicles are called perifollicular fibromas. Smaller, similar lesions around the penis are called pearly penile papules.

Treatment Because these lesions are benign, treatment is not necessary. Single lesions may be excised and groups of lesions of tuberous sclerosis may be excised with a CARBON DIOXIDE LASER or DERMABRASION to improve the appearance. Pearly papules on the penis are not usually treated.

angiokeratoma A condition resembling KERATOSIS, characterized by benign lesions that are usually soft and colored from pink to red-purple that are often found over bony prominences (such as hands and feet) of the body (especially in children and young adults). Sometimes they may be found on the scrotum or in groups on the legs and feet. Occasionally the lesions appear singly.

Angiokeratomas that occur as part of the rare fatal disease known as *angiokeratoma corporis diffusum* of Fabry (FABRY'S DISEASE) are a minor feature of the disorder; other symptoms include heart and kidney disease and high blood pressure. Patients with this variation usually die from heart or kidney failure. It is an X-linked recessive genetic disorder, which means that it is caused by a defect on the X chromosome usually leading to problems in males only. Women can be carriers of the defect, and half of those carrier's sons may be affected.

Treatment Angiokeratomas may be surgically removed.

angiokeratoma corporis diffusum See FABRY'S DISEASE.

angioma Small collection of blood vessels overlying and compressing the brain that may be associated with a PORT-WINE STAIN (this is known as STURGE-WEBER SYNDROME).

angiosarcoma See SARCOMA.

anhidrosis The absence of the ability to sweat. It may be caused by processes that control the sweating response, as well as certain skin diseases (PSORIASIS, atopic dermatitis), certain drugs (anticholinergics, quinacrine), dehydration, hypothyroidism etc. Many patients who can't sweat in some areas have a compensatory sweating response in other sweat glands.

In ANHIDROTIC ECTODERMAL DYSPLASIA there is a decrease or absence of sweating that most commonly is caused by an X-linked inheritance pattern (primarily affecting males). Hair may be sparse, light, coarse or strawlike, with sparse eyelashes and eyebrows and dental abnormalities.

Treatment Treatment is aimed at controlling the underlying cause. Those with untreatable anhidrosis should be careful when exposed to excessive heat, work or physical activity that would normally provoke intense sweating.

Complications Since the body relies on sweating to cool the body, the inability to sweat can lead to excessively high internal body temperatures.

anhidrotic ectodermal dysplasia A disorder, usually inherited, characterized by decrease or absence of sweating, decrease in scalp hair and eyebrows, and dental abnormalities. The classic, most common form is transmitted by an X-linked inheritance pattern predominantly affecting males. This condition is life-long, although patients can enjoy a full and productive life. See also HAIR, DISORDERS OF.

Symptoms Sparse, light, strawlike hair first appearing at birth or shortly thereafter. The abnormal hair pattern with a frontal upsweep suggests abnormal growth of the scalp during fetal development; eyelashes and eyebrows are often sparse. There is an absence of perspiration in infants, but the sweating abnormality may be undetected for years. Exercise is followed by flushing and fatigue, and an atopic dermatitis often accompanies this syndrome, together with allergic rhinitis and asthma. Patients with this condition may share similar facial features, including a depressed nasal bridge, pouting lips and protruding ears, with decreased activity of the tear ducts, nasal and salivary glands.

Treatment Acute hyperthermia should be treated with cool baths or sprays to help evaporate body heat. Patients should avoid drugs such as chlorpromazine, anticholinergics and diazepam that interfere with temperature control. The atopic dermatitis can be treated with antihistamines (such as hydroxyzine), emollients and topical corticosteroids.

animal bites Each year 2 million Americans get medical treatment for bites; in most cases the animal involved is a dog. If the skin has been broken by a bite, treatment depends on its depth and location and on what's known about the animal.

Treatment The area is first cleaned using an antiseptic. Medical treatment is essential. It includes an antibiotic (the best one in these cases is amoxicillin). Stitches may be required, but it's usually best for these wounds to heal without being sewn up to prevent any dangerous organism from getting trapped in the body. (Exception: bites on the face probably will need to be stitched to avoid disfigurement).

More than 25,000 Americans get a rabies vaccination each year.

ANSI sunglass standard A voluntary labeling program by the Sunglass Association of America, a group working with the Food and Drug Administration to provide consumers with uniform and useful labeling for nonprescription sunglasses. The ANSI standard is found on a label attached to sunglasses, describing how much and which types of UL- TRAVIOLET RADIATION is blocked out.

anthralin preparations A topical prescription compound used to treat PSORIASIS (a skin disease caused by excess skin cell production). Available as a cream or ointment, anthralin works by slowing the skin cell multiplication rate; its effects may be increased by using ultraviolet light treatments. Anthralin is applied to the skin and left on for a short period of time or overnight (depending on doctor's orders).

Anthralin should not be applied to raw or blistered areas of the skin. Even so, anthralin commonly causes redness and irritation. The skin around patches of psoriasis can be protected from inflammation by applying petroleum jelly or zinc oxide paste before using the anthralin. The higher-strength compounds are particularly troublesome for irritation and skin staining; lower strength compounds have been developed that make this therapy more tolerable. Because anthralin can stain skin, hair and clothing, users should wear gloves and old clothes when applying the drug.

anthrax This serious bacterial infection affects livestock, but it can occasionally spread to humans where it causes skin infection. Anthrax (even in cattle) is rare today largely because of a vaccine, but some serious epidemics have occurred among herds and humans in developing countries because of ineffective control programs.

Causes Anthrax is caused by the bacterium *Bacillus anthracis,* which produces spores that can remain dormant for years in soil and animal products. When reactivated, the bacterium can infect animals that graze on contaminated land. Anyone can contract the disease who eats the affected meat, or handles or inhales spores from animals that died from the disease.

Symptoms The most common symptom is a raised, itchy area at the site of entry, progressing to a large blister and then a black scab with swelling of surrounding tissue.

Treatment Anthrax is curable in the early stages with penicillin but can be fatal in advanced stages.

antibacterial drugs A group of drugs used to treat infections caused by bacteria. These drugs act in the same way as antibiotic drugs, but unlike antibiotics they have always been produced synthetically. The largest group of antibacterial agents is the sulfonamides.

Antibacterial ointments contain combinations of the "nonabsorbable" antibiotics (bacitracin, neomycin, polymyxin B and gramicidin). While these may help for mild skin wounds, more extensive bacterial skin infections require systemic antibiotics.

Bacitracin is effective against organisms including *Streptococcus, Staphylococcus* and pneumococcus. Neomycin is effective against most gram-negative organisms (gram staining is a way of identifying bacterial cells). It is about 50 times more active against *Staphylococcus* than bacitracin, but bacitracin is 20 times more active against *Streptococcus.* However, neomycin causes more allergic contact sensitivity than any other topical antibiotic.

Gentamicin, another antibacterial drug, is also effective against *Staphylococcus aureus* and group AB-hemolytic streptococci. While it may be used topically, it is no better than other drugs mentioned above and it may produce an allergic reaction.

antibiotic drugs A group of drugs used to treat infections caused by bacteria. Originally prepared from molds and fungi, antibiotic drugs are now made synthetically. Antibiotics help fight infection when the body has been invaded by harmful bacteria or when the bacteria present in the body begin to multiply uncontrollably. More than one kind of antibiotic may be prescribed to increase the efficiency of treatment and to reduce the risk of antibiotic resistance.

Many bacteria develop resistance to a once-useful antibiotic. Resistance is most likely to develop if a person fails to take an antibiotic as directed, during long-term treatment. Some drugs, known as broad-spectrum antibiotics, are effective against a wide range of bacteria, while others are useful only in treating specific types.

Antibiotics in acne treatment Topical antibiotics (tetracycline, erythromycin, clindamycin and meclocycline) have an antibacterial effect when applied to the skin, in much the same way as BENZOYL PEROXIDE—except they are probably less effective. A relatively new preparation that combines erythromycin and benzoyl peroxide in a gel is probably more effective together than either preparation alone.

Systemic antibiotics can be very effective in the treatment of acne, despite the fact that acne is not a bacterial disease. In fact, 10 percent of all tetracycline sold in the United States is used to treat acne. It is believed that systemic antibiotic treatment probably prevents the development of additional inflammatory lesions. Erythromycin is as effective as tetracycline and does not have to be taken without food. Minocycline is also effective but is more expensive.

Side effects Because these agents may kill "normal" bacteria naturally present in the body, fungi may grow in their place, causing oral, intestinal or vaginal candidiasis (thrush). Some patients sometimes experience a severe allergic response, causing facial swelling, itching or breathing problems.

Types Some of the most well-known antibiotics include the penicillins (amoxicillin, penicillin V and oxacillin), the aminogylcosides (gentamicin and streptomycin), the cephalosporins (cefaclor and cephalexin), the tetracyclines (doxycycline and oxytetracycline), erythromycin and neomycin.

anticoagulation syndrome (coumarin necrosis) A condition characterized by lesions beginning between three and 10 days after the administration of a coumarin drug (such as dicumarol or warfarin) that occurs occasionally in young women. Coumarin is administered as an anticoagulant (blood thinner) to treat disorders in which there is excessive clotting, such as thrombophlebitis and certain heart conditions. Once the lesions begin to appear, their course is progressive regardless of whether the drug treatment is stopped.

The lesions begin as minute spots or blue or purple hemorrhagic patches (usually on the lower fatty areas of the body), quickly followed by tissue death, which can extend into the deep subcutaneous fat; the resulting ulcer may not heal for months.

Coumarin necrosis has been associated with protein C and protein S deficiency. Heparin necrosis also can occur without the use of coumarin drugs.

Treatment There is no effective treatment. When the breast or penis is involved, amputation is recommended; other areas may require surgical debridement and skin grafts.

antifungal/anti-yeast agents A group of drugs prescribed to treat infections caused by either fungi or yeasts (and sometimes both in one product) that can be administered directly to the skin or taken orally or by injection. They are commonly used to treat different types of TINEA, including ATHLETE'S FOOT, JOCK ITCH and SCALP RINGWORM. They are also used to treat THRUSH and rare fungal infections such as CRYPTOCOCCOSIS.

Side effects Agents applied to the skin, scalp, mouth or vagina may sometimes increase irritation, and antifungal agents given by mouth or injection may cause more serious side effects, damaging the kidney or liver.

Types Antifungal agents are available as creams, injections, tablets, lozenges, suspensions and vaginal suppositories. The most common antifungals include AMPHOTERICIN B (IV only), cyclopirox, clotrimazole, naftidine,

terbinefine ECONAZOLE, GRISEOFULVIN (by mouth only), itraconazole (by mouth and IV only), fluconazole (by mouth and IV only), ketoconazole, miconazole and TOLNAFTATE. While amphotericin B is the standard drug for treating fungal infections, it is usually given in the hospital because of the danger of side effects. On the other hand, itraconazole and fluconazole are the two most recently approved drugs to enter the antifungal arsenal. These two cause fewer side effects and can be taken orally on an outpatient basis.

Nonprescription creams such as Monistat 7 and Gyne-Lotrimin may be helpful in remedying candidal vaginal yeast infections, but fatal candidal infections affecting the brain, kidney or other organs may occur in immuno-compromised patients in the hospital.

Anti-yeast agents, such as nystatin, do not kill most fungi, but most antifungals kill yeasts as well—except for griseofulvin. Drugs that are used for both systemic fungal and yeast infections include fluconazole, ketoconazole, amphotericin-B and itraconazole.

antihistamines A family of drugs used to treat allergic conditions, such as itching and hives. The drugs work by blocking the action of histamine, a chemical that is released during an allergic reaction. Examples of antihistamines include diphenhydramine, promethazine, terfenadine, chlorpheniramine, etc.

Without drug treatment, histamine dilates small blood vessels, causing redness and swelling; antihistamines block this effect, while preventing the irritation of nerve fibers that would otherwise cause itching. They are the most effective treatment for hives.

Adverse effects Some antihistamines cause drowsiness and dizziness, but new antihistamines such as Seldane and Claritin do not enter the brain and thus do not cause dizziness. Other possible symptoms include appetite loss, nausea, dry mouth, blurry vision and problems in urination. Because older antihistamines have a sedative effect, they may also be used to induce sleep; patients taking these types of antihistamines should not drive or operate heavy machinery until the effects wear off.

anti-inflammatory drugs A family of drugs used to help decrease inflammation and pain. This class of drugs includes the nonsteroidal anti-inflammatory drugs (NSAIDS) and the CORTICOSTEROIDS, both of which fight inflammation.

The NSAIDS are a group of chemically diverse drugs widely used to treat inflammation, which is one of the body's defense mechanisms in response to infection and certain chronic diseases (such as rheumatoid arthritis). They include ibuprofen (Motrin, Rufen, Advil, Medipren, Nuprin), fenoprofen (Nalfon), meclofenamate (Meclomen), naproxen (Anaprox, Naprosyn), sulindac (Clinoril), indomethacin (Indocin), tolmetin (Tolectin), mefanamic acid, piroxicam (Feldene), oxyphenbutazone and phenylbutazone.

On their own, NSAIDS are not very toxic, but they should not be used by people with gastrointestinal disease, peptic ulcers or poor heart function. They should not be taken with other nonsteroid painkillers or other anticoagulants (blood thinners), because bleeding time may be prolonged while on NSAIDs. Antacids and aspirin may also reduce the effectiveness of an anti-inflammatory drug.

The corticosteroids are a group of drugs used primarily to treat inflammation that are similar to natural corticosteroid hormones produced by the adrenal glands. Skin diseases treated with these drugs include eczema, acne, PEMPHIGUS, PSORIASIS, ALOPECIA, DERMATITIS, LICHEN PLANUS, ROSACEA, ERYTHEMA MUITIFORME etc. They include cortisone, prednisone, prednisolone, hydrocortisone, dexamethasone, beclomethasone etc.

When taken in high doses for a long time, adverse effects can include tissue swelling, high blood pressure, diabetes mellitus, peptic ulcer, Cushing's syndrome, excess hairiness and susceptibility to infection.

antimalarial drugs Also called antiprotozoals, this is a group of drugs used to treat malaria. The two most common used in dermatology are hydroxychloroquine and quinacrine. These drugs have been helpful in treating skin symptoms of malaria, LUPUS ERYTHEMATOSUS, PORPHYRIA and skin lesions in DERMATOMYOSITIS.
Adverse effects Hydroxychloroquine and chloroquine may produce retinal damage; other possible side effects include aplastic anemia (a type of anemia caused by a decrease in bone marrow production of all types of blood cells) or leukopenia. Quinacrine may produce a yellowing of the skin. Any antimalarial drug may cause the hair to gray; some patients also experience a bluish-black discoloration of the inside of the mouth and skin under the fingernails that improves when the drug is stopped. Infrequent side effects include HIVES, EXFOLIATIVE ERYTHRODERMA and a worsening of PSORIASIS.

antiperspirants Metallic salts designed to be applied to the skin to control excessive unpleasant odor by reducing the production of sweat. They contain aluminum or aluminum-zirconium salts that block the eccrine and apocrine sweat ducts, obstructing delivery of sweat to the skin's surface. These products also remove bad-smelling odors because they create a drier environment that reduces the number of odor-causing bacteria. Shaving hair under the arms reduces odor, since hair increases the surface area for the production and release of odor-causing chemicals. They are more effective than deodorants, which simply remove bad-smelling odors. Some deodorants also contain antiperspirants.

Commercially available antiperspirants reduce underarm sweating by 20 to 40 percent; their effectiveness can be increased by applying in the morning and at bedtime. Antiperspirants should not be applied to moist or irritated skin, nor should they be used soon after shaving.

For those with extreme body odor problems, physicians may prescribe aluminum chloride hexahydrate, 20 percent solution in absolute alcohol (DRYSOL), for use on underarms, palms or soles. Drysol is applied at bedtime under a plastic film, but it may cause irritation if used often. See also SWEAT AND THE SKIN; SWEAT GLANDS; SWEAT GLANDS, DISORDERS OF.

antipruritic agents Drugs used to treat itching; however, generalized itching is not easy to treat unless the underlying condition is identified. Oral antihistamines are often prescribed, but they are most effective when the underlying condition involves the release of HISTAMINE (a chemical released during an allergic reaction that causes inflammation and itching, such as in HIVES).

Alternatively, some patients' itching may lessen with use of the new drugs pramoxine and doxysin, or with a preparation containing menthol, phenol or camphor. Menthol eases itching because of the cooling feeling it produces; phenol temporarily numbs nerve endings in the skin. Camphor has a local anesthetic effect.

Less often, preparations of SALICYLIC ACID or COAL TAR may be used. Shake lotions of CALAMINE may also reduce itching.

Over-the-counter preparations containing benzocaine or diphenhydramine should be avoided, since either may produce an allergic skin contact response.

antiseptic cleansers Chemicals designed to prevent infection that are applied to the skin to destroy bacteria and other microorganisms. The use of antiseptics to prevent infection (antisepsis) is not the same thing as the creation of a germ-free environment (asepsis). Antiseptics are milder than disinfectants which are used to decontaminate objects but are considered too strong for skin.

Antiseptic fluids are usually used to bathe wounds; antiseptic creams are applied to wounds before being bandaged.

Two commonly used antiseptics are iodine and chlorhexidine compounds; others include HYDROGEN PEROXIDE and thimerosal. *Chlorhexidine* is an antiseptic effective against many yeasts, fungi and both gram-negative and gram-positive bacteria. Well-tolerated by most people, it is quick-acting and effective for a long time. Antiseptic *iodine compounds* (such as the brownish yellow povidone-iodine) are effective against bacteria, fungi, yeasts, viruses and protozoa. However, they take longer to work than other antiseptics and may be ineffective in the presence of blood.

While *hexachlorophene* has been widely used in the past (effective against many gram-positive organisms such as *Staphylococcus*), it has also been associated with neurotoxicity. Because hexachlorophene is less safe than other agents such as chlorhexidine and iodine compounds, its use is regulated by the U.S. Food and Drug Administration.

antioxidant beauty products The newest anti-aging products contain the antioxidant vitamins E and C, and BETA-CAROTENE. They theoretically work by destroying free radicals (oxygen molecules that break down collagen, causing wrinkles and sagging). See VITAMIN E, VITAMIN C.

antiviral agents A group of drugs used to treat viral infections; one of the best-known of these drugs is ACYCLOVIR, prescribed for the treatment of various forms of HERPES, and AZT (zidovudine), prescribed for the treatment of AIDS. Until the development of acyclovir and AZT, no effective antiviral agents existed.

To this point, no drugs have been developed that eradicate viruses and cure the illnesses they cause. This is because viruses live only within cells; a drug capable of killing a virus would also kill its host cell. New antiviral agents interfere with viral replication or otherwise disrupt chemical processes of viral metabolism; some prevent viruses from penetrating cells. They are effective treatments for a variety of infections.

Newly developed antivirals, including acyclovir, famcyclovir and volcyclovir are especially effective in treating herpes family infections. Antiviral drugs reduce the severity of the herpes symptoms and perhaps shorten the course of the infection, but the drugs cannot eliminate the virus completely. Recently, scientists have been testing several varieties of a vaccine that appears to lessen the severity of herpes attacks. The vaccine is a combination of alum and a genetically engineered protein, glycoprotein D (gD2), that sits on the outer surface of HSVII (herpes simplex, type II virus) and is targeted by the body's immune cells.

AZT, a drug used in the treatment of AIDS, works by interrupting the replication cycle of the HIV virus, and has demonstrated effectiveness in delaying the progression of HIV infection.

Side effects Antiviral drugs have a variety of side effects. Creams and ointments may irritate skin, while oral antiviral drugs can cause side effects ranging from nausea and dizziness to bone marrow suppression and kidney problems.

aplasia cutis The medical name for the congenital absence of small areas of skin, these localized birth defects are found on the back of the scalp, although they may occur anywhere on the scalp (rarely, on the face, trunk or limbs). At birth, the affected area may be covered by a tough, smooth membrane or it may be raw, ulcerated and crusted.

On the scalp, the areas tend to be hairless with sharp margins that heal slowly, eventually replaced by a flat or hypertrophic scar. Occasionally, there may be a secondary infection or hemorrhage. Once in a while, there may be an underlying defect in the bone that will heal on its own during the baby's first two years of life. The defect may be inherited, but it usually appears spontaneously. It is sometimes seen with syndromes such as the chromosome disorder trisomy 13.

Treatment Treatment should be conservative, but surgical excision of poorly healing lesions or unsightly scars are effective at easing cosmetic problems.

apocrine glands See SWEAT GLANDS.

apocrine bromhidrosis See BROMHIDROSIS.

arginosuccinicaciduria A rare genetic disorder caused by a deficiency of the amino acid arginosuccinase, causing sparse, dull, short and fragile hair with frayed ends that looks like broom ends pushed together. Patients develop seizures and coma and subsequently die. This disorder is an autosomal recessive disorder; this means that a defective gene must be inherited in a double dose to cause the abnormality. Generally, both parents of an affected person are unaffected carriers of the defective gene. Each of the children has a one in four chance of being affected, and a two in four chance of being a carrier.

Treatment Some patients benefit from a low-protein diet with arginine supplements or additions of keto analogues of essential amino acids.

argon laser A tube that contains argon gas energized by a power source (such as electricity). The resulting beam of light is up to 10 million times more powerful than the sun, and is absorbed by different types of substances in the skin, including melanin pigment and hemoglobin in blood vessels.

The argon laser is a good choice to treat vascular lesions because the red color of the blood absorbs the blue-green color of the argon laser beam. PORT-WINE STAINS may be considerably lightened with this type of treatment, as will TELANGIECTASES, SPIDER ANGIOMAS, venous lakes and certain pigmented lesions (such as LENTIGINES).

Until the late 1980s, the argon laser was the treatment of choice for port-wine stains; hemoglobin selectively absorbed the laser's light in the dilated blood vessels of these birthmarks. However, the therapy is limited by a substantial rate of scarring. The continuous laser energy dissipates into the surrounding dermis, causing thermal damage. Less-than-optimum treatment results in pale, immature port-wine stains. Moreover, the extent of clearing and rate of scarring are primarily dependent on the technique and experience of the operator.

However, more selective blood vessel damage can be obtained by using a wavelength that is more selectively absorbed by hemoglobin and delivered in a pulse shorter than the cooling time of the abnormal vessel, such as the pulsed dye laser.

There is some danger in using lasers. Because the beam generates heat, there is some risk of fire, especially on surgical dressings. Wet dressings placed around the surgical site will protect nearby normal tissue, reducing the chance of fire. Protective goggles are essential, and must be worn by the patient and all medical personnel.

artificial skin Synthetic skin, often used to treat burn victims, is capable of preventing infection and reducing fluid loss while not inducing an immune rejection response.

Some of the newest types of this artificial skin include a biodegradable skin substitute developed at the Massachusetts Institute of Technology called "stage I" and "stage II" skin. Composed of calf collagen, a complex sugar obtained from sharks, and silicone rubber, this artificial skin is stitched in place where the patient's own tissue-producing cells travel to the area and produce a new layer of skin. Within three weeks, the artificial skin is removed and the new skin layer (called a "neodermis") forms a base over which SKIN GRAFTS can be placed. Within several days, a completely new epidermis has formed.

Stage II skin uses the same basic stage I membrane, but the patient's own skin cells are seeded within the membrane. The advantage of this is that dermis and epidermis are made at the same time, eliminating the need to graft the patient's skin in a second surgical step. See also ALLOGRAFT, PINCH GRAFT.

ascorbic acid deficiency See SCURVY.

ashy dermatosis Another name for ERYTHEMA DYSCHROMICUM PERSTANS.

asteatolic eczema See ECZEMA.

astringents Substances that cause skin tissue to dry and shrink by reducing its ability to absorb water. Astringents are widely used in skin tonics, but they may cause burning or stinging when applied.

While old-fashioned astringents were used to dry out the skin in the treatment of ACNE they also stripped the skin of essential moisture (usually because of a high alcohol content). Today, there's a new type of toner that not only cleanses less harshly than some of the old products but can lightly exfoliate, soothe, refresh and leave skin soft and hydrated instead of dry and taut. These products are often marketed under a variety of names, including "toners," "clarifiers," "refreshers," "lotions," and "purifiers." While all may be more or less interchangeable, in general toners tend to be lighter and less drying than astringents because they usually contain lower concentrations of alcohol.

Dermatologists suggest that consumers with dry or delicate skin should avoid alcohol, witch hazel, SALICYLIC ACID, acetone and RESORCINOL; these products are more appropriate for less sensitive, oilier skin.

Many dermatologists advise patients to avoid alcohol, which dries the skin and actually increases oil production as glands are stimulated to compensate for excess dryness. Still, while alcohol may dry the skin temporarily, it does not cause any longer-term damage.

Those astringents or toners without alcohol rely on natural ingredients to cleanse and refresh the skin, using "botanicals" (naturally derived elements). Botanical extracts may include lavender, grapefruit seed and orchid, and serve different functions, soothing or stimulating the skin.

athlete's foot A common condition causing the skin between the toes (usually the fourth and fifth toes) to itch, peel and crack and resulting in diffuse scaling and redness of the soles and sides of the foot. Associated with wearing shoes and sweating, the condition is rare in young children and in places of the world where people do not wear shoes.

Itchy skin on the foot is probably not athlete's foot if it occurs on the top of the toes. If the foot is red, swollen, sore, blistered and oozing, it is more likely the result of some form of contact dermatitis, although inflammatory fungal infections can sometimes look like this.
Causes Athlete's foot is usually caused by a fungal infection and is called *tinea pedis;* secondary infection in skin cracks is caused by bacteria.
Treatment The condition may clear up without any attention, but it usually requires treatment. An untreated fungal infection can lead to bacteria-inviting cracks in the skin. It is important to keep the affected area dry,

wearing dry cotton socks or sandals. Even better—keep the foot uncovered. Most infections can be cured by applying the antifungal cream Lotrimin two or three times daily. Possible side effects include occasional skin irritation; antifungal oral or injected drugs may cause serious side effects including liver or kidney damage.

When the acute phase of the infection passes, remove dead skin with a bristle brush in order to remove the living fungi. Be sure to wash away any bits of the skin. In addition, scrape underneath toenails every two or three days with an orange stick or toothpick.
Prevention Disinfecting the floors of showers and locker rooms can help control the spread of infection. Once an infection has cleared up, continue using antifungal cream now and then—especially during warm weather. Avoid plastic or too-tight shoes, or any type of footwear treated to keep out water. Natural materials (cotton and leather) and sandals are the best choices, while wool and rubber can make a fungal problem worse by trapping moisture.

Air out shoes regularly in the sun, wiping inside of shoes with a disinfectant-treated cloth to remove fungi-carrying dead skin. Dust the insides of shoes with antifungal powder or spray. If you perspire heavily, change your sox three or four times daily. Wear only natural white cotton socks, and rinse them thoroughly during washing.

Air dry feet after bathing, then apply powder. Always wear sandals or flip-flops in public bathing areas. See also DERMATITIS, CONTACT.

atrophic papulosis, malignant See DEGOS' SYNDROME.

atrophie blanche Unusual types of white scars with red macules and spidery red veins resembling chili peppers. This type of scar, which is usually found on the tops of the feet, ankles and legs, is the final result of lower leg ulcers.

Treatment Combinations of aspirin and dipyridamole, which affect the formation of platelets, have been helpful in the treatment of the ulceration of causes some cases of atrophie blanche. Other treatments have included the administration of phenformin, ethylestrenol and pentoxifylline. See also LIVEDO VASCULITIS.

attar of roses An extract of roses used to perfume products that may cause allergic reactions in sensitive consumers.

atypical nevi (dysplastic nevi) Atypical moles that are markers for an increased risk of MALIGNANT MELANOMA. Researchers suggest that almost 7 percent of Caucasians in the United Staets have atypical nevi, and half of their close relatives may also be affected.

There are two types of atypical nevi: familial and sporadic. The significance of familial nevi is clear: Those who have dysplastic nevi *and* a family history of melanoma (two or more close blood relatives) have an almost 100 percent lifetime risk of developing melanoma. No one knows the true significance of sporadic atypical nevi. Although such patients with large numbers of atypical nevi also appear to be at increased risk for the development of malignant melanoma, the risk appears to be less than for those in the familial group (an estimated lifetime melanoma risk of 6 percent). It is believed that about 50 percent of the populace has at least one of these lesions. Melanoma warning signs include moles that are often asymmetrical (one half looks unlike the other), having irregular or hazy borders, variegated and of irregular color, with a diameter slightly larger than that of a pencil eraser.

Although atypical nevi continue to develop as the patient grows older, the lesions tend to remain stable. Only a small number of these spots ever undergoes malignant transformation.

Symptoms Atypical nevi are found most often on the back, chest, abdomen and extremities, but they may also occur on unexposed areas (scalp, buttocks, groin or breasts). They differ from ordinary acquired nevi in several ways: first, atypical nevi tend to occur in larger numbers than ordinary nevi—often more than 100. In addition, these nevi are often larger than the ordinary variety, and they will often measure more than 1 cm. Although ordinary nevi usually have stopped appearing by early adult life, atypical nevi continue to develop into adulthood.

Atypical nevi also tend to differ from ordinary nevi in appearance. They tend to have irregular contours with irregular pigmentation. In addition to shades of brown, atypical nevi may be red or pink—colors not normally found in ordinary nevi. When these atypical characteristics are pronounced it may be difficult to tell the difference between an atypical nevus and a superficial spreading malignant melanoma.

Cancer prevention If your doctor diagnoses atypical nevi, you should discuss your family history and have close relatives examined for any sign of nevus or melanoma. Patients who have both atypical nevi and close family members with malignant melanoma should have regular skin exams (as often as every four to six months) and supplement medical checkups with self-examinations; full-body photographs may help an individual to more easily spot changes in moles. Reduce sun exposure and use sunscreens with a high SPF. Consider an eye exam, since moles may also affect the eyes.

Treatment The most abnormal-looking lesions should be excised and examined microscopically. If very unusual, other odd-looking moles should be removed.

augmentation mammoplasty See MAMMAPLASTY.

aurothioglucose An oil-based form of gold salts used in GOLD THERAPY for the treatment of PEMPHIGUS. (See also GOLD SODIUM THIO-MALATE.)

Auspitz's sign Pinpoint bleeding that occurs when the scale of a lesion of PSORIASIS is forcibly removed.

autograft Tissue graft taken from one part of the body and placed on another part of the same patient; burn repair is often done by grafting strips of skin taken from elsewhere on the body (usually the upper body or thigh, called the "donor site"). Unlike ALLO-GRAFTS, autografts are not rejected by the body's immune system. See also SKIN GRAFT, PINCH GRAFT.

azathioprine The generic name for Imuran, this is an anti-cancer drug used in the treatment of severe autoimmune diseases when other drugs fail to slow the progression of the disease or to improve symptoms. It is particularly effective in conjunction with corticosteroids such as prednisone or cortisone in the treatment of bullous disorders such as PEMPHIGUS. It is also frequently used to prevent rejection of grafted organs such as the kidneys, liver and heart.

The drug works by reducing the efficiency of the body's immune system by preventing lymphocytes (a kind of white blood cell) from multiplying. Lymphocytes destroy proteins not usually found in the body, but in autoimmune disorders they attack proteins that the immune system interprets as foreign. *Adverse effects* Adverse effects include abnormal bleeding and increased susceptibility to infection as a result of reduced blood cell production. There may be nausea and vomiting, diarrhea, fever, hair loss and skin eruptions. In animals, this drug causes birth defects. Temporary chromosomal abnormalities when using this drug have also been reported. Long-term use increases the risk of skin cancer, a frequent side effect in kidney transplant patients.

azelaic acid A depigmenting agent originally identified as the cause of HYPOPIGMEN-TATION associated with the fungus infection TINEA VERSICOLOR (a common skin condition producing pigmented flaking skin patches). Azelaic acid has been shown to kill abnormal MELANOCYTES (melanin-producing cells). It is also being studied as a possible treatment for malignant melanoma (a deadly form of skin cancer). See also MELANOMA, MALIGNANT.

azulene A chamomile extract used in face and body creams, sunburn remedies, burn ointments, and bath salts.

B

bacterial skin infections Also known as pyodermas, this type of infection can be caused by a wide variety of bacteria. Most cases are caused by either *Staphylococci* or *Streptococci*. The most common of all the skin infections is IMPETIGO, a highly contagious infection of the topmost layers of the skin causing itchy, red and blistering patches and honey-colored crusts. Most often appearing in childhood, impetigo is usually caused by *Staphylococci*.

Staph organisms also cause FOLLICULITIS, an infection near the openings of hair follicles that resembles ACNE and can spread if untreated. It often occurs after repeated trauma to the area of skin from shaving, or following soaking in contaminated hot tubs and whirlpools.

When bacteria cause infection in deeper layers of the skin, they may result in BOILS, or furuncles: hot, inflamed lesions appearing on the face, scalp, underarms and buttocks that may look like an infected pimple. Larger and deeper than boils are CARBUNCLES, abscesses filled with pus and bacteria that are often extremely painful. Boils and carbuncles should never be squeezed, since the bacteria may be forced into the blood, causing widespread blood poisoning.

A most serious strep skin infection is CELLULITIS, usually appearing on the legs and characterized by high fever, weakness, shaking chills, pain, lymph gland swelling and spreading warm redness of the skin. If deep swellings appear on the face, the condition is diagnosed as the potentially fatal ERYSIPELAS.

In general, bacterial skin infections usually respond well to oral antibiotics. Strep infections respond very quickly to penicillin and its derivatives, but staph infections may not; for this reason, physicians usually prescribe dicloxacillin or erythromycin to treat staph infections. All types of antibiotics usually require a 10-day course for a complete cure.

In addition to oral antibiotics, topical treatments may include applying warm compresses of tap water or BUROW'S SOLUTION to the affected area, or using topical over-the-counter antibiotics.

See also GROUP B STREPTOCOCCI INFECTIONS, IN INFANTS; NECROTIZING FASCIITIS; ERYSIPELAS.

bags under eyes Loose, baggy skin under the eyes is the result of a gradual loss of skin elasticity due to aging, or because of an irreversible inherited condition called blepherochalasis. Puffy lower eyelids also can be caused by lack of sleep, stress or illness. The swelling can be reduced by applying dampened cotton pads, CHAMOMILE teabags dipped in cool water, or cucumbers and lying down for 10 minutes.

Once the bags have formed, they can be covered up with makeup or surgically removed using the surgical technique called BLEPHAROPLASTY.

baking soda A water-soluble powder used in baths for itchy skin, as a soothing soak for irritated skin conditions and as a simple tooth cleanser. Mixed with a bit of water into a paste, it can ease the pain of insect stings.

baldness Absence of hair on the scalp. See also ALOPECIA AREATA.

balneotherapy Method of treatment of disease by bathing (usually in mineral hot springs) once considered as fashionable "water cures."

bamboo hair Abnormal hair shafts in Netherton's syndrome, a genetic disorder characterized by roughened scaly skin. Hair (most noticably on the head) looks like ball-and-socket joints; spontaneous remission may occur in adolescence.

barber's itch The common term for *sycosis vulgaris,* meaning inflammation of the beard area. The condition is caused by infected hair follicles (usually with *Staphylococcus aureus* bacteria) picked up from infected razors and towels. Pus-filled blisters or boils develop around the follicles, sometimes causing severe scarring unless treated. Treatment is usually with antibiotic drugs; growing a beard may help prevent recurrence. See also PSEUDOFOLLICULITIS BARBAE.

basal cell Small round cell found in the innermost part of the EPIDERMIS, where the rest of the epidermal cells derive.

basal cell carcinoma Basal cell carcinoma is the most common form of skin cancer, affecting more than 500,000 Americans each year. One out of every three new cancers is a skin cancer, and 83.5 percent of these is a basal cell carcinoma. If untreated, the growth invades and grows deeper into surrounding tissues, but fortunately this type of cancer almost never spreads to other parts of the body.

Incidence Until recently, those most likely to get basal cell carcinoma were older people (especially men) who have spent a great deal of time outdoors. The incidence increases significantly in those with outdoor occupations and those who live in sunny climates; in Queensland, Australia, more than half the local white population has had a basal cell carcinoma by age 75. The number of new cases has risen sharply in the last decade because of the thinning ozone layer and extensive sunbathing. In addition, younger and younger people are being diagnosed with the disease. Today, almost as many women as men are getting basal cell cancer.

Causes Chronic overexposure to sunlight is the cause of 95 percent of all basal cell carcinomas. In a few cases, contact with arsenic, exposure to radiation and complications of burns, scars or vaccinations are contributing factors.

Symptoms More than 90 percent of this type of cancer is found on the face, often at the side of the eye or on the nose or other exposed area of the body, although it can appear in any location. The five most typical characteristics of basal cell carcinoma are very different from each other, and often two or more features are found in one tumor. Basal cell carcinoma may be:

· an open sore that bleeds or oozes, remaining open for three or more weeks
· a reddish patch or irritated area (often on the shoulder, chest, arms or legs) that may itch or hurt, or cause no sensation at all
· a smooth growth with an elevated, rolled border and indented center, developing tiny blood vessels on the surface as it grows
· a shiny bump that is pearly or translucent, often pink red or white, tan black or brown
· a scar (white, yellow or waxy) with poorly defined borders; the skin itself looks shiny and taut. This last sign is less frequent but may indicate an aggressive tumor

Diagnosis/treatment A diagnosis of basal cell carcinoma is made after physical examination and biopsy (removal and examination of a small piece of tissue). If tumor cells are found, the growth can be removed by surgery or destroyed by radiation. The treatment is based on type, size and location of the tumor and on the patient's age and health, but it can almost always be performed on an outpatient basis. Local anesthetics are used and not much pain is felt.

Surgical removal The most common treatment is simple excisional surgery. The physician simply removes the entire growth and an additional border of normal skin as a safety margin. The site is then stitched closed and the tissue is sent to the lab to determine if all malignant cells have been removed.

Alternatively, the surgeon may perform *electrosurgery* (CURETTAGE AND ELECTRODESICCATION) in which cancerous tissue is scraped from the skin with a curette (sharp ring-shaped device) and an electric needle burns a safety margin of normal skin around the tumor at the base of the scraped area. This technique is repeated twice to make sure the tumor has been completely removed.

With CRYOSURGERY, the physician does not cut the growth but instead freezes the lesion by applying LIQUID NITROGEN with a special spray or a cotton-tipped applicator; this method doesn't require anesthesia and produces no bleeding. It is easy to administer and is the treatment of choice for those who have bleeding disorders or are intolerant to anesthesia.

Laser Surgery is used to focus a beam of light onto the lesion either to excise it or destroy it by vaporization. The major advantage of this technique is that it seals blood vessels as it cuts.

Mohs surgery (microscopically controlled surgery) involves the removal of very thin layers of the malignant tumor, checking each layer thoroughly under a microscope. This is repeated as often as necessary until the tissue is free of tumor; this method saves the most healthy tissue and has the highest cure rate; it is often used for tumors that recur and for tumors in areas where basal cell carcinomas are known to recur after other treatment techniques (nose, ears and around the eyes).

Radiation therapy In radiation therapy, x rays are directed at the malignant cells; it usually takes several treatments several times a week for a few weeks to totally destroy a tumor. Radiation therapy may be used with older patients or with those in poor health.

Drug treatment Researchers are now studying the possible use of interferon, a genetically engineered product of the human immune system, as a possible treatment of some basal cell carcinomas. Interferon interferes with viral multiplication and increases the activity of natural killer cells (types of lymphocytes that make up part of the body's immune system).

Outlook When removed early, basal cell carcinomas are easily treated, but the larger the growth the more extensive the treatment. While this type of skin cancer almost never metastasizes, it can destroy surrounding tissue. Since removal of a tumor scars the skin, large tumors may require reconstructive surgery and skin grafts.

If a patient is diagnosed with one basal cell carcinoma, there is a greater chance of developing others over the body in the future. Even though a basal cell carcinoma has been removed, another can develop in the same place (or nearby), usually within the first two years after surgery. Basal cell carcinomas on the scalp, nose and sides of the nose and around the ears are particularly problematic. If the cancer recurs, the physician may recommend a different type of treatment the second time, most likely Mohs surgery. Therefore, it is important to examine the surgical site periodically.

Bazex syndrome This is a rare eruption of the nose, ears and extremities associated with cancer of the lungs, esophagus and tongue or the gastrointestinal tract.

Symptoms Symptoms begin on the hands and feet with scaling bluish red plaques; severe nail problems may include flaking and shedding of the nail itself, followed by involvement of the ear, nose bridge, elbows and knees. The skin symptoms, which look much like PSORIASIS, may appear before a tu-

mor is diagnosed and can predict the malignancy with almost 100 percent accuracy.
Treatment The skin lesions fade away when the tumor is removed. Symptoms may also be treated with keratolytics and topical steroids.

Beau's lines Temporary horizontal depressions across the nails that appear during certain acute infections such as MEASLES and MUMPS or inflammatory conditions such as inflammatory bowel disease or Lupus, or after a heart attack. The depression first appears at the cuticle a few weeks after the underlying disease begins and slowly moves out to the end of the nail as the nail grows over a period of months. When this condition appears during a systemic disease, all of the fingernails and toenails are likely to be affected. If only one or two nails are affected, the condition is probably caused by trauma or cold.

bedbugs These flat, wingless brown insects live in floors and furniture (especially beds) during the day, coming out at night to bite their human hosts. While they rarely transmit disease, their bites may become infected. Usually the bug sucks blood from several nearby sites, resulting in a group or cluster of lesions.

Soon after the bite, the victim experiences an itchy, burning wheal with a central hemorrhagic mark, which helps differentiate this from an ordinary wheal. The bedbug lesion may become reddened and firm or develop into a blister (especially in children). The wheal may subside soon, or it may last for several hours. They appear most often on the back, neck, face, ankles, wrists, buttocks or wherever the body touches the bed.

Bedbugs can be killed with a variety of insecticides, including malathion, lindane, pyrethrins and DDT.

bedsores A type of ulcer (also known as decubitus ulcers or pressure sores) that develop on the skin of bedridden, unconscious or immobile patients. They often affect victims of stroke or spinal cord injuries; constantly wet skin caused by incontinence may also be a factor. Common site of breakdown includes the shoulders, elbows, lower back, hips and buttocks, knees, ankles and heels.
Symptoms Bedsores begin as red, painful areas that turn purple before the skin breaks down, eventually turning into open sores. Once the skin is broken, the sores often become infected, enlarge, deepen and are very slow to heal.
Treatment Deep chronic ulcers may require treatment with antibiotics, packing with plastic foam and sometimes even PLASTIC SURGERY.
Prevention It's a far better idea to prevent a bedsore from developing than to try to treat one already in existence. Once a bedsore has developed, it will heal only if the pressure on the damaged skin is minimized. To prevent sores, a patient's position should be changed at least every two hours; it is important to wash and dry pressure areas carefully (especially if there is incontinence). Barrier creams may also further protect the skin.

A ripple bed mattress may help prevent bedsores by stimulating circulation; this rippling effect is created by pumping air in and out of the mattress. Cushions and pillows may relieve pressure (place them between the knees and under the shoulder). A sheepskin under the buttocks and booties under the heels may also relieve pressure.

bees and wasps More than half of all deaths due to venomous animals are a result of stings by bees and wasps. The Hymenoptera order includes three families: honeybee and bumblebees; wasps, hornets and yellow jackets; and several species of ants.

After being stung, the victim may have either an immediate (within two hours) or delayed reaction. Immediate reactions are the most common, and include local swelling, reddening, pain and itching, which usually subsides within a few hours. However, in some patients with hypersensitivy to venom, the local reaction is marked by more severe and prolonged swelling and redness, with systemic reactions ranging from mild to fatal. Anaphylactic reactions (with breathing problems and internal swelling) usually occur within the first 10 to 30 minutes after the sting. The faster a reaction materializes the more severe it is.

Treatment Ice, elevation and oral antihistamines minimize local pain and swelling. In the case of a delayed local reaction appearing after 24 hours, a five-day course of systemic steroids may help. In honeybee stings, scrape the stinger and attached venom sac from the skin; don't use forceps, because pressure on the sac can inject more venom.

Highly allergic individuals should carry an emergency kit including a tourniquet, syringe, epinephrine and antihistamine. Those who have had several severe reactions should consider hyposensitization; IMMUNO-THERAPY with venom is 95 percent effective in eliminating serious allergic responses.

beeswax A substance secreted by bees to build the walls of their cells, it is also used by cosmetic manufacturers as an emulsifier to soften and protect the skin. Without emulsifiers, the cosmetic would separate, leaving the solids at the bottom and the liquid ingredients at the top. Beeswax has caused allergic reactions in some sensitive people.

Behcet's syndrome A rare disorder causing among many other symptoms, skin rashes and recurrent mouth ulcers. Attacks often last for several weeks and often recur. Eye involvement may cause blindness and central nervous system involvement may be fatal. The syndrome was first described by Turkish dermatologist Hulusi Behcet (1889–1948).

Rare in the United States, the disease is more often found in some Middle Eastern countries and Japan, and is five times more likely to occur among men. The syndrome may become chronic in some patients.

Symptoms A variety of skin lesions throughout the body have been associated with the disease (papules, vesicles, pustules, abscesses, subcutaneous thrombophlebitis and nodular lesions). After puncturing the skin with a needle, the skin becomes inflamed and develops a small pustule. Other symptoms of the syndrome include genital, mouth or intestinal ulcers, eye inflammation, arthritis, venous thrombosis, arterial aneurysms and neuropsychiatric symptoms.

Cause Its cause is unknown, although some experts believe the disease could be caused by a virus, a clotting problem, an autoimmune disorder or heredity.

Treatment Oral and genital ulcers may be treated locally, although this won't prevent new ulcers from forming. Topical corticosteroids may cut down on inflammation; topical anesthetics may ease pain. In severe cases, systemic anticancer drugs, corticosteroids or immune suppressors (especially azathioprine) may be prescribed, but treatment is difficult. Treatments that are sometimes effective include colchicine or levamisole. The disorder can be fatal depending on which organ system is involved. The eyes and central nervous system pose the greatest risk if affected.

benign skin cancer See SKIN TUMOR, BENIGN.

benzoic acid A preservative used in skin care products that generally is not considered to be irritating, although it may cause an allergic reaction in consumers who are sensitive to similar chemicals.

benzophenone A SUNSCREEN that blocks both UVA and UVB light.

benzoyl peroxide An antibacterial agent that is considered to be the most effective non-prescription ACNE treatment, markedly suppressing the bacterium *Propionibacterium acnes* associated with acne. This extremely effective topical antibacterial agent draws peroxide into the pore where it releases oxygen, killing the bacteria that can aggravate acne. Benzoyl also suppresses fatty acid cells that irritate pores and heps to unplug comedones. It is most effective for patients with inflammatory acne; by inhibiting bacteria, it decreases the inflammation in the skin.

Benzoyl peroxide is sold in strengths ranging between 5 and 10 percent, but dermatologists usually advise patients to start with a 5 percent product, since the lower concentration is just as effective and less likely to cause irritation. Most over-the-counter products contain benzoyl peroxide in a lotion base; the prescription items contain the chemical in a gel base. A fairly new prescription preparation combining 3 percent erythromycin with a 5 percent benzoyl peroxide in a gel base may be more effective than either component by itself.

Caution Because the skin absorbs benzoyl peroxide, it should not be used by pregnant or nursing women unless directed by a physician. Its safety for children under age 12 has not been established. Because benzoyl peroxide is a bleach, it will discolor most fabrics and hair.

Over-the-counter cleansers that contain benzoyl peroxide include Fostex 10% Wash (liquid), Fostex 10% (bar), Oxy 10 Wash, Pan-Oxyl 5% and PanOxyl 10%. Non-prescription lotions include Acne-10, Benozyl 5, Benozyl 10, Clearasil 10%, Dry and Clear (5%), Loroxide (5.5%), Oxy 5, Oxy 10, and Vanoxide (5%). Nonprescription creams include Acne-Aid (10%), Clearasil Maximum Strength (10%), Cuticura Acne (5%), Dry and Clear Double Strength, Fostex (10%) and Oxy 10 Cover. Gels include Clear by Design (2.5%), Del Aqua-5, Del Aqua-10,

Fostex 5%, Fostex 10%, Xerac BP5, and Xerac BP10.

Adverse effects While most people experience some mild burning, itching or peeling, benzoyl peroxide can produce a stronger reaction in some people with very sensitive skin (especially those with very fair skin). It is normal to experience a warm or stinging feeling, with some dryness or peeling, but if the skin turns very red, or there is pain, a lot of scaling and swelling, then an adverse reaction has occured and use should be discontinued.

The stronger the preparation, the greater the chance of a reaction. Benzoyl peroxide should never be applied near the eyes, where it can cause swelling and irritation; some women are also sensitive around the nose and mouth. Wash hands thoroughly after using the product and never rub your eyes with contaminated fingers.

Some studies have reported that benzoyl peroxide may be carcinogenic, although this conclusion is controversial and inconclusive.

berloque dermatitis See DERMATITIS, BERLOQUE.

bergamot oil See OIL OF BERGAMOT

beta-carotene It may be possible to shield the body's immune system from harmful UVA rays—and reduce the risk of skin cancer—by supplementing the diet with beta-carotene, according to some researchers. Scientists at Cornell University and Hoffman-LaRoche, Inc. tested 24 healthy men on a low beta-carotene diet for 28 days. Part of the group got 30-milligram supplements of carotene and the others got a placebo; then, the whole group was exposed to UVA light 12 times over two weeks. Blood tests were taken to measure the men's carotene level and also to see how their immune system reacted to various types of disease-causing antigens. (The antigens were "deactivated" so they would not make the men sick, but would still trigger a measurable immune response on the skin).

The men with low blood levels of beta-carotene showed a weakened immune response to the antigens, but the men who got the carotene supplement maintained a strong immune system.

biotin deficiency A lack of this water-soluble vitamin important in amino acid metabolism has been purported to cause fissured lips; red, tender tongue; and reddening and dryness of mucosal surfaces. In infants, a lethal form of biotin deficiency may cause a generalized SEBORRHEIC DERMATITIS or ICHTHYOSIS; a different form of infant biotin deficiency may cause diffuse reddening, scaling and crusting at skin junctions and mucosal surfaces together with hair loss.

Treatment The intravenous administration of biotin is an effective treatment for this condition.

Cause Although rare, it can occur when raw egg whites are ingested or with total parenteral nutrition (feeding by tubes or injection) without biotin supplements.

birth control pills There are a number of skin problems that have been associated with the use of birth control pills, including ACNE, hair loss and blotchy pigmentation. It also can be associated with ERYTHEMA NODOSUM. Many varieties of the birth control pill (such as Norlestrin, Norinyl, Ovral and Loestrin) can aggravate acne and can also increased sensitivity to the sun, resulting in swelling of skin that has been exposed to the ultraviolet rays. Because of hormonal changes, hair may be lost while taking the pill or after the pill has been stopped. Women who develop skin problems while using birth control pills may be able to have their prescriptions changed to a different type of pill.

Pills with slightly higher estrogen levels, such as Demulen and others with 50 mg. of estrogen, may actually improve acne.

Between 5 and 30 percent of women taking the pill develop a blotchy, heightened skin color on their face, regardless of whether their prescription contained primarily estrogen or progesterone. This darkening, called melasma or CHLOASMA, also is often seen during the last trimester of pregnancy, although it also appears in women who are neither pregnant nor taking birth control pills. Exposure to the sun will make this darkening worse. When the pill is taken for longer periods of time and at higher dosages, skin changes are likely to be noticeable. Bleaching the skin with HYDROQUINONE-containing products is the effective treatment.

birthmarks An area of discolored skin present at birth; the most common birthmarks are MOLES (also called melanocytic nevi), which are malformations of pigment cells. Strawberry marks are bright red, spongy and protuberant; PORT-WINE STAINS are purple-red, flat and often cover large areas. Both strawberry marks and port-wine stains are malformations of blood vessels.

True strawberry (capillary) HEMANGIOMAS all clear by age 7, although they may leave an unsightly scar. Port-wine stains never clear. In a few cases (referred to as the STURGE-WEBER SYNDROME) port-wine stains are associated with abnormalities in the blood vessels of the brain.

Unattractive moles can be removed in late childhood through adulthood by plastic surgery. Port-wine stains can be lightened significantly using laser treatment.

The relatively newly developed pulsed dye laser is highly effective at lightening port-wine stains and treatment can be started within the first few weeks of life. See also STRAWBERRY BIRTHMARK.

bites and infestations Fly and mosquito bites may cause swelling and itching for several days and may lead to infection if sores are scratched open.

Treatment Because flies and mosquitoes can spread disease, wash the bite area with soap and water and then apply an antiseptic. To control itching, try a nonprescription antihistamine, calamine lotion and ice packs. Or try making a paste to spread over the bite out of: salt and water, baking soda (1 tsp. in a glass of water, place on bite for 20 minutes) or epsom salts (1 Tbs. in 1 quart of hot water; chill, then apply as above).

Prevention Try using insect repellents. *DEET* (N1N-diethyl-m-toluamide) is the most effective of all bug repellents. It may be used in children but should not be applied to infants. Keep out of eyes, and follow instructions on the package. New preparations combine sunscreen and a bug repellant in one cream.

bisulfites The mildest permanent waving solution used for body waves and color-treated hair contain this agent.

blackheads A dark semisolid plug of greasy sebum blocking the outlet of an oil-producing gland in the skin, most commonly found on the face, chest, back and shoulders. They are associated with increased sebaceous gland activity, which is normal in adolescents, and are often characterized by certain types of ACNE. The black color is not dirt, but a reaction that occurs when the plug mixes with air and skin pigment.

Treatment Salicylic acid and Retin-A are particularly effective treatments for blackheads, but benzoyl peroxide may also be effective. Blackheads may be gently squeezed; cosmetologists may also remove blackheads.

black skin Black and white people have the same number of pigment cells; however, blacks have larger pigment granules within the cells that are completely filled with pigment whereas whites have smaller pigment granules. A major difference between black and white skin is that after an injury, black

Cross section of Blackhead

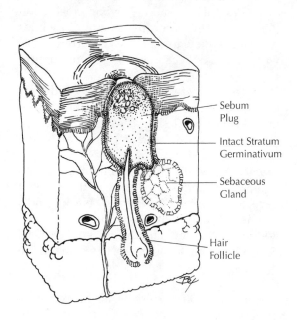

Sebum Plug

Intact Stratum Germinativum

Sebaceous Gland

Hair Follicle

skin tends to change color when it heals (either darker or lighter).

Dark skin may run the gamut from pale olive to blue-black, together with varying tones of reds and yellows. In general, black skin is tougher, thicker and smoother than white skin, with more sweat glands and larger oil glands. Skin tones can be uneven, appearing darker around the forehead and mouth and lighter on the cheeks and lower lip.

Pigmentation problems are more likely to occur with darker skin, and certain products that could lead to mottling—such as medicated soaps and products with irritants such as resorcinol—should be avoided. Likewise, chemical peels, dermabrasion and certain types of cosmetic surgery are not recommended for black skin, since injury frequently causes raised scars (keloids) or it may turn lighter or darker than the surrounding skin.

With a few exceptions, skin diseases affect blacks and whites about the same way. While disorders that cause hypopigmentation (lightened skin) occur just as often in whites and blacks, they are of more concern to those with dark skin because they are more noticeable.

However, there are a few skin conditions that occur more commonly in blacks. These include KELOIDS, flesh moles (DERMATOSIS PAPULOSA NIGRA), deodorant bumps and acne keloidalis.

Infancy At birth, a black infant has both lighter skin and straighter hair than it will have as an adult. A newborn black child's hair is soft and silky, becoming more curly within the first few months; the skin darkens as well. At birth, however the skin of the genitals, fingertips and earlobes is already dark.

More than 90 percent of all black babies are born with MONGOLIAN SPOTS, which appear on black skin as large, flat, blue-black lesions on the lower back or buttock. These lesions usually fade in early childhood, although some persist into adulthood. These benign lesions do not require treatment.

Neonatal pustular melanosis is a rash present at birth in about 5 percent of black infants (but only 1 percent or less of white infants). The rash consists of pinpoint dark brown and red pimples that eventually fade; no treatment is necessary.

The most common skin problem in black (as well as white) children is ACNE. While all races suffer about the same incidence of acne, black teens are more likely to experience hyperpigmentation (skin darkening) as a result of this condition. In addition, some treatments (such as strong peeling agents like vitamin A gel or 10 percent BENZOYL PEROXIDE) can inflame black skin and cause darkening.

During winter, black skin may appear "ashy." The outer horny layer of cells dries up and appears grayish, with a fine scale. It can be treated by using bath oil, using mild soap, or humidifying winter air in the home. Instead of directly lubricating the skin, it is better to wet the skin first and then apply lubricant.

Hair Hair (an appendage of the skin) is also different in blacks and whites. A black person's hair is oval and curved, and is curly all the way down into the root. Because of the curved nature of the hair, black men often experience "shave bumps" (or PSEUDOFOLLICULITIS BARBAE).

Aging black skin While white skin is at risk by middle age for skin cancer, the darker color of black skin provides more protection from the ultraviolet rays of the sun. Skin cancer is rare among black patients. This darker skin protection also guards against sun damage, which produces wrinkles.

As black skin ages, however, the oil glands become less active and dryness becomes a problem. At this time, some older patients encounter guttate hypomelanosis, the appearance of small white round confetti-sized spots on the lower legs and body (but not the face), which gradually enlarge and spread.

black widow spider One of two poisonous spiders in the United States, the bite of the black widow can cause a numbing pain at the site, but little serious problems for adults; however, children often react badly to a black widow bite and should see a physician if this type of bite is suspected. Most spider bites occur in southern California. Black widow spiders are found under or between rocks, under loose bark, around outdoor water faucets and in woodpiles, garages, basements, garbage cans and sheds, under toilet lids and in cushions.

The bite produces two tiny puncture marks and may cause a slight swelling, followed by a dull pain increasing in intensity, peaking in up to three hours and continuing for 48 hours. The venom of the black widow spider is a neurotoxin that destroys nerve endings and causes an ascending paralysis.

In the past, bites from these spiders caused a number of deaths, especially during swarms recorded in Spain and Sardinia in the mid-1800s. The most common and deadly bites are on the genitals.

Treatment Best obtained in an emergency room, treatment usually includes intravenous calcium (for muscle cramping), antivenom, or both. The wound should be cleaned and disinfected, followed by a tetanus shot if needed.

bleaching   creams Nonprescription cosmetic bleaching creams do not change the color of the skin that may be darkened as a result of hormonal imbalances, chemicals, sun exposure etc. Instead, they prevent the formation of melanin.

A variety of substances has been used in the past to bleach the skin, including lemon juice, tea and salicylic acid. AMMONIATED MERCURY was used until 1974, when the U.S. Food and Drug Administration barred the sale of creams containing this substance because of its toxicity and the incidence of allergic reactions.

The agent HYDROQUINONE can sometimes be successful as it both helps to prevent new melanin production and bleaches existing pigment. It may be purchased over the counter in concentrations of 2% or less. Higher prescriptions require a prescription. Hydroquinone may be prescribed in combination with RETINOIC ACID (to enhance penetration) and a corticosteroid (to reduce irritation). It may require several months' treatment before a good response is achieved. Rarely, hydroquinone can trigger an allergic response or irritation in some people or produce a mottled appearance.

Monobenzoyl ether of hydroquinone (Benoquin) should never be used to bleach the skin because it destroys melanocytes and leaves permanent disfiguring white spots (it should only be used for patients with extensive VITILIGO in an effort to bleach their re-

maining unaffected skin so that they will be uniformly colored).

Prescription products containing hydroquinone include Eldopaque Cream, eldoquin, Eldopaque Forte (4 percent hydroquinone), Solaquin Forte (4 percent hydroquinone, PABA ester, benzophene) and Melanex (3 percent hydroquinone).

Nonprescription products include Esoterica Cream, Atra HCQ Kit (4 percent hydroquinone, 1 percent hydrocortisone) and Ambi (2 percent hydroquinone, PABA ester).

Combined medications include hydroquinone 4 percent and salicylic acid 2 percent; hydroquinone 2 percent or 4 percent, hydrocortisone 2 percent and tretinoin cream 0.05 percent applied sequentially; hydroquinone 4 percent, tretinoin 0.1 percent and dexamethasone 0.1 percent applied sequentially.

Trichloroacetic acid may be effective in light-skinned people, but it should not be used on black skin. This highly caustic agent must be used with great caution to avoid instant tissue necrosis and permanent scars. In mild concentrations, it can be painted on pigmented lesions, which produces a mild lightening. The best concentration of this acid is one which produces lightening without excessive injury to the skin.

Alteratively, gentle freezing with liquid nitrogen to treat localized colored spots may be effective by decreasing the amount of color. Melanocytes are particularly sensitive to destruction using this technique. This process does not work in those with dark or black skin, however, because of the risk of permanent depigmentation.

bleb A tiny blister usually formed by injecting a small amount of fluid under the outer layer of the skin, such as in a tuberculin test.

bleomycin An antibiotic obtained from a soil fungus, bleomycin is an anticancer drug that is effective in treating WARTS that have not responded to other treatment.

Adverse effects Painful injections, localized swelling and the development of a hemorrhagic ESCHAR.

blepharoplasty   See EYELID LIFT.

blister   A raised oval or round collection of fluid within or beneath the outer layer of the skin. Blisters larger than a half inch in diameter are sometimes called bullae; small blisters are also called vesicles. Blisters that have been inadvertently pierced may be susceptible to infection. If you notice redness, swelling, heat or increased pain, or the drainage has an odor or is not clear, then the blister has become infected.

Cause A blister appears after minor skin damage when serum leaks from blood vessels in underlying skin. The serum is usually sterile, and the blister provides valuable protection to the damaged tissue.

Blisters often appear after burns, sunburn and friction (such as damage to hands from using a rake without gloves or as a result of wearing tight shoes). There are a number of skin diseases that can also cause blisters, including ECZEMA, IMPETIGO, EPIDERMOLYSIS BULLOSA, PORPHYRIA, ERYTHEMA MULTIFORME, and the bullous diseases of PEMPHIGOID, PEMPHIGUS and DERMATITIS HERPETIFORMIS.

In addition, small blisters develop in the early stages of many viral infections, including CHICKENPOX, SHINGLES and HERPES SIMPLEX; these blisters contain infectious particles capable of spreading the infection.

Treatment A blister should not be disturbed, but be left to heal on its own. It may be pierced at the edge using a sterile needle, allowing the fluid to slowly seep out. Never unroof a blister, as the roof protects against infection. However, patients with large, troublesome or unexplained blisters should seek medical advice; some experts believe that a large blister on a weight-bearing area almost always has to be pierced.

Otherwise, try applying a moleskin pad (available at drug stores) cut to resemble a doughnut with the blister in the middle; the moleskin will absorb the friction of daily activity.

If a blister inadvertently bursts or gets pierced, do NOT remove the skin over the top of the blister. Left intact even after the blister has been drained, this skin flap will act as a type of Band-Aid; it will eventually harden and fall off by itself.

Triple antibiotics (such as Neosporin) may eliminate bacterial contamination, whereas iodine or camphor-phenol slow down healing.

Prevention Always wear socks with shoes, and gloves on hands when working with tools. Powder your feet if you're wearing new shoes. If you're worried about getting blistered feet, try coating blister-prone areas with PETROLEUM JELLY or DIAPER RASH ointment (such as A&D ointment) to cut down friction.

While there is currently controversy over the kind of sock material that best prevents blisters, current research suggests that acrylic spun fibers may actually be better than cotton in the presence of water. Wearing two sets of different materials on each foot with properly fitted shoes helps prevent blistering.

blistering disorders   Blistering (or bullous) diseases are not common, but they are very dramatic and can be quite serious. Many of these diseases are triggered by problems in the immune system, which is responsible for producing the blisters.

Among the blistering disorders are PEMPHIGUS, DERMATITIS HERPETIFORMIS and the PEMPHIGOID group (bullous pemphigoid, HERPES GESTATIONIS, cicatricial pemphigoid, epidermolysis bullosa acquisita and linear IgA dermatosis).

Bloch-Sulzberger syndrome This is a disorder of pigmentation (also known as *incontinentia pigmenti*) that is probably transmitted as an X-linked dominant disorder that is usually lethal to male fetuses, and occurs in female infants of all races who carry the trait. It is sometimes associated with multiple defects of the central nervous system within the first month of life. Most affected individuals exhibit numerous skin symptoms.

Symptoms Streaks of red papules or vesicles over the arms, legs and trunk in a swirled or marbled pattern. Over a period of weeks, the swirls evolve into papules that eventually heal, leaving a brown-gray hyperpigmented discoloration.

Treatment There is no effective treatment; the child rapidly passes through the stages of the disease, and the lesions are usually gone by the age of two. The unusual pigmentation usually fades by age 20.

Bloom's syndrome This inherited syndrome is characterized by an intense sensitivity to light beginning in infancy, which causes reddening, blistering and eventually persistent areas of reddened skin and TELANGIECTASIA on the face and hands. At birth, there is proportionate dwarfism; adults are short, with normal intelligence and sexual development, although males often have small testes.

The condition is found most often among Ashkenazi Jewish men originally from southeastern Poland and northwestern Ukraine. While Bloom's syndrome is characterized by many chromosomal abnormalities, the basic genetic defect is not known.

Because of the sensitivity to sunlight, the risk of skin cancer increases significantly with this syndrome.

Treatment Topical SUNSCREENS will prevent the sunburn reaction and decrease sun damage.

blush An involuntary reaction to unwanted attention sends blood rushing to the face, neck, upper chest and ears. When a person is embarrassed or tells a lie, the body experiences this as stress, and involuntarily heats up. As a result, the hypothalamus (the body's temperature regulator) directs heat to the face, the site of the most capillaries (tiny blood vessels that let heat escape). The result? A red blush.

Some women during menopause also experience blushing due to changes in hormonal activity; facial flushing also occurs with the carcinoid syndrome (a rare condition characterized by facial flush, diarrhea and wheezing caused by an intestinal or lung tumor).

Four out of five people have the tendency to blush, but how easily this occurs also depends on a person's genetic makeup. The way to stop a telltale blush is to sip cold water to head off the body's response to heat.

This nonverbal sign of embarrassment and apology is understood in all human cultures, and studies have shown that those who appear embarrassed are found more likeable. To test onlookers' response to a person who blushes, investigators staged a potentially embarrassing accident by having an actor knocking over toilet paper rolls with two versions: in one version the actor restacked the rolls without a care in the world. In the other version, he appeared embarrassed. Onlookers who saw the embarrassed version found the man more likeable.

Researchers conclude that those who don't show signs of embarrassment after a blunder send a disturbing message—either they are unfazed because they are accustomed to their own incompetence or because they don't care about the rules of behavior. Blushing asks onlookers: "Please forgive me. I'm not usually like this."

blusher A type of colored cosmetic designed to give the face a healthy-looking glow.

Blushers come in four basic types: powder, cream, liquid and gel.

Powder blushers have a soft finish and can be used to produce as much or as little color as desired. Powdered products work well on any skin characteristic, especially for those with oily or combination skin. Powder blushers should be applied with a fluffy brush over foundation or directly on bare skin.

Cream blushers are good choices for those with normal or dry skin; they camouflage fine lines and wrinkles better than powder products. However, creams must be applied carefully or they will streak. Blend a bit of moisturizer into the blusher, then smooth onto cheeks using a moistened cosmetic sponge for more control. Apply in a soft arc along the cheekbones, blending edges until there is no obvious line. Never apply in a circle, because the color will look artificial.

Liquid blushes (also called "color rubs") are sheer and can be used to color cheeks or as an all-over facial tint. They work best for dry or normal skin, where they should be blended onto the skin with fingertips, working quickly for even coverage and a sheer finish.

Gel blushers are more transparent than liquid products, and they work best on normal or dry skin. They must be applied gently with fingertips because they streak easily; they can also be used for total facial tint.

For an idea of where to apply blusher, place your index and middle fingers in a "v" formation over your cheek, touching the top and bottom of the ear. Avoid applying too much blusher close to the nose or too close to the eyes. Blusher too high or too low on the cheek can look unnatural; it's always easier to add more than take some away.

The color of blusher should complement skin tone. Fair-skinned blondes look best with beige-pink to coral shades; fair-skinned brunettes are better in rosy to pale pink shades. Olive skin looks best with reddish bronze, soft rose or coral shades, and black skin is best with a sheer tint of soft pink, pink-mauve or blue-red (dark mauve blush tends to emphasize ashiness).

Bockhart's impetigo See IMPETIGO, BOCK-HART'S.

boil An inflamed pus-filled section of skin (usually an infected HAIR FOLLICLE) found often on the back of the neck or moist areas such as the armpits and groin. A boil that is much larger is called a CARBUNCLE.

Boils are usually caused by infection with the bacterium *Staphylococcus aureus*, which invades the body through a break in the skin, where it infects a blocked oil gland or hair follicle. When the body's immune system sends in white blood cells to kill the germs, the resulting inflammation produces pus. A boil begins with a red, painful lump that swells as it fills with pus, until it becomes rounded with a yellowish tip.

Cross section of Boil

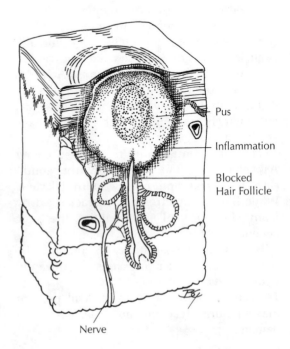

Pus

Inflammation

Blocked Hair Follicle

Nerve

The boil may either continue to grow until it erupts, drains and fades away, or it can be reabsorbed by the body. Recurrent boils may occur in people with known or unrecognized diabetes mellitus, or other diseases involving lowered body resistance.

Complications More seriously, bacteria from a boil may find its way into the blood, causing blood poisoning; for this reason, doctors advise against squeezing boils that appear around the lips or nose, since the infection can be carried to the brain.

Signs of a spreading infection include generalized symptoms of fever and chills, swelling lymph nodes, or red lines radiating from the boil.

Treatment Bursting a boil might spread the infection. Instead, apply a hot compress for 20 minutes every two hours to relieve discomfort and hasten drainage and healing. Change the compress for a new hot one every five minutes during the 20-minute intervals. After treating a boil, wash hands thoroughly before cooking to guard against staph infection getting into food.

It may take up to a week for the boil to break on its own. To further reduce the chance of infection, take showers, not baths. If the boil is large and painful, a physician may prescribe an antibiotic or open the boil with a sterile needle to drain the pus. Occasionally, large boils must be lanced with a surgical knife; this is usually done using a local anesthetic.

Prevention Some experts note that boils are usually infected cysts, and recommend leaving these cysts untouched, or having them lanced by a physician. For patients prone to boils, some experts recommend washing the skin with an antiseptic soap. Take showers to lessen the chance of spreading the infection.

borate While sodium borate may act as an abrasive in removing superficial ACNE lesions, it probably does not effectively remove primary lesions of acne since those are deeply rooted in the follicles, according to an advisory panel of the U.S. Food and Drug Administration. The panel also found that it had not received enough clinical evidence to support the effectiveness of BORIC ACID and sodium borate as acne treatments.

borax A white, odorless mineral that is a mild cleanser and antiseptic. It is most often used as an emulsifier in cold cream, but it also is included in mouthwashes, vanishing creams, bath salts, eye lotions, cleansing lotions and scalp lotions. It has not been found to cause allergic reactions.

boric acid An antiseptic, bactericide and fungicide prepared from sulfuric acid and natural BORAX. It should not be ingested or inhaled, and should not be used on babies. Boric acid has been used in talcum powders in the past. Boric acid was once used as a dressing for wounds and burns, but after a number of people died following excessive absorption of boric acid in extensive wounds, borax fell out of favor as a salve for burns. Borax is no longer included in the manufacture of baby products.

botox (botulinum A toxin) A purified form of the toxin that causes botulism that has been studied as a possible wrinkle remover. In studies at Columbia Presbyterian Hospital, the substance was injected into the faces of 200 patients interested in smoothing their skin. Botox temporarily and partially paralyzes the muscles beneath frown lines and crow's feet, preventing them from contracting fully. The result, scientists say, is a smoother, less furrowed face that lasts between three and six months. Experts have found a reduction in wrinkling of between 50 and 90 percent; almost nine out of 10 patients in the study chose to continue the treatments.

The only side effect researchers reported was a feeling of heaviness in the face of five patients for a few weeks.

The technique does have its critics, who charge that the slackened muscles can give a blank, lifeless look. In the hands of inexperienced practitioners, botox treatments could paralyze a person's face.

bouba   See YAWS.

Bowen's disease   This precancerous condition is a synonym for SQUAMOUS CELL CANCER in situ, causing a scaling, reddish pink slightly raised growth (usually on the face or hands). The disease is more often found among men with fair skin; chronic sunlight exposure is the primary cause. Chronic ingestion of inorganic arsenicals also causes Bowen's disease, although this is rare today. About one-third of these patients have multiple lesions.

Squamous cell cancers that occur as a result of Bowen's disease are usually more aggressive than those from ACTINIC KERATOSES. It is not uncommon for the cancer developing from Bowen's disease to spread to the lymph nodes.

In addition, some studies suggest that patients with Bowen's disease may develop other premalignant and malignant tumors, such as actinic keratoses, BASAL CELL CARCINOMAS and adnexal carcinomas.

Bowen's disease lesions on mucosal surfaces have a different appearance and biologic potential; when they occur on the penis they are called erythroplasia of Queyrat (usually in uncircumcised males); they occur less frequently on the vulva. These lesions are bright red with a velvety, glistening surface. While microscopically identical to Bowen's disease, these lesions have a higher rate of malignant transformation and the resulting squamous cell carcinomas are more aggressive than those arising from ordinary Bowen's disease.

Treatment   The condition is treated by surgically removing the diseased patch of skin, or destroying it by freezing or cauterization. Once removed, these skin conditions do not return.

breast enlargement   See MAMMOPLASTY.

breast lift   See MAMMOPLASTY.

breast reduction   See MAMMOPLASTY.

bromhidrosis   A condition caused by apocrine sweat that has become foul-smelling because of bacterial decomposition. See also SWEAT GLANDS.

bromoderma   A pustular skin eruption due to ingestion of bromides. Bromides, once prescribed as a sedative, are no longer administered because of their unpleasant side effects—including ACNE. The acne would fade once bromides were discontinued.

brown recluse spiders   The bite of two species of the *Loxosceles* family cause severe skin tissue necrosis (tissue death) and extensive sloughing of the skin at the site of the bite, which may also be accompanied by generalized symptoms.

The United States species of this deadly spider, *L. reclusa* (or the Missouri brown spider), lives in about half of the states, although it is most often found in the central and south central U.S. Ounce for ounce, the venom of this spider is more deadly than that of many poisonous snakes. It is believed that the spider was mistakenly imported to this country in fruit crates and vegetables within the last 50 years; since then it has been making its way steadily north and west. The secretive spiders get their name from their fondness for dark, secret storage spaces, under boxes and in closets. While these spiders are not aggressive and will try to escape when cornered, if trapped they will bite. The venom of the female is more deadly than that of the male. Its brown to fawn-colored body is about a ½ inch long, with a dark brown violin-shaped marking.

Symptoms Reaction to the brown recluse bite varies considerably from one person to the next, depending on the amount of venom injected, the patient's age and health. Basically, the bite can cause a skin injury ranging from a small papule to a huge necrotic ulcer, together with a systemic reaction. Severe systemic reactions and death occur most often in children, but even this is rare.

The bite of this spider causes little pain at first, but within eight hours the pain is often severe, and the area of the bite will become red. The local skin reaction may be minor, with mild itching and a plaque or a small area of dead tissue that heals by itself within five days. Still, brown recluse spider venom contains a substance that is very destructive to tissue; in more severe cases, a blue-gray halo is seen at the bite site, followed in 18 hours by a small blister and surrounding area of redness and swelling. Eventually, the blister ruptures, and within a week the skin cells in the area begin to die, with a thick black scar on the base that slowly separates over several weeks. In a small number of patients, the ulcer doesn't heal for a months.

The bite can also cause systemic reactions of fever, chills, weakness, nausea and vomiting, joint pain and a generalized rash. If the bite is fatal, the victim usually dies within the first 48 hours as a result of kidney failure.

Treatment There is no specific antivenin, although antivenin for other species of brown spiders of South America could give protection. Small bites may require just cold compresses, elevation, painkillers and a tetanus shot. DAPSONE may prevent necrosis, and although corticosteroids are sometimes used for larger lesions, their usefulness has not been proven. Antibiotics may prevent infection. In addition, antihistamines and muscle relaxants may provide some relief. Exchange transfusions in which nearly all the patient's blood is replaced by a donor's blood may be attempted.

Immediate excision of the bite area may be the only way to prevent the massive necrosis caused by this spider, although not all experts agree on this treatment. Most physicians will not touch the lesion until all the destruction has been done, sometimes as long as 40 weeks after the bite.

Skin grafts may be necessary to heal the ulcer. If a brown recluse bite is suspected, a physician should be consulted at once.

bruise A deep blue or black discoloration on the skin following trauma, caused by bleeding under the skin. Initially the bruise looks blue or black; as the hemoglobin begins to break down, the bruise turns yellow. While most bruises occur after a bump, they may also follow a period of heavy exercise; exercise sometimes causes tiny tears in blood vessels below the skin, allowing blood to seep out.

Easy bruising may also be a sign of disease, especially blood disorders such as anemia. In addition, some drugs (such as aspirin and other blood thinners) may lead to increased bruising; other drugs, such as anti-inflammatory agents, antidepressants or asthma drugs may interfere with blood clotting under the skin. AIDS can also cause purplish bumps that *seem* to be bruises that don't fade. Substance abusers also may find they have an increased susceptibility to bruising.

Some studies suggest that patients who lack vitamin C in their diets tend to bruise more easily and their wounds heal more slowly. This may be due to the fact that vitamin C helps build supportive COLLAGEN around blood vessels in the skin, which helps protect the vessels from rupture. For those who bruise easily, some experts suggest 500 mg. of vitamin C three times a day to help build collagen (although vitamin C is not toxic, patients taking high doses of vitamin C should consult with their physician).

Treatment The discoloration of a bruise can be minimized by immediately applying cold, to keep down the swelling and constrict blood vessels, which helps to decrease the internal bleeding. Apply an ice pack at 15-minute intervals immediately after the bump for the first 24 to 48 hours. If you are in a location without ice, you can also use a clean cold soda can, applying it for five to 10 minutes every 15 minutes. After 24 hours, use heat to dilate the blood vessels and improve circulation.

Prevention Recent studies suggest that those who don't get enough vitamin C tend to bruise more easily, and their wounds heal more slowly. This may be due to the fact that vitamin C helps build up supportive tissue around blood vessels. Those who bruise easily may find that 500 milligrams of vitamin C taken three times a day to build collagen may be effective. Although vitamin C is not considered to be toxic, experts advise patients to get their physician's okay before using high doses of vitamin C.

bubble bath Detergent cleansers containing ingredients capable of making bathwater foam. These products can be irritating to mucous membranes and the skin if used in too great a concentration, especially in people with dry skin or ECZEMA because these detergents tend to dry out the skin. Be sure to swirl the bubble bath throughout the water, and use a moisturizer after the bath. The drying or irritating effect of bubble bath can be prevented by adding bath oil (such as Nivea oil or Lubriderm oil) to the bath water.

bubo Swollen and inflamed lymph node, (particularly in the axilla or groin) due to BUBONIC PLAGUE, tuberculosis, SYPHILIS, etc.

bulla A large fluid-filled BLISTER, usually 2 cm. or more in diameter.

bubonic plague The most common form of PLAGUE, characterized by the appearance of a BUBO (swollen lymph node) in the groin or armpit early in the illness. Plague is primarily a disease of rodents, and is transmitted from rodents to humans by flea bites. After the bite, the bacteria spreads through the body to the lymph nodes, which become painful and enlarged.

Treatment Streptomycin should be administered to treat this disease.

burns Every year, about 2 million Americans are burned or scalded badly enough to require medical care; about 70,000 are hospitalized. This type of injury is most common among children and the elderly and are usually due to preventable accidents in the home. Because the skin is a living tissue, temperatures that even briefly reach 120° F will destroy its cells.

Burns can be caused by contact with hot substances, flames, chemicals, radiation (in sunlight, x rays, or ionizing radiation). While most accidental burns are visible almost immediately after the accident, burns from sunburn may appear several hours to a day later. It may be 10 to 30 days before the full effects of ionizing x-ray irradiation burns appear.

Severity of burns The severity of a burn depends on two factors: how deep the tissue destruction has penetrated, and the amount of body surface that has been affected. Burn recovery is also influenced by the age and general health of the victim, the location of the burn and any other associated injuries.

Traditionally, physicians have characterized burns as first-, second- or third-degree, depending on the depth of skin damage. By accurately estimating the extent of damage, the physician can best determine the appropriate treatment.

First-degree burns This type of minor burn affects only the epidermis (top layer of skin), causing reddening but no blisters or swelling. Typically, pain ebbs within 48 to 72 hours, and the burn heals quickly without scars, although the damaged skin may peel off in a

Degree of Burn

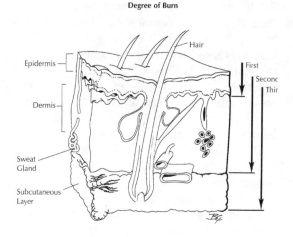

day or two. A sunburn is an example of a first-degree burn.

Second-degree burns This type of burn destroys the skin on a deeper level, creating redness and blisters; the deeper the burn, the more blisters, which increase in size within a few hours after the injury. However, some of the dermis (deep layer of the skin) remains, so that this type of burn can usually heal without scarring as long as there has been no accompanying infection. Second-degree burns may be extremely painful. How well a second-degree burn heals depends on the amount of skin that has been damaged.

However, in very deep second-degree burns, the healed skin may resemble scars from a third-degree burn. These deeper burns take longer to heal—often up to a month or more—and the healing epidermis is extremely fragile. In fact, some of the worst burn scars are caused by these very serious second-degree burns.

Third-degree burns This is the most serious type of burn, which destroys all the layers of the skin. If the burn is very deep, muscles and bones may also be exposed. The affected area will look white or charred, and even if the burned area is only small, it will require special treatment and skin grafts to help prevent serious scarring.

In this type of burn, there is no pain because the pain receptors have been destroyed along with the rest of the dermis and blood vessels, sweat glands, sebaceous glands and hair follicles. Fluid loss and metabolic problems in these injuries are profound.

These burns always heal with scarring. Extensive third-degree burns require aggressive treatment in a hospital burn unit, and the mortality rate is significant.

Fourth-degree burns Occasionally, burns even deeper than a full thickness of the skin occur, such as when a part of the body is trapped in flame—or in an electrical burn. These deep burns enter the muscle, fascia and bone and are also called "black" or "char" burns (because of the typical color of the burn). If a fourth-degree burn involves more than a very small area of the body, the prognosis is very grave, since these deep burns can release toxic materials into the bloodstream. If the burn involves a small area, it should be excised down to healthy tissue; a charred large area on an extremity usually requires amputation.

Electrical burns Electrical accidents can cause several different types of burns, including flame burns caused by ignited clothing, electrical current injury or electrothermal burns from arcing current. Sometimes all three types of burns will be found in one victim.

Flame burns from ignited clothing may be the most serious part of the wound. An electric current injury is characterized by focal burns at the point where the current entered and left through the skin. Once an electric current enters the body, its path within the body is determined by tissues with the least resistance. Bone offers the most resistance to electrical current, followed in descending order by fat, tendon, skin, muscle, blood and nerve. The path the current takes determines whether the victim will survive, since current passing through the heart or the brain stem will result in almost instantaneous death from ventricular fibrillation. As current passes through muscle, it can set off severe spasms that can fracture or dislocate a bone. Although bone does not conduct the current well, it stores the heat from the electricity and can damage surrounding muscles.

Electrothermal (flash or arc) burns are heat injuries to the skin that occur when high-tension electrical current touches the skin, causing intense, deep damage. Damage is severe because the arc carries temperature of about 2,500° C—hot enough to melt bone.

Skin at both the entry and exit of the current is usually gray, yellow and depressed; there may be some charring. All of these wounds must be debrided.

Extent of burn When a health care worker estimates a burned patient's injuries in a percentage ("a burn over 60 percent of the body," for example) the percentage isn't simply a guess. Health care workers use a "rule of nines" to estimate the amount of body area affected by a burn. The percentage figure is computed by dividing the body into sections: 9 percent to the head and neck, 9 percent to each arm, 18 percent to each foot and leg, and 18 percent each to the front and back of the trunk. The remaining 1 percent makes up the perineum (the region of the body between the anus and the urethral opening). This rule is more accurate for adults, but less reliable in children, whose body proportions are different.

Effects Because a burn destroys a large area of skin, it also disrupts fluid balance, metabolism, temperature and immune response. Fluid is lost in part by oozing from blisters (called a "weeping burn") and also from dilation of blood vessels that leak fluid into the area beneath the burned skin 36 to 48 hours after the injury. After this period, the fluid is slowly reabsorbed by the body. This fluid and salt loss can be significant, depending on the percentage of the burn.

While there is not much weeping from second- and third-degree burns, the underlying fluid loss is extensive; there may even be fluid loss from remote capillaries in unburned tissue (such as the lungs). If fluid loss is not reversed within an hour after the burn, the fluid loss begins to interfere with organ function and shock sets in. Once the fluid loss reaches a critical level, the circulatory shock becomes irreversible and nothing can be done to save the patient's life.

Burn victims also experience an increase in the metabolic and oxygen use rates. This metabolic increase is at first fueled by glycogen stored in the liver and muscles, but when these stores are depleted the body begins to break down its own protein structures. This metabolic response reaches a maximum level in burns of more than 40 percent.

Most burn patients die from infections of the skin, bloodstream and lungs, in part due to a weakened immune system.

Treatment It is only since World War II that treatment of burns has made much progress.

In fact, since ancient times physicians knew very little about proper burn management technique. Emollients with unusual ingredients were often placed on the burn, and bleeding was a popular treatment for burns throughout the Middle Ages. Until the mid-1940s, the best treatment that could be offered was to wash the burn with soap and water, leaving it exposed to the air.

Generally, first-degree burns can be treated with proper first aid. Second-degree burns covering more than 15 percent of an adult's body, or 10 percent of a child's body, or burns of the face, hands or feet require prompt medical attention. All people with third-degree burns should get immediate medical help.

First/second-degree burn treatment First, flush burns with plenty of cold (not ice) water for 15 to 30 minutes; if the burn was caused by hot grease, battery acid, etc., remove saturated clothing, wash the grease off the skin and then soak the burn in cold water. If clothing sticks to the skin, *don't pull it off—*

rinse over the clothing and go to the emergency room. If a first- or second-degree burn is smaller than a quarter on a child, or smaller than a silver dollar on an adult, the burn can probably be treated at home. Any burn on an infant, a person over 60 or a large burn should be treated by a professional.

Never put butter on a burn, since the fat can hold in the heat and actually worsen the burn, possibly causing infection.

After rinsing with cold water, wrap in clean dry gauze and leave the wound alone for 24 hours. Avoid applying antiseptics or other irritating substances. A good way to remember how to treat a first-degree burn is not to put any substance on your burn that you would be afraid to put into your eye.

Wash the burn with soap and water or a mild Betadine solution. Several days later, you can apply the sap from a fresh piece of aloe plant or an aloe cream to ease the pain. Do not use aloe if you are taking prescription blood thinners, or if you have any heart problems.

Third-degree burn treatment A third-degree burn should be seen by a physician as soon as possible. These wounds should not be plunged into water, since cool water may worsen the circulatory shock that often accompanies severe burns. Instead, cover the injury with a bulky sterile dressing or with freshly laundered bed linens. Clothing stuck to the wound should not be removed, and don't apply any ointments, salves, sprays, etc. Elevate burned feet and legs and raise burned hands above the level of the heart. Closely monitor breathing, and give artificial respiration if breathing stops.

Your doctor will either lightly dress these burns with an antibacterial dressing or leave them exposed to enhance healing. Every effort is made to keep the skin germ-free by reverse isolation nursing. If necessary, painkillers and antibiotics are prescribed and intravenous fluids are given to offset fluid loss. Extensive second-degree, and all third-degree

burns are treated with early skin grafts to minimize scarring. Extensive burns may need repeated plastic surgery.

Complications Despite the widespread use of antibacterial agents, infection remains one of the most serious complications of burn wounds. Acute gastrointestinal ulcers often complicate recovery. Children are also prone to developing post-burn seizures, probably from electrolyte imbalances, low oxygen blood levels, infection or drugs. Youngsters are also prone to high blood pressure after a burn injury, probably related to the release of certain stress hormones after the burn.

Common complications of burn grafts are the formation of fibrous masses of scar tissue called HYPERTROPHIC SCARS and KELOIDS, especially in dark-skinned individuals. Direct pressure on inflamed tissue reduces its blood supply and collagen content, which can head off the development of these scars. This pressure can be provided by wearing a variety of special burn splints, sleeves, stockings and body jackets. Special cases may require body traction.

Prognosis Scars are the most common after effects of a serious burn and may require years of additional plastic surgery after skin grafting to release the contractures over joints. Unfortunately, despite modern cosmetic surgical techniques, burn scars are almost always unsightly and the results are almost never as good as the patient's pre-burn condition.

Burn scars should be carefully treated, even after they have completely healed. They should not be exposed to sunlight, and those areas of the skin exposed to the sun should be covered by sunscreen. Since deep burns destroy oil and sweat glands, the patient may need to apply emollients and lotions to prevent drying and cracking.

Recovery from serious burns may take many years. Patients may require extensive psychological counseling in order to adjust to disfigurement and physical therapy to regain or maintain mobility in damaged joints. See also CHEMICAL BURNS.

Burns United Support Groups A support group for burn survivors and their families that provides support services and information on burn care and prevention. The group conducts educational programs and childrens' services, and operates a speakers' bureau. Founded in 1986, the group has 80 members. For address, see Appendix A. See also AMERICAN BURN ASSOCIATION, INTERNATIONAL SOCIETY FOR BURN INJURIES, NATIONAL BURN VICTIM FOUNDATION, PHOENIX SOCIETY FOR BURN SURVIVORS, NATIONAL INSTITUTE FOR BURN MEDICINE.

Burow's solution One of the most common ASTRINGENTS for wet dressings, this clear, colorless substance is also known as aluminum acetate.

burrow An excavation by parasites in the STRATUM CORNEUM (topmost layer of epidermis) of differing sizes and shapes. See also SCABIES.

Buschke-Lowenstein tumor See WARTS.

Buschke-Ollendorff syndrome This genetic disorder, also known as osteopoikilosis with connective tissue nevus, is passed on to 50 percent of all offspring of an affected parent. This disorder is characterized by multiple raised yellow-orange skin PAPULES, with a marked increase of connective tissue within these lesions. The condition usually appears in the 20s or 30s, with nodules or plaques on the thighs buttocks or abdominal wall. No treatment is required. See also CONNECTIVE TISSUE NEVI.

butyl stearate One of the most common stearic acids used in cosmetics, such as nail polish removers, lipsticks and cleansing creams. Butyl stearate may cause an allergic reaction in sensitive consumers.

C

café au lait macule Pale, coffee-colored oval patches that may develop up to 3 inches across anywhere on the skin. While an individual such spot has no significance, the presence of six or more spots greater than 1.5 cm. may be a sign of NEUROFIBROMATOSIS, a hereditary disease of the nerve fiber sheaths. These spots are not related to ultraviolet radiation exposure, and may be present at birth or acquired later in life.
Cause The hyperpigmentation is due to increased MELANIN in the skin.
Treatment Laser therapy may be used to treat these patches.

calamine lotion A pink compound of ferric oxide and zinc oxide that is applied (as a lotion, ointment or dusting powder) to the skin. Calamine lotion cools, dries and protects skin that is irritated or itchy because of DERMATITIS, ECZEMA, POISON IVY, INSECT BITES or SUNBURN. It may also be combined with a topical local anesthetic such as benzocaine, or with corticosteroids or antihistamines, which reduce inflammation.

calcinosis cutis The condition in which abnormal amounts of calcium are deposited as nodules in the skin and connective tissue. Calcinosis is often associated with disorders of the connective tissue such as DERMATOMYOSITIS or SCLERODERMA.

callus An area of thickening of the stratum corneum caused by regular or prolonged pressure or friction, or if body weight is carried unevenly. It is the body's protective response to repeat friction. Found most often on the feet, they may occur anywhere on the body that experiences constant friction. A small focal callus with a hard core is called a CORN. Corns are often surrounded by callus. Initial thickening of the skin is a protective response, and the resulting callus is not painful unless very thick or fissured.

Some amount of callusing may be beneficial, especially for those who go barefoot a great deal or who perform a repetitive activity such as shovelling, gymnastics or weightlifting. Calluses protect the skin from heat, rough surfaces and cuts.
Treatment Often, it's best to leave a callus alone because of its protective capability. A painful or troublesome callus on the foot may be treated by a dermatologist or podiatrist, who can pare away the thickened skin in layers with a scalpel. But calluses caused by foot deformities almost always recur unless the underlying problem is corrected either surgically or by using a molded shoe insole.

For patients with a lot of callused tissue, some experts suggest soaking the feet in diluted chamomile tea, which will soothe and soften hardened skin. For those with bad calluses, treat the area daily after a warm bath by abrading lightly with a callus file or pumice stone followed by a moisturizing cream. Do not use this treatment on hard corns.
Caution: Patients with diabetes or those with reduced feeling in their feet should never treat themselves.

camouflage cosmetics Special types of cosmetics used for those with scars or discolored patches on the skin. The key cosmetic for camouflage is an opaque, heavyweight foundation (usually a cream) that is thicker than regular foundation and may be applied under regular foundation. Spread over an area with a skin problem, it can make many disfiguring marks (including BIRTHMARKS,

SCARS and even discoloration left by SUN-BURN) less noticeable. Both men and women can use these products that come in cream, powder and stick formulas. Today, the use of opaque ingredients such as titanium dioxide allow consumers to use lighter, more "breathable" coverup products.

The key to using any corrective makeup is to blend the edges into surrounding skin; the best results come from using products that are precisely matched to skin color. However, for some people a slightly darker shade will hide a defect more completely. Opaque foundations (also called concealing creams) are available in shades from pale ivory to dark chocolate, and may be found at cosmetic counters in large department stores.

If you are using a coverup product only on one small area, such as a birthmark on your cheek, always apply the coverage product under your foundation; once you apply a translucent foundation over it, it will seem as if the skin—not the makeup—is what is showing through.

Foundation cream is applied by first warming it in your hand and then applying with a finger or makeup sponge, using a pat-dab motion, beginning in the center of the area to be covered and blending outwards. Rubbing causes an uneven application. After five minutes, apply a special translucent setting powder; wait another five minutes and then brush away any excess. Apply regular makeup if desired.

When covering recent scars, always discuss the product safety with your dermatologist or surgeon first. In the first week or two after an accident or plastic surgery, it's best not to wear cosmetics at all, and it can take several weeks or months for the skin to heal completely.

For women interested in concealing dark shadows under the eye, the key is to use as little cover-up as possible. The best idea is to apply concealer under the dark circles, which are often caused by shadows cast by excess skin or fat below the eyes. Pat on small dots of concealer, blending upward into the darker area with light strokes of the fingertips. Avoid white under-eye concealer because it looks too unnatural.

It's also possible to change the color of the skin with these products. To neutralize a reddish complexion, start by applying a delicate pale green base; to improve a yellowing complexion, start with a peach or lavender base. A flesh-colored concealing cream or regular makeup base can then be applied over this.

If applied thickly enough, the opaque cream can also be an effective sunblock; a better choice is a cream that specifically includes a sunscreen.

camphor A volatile fragrant compound derived from an Asian evergreen tree that is used as an antiseptic in some skin care products because it feels soothing to the skin. It may also help stop itching and is a rubefacient (it reddens the skin). Camphor is absorbed almost immediately in the skin and it causes a feeling of warmth and then numbness. Camphor will not affect the outcome of an ACNE breakout, but it is helpful for chapped skin and as a counter-irritant in liniment rubs, where it warms and soothes sore muscles.

If inhaled for a long time, camphor can induce a severe headache.

cancer, skin See SKIN CANCER.

Candida albicans The yeast that causes the infection called CANDIDIASIS, often within the vagina or on other areas of mucous membrane (such as the inside of the mouth). The infection is also known as thrush or moniliasis.

candida infection A type of YEAST INFECTION by *Candida albicans*. The infection is also known as "thrush," moniliasis or candidiasis. *Candida* produces skin disease by invading the keratinized epidermis—rarely, in some forms of chronic infection of the skin and mucous membranes, the infection may invade the dermis and subcutaneous tissue.

The yeast that causes candidiasis naturally grows in both the vagina and the mouth, where it is usually kept under control by bacteria present in the body. However, the yeast may grow if the bacteria are destroyed, for example, as during antibiotic therapy, if the body's natural resistance to disease is affected (as in AIDS) or if a person is taking drugs that suppresses the immune system. The fungus may also flourish in the presence of some disorders (diabetes mellitus), during hormonal changes of pregnancy or while taking birth control pills.

Candidal infection of the penis, which occurs more often among uncircumcised males, may be transmitted from an infected partner. Similarly, it can also spread from the genitals or mouth to other moist areas of the body (such as the skin folds in the groin or under the breasts). It may crop up with diaper rash in infants.

Symptoms Infection of the skin of the mouth causes sore, white-colored raised patches which are usually asymptomatic. In skin folds or with diaper rash, it forms an itchy red rash with flaky white patches. There may be burning or stinging and itching in skin folds or other affected areas. The skin looks beefy red or scalded with an irregular margin; a chronic scaly form may occasionally occur.

Treatment Antifungal drugs (such as clotrimazole, miconazole, nystatin or econazole nitrate) will usually clear up the infection, but it may recur. Those with a tendency toward this type of infection should keep the skin dry. However, primary irritation or allergy rarely may occur due to topical medications and worsen the skin condition. Compresses with Burow's solution, plenty of air and infrared heat lamps to dry the affected parts may help. See also CANDIDA PARONYCHIA.

Yogurt (18 oz. daily serving), which contains lactobacillus acidophilus, reduces the colonization of the vagina and mouth and is effective in preventing recurrent yeast infections.

Candida paronychia Infection by the yeast *Candida albicans* affects the nails, causing red, tender, swollen fingertips in those who must frequently immerse the hands.

Treatment Soak the finger with Burow's solution for 10 minutes four times daily; topical imidazole antifungals in solution or cream are also helpful. Oral treatment may also be required.

See also CANDIDA INFECTION.

candidiasis See CANDIDA INFECTION.

canker sore A small painful ulcer on the inside of the mouth, lip or underneath the tongue that heals without treatment. Canker sores are *not* the same type of skin lesion as herpes simplex (also known as "cold sores" or "fever blisters"). You can tell the difference between the two by their appearance and location. Herpes often involves the skin of the lips, and cankers don't; herpes often strikes the gums, and cankers rarely do; and herpes is often accompanied by tender lymph glands in the neck.

About 20 percent of Americans at any one time experience a canker sore, commonly between ages 10 and 40. They are particularly common in children who wear braces. The most severely affected people have almost continuous sores, while others have just one or two per year. A canker sore is usually a small oval ulcer with a grayish white center surrounded by a red, inflamed halo, which usually lasts for one or two weeks. A canker sore should heal within two weeks. Only if the sufferer cannot eat, speak or sleep, or if the sore does not heal not within two weeks, medical help should be sought.

Cause Unlike herpes, cankers are not caused by a virus but are probably the result of bacteria or a temporarily malfunctioning immune system. Because hemolytic streptococcus bacteria have so often been isolated from canker sores, experts believe they may be caused by a hypersensitive reaction to the bacteria. Other factors often associated with a flareup include trauma (such as biting the inside of the cheek), acute stress and allergies, or chemical irritants in toothpaste or mouthwash. More women than men experience canker sores, which are more likely to occur during the premenstrual period and are also more likely to occur if other members of the family suffer from them.

Treatment While the ulcers will heal themselves, topical painkillers ease the pain; healing can be hastened by using a corticosteroid ointment or a tetracycline mouthwash.

For severe sores, the prescription drug Aphthasol has recently been approved: This drug's safety for those with impaired immune systems has not been studied.

Over-the-counter medications containing carbamide peroxide (Cankaid, Glyoxide and Amosan) may help. Other treatments include benzocaine, menthol, camphor, eucalyptol or alcohol, or pastes (such as Orabase or Zilactin) that form a protective "bandage" over the sore. For short-term pain relief, rinse with a prescription mouthwash containing 2 percent viscous lidocaine, an anesthetic.

Prevention No treatments can prevent canker sores. If you are prone to canker sores, try to avoid coffee, spices, citrus fruits, tomatoes, walnuts, strawberries and chocolates, toothpastes and mouthwashes. Brush teeth with baking soda for a month or two, and rinse your mouth with warm salt water.

capsaicin The active ingredient in hot peppers that produces an irritating effect when used on the skin; it has been found to ease the incessant itch of PSORIASIS. Capsaicin is believed to interfere with the substance P, the chemical in the body that transmits the "itch" impulse to the brain. When a patient applies capsaicin to the skin, the local nerves release a large amount of substance P, thus depleting the supply. The itch subsides because the body takes some time to build up the stores of the chemical again.

While capsaicin does not cure psoriasis, it can decrease the urge to itch, which, in turn, may shorten the duration of the outbreak since scratching can stimulate psoriasis. It also has been demonstrated to reduce the pain associated with SHINGLES.

The cream may burn or tingle when first applied to the skin, but this sensation should lessen over time. See also ZOSTRIX.

carbenicillin (trade names: Geopen, Pyopen) A synthetic penicillin, available by mouth or by intravenous injection, that is effective against a wide range of bacterial skin infections.

carbolic acid A caustic acid formerly used in chemical face peeling. Carbolic acid is too caustic for this purpose and is therefore no longer used in skin care.

carbolic soap A disinfectant soap with about 10 percent phenol used to treat oily skin.

carbon dioxide laser The most versatile laser, this instrument can be operated in either focused or defocused mode. When defocused, the target area is larger and the beam surface vaporizes the surface of the target and destroys cells instantly. The heating and destruction occur so quickly, in fact, that there is little heat conducted to adjacent cells, and the zone of injury is small and can be carefully controlled.

In the focused mode, the beam diameter narrows to just 0.1 mm; this intense beam is capable of cutting tissue, the depth and precision of which depends on the speed with which the laser beam is moved along the tissue. Because it produces heat, the laser actually sterilizes the cut as it goes, and seals blood vessels so that the surgical field is bloodless unless a large blood vessel is cut. Because the heat is concentrated on a small area, there is little tissue damage, so the tissue can be preserved and examined later.

The CO_2 laser can be used to treat a variety of benign or malignant skin conditions. And while warts can also be destroyed with this technique, the plume of smoke that the treatment generates may contain infectious particles.

There are, however, some risks associated in the CO_2 laser treatment. Because the CO_2 beam is invisible, the potential for damage to eyes is great; usually, a small red helium-neon laser is used with the CO_2 beam, so that its red light marks the area being struck by the CO_2 beam. Still, everyone in the room must wear special protective eye goggles.

Because the beam generates heat, there is also a risk of fire (especially on surgical dressings). Wet dressings placed over normal neighboring skin will reduce the chance of fire and of inadvertent damage to surrounding tissue.

carbuncle A cluster of boils (pus-filled inflamed hair roots) commonly found on the back of the neck and the buttocks that are usually caused by the bacterium *Staphylococcus aureus*. Carbuncles usually begin as single boils that spread, but they are less common than single boils. They primarily affect patients with lowered resistance to infection.
Treatment Carbuncles are treated by the administration of oral and topical antibiotics and hot compresses. These may relieve the pain by causing the pus-filled heads to burst; if this occurs, the carbuncle should be cov-

ered with a dressing until it has healed completely. Once the inflammation has been controlled, the lesion may be cut and drained. The cavity may then need packing with a petroleum jelly or iodoform dressing. In some cases, draining is not necessary if a 10-day course of antibiotics and topical antibiotics cures the infection.
Prevention Recurrent carbuncles are usually caused by autoinoculation (that is, patients carry the bacteria that causes carbuncles and constantly reinfect themselves). Regular washing with antibacterial soap (especially around rashes, irritations, shaving, or areas of heavy sweating) can help prevent reinfection. Also, wash your hands and launder bedding often.

carcinoma, basal cell See BASAL CELL CARCINOMA.

carcinoma, squamous cell See SQUAMOUS CELL CARCINOMA, SQUAMOUS CELL.

carnauba wax A type of wax derived from the pores of the Brazilian carnauba palm tree used to give cosmetics a more solid consistency. This wax is included in depilatories, creams, and stick deodorants. It has not been shown to induce an allergic reaction.

carotenemia Yellowing of the skin resembling JAUNDICE caused by excess carotene in the blood, most commonly found on the palms, soles of the feet and central third of the face, and in the sweat. Carotenemia does not usually affect the whites of the eyes, which helps distinguish it from jaundice.
Cause Excess ingestion of certain vegetables and fruits rich in carotene, or the result of therapy with BETA-CAROTENE for certain disorders (such as ERYTHROPOIETIC PROTOPORPHYRIA). Too much carotene in the blood may also be a symptom of hypothyroidism, diabetes mellitus, hypopituitarism or anorexia nervosa.

Treatment When carotenemia is caused by beta-carotene therapy or excess dietary ingestion, the skin returns to normal several months after the diet or therapy has stopped.

cartilage-hair hypoplasia A genetic disorder characterized by thin hair shafts with little or no pigment and short-limb dwarfism. Because of defects in the immune system, there may be other problems such as recurrent respiratory infections and severe SHINGLES. There is no known treatment. See HAIR, DISORDERS OF.

casein A whole-milk protein used in cosmetics as an emulsifier (especially in massage creams) that does not affect the skin's health in any way.

castor oil A vegetable oil derived from the castor bean. Used in many cosmetics as an emollient, it forms a hard film when dry. It is often used in lipsticks, but because of its unpleasant smell, it is not often found in other cosmetics. Because it is rarely associated with skin irritation or allergic reactions, it is used in some medical-grade creams and pastes, and several types of eyedrops.

catagen The brief stage of the hair growth cycle in which growth (anagen) stops and resting (telogren) starts. See HAIR, ANATOMY OF.

cat-scratch fever An illness following the scratch or bite of a cat that may involve a rash, probably caused by a small bacterium the exact identity of which is being investigated. Three-quarters of cases occur in children, most often in fall and winter. The cat itself does not appear to be ill.
Symptoms Between three to 10 days after a bite or scratch, the victim reports one or more swollen lymph nodes near the scratch, which may become painful and tender and occasionally discharge. After three to 10 days, a red round lump usually appears at the sight of infection. A small, infected blister sometimes develops at the original site of the skin wound; occasionally, there is fever, rash, malaise and headache.
Diagnosis/treatment The disease is diagnosed from a biopsy of a small sample of the swollen lymph node and from a skin test using a cat-scratch fever antigen. Painkillers may be needed to relieve fever and headache; a severely affected lymph node or blister may have to be drained. In most cases, the illness fades after one or two months, and the cat does not need to be destroyed.
Prevention Other than avoiding cats, there is no way to avoid the disease. However, cats only carry the infecting organism for a few weeks during their lifetimes, so the likelihood of being reinfected, or infected by just one pet in the home, is minimal.

causalgia A persistent burning pain (usually in an arm or leg) with red and tender skin over the painful area; conversely, the skin may sometimes be cold, blue and clammy. It is usually caused by nerve injury following trauma (such as gunshot wound, fracture or deep cut). The pain may become worse during times of emotional stress or by normal sensations (such as touch).
Treatment There is no guaranteed treatment, although sometimes pain may be relieved by severing certain nerves. Full recovery may take many months. A one-month trial of capsaicin cream applied three times daily may help.

cavernous hemangioma See HEMANGIOMA, CAVERNOUS.

cayenne pepper spots Tiny red spots often associated with inflammation of tiny blood vessels (capillaritis). These spots are seen typically in a group of conditions called progressive pigmentary purpura.

cellulite The so-called "dimpling" of the legs in women that is actually an imaginary condition used to describe an anatomically normal irregularity found in almost all women's skin. In fact, there is no such thing as "cellulite" itself; the appearance of dimpling simply occurs because the fat deposits in a woman's leg are different from those in a man's leg. In women, the subcutaneous fat appears in large channels, whereas men have connective tissue strands that hold in the fat, preventing the dimpling effect.

Although European clinics inject enzymes into the leg to "dissolve" this nonexistent substance, and topical aminophylline cream has recently been used in the U.S., there is no uniformly effective treatment for "cellulite" except for physical removal of fat (liposuction) or by decreasing the amount of fat in your legs through diet and exercise.

cellulitis A bacterial infection of loose connective tissue (particularly subcutaneous tissue) usually caused by B-hemolytic streptococci and staphlococci bacteria. Untreated, the disease may lead to bacteremia, septicemia or GANGRENE; facial infections may spread to the eye socket. Very rarely, cellulitis develops after childbirth and may spread to the pelvic organs. Before the development of antibiotics, cellulitis was occasionally fatal. Today, any form of cellulitis is likely to be more serious in those with compromised immune systems.
Symptoms Affected area (usually face, neck or limbs) is usually hot, tender and red, with associated fever and chills.
Treatment Antibiotics (penicillin, cephalosporins or clindamycin) must be taken for up to two weeks to clear the infection.

cerate An ointment or cream made with wax and oil.

chalazion Also called a meibomian cyst, this is a round, painless swelling on the eyelid. It is caused by an obstruction of one of the meibomian glands responsible for lubricating the edge of the eyelid. A large swelling may exert pressure on the cornea at the front of the eye, blurring the vision.
Symptoms The cysts can occur at any age. But they are especially common in people with ACNE, ROSACEA or seborrheic dermatitis. If the cyst becomes infected, the lid swells even more, becoming even more painful and red.
Treatment About one-third of the cysts fade without treatment. Compressing with hot compresses for 20 minutes, four times a day for several days is often effective. Large chalazions usually need to be surgically removed with local anesthetic.

chamomile An herb that scientists have found to have real value for hair and skin. A mild mixture of chamomile leaves produces an oily substance that is soothing to the skin, used most often by adding it to the bath. A solution of concentrated chamomile left on the hair for a few hours will lighten it by several shades.

chancre An ulcer (usually on the genitals) that develops during the first stage of SYPHILIS, usually appearing first as a dull red spot between three to four weeks after exposure. It can also appear on the lips or in the throat if oral sex has taken place. The spot gradually develops in a painless ulcer with a clearly defined firm, heaped up edge and a rubbery base. If the chancre is the result of a sexually transmitted infection (which is very common) the ulcer may be painful.
Diagnosis Microscopic examination of a smear of the chancre will reveal the spirochete, which causes the disease; blood test results are usually negative early in primary syphilis.
Treatment Penicillin injections almost always prevent primary syphilis from developing into more serious stages of the disease.

chapped skin Red, dry and cracked painful skin caused by low humidity (especially during fall and winter). Badly chapped skin should not be put in water; related washing removes the oil layer, allowing moisture in skin to evaporate. Instead of using soap, try soap-free skin cleanser that is rubbed on, worked into a lather and then wiped off—or wash skin with bath oil.

Treatment To treat chapped skin, avoid handwashing; use warm, not hot water in the bath; always add oil to the bath; pat dry, then apply body lotion such as Lubriderm, Complex 15, Moisturel, Eucerin, etc.

Chediak-Higashi syndrome A defect of pigment characterized by partial ALBINISM, PHOTOPHOBIA, silvery hair and susceptibility to infection. A few patients have white hair and skin, and some have nystagmus (involuntary eye movements). Most have blond or gray hair, blue eyes and fair skin.

Skin infections occur frequently and may be fatal, ranging from a superficial pyoderma (ulcer) to deep, slow-healing abscesses and ulcers that may cause scars.

The disorder has been observed not just in humans, but also in many different mammals, including cats, Aleutian minks, beige mice and even killer whales.

Treatment There is no known treatment. The use of 500 mg. of vitamin C three times a day is controversial. Patients should protect themselves against exposure to the sun, wearing protective clothing, ultraviolet blocking sunglasses and sunscreens.

cheilitis Inflammation, dryness and cracking of the lips and corners of the mouth that can be caused by downturned mouth, poorly fitting dentures, dental work, local infection, COSMETIC ALLERGY, sunburn, skiing or windburn. Apply vaseline (or other lip balms in stick form) hourly to ease the pain until the underlying cause is identified and treated. Avoid licking the lips.

cheiloplasty Cosmetic surgery to reshape the lips.

chemabrasion See CHEMICAL FACE PEEL.

chemical burns Although most industrial chemicals are relatively weak and require prolonged contact before visible changes occur, some (such as concentrated sulfuric acid) can be quite harmful. Almost any substance encountered in the workplace may become an irritant if exposure is frequent enough. Workers are usually exposed to many different potential irritants, and skin BURNS may be the accumulation of multiple exposures.

Treatment The irritant agent must be identified, and exposure to the skin eliminated. Severe cases may be treated with an oral corticosteroid such as prednisone. Topical steroids, which reduce inflammation, may be applied to the skin. High-potency topical corticosteroids are more useful when inflammation is moderate to severe; gel and cream preparations absorb moisture and help to dry oozing, weeping vesicular DERMATITIS.

chemical exposure and the skin Certain chemicals used in manufacturing are dangerous to the skin, but only to employees—not the general public. Workers should use appropriate protective clothing.

Another concern about chemical exposure is the effect of FREE RADICALS on the skin. Free radicals are unstable molecules that can disrupt healthy cells during metabolic processes, and are believed to speed up aging and even cause cancer. They are produced naturally in the body, but they also occur in cigarette smoke, nitrous oxide, ozone and toxic wastes.

As a result of these concerns about pollution, skin care companies have devised a range of pollutant-fighting treatments, some which prevent oxidation and others that just shield the skin from pollution. But experts disagree as to whether these products are just a fancy marketing gimmick or whether they represent serious skin safeguards; none has ever been studied.

Until more research has been completed, experts advise consumers to wash with mild soap and apply moisturizer, which creates an extra barrier against dirt and debris.

chemical face peel (chemabrasion) A deep, controlled, second-degree burn using a caustic chemical to repair facial damage such as acne scars or wrinkles caused by sun damage. A chemical peel is the only means of regenerating elastin or COLLAGEN (the skin's supportive tissue) lost to age and sun exposure. There are two major types of peels: superficial and deep.

While it may sound like a facial, a chemical peel is in fact surgery, using potent chemicals (glycolic acid, lactic acid, trichloroacetic acid, phenol and or resorcinol) that actually dissolves the top layer of skin, erasing irregular pigmentation, mild acne scars, crow's feet, fine cheek wrinkles and tiny vertical lines above the upper lip.

After the peel (depending on the peel's depth), a thick crust lasts for a week, and the purple-red skin color may take six months to fade away. It is a painful, emotionally difficult process to endure, but after the skin heals the result is pinker, tighter, smoother and relatively wrinkle- and blemish-free skin, which may remain younger-looking for 15 years or more.

On the other hand, a "surface" or freshening peel is more like a superficial facial, leaving the skin glowing for a week or two, but not going deep enough to erase scars or wrinkles.

The procedure is not for everyone. Subjects with dark or olive skin may end up with a blotchy appearance, and those with poor liver, heart or kidney function could be affected by the solution that strips away the upper layers of the skin, which is absorbed into the bloodstream.

Prospective patients of any peel, no matter how minor, should investigate the surgeon's ability and experience, since it takes a great deal of expertise to apply a good chemical peel. Consumers should ask whether the procedure comprises a large portion of the person's practice (one of the two or three procedures most often performed). Ask how many peels the doctor does a week, and how he or she learned the procedure.*

The cost of a peel ranges from $200 to $3,000 depending on the area of skin to be treated, the depth of the peel and the area of the country in which the dermatologist practices.

Chemical skin peels have been around for thousands of years, with women using everything from sour milk to wine residue to freshen their complexions. Since the 1950s, American women have gone to plastic surgeons and dermatologists for peels using phenol or trichloracetic acid. While these products are still used for those who need fairly deep chemical peels, newer milder, products are now on the market.

These new products, called ALPHA HYDROXY ACIDS, are available over the counter in concentrations of less than 10 percent, in beauty salons in concentrations of up to 40 percent, and in dermatologist's offices in concentrations up to 70 percent. These milder peels improve the skin's appearance by speeding up the shedding of dead skin cells, clearing up acne-prone skin, softening tiny lines around the eyes and mouth, smoothing dry skin and fading dark spots caused by sun or hormonal changes. See also DERMABRASION; GLYCOLIC ACID).

chemical pollutants and the skin The daily onslaught of smog, car exhaust and acid rain take their toll on building facades in Ameri-

---

*For a list of experts qualified to perform chemical peels, call the toll-free hotline of the American Society for Dermatologic Surgery at (800) 441-2737.

ca's cities, and some dermatologists believe chemical pollution can also harm your skin.

Some experts blame toxics for a range of problems from minor irritation to premature aging, although there have been few controlled studies of the problem. Some experts believe the increase in airborne toxicants contributes to the rise of skin cancer; others believe that ozone in smog can penetrate and damage the skin's outer layer. Others point to the effect of FREE RADICALS on the skin. Free radicals are unstable molecules that can disrupt healthy cells in a process known as oxidation; they have been linked to premature aging and cancer. They are produced naturally in the body, but they are also found in cigarette smoke, nitrous oxide, ozone and toxic waste.

Critics of this belief, however, point out that a person's skin was designed to keep *out* such harmful substances.

Just in case there might be truth to the concerns, experts advise patients to wash with mild soap and apply a moisturizer, which creates an extra barrier against dirt and debris. Washing the facial area thoroughly at the end of the day with soap or a soap substitute and water is also important.

chemosurgery See MOH'S SURGERY.

chicken pox This is a common childhood infectious disease characterized by a rash and fever that—prior to the development of a vaccine in 1995—affected about 3.9 million people each year in the United States. About 90 percent of cases occur in children under age 10, primarily in winter and spring.

Chicken pox is also known as varicella, after the virus (varicella-zoster, or VZV) that causes the disease. VZV is a member of the family of herpes viruses and is similar to the herpes simplex virus (HSV). The virus is spread by airborne droplets.

While an attack of chicken pox creates a lifelong immunity to the disease, the virus does not disappear. It remains dormant within a patient's nerve tissues after the attack. In later life, the virus can reactivate and cause an attack of herpes zoster (SHINGLES).

Most people throughout the world have had the disease by age 10, and chicken pox is rare in adults. When it does occur after childhood, it can be deadly. About 90 people in the United States die every year as a result of chicken pox, and another 9,300 must be hospitalized. The infection strikes hardest in infants, adults and those with immune system problems. Adults are much more likely to be hospitalized than children.

If possible, a child with suspected chicken pox should not be brought into a doctor's office where others may be exposed to the disease; it can be very dangerous to newborns or those with suppressed immune systems. The virus can be spread both through the air and by direct contact with an infected individual. Instead, contact a physician by phone and describe symptoms.

Symptoms The incubation period after exposure ranges from one to three weeks, and is followed by a rash on the body (torso, face, armpits, upper arms and legs, inside the mouth, and sometimes in the windpipe and bronchial tubes, causing a dry cough). The rash is made up of small, red, itchy spots that grow into fluid-filled blisters within a few hours. After several days, the blisters dry out and form scabs. New spots usually continue to form over four to seven days. *Patients are contagious five days before the rash appears and until all the skin lesions have crusted over* (usually about a week after they appear).

Complications Although children usually have only a slight fever, adults often experience fever, breathing problems and severe varicella pneumonia. In rare cases, children may develop this type of pneumonia or Reye's syndrome; they may also develop bacterial infections. Occasionally, chicken pox can lead to varicella encephalitis (an inflammation of the brain). Immunocompromised patients who are susceptible to VZV are at high risk for having severe varicella infections with widespread lesions.

Prevention The American Academy of Pediatrics recommends the new chicken pox vaccine (VARIVAX) for all children, teens and young adults who haven't had the disease. The vaccine, which has been used in Japan for some time, was approved by the Food and drug Administration in April 1995. Although its approval has met with some controversy, most pediatricians recommend the vaccine for their patients.

The vaccine is made from a live, weakened virus that, once injected in a human patient, creates a mild infection similar to natural chicken pox—but without related complications. The mild infection spurs the body to develop an immune response to the disease; these defenses are then ready when the body encounters the natural virus.

Although the vaccine is considered to be safe, it is still subject to debate. Proponents of the vaccine point out that it makes sense to vaccinate children because they are likely to suffer from chicken pox. Some researchers, however, are uncertain how long the vaccine confers immunity. Critics warn that although there has been no evidence of this to date, they worry that if the vaccine wears off later in life the adult could then be vulnerable to infection at an age when chicken pox can be serious.

Others are concerned about the possible link between the VZV and shingles. Since the virus belongs to the herpes virus group, critics worry that the vaccine might cauase periodic reactivation of the varicella-zoster virus and resultant cases of shingles. On the other hand, research so far indicates that the vaccine causes fewer (or no more) cases of shingles than does naturally contracted chicken pox.

Most doctors recommend the vaccine for all children, teenagers and young adults who haven't had chicken pox. One dose is needed for children up to age 12 (ideally given between 12 and 18 months of age); teenagers and adults need two shots, four to eight weeks apart. High-risk, susceptible patients may also obtain passive immunization with VZV immune globulin, which can abort or modify infection if administered within three days of exposure.

Treatment In most cases, rest is all that is needed for children, who usually recover within 10 days. Adults take longer to recover. Acetaminophen may reduce fever, and calamine lotion, baking soda baths and oral antihistamines ease the itch. Compresses can dry weeping lesions. Scratching should be avoided, since it can lead to bacterial infection of lesions and increases the chance of scarring; children may need to wear gloves during sleep to avoid nighttime scratching.

Never give aspirin to a child who has been exposed to (or has recently recovered from) chicken pox. Aspirin in these cases has been linked to the development of Reye's syndrome.

The drug ACYCLOVIR may be prescribed for chicken pox patients. It is usually recommended for people with chronic skin or lung disorders, in severe cases of chickenpox or for those with compromised immune systems. VZV is relatively resistant to acyclovir, and doses required for treatment are much larger than for other diseases. When taken within the first 24 hours, the drug may decrease the length of the illness and mitigate symptoms, but its cost and marginal effectiveness have prompted the American Academy of Pediatrics not to recommend it as a routine treatment.

chigger bites A bite from the chigger (or harvest mite) causes an intense, itchy swelling up to half an inch across. The swelling usually fades without treatment between three days to a week.

The female mites are attracted to warm moist areas of the body, such as the skin underneath sweat bands, where they burrow under the skin's surface.

The larvae of these mites of the genus *Trombidioidae* live outdoors throughout the southeastern United States, and they are especially active in the grass near trees in summer. They attach themselves to their victims' legs where they feed on blood. The swelling may progress to form a blister, and the itching can last for weeks.

Complications Secondary infection may occur as a result of scratching.

Prevention Wear close-fitting clothing with shirts tucked in and pants tucked into socks.

chilblains An injury of the skin tissue caused by cold, but not frozen, temperatures. Also known as "pernio," chilblains are most commonly seen on the earlobes, nose, fingers and toes of young women.

Itchy purple lesions occur after exposure to cold. These lesions may last from days to weeks, with burning, itching and pain. Repeated episodes of chilblains may lead to a chronic condition that persists throughout the winter.

Prevention Chilblains may be prevented by moving to a warm climate, or by wearing adequate clothing in cold temperatures. Severe lesions respond to bed rest and gentle rewarming in a 105 degree bath. The patient with chronic chilblains *must* avoid exposure to cold. The administration of vasodilating drugs may also give some help.

chin augmentation This surgical procedure is often performed together with NOSE REPAIR (rhinoplasty) in order to rearrange the facial balance, accentuating and flattering the neckline. The incision may be placed either inside the mouth or under the chin, which creates a pocket in the chin into which an implant can be placed. The wound is then closed with stitches and a tape bandage applied to the chin.

If the incision is in the mouth, antibiotics are administered to prevent infection, and a liquid diet is required for 48 hours to avoid getting food in the wound. Elevating the head prevents excess swelling and bruising, and the bandage is removed after the fifth day. Stitches are removed a week after surgery, and swelling usually subsides in the second week.

chloasma Also known as melasma, this is a condition often appearing during pregnancy in which blotches of pale brown skin pigmentation appear on the face. It may also occur in women who have been taking birth control pills or been exposed to too much sun. Occasionally, the skin darkening will appear in men or postmenopausal women. The tendency to develop chloasma may run in families.

Symptoms The pigmentation primarily appears on the forehead, cheeks and nose, sometimes merging to form the "mask of pregnancy" and is worsened by even brief exposures to sunlight. While it usually fades away over a period of time, in some patients it becomes permanent; it also tends to recur in successive pregnancies.

Treatment The condition may improve if the patient avoids sunlight or uses a strong sunblock and (if appropriate) changes the brand of (or stops using) birth control pills. In addition, some patients may respond to hypopigmenting agents containing hydroquinone or to the combination of tretinoin cream and hydroquinone. Chloasma in premenopausal women may improve after menopause, even without therapy.

chloracne An acne-like eruption caused by exposure to chlorinated hydrocarbon products. These lesions may occur in up to 95 percent of cases where toxic generalized symptoms (such as liver disease) are also present. Chloracne is caused when toxic materials cause the underlying sebaceous glands to atrophy, forming KERATIN-filled cysts. The hydrocarbon product most often associated with chloracne is 2,3,7,8-tetrachlorodibenzod-ioxin.

Chloracne has usually been associated with massive hydrocarbon exposure, such as in an industrial accident or contamination during the manufacturing process.

New chloracne lesions usually stop forming within six months after exposure, but existing lesions often take a long time to heal and may persist indefinitely.

Symptoms Numerous closed comedones with some inflammatory pustules and noninflammatory, straw-colored cysts. In addition to the usual acne areas, the ears may also be affected, and covered areas outside the usual acne distribution may be involved in severe cases.

Treatment Chloracne is often resistant to treatment, and does not respond well to systemic antibiotics and topical BENZOYL PEROXIDE. Topical derivatives of vitamin A, such as retinoic acid creams or gels (RETIN-A) may help. Oral vitamin A sometimes helps and sometimes does not; anecdotal reports indicate that ISOTRETINOIN (Accutane) may be effective. In some cases, acne surgery is the only effective treatment.

chlorophyll A chemical in the cells of green plants that absorbs light so that plants can synthesize food. It is widely used as an ingredient in deodorants, toothpastes and mouthwashes to protect against odor.

chromate, allergy to See ALLERGIES AND THE SKIN.

chromomycosis An invasive fungal infection of the top two layers of the skin in the feet and legs that almost always begins in the skin (often the site of trauma, or penetration of a foreign object), and is most common in the tropics. Also called chromoblastomycosis, chromomycosis is characterized by heaped up warty sores, usually on the legs. The infection may remain local, involve the entire extremity or become a generalized infection.

Cause This uncommon tropical infection includes a group of closely related molds that are found in the soil, affecting people involved in manual labor with soil or its products. While it is not clear why the infection occurs only in the tropics, it is believed that in colder climates, workers wear shoes, which protect feet from contracting chromomycosis. Still, even in the tropics this disorder is not common.

The condition is chronic and may last for years or decades, leading to the necessity of amputation, the development of ELEPHANTIASIS or SQUAMOUS CELL CARCINOMA.

Symptoms The infection begins with itchy, watery papules or an ulcer on the leg or foot, followed by foul-smelling plaques of the foot, ankle, knee, elbow or hand. The papule or ulcer slowly enlarges over months to years; as it spreads, the central area becomes scarred. Many patients develop secondary bacterial infections.

Treatment Bed rest, elevation of affected part and antibiotic therapy to control secondary infections are recommended. Surgical excision of the affected area, destruction of the affected tissue or drug treatment (potassium iodide, flucytosine, thiabendazole, ketoconazole and topical heat) may be successful.

chromosomal defects and skin disease Abnormalities in the human chromosome are often associated with prominent skin defects. Deletion of the short arm of chromosome 4 (4P) causes central scalp defects. An extra autosome (trisomy 8) causes short nails, excess skin on the back of the neck and no knee cap. Trisomy 10 causes congenital scalp defect and trisomy 13 causes scalp defects. Down's syndrome (trisomy 21) may cause ELASTOSIS PERFORANS SERPIGINOSA, unusual palmar creases, a shortened fifth finger, premature wrinkles, frequent alopecia (hair loss), and fissured and furrowed skin. Turner's syndrome (deficiency of one X chromosome or presence of an abnormal X) may cause congenital and persistent lymphedema, nevi, cystic hygromas, low hairline in back and increased skin aging. Klinefelter's syndrome (XXY) may be associated with leg ulcers.

chrysotherapy See GOLD THERAPY.

cimetidine (trade name: Tagamet) An antihistamine developed for the treatment of gastrointestinal ulcers, cimetidine is occasionally effective in the treatment of chronic HIVES and has recently been studied as a treatment for multiple WARTS in children.

In new research at Children's Memorial Hospital in Chicago and New York University, youngsters whose warts did not respond to more traditional treatment received three daily doses of the drug. Within seven weeks, many of the warts had become flatter and less visible and eventually disappeared completely in 80 percent of the children.

cinnamate A SUNSCREEN that blocks both ultraviolet-B (UV-B) and, less well, UV-A sun rays. Cinnamate is one of more than 20 chemicals that the U.S. Food and Drug Administration recognizes as safe, effective sunscreen ingredients. The success of the product depends on how well, how often and how consistently it is used. However, cinnamate can cause a contact and photocontact dermatitis.

ciprofloxacin (trade name: Cipro) An oral antimicrobial drug used to treat skin infections (among others).
Side effects Nausea and vomiting, diarrhea, abdominal pain, sun sensitivity and headache.

citric acid Chemical found in citrus fruits that is used as a grease-cutter in shampoos.

citronella A strong-smelling substance obtained from the *Cymbopogon nardus* grass of Asia, used as an INSECT REPELLENT and perfume. Some sensitive individuals may develop skin sensitivity to citronella.

clavus See CORN.

clay A mineral used in face and body powder, face masks and foundations that is particularly helpful for normal and oily skin, and ACNE conditions. It does not cause allergic reactions.

cleansing products While it is true that skin problems like ACNE have more to do with trapped oil and bacteria in the oil glands than oil on the skin's surface, cleansing agents can give a feeling of improvement because they do remove the surface oil. Skin cleansing can remove dirt, cosmetics, cellular debris, body secretions, sweat and microorganisms.

How often and how vigorously you clean the skin depends on skin type, daily activities and the environment. Washing alone is the most effective method of skin cleansing; while water alone removes many types of dirt, a soap or detergent helps to remove oils. In the United States, soaps account for about 90 percent of the toilet bars sold.

For normal skin, you should wash your face no more than twice a day with gentle cleansers. Avoid very hot water, and use a low-alcohol astringent or an alcohol-free toner after each washing.

For oily skin, wash three times a day and never use "gentle" or "rich" cleansers. You can use hotter water than people with other skin types; use an astringent with a high alcohol content after each washing, and exfoliate twice a week.

For combination skin, use the same regimen as those with normal skin; use astringent on nose, chin and forehead.

For sensitive skin, limit washing to once a day and use a very gentle cleanser and lukewarm water. Do not use abrasives such as washcloths, Buf-Pufs or grains and never rub with a towel. Never use toners or astringents with alcohol.

Abrasive cleansers/pads contain small gritty particles that mildly sand the skin. These are designed for people who want to scrub their acne away, but in fact most experts believe they are too irritating and are not that helpful.

Soaps, lotions and cleansers work about as well as abrasives but they aren't as harsh. All induce a mild exfoliation by helping to remove superficial skin cells, but they can't really remove the oil in the follicles. In some cases, soaps can be excessively drying and irritating.

Soap-free cleansers or emollients may be used by those with sensitive skin.

Astringents, fresheners, toners or refining lotions are usually composed of alcohol-in-water combinations used by those with oily skin to remove sebum or makeup. While many of these products are said to shrink pores, in fact it is impossible to permanently shrink pores. The pores may appear smaller as acne lesions are treated and oil and blackheads are removed.See also SOAP AND THE SKIN; COSMETICS; MAKEUP.

climatotherapy The use of climate in the treatment of disease. This type of therapy is especially popular in the treatment of PSORIASIS, which responds well to hot, dry climates. Many patients often visit Hawaii, Florida, Mexico and the Caribbean to clear their skin conditions by sunbathing, since natural sunlight in regular doses will often clear most cases of psoriasis.

As yet there are no climatotherapy centers for psoriasis in the United States; the most organized centers for psoriasis are located in the region of the Dead Sea between Israel and Jordan.

For more information about sunbathing and climatotherapy, contact the National Psoriasis Foundation for their educational booklet "Sunshine & Psoriasis" at 6600 SW 92nd Ave., Suite 300, Portland OR 97223, (503) 245-0626.

clindamycin An antibiotic drug used to treat ACNE and serious infections that haven't responded, or are resistant to, other antibiotics. Clindamycin is especially effective against most anaerobic bacteria, including *Propionibacterium acnes,* which are often responsible for acne. It is also an excellent agent against *Staphylococcus aureus* and streptococcal species.

clofazimine A dye used primarily in the treatment of LEPROSY. It is also effective in some patients with PYODERMA GANGRENOSUM, DISCOID LUPUS ERYTHEMATOSUS, ACNE FULMINANS and GRANULOMA FACIALE.

This drug has a remarkable lack of toxicity, and although there is no evidence of birth defects, it does cross the placenta and cause pigmentation in offspring.

Administered by mouth, the drug should be taken with meals or milk; about 70 percent is absorbed within the small intestine. For most skin conditions, the drug needs to be taken for at least two months before any benefit is seen.

The drug should not be taken during the first three months of pregnancy, in patients prone to diarrhea or recurrent abdominal pain, and in those with kidney or liver disease.

Adverse effects The most obvious side effect is pink, red or brownish black discoloration of the skin, especially in areas exposed to sunlight. Hair, sweat, sputum, urine and feces may also be discolored. These pigmentation side effects are related to dosage, however, and begin to fade when therapy is stopped. Other side effects include XERODERMA, ichthyosis, itching, sensitivity to sunlight, and acne-like skin eruptions. There may also be nausea and vomiting, abdominal pain and diarrhea.

cloxacillin A penicillin-type antibiotic used to treat staphylococcal infections. Do not take this drug with acidic fruits or juices, or aged cheese. Taken with alcohol, this drug could cause stomach irritation. Use with birth control pills may impair the efficacy of the contraceptive.

coal tar derivatives A thick, black substance commonly found as an ingredient in ointments and some shampoos, used to treat skin and scalp conditions such as ECZEMA, PSORIASIS and certain types of DERMATITIS.

Crude coal tar or coal tar solutions are available as over-the-counter and prescription preparations, depending on strength. In the treatment of psoriasis, it may be applied directly to the affected area or may be added to bath water for a daily body soak. It can also be used with topical steroids. It can reduce the size and redness of itchy patches.

In addition, the coal tar may be used with ultraviolet light (UV-B), followed by exposure to radiation treatments in resistant cases of psoriasis. The tar is partially removed from the skin before exposing it to UV-B light and then to radiation therapy. The treatments are given daily for three to six weeks, or may be done at home with a portable machine or natural sunlight.

Cockayne-Touraine syndrome An inherited form of dwarfism associated with sensitivity to sunlight that causes skin reddening and TELANGIECTASIA of nose and cheeks as well as cold, blue extremities. As patients age, the reddening clears, leaving mottled pigmentation, scarring and atrophy. There is no increased risk of skin cancer as a result of the syndrome. Other characteristics of the syndrome include long arms, large ears, sunken eyes, joint contractures, microceph-

aly, mental retardation, deafness, retinitis pigmentosa, optic atrophy and cataracts.

cocoa butter An oil extracted from roasted cocoa nut seeds used to soften and lubricate the skin, often used instead of wax or harder creams. It has the same emollient properties as any other vegetable oil, and it has not been associated with allergic reactions.

coconut oil A white saturated fat derived from coconuts that melts at body temperature and is used to smooth and lubricate the skin. Because it produces an excellent lather, it is often included as an ingredient in soap. Coconut oil can cause skin irritation in some sensitive individuals.

cold cream A pharmaceutical and cosmetic product—used to wash off makeup—of animal fat or mineral oil and a sodium salt with a dispersing agent to enhance its vanishing quality.

cold sore A small skin blister on the mouth usually found in a cluster, caused by the HERPES SIMPLEX virus (HSV). The viral strain usually responsible for cold sores is herpes simplex Type I (HSVI); up to 90 percent of all people around the world carry this virus.
Symptoms The first attack may not even be noticed, or it may cause a flu-like illness with painful ulcers on the mouth or lips (called gingivostomatitis). An outbreak is often signalled by a tingling in the lips, followed by a small blister that soon grows, causing itching and soreness. Within a few days the blisters burst, encrust and then disappear within a week. The virus then retreats along the nerve where it lies dormant in the nerve cell; in some patients, however, the virus is constantly reactivated.
Causes Cold sores tend to appear when the victim is under stress, exposed to sunlight, cold wind or another infection, or feels run down. Women tend to experience more cold

sores around their menstrual periods, but some people are afflicted at regular intervals throughout the year. People with compromised immune systems may experience prolonged attacks.

Treatment For mild symptoms, keep the sore clean and dry and it will heal itself. For particularly virulent outbreaks, the antiviral drug ACYCLOVIR or idoxuridine paint may relieve symptoms or briefly shorten the length of the outbreak by no more than one day, but there is no evidence acyclovir ointment is particularly helpful. Otherwise, there are a range of nonprescription drugs available containing some numbing agent (such as camphor or phenol) that also contain an emollient to reduce cracking. For patients with frequent outbreaks of HSV, acyclovir may be prescribed to be taken from seven to 10 days as soon as the patient feels tingling. This usually prevents the outbreak but doesn't prevent future outbreaks. In patients with very severe symptoms, daily acyclovir application is occasionally prescribed.

Some studies have suggested that zinc may help prevent outbreaks because the zinc interferes with herpes viral replication. Studies found that both zinc gluconate and zinc sulfate helped speed up healing time, but zinc gluconate was less irritating to the skin. Both zinc products are available at health food stores.

Sores can be protected with a dab of petroleum jelly (applied with a clean cotton swab); don't dip the swab that touched the affected area back into the jar.

collagen A tough natural constituent of connective tissue, collagen is the body's major structural protein, forming an important part of tendons, bones and connective tissues. The most common protein in the body, its tough insoluble nature is what gives skin its elasticity, and helps hold the cells and tissues together. Collagen makes up 77 percent of the fat-free dry weight of the skin. Injectable collagen is a natural animal protein made from the skin of cattle and injected into human skin to eliminate wrinkles or facial depressions. It has long been touted as a potent weapon against the appearance of aging.

Recent research has found that exposure to the sun's ultraviolet rays may significantly reduce collagen production, according to researchers at the University of Michigan in Ann Arbor. Studies there revealed that sun-exposed skin produced 56 percent less collagen than did skin that is normally covered up (such as skin over the buttocks).

To restore lost collagen, researchers have found that treating photodamaged skin with RETIN-A resulted in an 80 percent increase in collagen, whereas patches treated with a placebo cream showed a 14 percent collagen reduction. However, researchers note that the results of improved collagen after treatment with Retin-A were observable only under the microscope; the increase in collagen was not readily apparent to the naked eye. See COLLAGEN DISEASES; COLLAGEN INJECTIONS; LUPUS ERYTHEMATOSUS; SCLERODERMA.

collagen diseases There are two groups of diseases called COLLAGEN diseases; the true collagen diseases, and connective tissue diseases. True collagen diseases are rare and are usually inherited; they are usually caused by faulty formation of collagen fibers. True collagen diseases are characterized by slack skin and poor wound healing.

Connective tissue diseases are caused by a malfunction in the immune system that affects blood vessels, producing secondary damage in connective tissue. For this reason, these diseases are sometimes called collagen vascular diseases, and include rheumatoid arthritis, systemic LUPUS ERYTHEMATOSUS, PERIARTERITIS NODOSA, SCLERODERMA and DERMATOMYOSITIS.

collagen injection One of the less painful and conservative ways to temporarily remove wrinkles (superseded by Retin-A treatments). Dermatologists perform this treatment by injecting collagen derived from cowhide into the skin to minimize lines and scars, filling deep vertical wrinkles between the eyebrows, deep wrinkles running from mouth to nose, and forehead wrinkles.

It's now possible to use a person's own collagen for this procedure. Results last only between three and 18 months, averaging about six months. The price will vary depending on the part of the country where the procedure is carried out. Each nose-to-mouth crease requires a full syringe, and between a quarter to a half syringe of collagen is needed to fill furrows between the eyes.

Technique Tiny drops of thick collagen are injected with a fine needle underneath the skin to replace collagen lost by the body. During this injection, some patients may feel some stinging. The entire procedure may take between two and 10 minutes, and patients recover in about two to three hours.

After treatment, there may be some redness lasting up to 10 days; a few patients also experience bruising, temporary stinging, burning sensations, faint redness, swelling or excessive fullness. Other patients have no reaction at all.

Collagen is effective only when injected under the skin; applying collagen to the skin directly has no proven benefit other than as a moisturizer. A person's own collagen may be better tolerated than collagen from other sources.

Risks Because about 3 percent of the population is allergic to bovine (cow) collagen (developing a rash and swelling), physicians usually perform two separate skin tests and wait a month after each to be sure the patient has no allergic reaction. Other possible risks include contour irregularities, infection or local abscess.

Not everyone is a suitable candidate for collagen injections. They are not recommended for anyone with a history of immunological disorders such as LUPUS ERYTHROMATOSUS or rheumatoid arthritis. According to the U.S. Food and Drug administration (FDA), more studies are required to establish whether or not collagen is linked to certain connective-tissue disorders.

Benefits Collagen injections are a good choice for someone who wishes to avoid the risks of surgery and is not ready for a moderate or deep peel, dermabrasion, laser abrasion or a full face-lift. According to the FDA, collagen injections are safe, and the least likely of all the wrinkle-removal methods to develop complications.

collagenomas A rare connective tissue nevus (or birthmark) comprised of increased collagen, characterized by yellowish plaques up to several mm. in diameter that usually occur on the upper trunk and sometimes the arms and legs. Usually present at birth or shortly after, no treatment is necessary. See also CONNECTIVE TISSUE NEVI.

colloid millium A papular dermatosis that usually occurs on facial skin that has been extensively damaged by overexposure to the sun; the condition consists of degenerated COLLAGEN.

collodian baby At birth, these infants are enclosed in a taut yellow-pink cellophane-like membrane that may temporarily distort facial features (especially the ears, lips and eyelids). They are usually afflicted with LAMELLAR ICHTHYOSIS (a skin disorder characterized by rough, reddened, scaling skin). The membrane may be perforated by LANUGO (downy fetal hair) and scalp hair. Shortly after birth, the membrane begins to crack and peel, revealing underlying red skin; it may take several weeks for the membrane to be completely shed, and a new membrane may form temporarily.

Infants born with collodion membrane rarely have normal skin after shedding. Patients with this condition will have lifelong scaling and dry, rough skin.

Although often born prematurely, collodian babies are otherwise healthy. More severely affected babies may lose hair or nails, and have some problems in eating and breathing. These babies often have secondary bacterial and fungal infections because their skin must be softened by high humidity in their isolettes, which leads to infection.

Treatment At birth babies should be kept in a humid environment. Experimental use of oral synthetic ISOTRETINOIN (Accutane) and etretinate (Tegison) appears promising, but long-term toxicity, especially in children, is unknown.

comedo Another name for BLACKHEAD (open comedo).

concealing creams See CAMOUFLAGE COSMETICS.

conditioner Products that use ingredients to change the surface structure of the hair, allowing it to be more manageable for combing and styling. These structural changes in the surface texture also provide hold, softness and sheen. Conditioners are made up of ingredients that cling to the hair cuticle—some conditioners penetrate and bind with the cuticle in a tight chemical bond. While shampoos and conditioners share many ingredients, their combinations and sequences vary widely.

Most conditioners contain basically the same ingredients: water, slip agents and lubricants (dimethicone and cyclomethicone), quaternary compounds, thickeners and more lubricants (stearyl alcohol, cetyl alcohol,

protein or balsam), humectants (propylene glycol, glycerin, sodium PCA, mucopolysaccharides, hyaluronic acid), preservatives, fragrance and coloring agents. Many conditioners also add more exotic "natural" ingredients to appeal to consumers.

There *are* differences between conditioners, depending on your hair's condition, and there are differences in amounts of specific ingredients (some of which are better than others).

Application Beauty experts caution that most consumers apply conditioner improperly. Instead of applying near the top of the head and working it toward the ends, consumers should bend over and apply conditioner to ends first, using little or none on the roots. By sparing the roots, you're lifting the roots instead of weighing them down.

condylomata acuminata A type of genital wart caused by infection with the human papilloma virus. Found throughout the world, the disorder is often seen in sexually transmitted disease clinics, since the warts are usually spread by sexual contact.

The WARTS primarily appear in the moist genital folds and creases, and while just one wart may appear, they are more commonly found in heaped-up bunches that form cauliflower-like masses. They are subject to injury and can bleed, although they are generally painless.

Giant condylomata acuminata can invade local tissue (BUSCHKE-LOWENSTEIN TUMOR), which may rarely develop into SQUAMOUS CELL CARCINOMA.

Prevention Because these warts are easily spread, sexual contact with affected individuals should be avoided.

Treatment There is no known treatment to specifically eradicate human PAPILLOMAVIRUS from the skin. The virus may survive even the most aggressive treatment (such as laser treatment). Recurrence, therefore, is common.

Treatment is aimed at physically removing warts in the patient, and in affected sexual partners. Condoms should be worn to help reduce transmission.

Most lesions in moist areas can be treated with podophyllum resin in tincture of benzoin, which is painted on the lesion by a physician and allowed to dry. It is then washed off four hours later. Extensive areas should not be treated at one time, since absorption of the resin can be toxic. For the same reason, pregnant women should not be treated.

The active chemical in podophyllum resin has been identified and is now available in the prescription product Condylax.

CRYOTHERAPY (freezing) with liquid nitrogen is often effective, and it is nontoxic and does not require anesthesia. CURETTAGE AND ELECTRODESICCATION may also be successful.

While alpha interferon is available for treatment of resistant cases, it is not frequently recommended because of its high likelihood of toxicity, low effectiveness and expense.

The CARBON DIOXIDE LASER and more conventional surgery may also be helpful in cases of extensive growths, especially for those who have not responded to other treatments.

In pregnant patients, cryotherapy is most effective. Birth control pills are believed to cause the warts to grow. Therefore, women taking birth control pills should stop taking the pills before the warts can be successfully treated.

congenital absence of skin See APLASIA CUTIS.

congenital disorders of the skin There are a range of skin disorders that can be present at birth. These include abnormalities of KERATIN such as ICHTHYOSIS; of pigment, such as CONGENITAL TISSUE NEVI and PIEBALDISM; of fat, such as lipodystrophy; of blood vessels, such as PORT WINE STAINS and HEMANGIO-

MAS; of nerves, such as NEUROFIBROMATOSIS; and TUBEROUS SCLEROSIS.

connective tissue diseases See COLLAGEN DISEASES.

connective tissue nevi A group of rare conditions (sometimes inherited) characterized by lesions and tumors of the connective tissues of the skin. The nevi are usually normal or slightly yellowish colored. They include ELASTOMAS, COLLAGENOMAS, SHAGREEN PATCH and BUSCHKE-OLLENDORF SYNDROME.
Treatment No treatment is necessary for most connective tissue nevi, since they don't cause any severe cosmetic defects. Surgical removal is occasionally performed.

Conradi's disease Also known medically as "chondrodysplasia punctata," this genetic disorder is characterized by skin abnormalities in 30 percent of patients, together with facial abnormalities and congenital cataracts. At birth, the skin is dry and cracked, especially around hair follicles; some hair loss may also occur. See also HAIR, DISEASES OF.

contact dermatitis See DERMATITIS, CONTACT.

contracture A deformity caused by shrinkage of scar tissue in the skin or connective tissue. They are common following extensive burns, and can result in restricted movement.

corn A small area of thickened skin (callus) with a hard core, usually found on the toe, caused by the pressure of a tight shoe. Patients with high arches suffer most from corns, because the arch increases the pressure on the tips of toes while walking. "Soft corns" are caused by the rubbing of two bones from adjacent toes; they remain slightly softer than "hard corns" because of foot perspiration. Women with wide feet who wear pointed shoes are vulnerable to getting corns.

Treatment First, change shoes if you develop painful corns; the corn may gradually disappear. Do not pare corns with a sharp instrument.

Until the corn disappears, a corn pad may be used to cushion surrounding skin from pressure. Make sure the pad is cut into the shape of a horseshoe, not an oval (which can make the corn bulge through the oval opening in the middle). Place the pad far enough behind the corn so it won't rub.

A nonprescription corn plaster (as a liquid, salve or disk) should be applied to the corn to shield it. Because the plasters contain harsh acids that may burn normal skin as well as the corn, patients should use with caution. If irritation develops, stop use for a day or two.

At the first sign of pain, massage a bit of lanolin to soften the corn; then place a pad on the area to relieve pressure. Wrap a toe with a few strands of lambswool or place a toe separator/spacer between the toes to keep the toes from rubbing together.

corn oil A vegetable oil that can be used as an emollient. Corn oil is not usually associated with allergic reactions.

cornstarch A starch derived from corn kernels, used as a nonabrasive powder for irritated skin. Although cornstarch may encourage fungal skin infections (especially in people with diabetes), some experts suggest using a powder made of cornstarch instead of talcum powder. Reports have linked talcum powder with cancer (inhaled talc in rats) and higher rates of ovarian cancer in women using talcum powder in the genital area, but experts at the National Institutes of Health conclude the data on talc are inconclusive.

corrosive chemicals Certain corrosive chemicals (such as oven cleaners, drain clean-

ers and dishwasher detergents) contain alkalizers, which can cause serious burns on the skin. Alkalizers (which have a pH of 11.5 or more) include potassium, sodium, ammonium and calcium; of these, potassium hydroxide is the strongest. When considering the danger from these products, the higher the concentration of these ingredients in the alkalizer, the more serious the burn caused.

While most people think of acids as corrosive, an alkalizer is even more so; acid walls off its burn, while an alkalizer actually *spreads* in the skin, dissolving tissue as it goes.

Treatment Any severe burn should be treated in the emergency room of your local hospital. For a mild alkalizer burn, immediately wash the affected area in lukewarm water for at least 15 minutes (preferably longer). Remove any contaminated clothes or jewelry, and (if eyes are involved) immediately remove contact lenses. If the alkaline substance is solid, scrub the skin to make sure all particles are removed and then use a weak acid (such as vinegar, lemon or orange juice diluted with four parts water,) to neutralize the alkaline that may be penetrated deeper in tissues.

Exception: calcium oxide, or quicklime. Quicklime tends to absorb water and creates slaked lime, which gives off heat. The quicklime should be removed *before* it comes in contact with water. Try oiling or greasing the skin before the lime is wet, then take a stream of water at high pressure to immediately remove oxide particles. Any lime left on the skin can cause burns. Then, seek professional help.

Corrosive burns can also be caused by *strong acids*, such as a toilet bowl cleaner (usually sulfuric or hydrochloric acid). Unfortunately, these acids are not usually listed on the container. If these products contact the skin, wash with large amounts of lukewarm water for 15 to 30 minutes—avoid applying salves and ointments to the burn and seek medical help.

corticosteroids Developed more than 30 years ago, the first topical corticosteroid revolutionized dermatologic therapy with their strong anti-inflammatory properties; stronger and stronger compounds have been developed ever since. The corticosteroids are a group of hormones similar to the natural hormones produced by the cortex of the adrenal glands.

They are used both topically and systematically to treat a wide variety of skin disorders from mild ECZEMA to widespread blistering disorders such as PEMPHIGUS. Their broad anti-inflammatory effects are the basis for both the therapeutic benefits and the adverse reactions associated with topical use of these drugs.

Applied in the form of creams, ointments, lotions and aerosols, their absorption is increased if the drug is applied when the skin is moist (such as right after bathing). Absorption of topical corticosteroids also varies with body location; absorption is greater through the layers of skin on the scalp, face and genital area than on the forearm; as a result, these areas are more susceptible to the side effects of the drugs than other sites. Excessive use of over-the-counter topical steroids (especially on large areas of inflamed skin) can lead to increased side effects and decreased therapeutic effects.

Furthermore, some skin problems may be masked or worsened by using topical corticosteroids. Infections and infestations (especially CANDIDIASIS, IMPETIGO and SCABIES) may be either promoted or hidden, and ROSACEA may be exacerbated by topical corticosteroids.

Adverse effects The incidence of adverse effects depends on dosage, the form of the drug and how long it was administered. Side effects are uncommon when given as a cream or by inhaler because only small amounts of the drug are absorbed into the blood. Infants and children have a greater risk of developing adverse effects, and should be treated with topical corticosteroids of low potency.

Acute side effects can include atrophy and thinning of the skin, especially when used on the skin of the face.

Tablets taken in high doses for long periods may cause tissue swelling, high blood pressure, diabetes mellitus, ulcers, HIRSUTISM (excess hairiness) and (rarely) psychosis. High doses also increase the susceptibility to infection by interfering with the body's immune system. Because long-term use of these drugs suppresses the production of natural corticosteroid hormones, sudden withdrawal of the drug may lead to collapse, coma and death. Corticosteroid dosages should always be tapered off in decreasing amounts.

cortisone A synthetic CORTICOSTEROID drug used to reduce inflammation in severe allergic, rheumatic and connective tissue diseases, among other things.

Adverse effects High doses for long periods of time can cause swelling, high blood pressure, diabetes, excess hairiness and inhibited growth in children. They can also interfere with the immune system, leaving the patient vulnerable to illness. Sudden withdrawal of the drugs may lead to collapse, coma and death.

cosmetic acupuncture A specialized type of acupuncture designed to help tighten up facial muscles and stimulate good circulation in facial skin. This type of acupuncture works on the same basis as any other type: the special needles supposedly release energy channels and affected areas are stimulated to heal themselves. There is no scientific evidence of its effectiveness.

Technique In this process, needles are inserted into acupuncture points on the face (and sometimes on the body), followed by a moisturizing facial massage. Several treatments are usually required for best results.

cosmetic allergy About 6 percent of all allergic skin reactions are linked to cosmetics, although this number is declining because of more sophisticated testing of cosmetic products.

While "HYPOALLERGENIC," "allergy-tested" or "dermatologist-approved" labels seem to indicate a safe choice for those allergic to cosmetics, in fact these labels are not regulated by the government and don't guarantee that the product they're on is any more extensively tested than any other cosmetic.

The Food and Drug Administration has not established a legal definition of such terms as "hypo-allergenic" and while only a few products may actually be labeled "dermatologist tested," in fact most cosmetic safety testing is performed by dermatologists who work for private cosmetic-testing labs.

Experts do agree that even the best products labeled "hypo-allergenic" do not guarantee than *no one* will experience a reaction; the label simply means that these products are *less* likely to cause an allergic reaction.

Hypo-allergenic means that a manufacturer has tried to eliminate as many of the known common sensitizing ingredients as possible (such as flavorings, some preservatives and fragrances) and has tried to cut out manufacturing byproducts that might contaminate the final product. Manufacturers also work closely with dermatologists to find out the source of allergies to their products by providing samples of the individual ingredients for testing.

Those with highly sensitive skin should choose products that are labeled "fragrance free," since many studies have determined that it is the fragrance in a product that *most often* causes an allergic reaction. However, consumers should understand that "unscented" is *not* the same as "fragrance free"— an unscented product often contains masking fragrances to neutralize unpleasant odors.

As a general rule, all consumers should apply cosmetics carefully near the eye, since this area is the most vulnerable to an allergic reaction, due to the thin, sensitive nature of the skin here.

If you suspect you may be allergic to a product, bring it (along with package and ingredients label) to your dermatologist. A new program cosponsored by the American Academy of Dermatology allows any board-certified dermatologist to obtain help from most cosmetic companies in determining the ingredients list of specific products.

cosmetics Preparations that are applied to the skin to enhance appearance. Since earliest times, women have been applying vegetable dyes and color pigments to their faces, pounding out preparations from leaves and flowers and natural ores. In 1992, Americans spent $3.5 billion on skin-care products alone—a 5.5 percent increase over 1991, according to the cosmetic consulting firm Kline & Co. At best, most cosmetics are only helpful in improving appearance; others are actively harmful to the skin.

Cosmetics are not drugs, which are products that change the function or structure of the skin. For example, a deodorant isn't a drug because it doesn't alter the body's sweating, it simply adds a perfume. But an antiperspirant *is* a drug, because it affects the function of the skin in order to decrease the amount of sweat.

While cosmetics and drugs are regulated by the U.S. Food and Drug Administration, very little is spent on investigating cosmetics. While cosmetics are loosely regulated, they must list ingredients on the label, although they don't give details on concentration or purity. For more information on cosmetics call the FDA hotline at (800) 270-8869.

Ingredients Cosmetics are made up of a variety of substances, including preservatives, stabilizers, emulsifiers, antioxidants etc. Preservatives are included in order to extend a product's shelf life. Most preservatives are divided into two types—antimicrobial agents and antioxidants. Antimicrobial agents, which work by inhibiting the growth of microbacteria and fungi in the cosmetic, include organic acids, alcohol, aldehydes, essential oils, ammonium compounds, mercury agents, phenolic agents and acid agents. Antioxidants work by reducing oxidation and destruction of fats and oils in the product; they include both organic and inorganic agents. Preservatives are so important to the ingredients of cosmetics that preservative-free cosmetics would have to be kept in the refrigerator.

Cosmetics also contain some unusual ingredients. Squalene, used in moisturizers for its antibacterial qualities, originates in olives and sharks' livers. The red color found in many cosmetics is derived from carmine (crushed shells from a beetlelike slug). Some frosted eye shadows contain guanine, (crushed fish scales). While ambergris (material coughed up by whales) was once coveted as a fragrance fixative, cheaper fixatives are used today.

Contamination Cosmetics should never be shared with anyone else. Bacteria, viruses and fungi can all flourish in makeup. (There are no known cases of AIDS transmitted via cosmetics, however).

To counter the risk of infection, stores that once offered communal lipsticks and eye pencils are now using safer sampling products. For example, some companies now offer one-time-use tubes of mascaras; other companies provide sterile swabs and sponges for consumers eager to sample the latest makeup shades. Some stores forbid their clerks to apply lipstick directly, even on someone's hand; instead, they use a new applicator for each customer. If consumers can't find single-use makeup samples or fresh applicators, they should bring cotton swabs or applicators from home.

Choosing cosmetics Experts recommend that consumers should analyze their skin type be-fore buying skin-care products. Always read labels to find out what ingredients are included. While hypoallergenic products have the simplest formulations, there is no guarantee that a reaction will not occur.

See also HYPOALLERGENIC; PH; MAKEUP.

cosmetic surgery Operations performed to improve the appearance, instead of improving function or treating disease. Individuals seek out cosmetic surgery for a wide range of reasons, for example, to appear younger, to reduce too-large breasts or resculpt a nose.

Cosmetic surgery can include operations of the brow and upper face and eyebrows to remove signs of aging; mid-face lift, to lift and restructure the mid-face; neck and chin (segmental meloplasty), to remove sagging excess neck skin and/or rebuild the chin; full FACE-LIFT (rhytidectomy) to lift the whole face; eyelids (blepharoplasty); nose (rhinoplasty) to reduce or reshape; abdomen (abdominal lipectomy) to remove excess fat tissue and skin; breast reduction/augmentation, to change the shape of the breast; ears (otoplasty) to pin back ears or change their shape; LIPOSUCTION, to remove excess fat; DERMABRASION, laser resurfacing and chemical peels, to improve the appearance of the complexion.

Those who are contemplating cosmetic surgery should ask themselves the reasons why they want the operation, whether expectations for results are realistic, whether they can afford the procedure and whether they will be able to put up with the pain and other aftereffects.

Before a cosmetic operation, a responsible surgeon will ask you all the above questions, consult your medical history and ask you about other surgeries. All options will be presented, and the surgery itself will be explained in detail. See also ARGON LASER; CARBON DIOXIDE LASER; CHEMICAL FACE PEEL; COLLAGEN INJECTIONS; EYELID LIFT; FAT TRANSPLANTS; FIBREL; FREE-FLAP SURGERY; LA-

SER TREATMENT; NOSE REPAIR; MAMMOPLASTY; LASER RESURFACING.

coumarin (coumadin) necrosis Another name for an anticoagulation syndrome, this severe reaction to the anticoagulant drug coumarin occurs infrequently, usually in young women. The reaction begins between three and 10 days after beginning treatment with a coumarin drug such as dicumarol or warfarin. Neither stopping nor continuing the drug changes the course of the lesions, once they appear. They begin as tiny red spots or a blue-purple hemorrhagic patch, quickly followed by necrosis (tissue death), which can extend deep into the subcutaneous fat and take months to heal. About 80 percent of the lesions occur on the lower body, such as the thighs, abdomen and breasts (especially in areas filled with subcutaneous fat). The condition has been associated with a lack of protein C, a vitamin K-dependent plasma protein that interferes with blood clotting. See also HEPARIN NECROSIS.

Council on Electrolysis Education A professional group for electrologists that sponsors educational programs and research the field of ELECTROLYSIS; establishes criteria for accreditation and certification; maintains a speakers' bureau; and compiles statistics. Founded in 1972, the group sponsors an annual seminar in March. For address, see Appendix D; see also AMERICAN ELECTROLOGY ASSOCIATION; INTERNATIONAL GUILD OF PROFESSIONAL ELECTROLOGISTS; NATIONAL COMMISSION FOR ELECTROLOGIST CERTIFICATION; SOCIETY OF CLINICAL AND MEDICAL ELECTROLOGISTS.

Cowden's disease An inherited skin disease that appears in childhood or puberty, characterized by shiny papules on the face, palms, tongue and in the mouth area. There is also a strong association between Cowden's disease and the development of breast cancer in women, and thyroid and gastrointestinal cancer in males and females.

Cowden's disease is an autosomal dominant disorder, which means that only one defective gene (from one parent) is needed to cause the syndrome. Each child of an affected person usually has a 1 in 2 chance of inheriting the defective gene and of being affected, and a 1 in 2 chance of being unaffected.
Prevention Some experts suggest that bilateral preventive mastectomies should be carefully considered for women with a strong personal or a strong family history of Cowden's disease.
Treatment Facial lesions can be removed with electrocautery by surgery or with laser therapy.

crab lice See LICE.

cradle cap A harmless, common skin condition in infants in which thick yellow scales form in patches over the scalp. It is a form of SEBORRHEIC DERMATITIS, which may also occur on the face, neck, behind the ears and in the diaper area. Without treatment, it may persist for months but, when properly cared for, usually fades away within a few weeks.
Treatment Wash the baby's hair with baby shampoo or a mild anti-dandruff shampoo once a day; after lathering, massage the scaly scalp with a soft toothbrush for a few minutes. For very crusty conditions, rub olive or mineral oil into the baby's scalp an hour before you shampoo. The oil loosens and softens the scales, which can then be washed off. Be sure to wash out all the oil, because if this is left in the hair it could aggravate the problem.

This treatment may need to be repeated for several days until all the scales are washed off. Brush baby's hair daily with a soft-bristle brush; this will also help loosen scales that can then be removed with a fine-tooth comb. Consult a physician if the skin looks inflamed or the condition worsens. A mild corticosteroid solution or cream may be prescribed until the condition clears.

cream, cleansing An emulsifier that is really a soap, and therefore more alkaloid than the pH of the skin. Cleansing creams are all basically variations on old formulas containing borax, water, mineral oil and beeswax. Cleansing lotions and aerosol foams are basically variations of the same product in a different format.

Soap and water are better at removing oily dirt from the skin, but cleansing creams are better at removing oily makeup. Because of their alkalinity, cleansing creams can be irritating to sensitive skin. See also COSMETICS; MAKEUP; SOAP AND THE SKIN.

CREST phenomenon Acronym for a condition that manifests the symptoms of "calcinosis, RAYNAUD'S PHENOMENON, esophageal dysmotility, sclerodactyly and TELANGIECTASIA." It is found in a group of patients with progressive SYSTEMIC SCLEROSIS.

Cronkhite-Canada syndrome Absence of the fingernails and toenails associated with diffuse hyperpigmentation of the palms and parts of the fingers, and gastrointestinal polyps.

Cross-McKusick-Breen syndrome A disorder featuring lack of pigmentation, with mental retardation, short stature, writhing movements and gingival fibromatosis. Patients with this syndrome should avoid the midday sun and use UVA-UVB sunscreen. Sunglasses will help combat photophobia. While neither beta-carotene nor PUVA can offer solar protection, beta-carotene may help improve skin color.

crotamiton cream (trade name: Eurax lotion) A treatment for SCABIES that is not particularly effective. Experts suggest that five daily applications may be better than the two

currently recommended, but current data are not conclusive. It toxicity is unknown; it is applied to the whole body below the neck, left on for 48 hours and then washed off.

cryosurgery The surgical destruction of tissue using below-freezing temperatures.

The standard agent for this type of surgery is liquid nitrogen at $-195.6°$ C. Carbon dioxide is less often used. The liquid nitrogen is applied to the skin with a cotton-tipped applicator or via a Cryospray unit for five to 30 seconds, depending on the diagnosis. Cryotherapy precludes the need for anesthesia, which makes the procedure simpler than cold steel surgery. Dressings are usually not required after treatment. The area is washed twice daily with mild soap and water followed by application of an antibiotic ointment to prevent bacterial infection. Most lesions are red and scaly for several days to a few weeks, eventually crumbling away and leaving a smooth surface behind. A blister may form and may cause mild discomfort.

Because it involves minimal scarring, it is especially helpful for cosmetic reasons.

The most common use of cryotherapy is for the treatment of LENTIGINES (liver spots), SEBORRHEIC KERATOSES, ACTINIC KERATOSES, WARTS and MOLLUSCUM CONTAGIOSUM. Skin cancers, such as basal cell carcinoma and some in-situ squamous cell carcinomas, also may be treated with cryotherapy. Some lesions may require more than one treatment (usually spaced three weeks apart).

Complications may include hypopigmentation or, less often, scarring.

Some malignant lesions (basal cell or squamous cell carcinomas) treated with aggressive cryosurgery have reported cure rates of 95 percent.

cryptococcosis A rare fungal infection caused by inhaling *Cryptococcus neoformans*, found throughout the world, especially in soil contaminated with pigeon droppings. Although it usually affects adults, infection can occur at any age, especially among those already ill with cancer, such as leukemia or lymphoma, or those who have suppressed immune systems (such as patients with AIDS). Infection with this fungus is unusual in patients who are otherwise healthy. Untreated, this infection may be progressive and fatal.

Symptoms While meningitis is the more usual and serious form of the disease, it also can cause a range of granular lesions, including ulcers, abscesses, tumors, papules, nodules, and draining sinuses into the skin, lungs, etc.

Treatment Fluconazole freely passes through the central nervous system and is the drug of choice; intravenous AMPHOTERICIN B and oral FLUCYTOSINE also may be helpful.

cucumber As a fresh vegetable or in extracts, the naturally acidic cucumber contains vitamin C and CHLOROPHYLL; slices of cucumber can be helpful in soothing tired, puffy eyes. While the fresh cucumber can be beneficial, heavily processed commercial extracts don't usually contain any beneficial ingredients.

curettage and electrodesiccation The removal of tissue with a sharp instrument called a curet is called curettage. This is often followed by electrodesiccation, a form of electrosurgery in which tissue is destroyed by burning with an electric spark. Bleeding can also be stopped by electrodesiccation.

In the procedure, the bulk of a lesion is first removed with a curet under local anesthesia and the base is destroyed afterwards with electrodesiccation. Because the current does not penetrate very deeply, scooping out tissue with a curet increases the efficiency of the procedure. Curettage is often used to remove WARTS, SEBORRHEIC KERATOSES and BASAL CELL CARCINOMA.

For treating most basal and some squamous cell cancers, the procedure is usually repeated three times.

cutaneous atrophy The medical term for thinning of the skin. It is a normal part of aging resulting in the loss of substance from the first two layers of the skin. In this condition, the skin is thin, easily wrinkled and fragile, with blood vessels showing through the skin. Multiple bruises (called Bateman's purpura) are also common, and minute tears in the skin on the backs of the hands and forearms may cause scars. This condition is most likely to occur in areas of aged skin exposed to excessive amounts of sunlight. Atrophy may also result from some inflammatory skin conditions such as syphilis or as a type of scarring.

cutaneous diphtheria A bacterial infection common in the tropics, but also found in Canada and the southern United States. It is caused by the organism *Corynebacterium diphtheriae*, normally found in the mucous membranes of the nose and throat and probably on human skin.

Symptoms Superficial ulcers on the skin with a gray-yellow or brown-gray membrane in the early stages that can be peeled off; later, a black or brown-black scab appears, surrounded by a tender inflammatory area.

Treatment Antibiotics and specific antitoxins are useful. Oral penicillin V potassium is effective in mild cases. While the antibiotics will inhibit the growth of the bacteria, diphtheria antitoxin is required to inactivate the toxin.

Prevention Today, diphtheria in the U.S. and other developed countries is extremely rare because the triple DPT vaccine (against diphtheria, pertussis and tetanus) is given routinely to children in the first year of life.

cutaneous focal mucinosis See MUCINOSES.

cutaneous infections, noninvasive See TINEA.

cutaneous tag See SKIN TAGS.

cuticle A layer of solid or semisolid material that covers the EPITHELIUM.

cutis The skin.

cutis hyperelastica The medical name for EHLERS-DANLOS SYNDROME.

cutis laxa A group of genetic or acquired diseases of the connective tissue that is characterized by loss of normal skin elasticity, resulting in skin abnormalities. In cutis laxa, the looseness of the skin may either be generalized or localized.

Generalized cutis laxa, also called generalized elastolysis, is characterized by loose folds of skin on the sides of the face, leading to sagging jowls and a bloodhound appearance. It appears around puberty or later. Changes appear in connective tissues in other parts of the body, leading to pulmonary emphysema, gastrointestinal tract and bladder problems and multiple hernias. In its most severe form, the saggy skin over the entire body (not just sun-exposed areas) produces a striking appearance of old age; these patients do not survive infancy. Other patients may live to adulthood with various disabilities.

Congenital forms of cutis laxa are characterized by loose, pendulous skin present at birth or shortly thereafter, giving the child a prematurely aged appearance. The skin can be pulled up but will not spring back when released. Multiple organs may be affected because of the defect in supporting structure.

Localized forms of cutis laxa may be hereditary, and may occur only in certain areas of the body as an independent disorder or as a part of the generalized form of the disease. The localized form may be the only expression of the disease, or it may be a precursor for later development of a more widespread form. Blepharochalasis (abnormal looseness of the eyelids) may result from aging or may begin early in life. In the localized form, there may be coin-sized areas of loss of tissue in the skin, with outpouching of underlying tissue. These patches may appear spontaneously, or after the skin has been injured by inflammation or disease (such as SYPHILIS, ERYTHEMA MULTIFORME, ACNE, HIVES, CHICKEN POX etc.) Lesions will continue to appear throughout life, although most appear during childhood and adolescence.

Treatment There is no helpful treatment for either the generalized or the localized form of cutis laxa. Any attempt at surgical tightening is followed by prompt reappearance of the skin folds.

Patients with the localized form should avoid injury that could lead to inflammation and new lesions. Unattractive lesions can be surgically excised, but the wounds may not heal well and the scars may spread and gape.

cutis marmorata telangiectatica congenita Also known as van Lohuizen's disease, this congenital circulatory disorder causes an exaggerated network marbling (fixed LIVEDO RETICULARIS) of the skin of the trunk, legs and arms, face, and scalp. The demarcation between normal and abnormal skin is sharp and often seen at the midline. In addition, ulcers may appear on the affected skin. The condition usually improves with time.

Other symptoms include atrophy of the soft tissues and bones of the affected part. Other developmental abnormalities can also occur. HEMANGIOMAS and areas of NEVUS FLAMMEUS may be associated with this disorder.

This disease should not be confused with CUTIS MARMORATA, which is the term used to describe the normal transient physiological reaction of mottled blue skin in reaction to the cold that is seen in about half of all normal children and adults.

Treatment Only local treatment is needed if complications such as ulcers develop.

cyanosis Bluish discoloration of the skin due to an excess of deoxygenated hemoglobin in the blood, most easily seen in the nail beds of fingers and toes, and on lips and tongue. It occurs most often when blood flow through the skin slows down because of cold; however, this type of cyanosis is not serious and doesn't indicate any underlying disease.

In other instances, though, cyanosis can be a serious symptom of disease. It may indicate poor blood circulation in the extremities, in which fingers and toes turn blue even when the environment is fairly warm. Cyanosis may also be a sign of heart problems (such as heart failure) or fluid in the lungs. Cyanosis present at birth might be a sign of congenital heart disease in which some of the blood does not reach the lungs to pick up oxygen but instead goes directly to the rest of the body.

cyclophosphamide The generic name for Cytoxan and Neosar, this is an anticancer drug that has been used with some success in those with PEMPHIGUS and BULLOUS PEMPHIGOID. Other skin diseases that may respond to this drug include LUPUS ERYTHEMATOSUS, and PYODERMA GANGRENOSUM and in some types of vasculitis, such as Wegener's granulofosus. Patients with advanced forms of MYCOSIS FUNGOIDES have been treated with chemotherapy combinations including cyclophosphamide.
Adverse effects The common side effects are hair loss, nausea, vomiting and caused by irritation of the bladder cystitis, by drug metabolites. Cystitis may be avoided if the patient drinks plenty of water shortly before and up to two hours after taking the drug orally followed by frequent urination. Less common side effects include mouth ulcers, increased discoloration of skin and nails, hair loss, jaundice, clotting abnormalities, the complete absence of sperm, or lack of ovulation. This drug causes birth defects.

cyclopiroxolamine The generic name for Loprox, this is a topical agent used to treat fungus infections. It works by inhibiting the growth of dermatophytes (microscopic fungi), *Candida albicans* and the agent causing TINEA VERSICOLOR (a type of ringworm).

cyclosporine An immunosuppressant drug derived from soil fungus that suppresses the body's natural defense against abnormal cells. Introduced in 1984, it is used primarily to prevent and treat organ transplant rejection. It is also helpful in the treatment of skin diseases such as recalcitrant PSORIASIS, PEMPHIGUS VULGARIS, GRAFT-VERSUS-HOST DISEASE, and BEHCET'S SYNDROME. Benefits from cyclosporine have also been reported in patients with severe atopic DERMATITIS, ALOPECIA, ICHTHYOSIS VULGARIS, EPIDERMOLYSIS bullosa acquisita, PYODERMA GANGRENOSUM, systemic LUPUS ERYTHEMATOSUS, cutaneous T-cell lymphoma and SARCOIDOSIS.
Adverse effects Because cyclosporine interferes with the immune system, patients treated with this drug are more susceptible to infection. Any flu-like illness or localized infection requires immediate medical attention. Because cyclosporine is metabolized primarily by the liver, patients with liver disease may experience problems with this drug.

In addition, the drug has been found to cause kidney problems; therefore, regular kidney function monitoring is necessary for anyone being given this drug. If signs of kidney damage appear (such as protein in the urine), the dosage needs to be reduced or other drugs may be substituted. In many people, kidney problems disappear after the drug is stopped, but some people experience irreversible kidney damage from use of cyclosporine.

Other side effects may include high blood pressure, gastrointestinal problems, fatigue, development of secondary cancer (primarily lymphomas) and infections. Another fairly common side effect is swelling of the gums and hirsutism.

cyst A closed cavity or sac containing a liquid or semisolid material beneath the skin. Cysts may be caused by a variety of reasons; those affecting the skin may be caused by a blocked duct leading from a fluid-forming sebaceous gland to the skin gland. While these cysts are benign, they may become unsightly and may be surgically removed. Other types of skin cysts include dermoid cysts, a type of skin cyst that may contain particles of hair follicles, sweat glands, nerves and even teeth. Dermoid cysts are found in parts of the body that fused during fetal development. Sometimes a dermoid cyst may appear after an injury. Treatment is surgical removal.

cytotoxic drugs, skin side effects of Anticancer drugs that kill or damage cells may also cause HYPERPIGMENTATION (darkening of the skin). While cytotoxic drugs primarily affect abnormal cells, they can also damage or kill healthy cells, especially those that multiply rapidly such as in the skin.

Cytotoxic drugs that may affect the skin include BLEOMYCIN, which causes the skin to become deeply tanned because of pigment cell stimulation. In addition, cyclophosphamide and melphalan can cause bands of hyperpigmentation of the skin and in the nails (MELANONYCHIA).

cytotoxic drugs for skin diseases There are several cytotoxic drugs that can be used in the treatment of a variety of skin diseases. These include AZATHIOPRINE (Imuran), CYCLOPHOSPHAMIDE (Cytoxan), HYDROXYUREA (Hydrea) and METHOTREXATE.

D

Damien Dutton Society for Leprosy Aid A group of religious leaders and laypeople interested in helping sufferers of Hansen's disease (LEPROSY) that provides relief, research and recreation to patients all over the world. Founded in 1944, the society has 30,000 members and publishes the quarterly newsletter *Damien-Dutton Call.* Its annual meeting is always held in Bellmore, N.Y. For address, see Appendix D; see also AMERICAN LEPROSY FOUNDATION; AMERICAN LEPROSY MISSIONS.

dandruff A very common, harmless condition (also called seborrhea) in which the scalp sheds dead skin, producing unattractive white flakes in the hair that often fall onto the collar and shoulders. When it worsens into an itchy, inflamed scalp rash, it is called seborrheic dermatitis (see DERMATITIS, SEBORRHEIC), and is also found on the face, back and chest.

Treatment While no cure for dandruff exists, consumers find some relief with frequent shampooing; the more often you shampoo, the easier it is to control dandruff. Because dandruff is often caused by an oily scalp, a mild nonmedicated shampoo may be enough to control the problem.

If the mild shampoo is not effective, try using an anti-dandruff product. Those with selenium sulfide or zinc pyrithione offer the quickest results by slowing down the rate at which scalp cells multiply, but no matter which type of anti-dandruff shampoo you use, don't rinse the lather off too quickly. Lather up as you begin your shower, leave it on until the very end and then rinse; lather and rinse again.

Products with salicylic acid and sulfur loosen up the dandruff so it can be washed away, while antibacterial shampoos reduce bacteria on the scalp. Very stubborn cases may respond to tar shampoos, which work by slowing down cell growth; leave the tar lather on the hair for up to 10 minutes so the tar can work.(Please note that blond or silver hair may be stained by tar compounds.)

More and more dermatologists prescribe antifungal shampoos (such as Nizoral 2% shampoo) to curb flaking by controlling the growth of a yeast that occurs naturally on the scalp. Other choices include a corticosteroid cream or lotion to apply to the scalp.

dapsone (4,4′-diaminodiphenyl-sulfone) An antibacterial drug that has been used to treat resistant ACNE, LEPROSY and DERMATITIS HERPETIFORMIS. Results with this drug, the most often-used of the sulfones, have been variable, but in some cases there have been excellent results. Its mechanism of action is unknown, although it is known to interfere with neutrophil function. Other diseases that may be treated with dapsone include bullous diseases and PYODERMA GANGRENOSUM.

The introduction of the sulfones in the 1950s had a dramatic impact on the treatment of leprosy. Of these, dapsone was the first safe and effective drug available, killing the bacteria (*Mycobacterium leprae*) and eliminating the need for patient isolation. Although resistance to dapsone is becoming widespread, it remains the drug of choice in the treatment of leprosy in conjunction with other medication.

Adverse effects The adverse effects of this drug tend to be dose-related, and adverse effects are uncommon with low doses. Concerns over safety may have been exaggerated by the high doses used in some early studies, according to some experts.

Severe allergic reactions may occur, including TOXIC EPIDERMAL NECROLYSIS and STEVENS-JOHNSON SYNDROME. Other side effects may include nausea, vomiting and rarely, damage to the liver, red blood cells and nerves. There may also be sensory and motor neuropathy that can be significant. During long-term treatment, blood tests are conducted to monitor liver function and the red blood cell level.

Neurological symptoms (such as psychosis) are believed to be dose-related; those with a history of psychiatric problems may be more likely to develop mental problems on this drug.

The cases of agranulocytosis (deficiency of blood cells due to bone marrow damage) seen among troops in Vietnam taking dapsone to prevent malaria could have been caused by concurrent use of other antimalarial drugs. According to reports, millions of patients have been successfully treated with dapsone for years with relatively low rates of toxic side effects.

Darier's disease Known medically as keratosis follicularis, this is a disorder of keratinization (the process where by cells become horny as they approach the surface of the skin); it affects the skin, mucous membranes and nails. An uncommon inherited disease, this disorder usually begins in childhood or adolescence and gets worse following exposure to ultraviolet radiation.

Patients are also at risk for secondary bacterial infection and for serious, widespread viral skin infections usually due to the herpes simplex virus.

While the disease comes and goes, there is a tendency for it to become more severe over time.
Symptoms Itchy, greasy, foul-smelling brown papules form plaques on scalp, ears, face, neck and upper trunk—these lesions are often induced by sunlight. Distinctive nail changes include fragile, short and relatively wide nails with notching, ridging and red and white linear streaks.
Treatment Patients should avoid sun exposure and use sunscreen. Secondary infections should be treated with antibiotics. Wet compresses and tap water soaks can help lessen odor and crusts. Synthetic retinoids (Tegison or Accutane) often induce remission, but chronic use is often necessary to prevent relapse. Because many patients on long-term retinoids have developed diffuse skeletal abnormalities this chronic administration is rarely justified.

Deep dermabrasion followed by skin grafts may help some patients with severe problems.

Darier's sign Itching and hives that occur after stroking or rubbing lesions of URTICARIA PIGMENTOSA.

Darier-White disease See DARIER'S DISEASE.

decubitus ulcer Another name for BEDSORES.

Degos' disease The common name for malignant atrophic papulosis, this is a rare, often-fatal disease, occurring most often in men, characterized by porcelain-white skin lesions (from five to more than 100) in the skin and gastrointestinal tract. Half the patients with this disease develop these lesions in the gastrointestinal area, which results in loss of blood to the area and subsequent tissue death in weeks or years; these complications are usually fatal.
Treatment There is no effective treatment.

delusion of bromhidrosis The psychotic belief that a person's own body odor is profoundly offensive. This problem usually occurs during adolescence, often in conjunction with fastidious habits and no body odor. These patients usually show an ambivalent sexuality and little emotion. Outlook is very poor for these patients, who often go on to develop schizophrenia.

Treatment There is no published data regarding the treatment of this disorder with pimozide, the drug used to treat Tourette's syndrome and DELUSIONS OF PARASITOSIS. The patient's delusion must never be reinforced.

delusions of parasitosis The erroneous belief that the skin is infested with parasites. Most of these patients suffer from some type of mental disorder, such as psychosis or an obsessive-compulsive disorder.

Patients may report feelings of bugs crawling within the skin, and will go to extraordinary lengths to remove the bugs. They may try to rid themselves of "parasites" by washing often, applying insecticides or parasiticides, avoiding others to contain the "contamination." Some patients may paint their homes, destroy "infested" bedcovers, and call on pest control companies for help.

Also called acarophobia or parasitophobia, it is classified as a hypochondriacal psychosis. While treatment for parasitic delusions was once thought to be hopeless, a few patients have recovered.

Symptoms While there is no evidence of skin problems, these patients may insist there is; some puncture the skin with fingernails or needles to dig out the "parasites." These "insects" are then produced (usually bits of skin, hair, crusts, and other debris). Patients usually reject any suggestion that the parasites are not real with scorn or disbelief, and refuse to seek psychological counseling.

Complications Chronic attempts to clean the skin may cause tissue breakdown; isolation to prevent "contamination" may result in psychological problems. Suicide is possible.

Treatment Some experts recommend confronting the patient with the delusion, but others counter that confrontation can be disastrous since the patient is absolutely sure of the infestation. The patient's belief should never be treated as factual, and antiparasitic lotions shouldn't be administered. Depression or other psychological problems should be treated.

Pimozide (a drug used to treat Tourette's syndrome) may help control, but not cure, the disorder, although side effects include irreversible tardive dyskinesia, EKG abnormalities, drowsiness and sometimes death. Still, chronic administration of pimozide allows many patients to live normal lives.

Demodex folliculorum A mite found in the hair follicles and sebaceous secretions (especially in the face and nose). The mites usually cause no problems but may occasionally cause a folliculitis called demodex folliculitis.

deodorant A modestly effective substance designed to be applied to the skin to control unpleasant odor, usually containing antimicrobial agents; it may also contain fragrance to disguise odor and antiseptics to destroy bacteria. Deodorant is a useful help against body odor caused by bacteria in decomposing sweat on the skin, but is less effective than ANTIPERSPIRANTS. See also SWEAT GLANDS; SWEAT GLANDS, DISORDERS OF; DRYSOL.

depigmentation The removal of PIGMENT (usually MELANIN). "Depigmented" refers to the absence of pigment (usually melanin).

depigmentation, chemically induced A variety of chemicals (mostly derivatives of phenol or hydroquinone) can produce depigmentation of the skin that looks very much like VITILIGO. Progressive depigmentation beginning on the hands and spreading to other parts of the body may be caused by exposure to phenolic compounds, especially if the patient works in the plastics and rubber industries, or uses germicidal agents.

Treatment First, the patient should be protected from further exposure to industrial cleaning solutions, germicidal agents, rubber products or depigmenting medications. It may be possible to repigment hair-bearing skin with PUVA.

depigmentation disorders Any of the disorders resulting in absence of pigment cells from the skin, too few melanosomes, or improper melanin synthesis.

Disorders of congenital depigmentation due to absence of melanocytes include PIE-BALDISM, ALBINISM and WAARDENBURG'S SYNDROME. Disorders involving acquired depigmentation caused by the absence of melanocytes include VITILIGO, post-traumatic depigmentation and chemically induced depigmentation. See also DEPIGMENTA-TION, POST-TRAUMATIC and DEPIGMENTATION, CHEMICALLY INDUCED.

depigmentation, post-traumatic Any physical, chemical or infectious agent that destroys the EPIDERMIS (outer skin layer) will also destroy the pigment cells along the basal skin layer. Normally, skin is repigmented as pigment cells proliferate and migrate from hair bulbs and adjacent skin. If an injury destroys the hair bulbs or other nearby skin, the normal reservoir of new pigment cells is destroyed. That skin will probably remain permanently white.

Injuries that cause this type of depigmentation include burns, radiation, deep lacerations or abrasions. Likewise, any infections that leave deep scars (such as herpes zoster or CHICKEN POX) often leave depigmented areas. Many lesions of discoid LUPUS ERYTHE-MATOSUS may be permanently depigmented.

Pigment cells are particularly vulnerable to injury from cold; freezing the epidermis by CRYOTHERAPY may cause a temporary depigmentation, but new pigment cells will eventually migrate into the area. Therefore, minor lesions in dark-skinned patients should be treated with cryotherapy with great caution.

Deep freezing to destroy basal cell epithelioma or SQUAMOUS CELL CARCINOMA may also leave an area of permanent depigmentation, since pigment cells in the hair bulbs are destroyed.

depigmenting agents Pigmentation may be reduced through the use of a range of agents, including HYDROQUINONE, monobenzyl ether of hydroquinone or AZELAIC ACID. See also DEPIGMENTATION, CHEMICALLY INDUCED.

depilatory A chemical agent for removing or destroying hair, such as barium sulfide, that is available in a cream or paste. Depilatories are used for cosmetic purposes and for the treatment of HIRSUTISM. They dissolve the hair at the skin's surface but do not affect the hair's root. Hair grows back within a few days; therefore, they are only a temporary solution to hair removal.

Depilatories should not be used immediately after a hot bath or shower, since heat increases blood flow to the skin, opening skin pores and increasing the amount of chemical absorbed into the body.

Today, the most popular chemical depilatories are made of thioglycolates combined with calcium hydroxide. Older depilatories contained alkaline earth sulfides that had an unpleasant odor and irritated the skin. They are still used, however, by some black men to remove beard hair.

Although chemical depilatories offer a smoother skin surface than shaving, only about 1 percent of American women use them exclusively for hair removal; 8 percent of American women use depilatories in combination with other methods. Many consumers consider them expensive, slow and irritating to the skin, with an unpleasant odor.

Adverse effects Chemical depilatories may cause an allergic reaction characterized by swelling and inflammation, and are not usually recommended for use on the face. Because the chemical structure of the KERATIN of the top-most skin layer resembles hair chemically, depilatories should not be left on the skin too long or they will cause irritation. See also HAIR REMOVAL; ELECTROLYSIS.

dermabrasion Surgical removal of the surface layer of the skin by high-speed sanding to reduce pitted scars of ACNE, improve appearance of raised scars or to remove tattoos. Dermabrasion is the most dramatic resurfacing technique that dermatologists can use, and it leaves the skin relatively smooth.

In the procedure, the skin is numbed with a local anesthetic and, using an abrasive wheel, wire brush or diamond fraise rotating at high speeds, the dermatologist removes layer after layer of skin to reach the smooth skin underneath scars, and remove precancerous lesions, broken blood vessels, wrinkles and tattoos. The skin heals in about two weeks, although the full effect of the treatment is not apparent for two months. While pain is not considered to be a problem, many patients are bothered by the red, raw appearance of the skin for about 10 days after the procedure.

As with other types of facial peels, dermabrasion may cost several thousand dollars. For a list of dermatologists qualified to perform dermabrasion, call the toll-free hotline maintained by the American Society for Dermatologic Surgery at (800) 441-2737.

dermaplaning A process that scrapes away dead cells before a facial peel. Dermaplaning is far less aggressive than DERMABRASION, which sands away the outer layer of skin (epidermis) and the superficial dermis to smooth down scars.

In dermaplaning, the physician uses a Teflon-coated scalpel to gently scrape away only the outermost epidermis. The technique, which feels something like a fingernail scraping the skin, makes a mild peel more effective because it allows the chemicals to get beneath and fully penetrate the skin's surface. See also CHEMICAL FACE PEEL.

dermatitis The general term used to refer to a group of inflammatory conditions of the skin ("derm" meaning "skin" and "itis" meaning "inflammation of"). While people often use the terms ECZEMA and dermatitis interchangeably, eczema is actually dermatitis in its advanced stages, with blisters, fissures, oozing, crusting, scabbing, thickening, peeling and discoloration. While there are a wide variety of dermatitis conditions, the three main categories: atopic, contact and seborrheic. See DERMATITIS, ARTEFACTA; DERMATITIS, ASTEATOTIC; DERMATITIS, ATOPIC; DERMATITIS, BERLOQUE; DERMATITIS, CEMENT; DERMATITIS, CONTACT; DERMATITIS, EXFOLIATIVE; DERMATITIS, HAND; DERMATITIS, HERPETIFORMIS; DERMATITIS, IRRITANT CONTACT; DERMATITIS, NICKEL; DERMATITIS, NUMMULAR; DERMATITIS PAPULOSA NIGRA; DERMATITIS, PERIORAL; DERMATITIS, SEAWEED. See also ACNE KELOIDALIS; ALLERGIES AND THE SKIN; CRYOSURGERY; DIAPER RASH; DRY SKIN; GOURGEROT-BLUM SYNDROME; OIL OF BERGAMOT; SALYCYLIC ACID; SULFUR.

dermatitis, allergic See ALLERGIES AND THE SKIN.

dermatitis artefacta Any self-induced skin condition, ranging from a mild self-inflicted scratch to severe and extensive mutilation by a disturbed patient. Also called factitial dermatitis, the skin damage with this problem may range from ulcers, blisters or scratches, and often exhibits an asymmetrical or bizarre pattern that does not resemble any normal skin disease.

The problem occurs more often in women and is part of a general syndrome in which patients (often quite intelligent) cannot deal with emotional stress and react by mutilating themselves. Their actions are the result of an inner compulsion, and they may not be aware of what they are doing.

Various methods of causing lesions include applications of caustic substances (silver nitrate or phenol), injection of foreign material, burns, beating or pricking the skin with a pin.

Symptoms The well-defined lesions may include erythema, blisters, ulcers, abscesses, swelling, superficial GANGRENE and purpura. They are unlike lesions of recognized skin diseases and appear with no set pattern.

Treatment The treating health care expert is often regarded as an adversary, and treatment can be difficult because on a deeper level these patients do not really want to get better. Patients can be difficult, manipulative, evasive, untruthful and ungrateful. Often, they are either unaware of, or they conceal, the real nature of their lesions.

Patients should not be directly confronted about the cause of their lesions, instead this information should be conveyed indirectly. Medication (such as tranquilizers) has little effect. The prognosis is good in those patients who have suffered only a brief, traumatic experience, but is not good in those who are chronic sufferers. These patients tend to be immature and may adopt the production of self-induced lesions as a way of life.

dermatitis, asteatotic Also known as "winter itch" or eczema craquelé, this disorder is characterized by DRY SKIN. This type of eczema is often seen in elderly individuals. It becomes more severe and affects more people as winter progresses. The condition is caused by low humidity and indoor heat. Moisturizers may provide some relief.

dermatitis, atopic Also known as atopic eczema, this condition is a chronic superficial inflammation common in infants, often appearing between two and 18 months of age. It tends to occur in those with an inherited tendency to develop allergy and is found in 10 percent of the population. It is usually associated with asthma, hay fever or allergic rhinitis, and it may affect as many as 7 to 24 of every 1,000 individuals. The highest prevalence is in children.

Typically, the condition begins in the first year of life in about 60 percent of cases, and before age 5 in 85 percent. The disease fades away in about 40 percent of individuals by adulthood, although patients with severe diseases are more likely to have a persistent course.

Although there is no cure, the long-term prognosis is good; spontaneous remission occurs in almost half of all patients by age 15. Those who may go on to struggle with persistent disease often have a family history of atopic dermatitis, associated asthma or hay fever and late onset of severe disease.

Symptoms In acute cases, this form of eczema is characterized by a mild, very itchy rash on the face, inner elbow creases and behind the knees, with red, scaling skin and pimples. If scratched, the pimples leak a clear liquid, forming large weeping areas; infection may occur if the condition appears in the diaper area. Adults usually experience symptoms on the back of the neck.

Atopic dermatitis tends to wax and wane; in chronic stages, there is scaling and skin color changes. Most patients improve during the summer and worsen during the winter, which is probably related to humidity and temperature.

Treatment Adequate hydration of the skin and avoiding irritants may be all that is required in those with mild cases. Irritants include wool clothing, strong detergents and water. Irritants can be avoided by using a mild detergent (such as Ivory Snow flakes or Dreft), by avoiding wool and adding bath oil to bath water. Emollients such as white petrolatum should be applied immediately after bathing, and topical corticosteroids and tar preparations are useful.

In acute cases, a medium-potency topical corticosteroid lotion or cream should be applied after bathing or after applying aluminum acetate or saline compresses.

For chronic cases, potent topical corticosteroids should be applied right after bathing; soaking or using compresses of water-soluble tar preparations may decrease the need for topical corticosteroids.

Adequate doses of antihistamines can control itching and prevent scratching, which could lead to secondary infection. With severe involvement, a short course of systemic corticosteroids may be needed; however, the risks of systemic corticosteroids limit their use in long-term treatment.

Oral antibiotics are helpful in infections of eczematous skin, a frequent complication in itchy children.

Gamma interferon and thymopoetin are two experimenal treatments being studied in atopic eczema.

dermatitis, berloque A type of phototoxic contact dermatitis causing an irregular hyperpigmentation usually found on the neck. Berloque (French for "pendant" or "droplike") dermatitis is caused by perfumes that contain OIL OF BERGAMOT, a naturally occurring photosensitizer (PSORALEN). After exposure to the sun, macular hyperpigmentation with sharp margins and streaks begins to appear, with very little reddening, on the neck or hands.

Exposure to certain concentrated plant juices (such as limes) that contain psoralens and subsequent exposure to the sun may produce a more severe reaction producing painful redness and blistering.

The reaction usually appears within 24 hours after sun exposure, peaking within 48 hours.

dermatitis, cement See ALLERGIES AND THE SKIN.

dermatitis, contact An inflammation of the skin caused by an allergic reaction to direct contact with a substance to which a person is sensitive. Usually an itchy or scaly rash erupts at the point of contact, which can be anywhere on the body. While the immune system normally protects against bacteria and viruses, an allergic response causes the immune system to overreact to usually harmless substances like dyes or metals.

Causes Substances that are often implicated in contact dermatitis include metals (especially nickel); dyes and chemicals in clothing, furs, shoes, hair products, rubber compounds, paints, textiles, ink and paper; cleaning products, detergents; cosmetics, perfumes, shaving lotions; POISON IVY; and insecticides. Formaldehyde is a potent antimicrobial that causes many cases of contact dermatitis, and is found in industry, medicine, the home (as a preservative) in permanent press clothes, newspapers etc. Formaldehyde-releasers are used as preservatives in cosmetics and industrial products and are often masked by other names.

Chromates Chromium (in the form of chromates) is the most common cause of contact dermatitis in men, usually from exposure on the job. Because chromates are common, they are often hard to avoid. A main source is cement, effecting those in the building trades. Leather that has been tanned with chromate may also cause contact dermatitis on the feet of sensitive individuals.

Symptoms, which often resemble NUMMULAR ECZEMA, are scaling, redness and dryness. They may take years to improve, even after contact is avoided. In fact, most severely affected people never fully recover, probably because of the prevalence of chromates in everyday life. Workers with only a mild or moderate problem may remain on the job if they can avoid the substance, but a change in the work area doesn't guarantee the dermatitis won't recur. By adding ferrous sulfate to cement, the chromate becomes less sensitizing and this may be a breakthrough in preventing occupational chromate allergy.

Rubber A hypersensitivity to rubber may be suspected if the patient has a history of direct skin contact with a rubber product. There are many rubber chemicals that may produce allergy, especially those contained in disinfectants and preservatives in industrial processes (tetramethylthiuram disulfide and 2-mercaptobenzothiazole and thiourea derivatives). Because of the large number of different allergenic chemicals, it is not easy to perform patch testing for this problem. It is also common to find cross-reactions between related chemicals.

Topical medications About a third of all dermatology patients with a contact allergy will test positive for sensitivity to some type of ingredient in topical drugs or cosmetics. The most common include lanolin, neomycin, local anesthetics, formaldehyde, and preservatives (such as parabens or benzoisothiazides).

Lanolin, a skin cream product derived from sheep fleece, causes a reaction in some people. There is an artificial, hypoallergenic lanolin derivative now available.

Neomycin is a widely used topical antibiotic that may cause a contact dermatitis. The risk of allergy decreases when the antibiotic is used only for simple cuts or surgical wounds. It may be hard to diagnosis neomycin allergy, since the dermatitis is not vesicular or bullous but appears to be an aggravation of preexisting dermatitis (especially in stasis dermatitis).

Parabens are widely used preservatives found in foods, drugs and one-third of all cosmetics. Considering how widespread they are, sensitization to the parabens is low. Although hypersensitivity usually occurs when a person contacts the allergen with any part of the body, parabens may be tolerated on normal facial skin but may cause dermatitis on eczematous skin.

Symptoms Contact dermatitis usually starts as an itchy red rash, evolving into blisters with cracking and peeling skin. The severity of this type of dermatitis depends on the particular substance, and how sensitive a person is. Symptoms should subside within a few days or weeks if the offending substance is avoided, although some kinds of dermatitis can become chronic.

Once an allergic reaction to a substance has occurred, a person can become sensitized; even the briefest subsequent contact will probably set off another attack.

Diagnosis Allergy patch tests may be helpful in determining the substances that are provoking the reaction. In the test, a physician exposes small areas of skin to a variety of known allergens, observing the skin for development of a reaction.

Treatment Mild cases of contact dermatitis do not require treatment, but frequent or severe outbreaks should be referred to a physician. Topical medications (calamine lotion, antihistamines or over-the-counter cortisone creams) usually ease symptoms. Hydrocortisone cream (in 0.5 percent strength) is available without a prescription; stronger creams, which are necessary for cases of significant contact dermatitis, can have serious side effects and are available only with prescription.

It's a myth that patients with dermatitis should avoid bathing; *regular* bathing is now seen as a way to reduce infection and soothe irritated skin (make sure water is not too hot or cold). Try adding two cups of colloidal oatmeal (available in drugstores) or baking soda to the bath.

Individuals allergic to antiperspirants—specifically the metallic salts (such as aluminum chloride, aluminum sulfate and zirconium chlorohydrate) that are the active ingredients—should avoid them. Sensitive consumers should look for products with anti-irritants such as zinc oxide, magnesium oxide, allantoinate, aluminum hydroxide or triethanolamine.

In severe cases of weeping sores, cold milk compresses may help soothe the itching of contact dermatitis. Calamine lotion with menthol or phenol may be another good choice to help a dry oozing rash. See also DERMATITIS, NICKEL.

dermatitis, diaper See DIAPER RASH.

dermatitis, exfoliative A severe, extensive inflammatory condition (also known as erythroderma) that causes scaling and redness of all the skin of the body. An uncommon disorder, it is three times more common in men than women. Average age at onset is 50 years.

Drug reactions are the most common cause of exfoliative dermatitis, responsible for about 40 percent of cases. Common medications associated with this disorder include sulfonamides and penicillin; less commonly, antimalarials, barbiturates, allopurinol, nonsteroidal anti-inflammatory drugs, diphenylhydantoin and gold are suspected to trigger this disorder. Once the offending drug is no longer administered, the skin lesions will often clear within weeks.

In 30 percent of cases, the disorder is due to preexisting skin conditions—most commonly, PSORIASIS or atopic dermatitis. Other associated skin conditions include LICHEN PLANUS, REITER'S SYNDROME, PITYRIASIS RUBRA PILARIS, PEMPHIGUS, allergic contact dermatitis or stasis dermatitis. Most people suffering from this condition will usually find their exfoliative dermatitis clearing within weeks to months after effective treatment is begun, although recurrences are common.

Up to 20 percent of erythroderma is caused by cancer (usually either lymphomas and leukemias). Approximately 10 percent of cases have no known cause.

In those without a known etiology, the disease lasts on average about five years. Intermittent flare-ups are frequent.

Symptoms While the causes of exfoliative dermatitis may vary, the symptoms are the same: generalized redness, warmth, swelling, itch, thickened and scaling skin that begins in one small area and spreads across the skin within days to weeks to months. While the mucous membranes are not usually affected, the palms, soles, scalp and nails are often involved. Other common systemic complaints include chills or fever, dizziness on standing up, dehydration, enlarged lymph nodes and swelling.

Because of the profound effect this disorder has on the metabolic system, the basal metabolic rate may rise by as much as 50 percent above normal, resulting in huge increases in exfoliation that may cause malnutrition (caused by the protein loss in the flaking skin).

Death rates in the past have been as high as 30 percent, and are related to infection. Death from erythroderma has become rare with medical advances.

Treatment Hospitalization may be required to stabilize fluid volume and temperature and to treat added infection. Nutritional supplements and medication to control itching may be required. Steroids, emollients and moisturizing baths may make the patient more comfortable. Failure to implement these supportive treatments may require administration of methotrexate and retinoids.

dermatitis, hand Also known as "hand eczema," this condition is usually caused by exposure to detergents, cleansers or dishwashing soap, although in some a specific cause may never be found. It is restricted to the hands, with little dermatitis elsewhere, and afflicts between 4 and 8 percent of the population.

There may be many different causes behind the development of this condition. *Contact dermatitis* is the most common type of hand dermatitis, which can produce an irritant or allergic eczematous reaction. *Irritant dermatitis* accounts for about 70 percent of contact hand dermatitis; detergents, soaps and solvents are the most important causes.

Contact allergic hand dermatitis is seen in between 25 and 30 percent of cases. A preexisting irritant dermatitis can predispose an individual to the development of allergy. Contact allergic hand dermatitis usually evolves into chronically thickened skin that can't be distinguished from that caused by irritant dermatitis. The primary offenders behind the allergic type of hand dermatitis are nickel, chromate, rubber compounds, paraphenylenediamine and parabens. Nickel allergy, affecting about 5 percent of the population (mostly women), is caused by costume jewelry, coins, handles, pens, surgical instruments and kitchen utensils, any of which can be associated with hand dermatitis. Those with a chromate sensitivity can develop hand dermatitis from exposure at work (especially to cement, leather, paint, and photography dyes). Chemicals added to rubber (such as mercaptobenzothiazole and thiuram) cause rubber sensitization, producing hand dermatitis through contact with rubber gloves and tubing. Paraphenylenediamine is found in azo dyes, and often is a problem among hairdressers. Paraben-sensitive patients may find they are sensitive to many topical medications, cosmetics and foods. (See also ECZEMA.)

Symptoms The condition is characterized by itchy blisters up to an inch across on the palms, with dry cracked skin across the hands. The *acute* stage is characterized by dry blisters and redness; in the subacute stage the skin is red and scaly. Chronic hand dermatitis is characterized by thick, scaly and dry skin with more and more skin markings.

Treatment The condition usually improves if the patient wears cotton gloves under rubber gloves when touching any possible irritant; the hands should be thoroughly dried after immersion in water and an unscented hand cream or white petrolatum should be applied several times a day. If the condition is severe, topical corticosteroids may be prescribed for inflammation and antibiotics may be needed to combat infection.

dermatitis herpetiformis Also known as Duhring's disease, this is a rare chronic skin disorder in which clusters of tiny red itchy blisters appear in a symmetrical pattern on various parts of the body, especially the back, elbows, knees, buttocks and scalp.

The disease usually appears in people between the late 20s and early 40s, much more often in white males. It appears less often among blacks and is quite rare among the Japanese.

About half of these patients also experience gastric hypoacidity and gastric atrophy. Males have a higher frequency of lymphoma (cancer).

Treatment Oral DAPSONE or sulfapyridine usually improves the skin condition but has no effect on the problems occurring in the small intestine. Topical and systemic CORTICOSTEROIDS do not usually work. Removing foods containing gluten from the diet results in an improvement in skin condition and intestinal health, but this may take more than a year. Further, a wheat-free diet is expensive and especially difficult to maintain.

The skin condition has also improved following continuous treatment with PUVA (psorlens plus ultraviolet light A).

dermatitis, irritant contact Irritant contact dermatitis is a local inflammatory reaction (not an allergic reaction) caused by a single or repeated exposure to toxic chemicals. The appearance of lesions depends on the type of irritant which can range from a blistering reaction to a scaly, red thickened skin. An *acute case* may result after only one contact with a highly toxic irritant. Easily diagnosed, it often occurs after industrial accidents.

A *cumulative case* is more common than acute dermatitis and is caused by repeated contact with mild irritants over a long period of time. The first signs are usually dry, cracking skin with redness, scaling, papules, vesicles and thickening.

This type of dermatitis may involve a combination of irritants, set off by one highly toxic irritant (such as a caustic agent or a solvent). The irritation is sustained by subsequent use of detergents and soaps. Interestingly, the skin all over the body may become sensitized so that an acute condition on the hands can lead to increased sensitivity of the skin on the back.

Irritant contact dermatitis can be a difficult problem to treat, and may last for a long time. Moreover, it can lead to the development of allergic contact dermatitis (see DERMATITIS, CONTACT). People who have experienced atopic dermatitis (see DERMATITIS, ATOPIC) as children are more susceptible to developing irritant contact dermatitis as adults.

Because of the similarity between irritant and allergic contact dermatitis, patch testing can help distinguish between them.

dermatitis, nickel An itchy skin reaction following contact with nickel, probably the most common form of dermatitis. Nickel, a shiny stainless metal, is often used in surface plating of metal objects, such as buttons, costume jewelry and kitchen equipment. It is also an element in many alloys, and is widely used in dentistry.

It is found 10 times more frequently in women than men, and is often triggered by ear piercing. For some reason, having the ears pierced (using earrings with nickel posts) causes subsequent rashes to appear in other areas of the body whenever the person touches objects containing nickel. Necklaces, bracelets, belt buckles and other jewelry that have never before caused a problem may suddenly cause a rash after the ears are pierced.

Nickel dermatitis is also associated with an increased risk of developing dermatitis of the hand. Those at high risk for developing an occupational nickel allergy include those coming in regular contact with the metal: restaurant workers, hairdressers, nurses, cashiers and metal-industry employees.

Prevention If you have newly pierced ears, wear only gold or steel posts until earlobes heal (about three weeks). Surgical steel is the best choice, and is available in some types of earrings specifically designed for sensitive skin.

Perspiration plays a big role in nickel dermatitis because it leaches out the nickel in nickel-plated jewelry. So, it is best to avoid the heat when wearing this type of jewelry. Buy only high-quality gold jewelry that is at least 14-karat gold; the lower the karat, the higher the percentage of nickel.

A few dermatologists go so far as to warn highly sensitive patients to avoid foods containing traces of nickel (such as coffee, beer, tea, apricots, chocolate, nuts etc.).

dermatitis, nummular Also known as nummular eczema, this condition usually occurs in adults, causing circular, itchy scaly patches anywhere on the body, very similar to RINGWORM (tinea).

Treatment Corticosteroid ointments may be applied to affected skin to help reduce inflammation. Nonirritating materials (such as cotton) should be worn next to the skin. Moisturizers, bath or shower oil and antihistamines also may be effective.

dermatitis papillaris capillitii Another name for ACNE KELOIDALIS.

dermatitis papulosa nigra Groups of small, very dark seborrheic keratoses that develop on the faces of black persons. This disorder occurs earlier in life than seborrheic keratoses in fair-skinned patients.

In this disorder, the number of keratoses increases as time goes on, although the lesions do not carry a risk of malignancy. Unlike warts, they do not spontaneously disappear.

Treatment The lesions may be removed by a variety of methods, but their removal may be followed by changes in pigment. Hyperpigmentation often results following CRYOSURGERY, since melanin-producing cells are easily destroyed. While cautery may be better tolerated, this technique must be performed gently to prevent scarring. Hypopigmentation is also a risk. Light-brown-skinned people often get hypopigmentation after treatment. Sometimes physicians elect to treat only one lesion at first, to assess how the patient's skin responds to the treatment technique.

dermatitis, perioral Tiny pimples and pustules around the mouth and usually found in women in their 20s and 30s. These lesions leave no scars.

Cause Excessive use of corticosteroid creams, fluorinated toothpastes, moisturizing creams, cosmetics and birth control pills have been linked to perioral dermatitis, but often the cause is unknown.

Treatment Oral tetracycline can cure the problem within two to eight weeks, although some patients need repeated courses of treatment. Recurrences are not uncommon. Alternatively, topical antibiotics such as clindamycin or erythromycin, topical SULFUR or SALICYLIC ACID may be prescribed.

dermatitis, pigmented purpuric lichenoid See GOUGEROT-BLUM SYNDROME.

dermatitis, radiation See RADIODERMATITIS.

dermatitis, seaweed A rash of bumpy red lesions caused by marine algae in the ocean. It is found only on the skin under the loose parts of bathing suits, and has been reported only from northeastern Hawaii.

Treatment Calamine lotion and, occasionally, systemic steroids are effective. Careful drying afer bathing is a good way to prevent problems. Antihistamines reduce itch and topical emollients may provide relief from symptoms.

dermatitis, seborrheic An extremely common form of ECZEMA that causes scaling around the nose, ears, scalp, mid-chest and along the eyebrows, it is often misdiagnosed by non-physicians as DRY SKIN. However, the flaking from this type of dermatitis is *not* caused by dryness. It is believed to have a genetic link, although how it is inherited is not clear. It is most common in males after puberty, and its incidence increases with age. Seborrheic dermatitis has also been observed in patients with Parkinson's disease, mental retardation and a range of neurologic disorders. Use of some drugs (such as neuroleptics) has been associated with the skin problem.

Untreated, dandruff may progress to seborrheic dermatitis. There may be PSORIASIS-like plaques and secondary infections as a result of scratching.

Treatment Treatment is similar to other eczemas. Use shampoos containing tar, sulfur, salicylic acid or selenium daily. Hydrocortisone 1 percent cream will control the skin condition on the face and chest. If shampoos don't work, try a steroid solution such as fluocinolone 0.01 percent applied to the scalp one or two times a day. Alternatively, ketoconazole 2 percent cream twice daily to the affected area may also be helpful. Systemic antibiotics may also be useful.

dermatofibroma A type of benign tumor arising from connective tissue cells, this skin NODULE is found most often on the arms and legs. Also known as histiocytoma cutis, it is composed of fibroblasts, COLLAGEN, capillaries and histiocytes.

Many patients with this type of skin lesion report some type of preceding trauma, such as an insect bite, scratch or a minor skin puncture. They occur at any age, although they usually appear in early adulthood through middle age. Most patients have only one or two lesions; infrequently, there are many tumors. Most of the lesions are slightly elevated and firm, although some may be depressed below the skin's surface. They may range in color from dusky pale to medium- or pinkish brown, with a smooth or rough surface. When squeezed, the skin over a tumor often dimples. Tumors may continue to grow slowly, once formed.

Treatment Because these tumors are completely benign, no treatment is necessary, although if the patient desires, they can be excised.

dermatofibrosarcoma protuberans An invasive tumor that, after excision, tends to recur in up to 75 percent of cases, although the malignancy rarely spreads to other parts of the body. More common in men in their 30s, these tumors usually appear on the upper trunk and shoulder.

Symptoms The condition begins as a slow-growing firm nodule, ranging from brown to dusky red.

Treatment After excision of large tumors, a SKIN GRAFT may be often necessary.

dermatoglyphics Patterns of skin ridges on the fingers, palms, toes and soles.

On the fingers, ridges occur in patterns of loops, whorls, arches and compounds (combinations of the first three). Fingerprint classifications are based on an analysis of these ridges. Fingerprints are accepted as a legal identification since no two individuals share the same pattern of ridges—not even identical twins.

dermatographia Literally "writing on the skin," this produces HIVES induced by mod-

erately firm stroking or scratching of the skin with a dull instrument that can last up to 30 minutes. This is a form of chronic hives that may be inherited and usually persists for life. Antihistamines (especially hydroxyzine) may help.

dermatologist A physician who specializes in diagnosing and treating skin problems. Dermatologists spend at least one year after medical school in a hospital practicing general medicine, then go on to complete at least three years in advanced training in dermatology. Dermatologists are experts in all aspects of the skin, including hair, nails and mucous membranes, and treat skin problems with medicine or surgery. They are carefully trained to understand how diseases of the skin can be related to many other, more general medical conditions.

Dermatologists treat common skin disorders such as ACNE, ECZEMA and PSORIASIS. They also diagnose and treat skin growths, warts, cysts and tumors. While all dermatologists treat skin cancer, some have extra training in the surgical management of skin cancer and limit their practice to the treatment of this disease. Others have expertise in skin laser surgery, while still others perform skin resurfacing with chemical peels, dermabrasion or laser skin resurfacing.

Many dermatologists perform some COSMETIC SURGERY. For example, they can remove moles, destroy small capillaries on the face and remove brown spots. Some inject COLLAGEN or fat to smooth out facial creases and WRINKLES. FACE-LIFTS or breast augmentations are less often performed by dermatologists.

Some dermatologists supply patients with lotions and creams that are tailored to each patient's skin care needs.

dermatology The study of a vast field of knowledge about the physiology and pathology of the skin and its appendages (hair, nails, sweat glands and oil glands). Robert Willan in England (1757–1812) was the first to publish and classify information about skin disease, which was further explored by Jean-Louis Alibert (1768–1837) in Paris, who considered each dermatosis as a specific branch of dermatology. But it was not until the discovery of the microscope that dermatologists were able to see the skin in all its structural and cellular detail. At the same time, the infant science of bacteriology revealed the secrets of infectious diseases like IMPETIGO and BOILS. By 1906 the spirochete causing SYPHILIS had been isolated, and in 1914 pellagra was shown to be a simple nutritional deficiency, although the missing vitamin (nicotinic acid) was not identified until the 1930s.

Today, the field of dermatology includes the investigation of disease (such as examining skin scrapings under a microscope), diagnosis and treatment, ranging from application of creams and ointments to dermabrasion, liposuction, surgical excision and laser surgery. In fact, dermatologists perform a wide variety of surgery in the treatment of skin diseases, from sophisticated plastic surgical excisions to Mohs' technique for histological tracking of the furthest reaches of skin cancer. The newest surgical techniques include liposuction for skin contour control and the use of lasers for treating a variety of skin growths and marks, including tattoos and PORT-WINE STAINS.

Dermatology Foundation A foundation for members of national and regional dermatological societies and board-certified dermatologists that raises funds to help control skin disease through research, improved education and better patient care. The group stimulates interest of graduate physicians in academic dermatology, and supports basic and clinical investigations.

Established in 1964, the foundation has 3,300 members. Its publications include the quarterly *Dermatology Focus*, a membership activities newsletter that produces research articles and lists recipients of foundation awards, fellowships and grants; the quarterly *Progress in Dermatology*, a bulletin containing research reports; and an annual report, *Stewardship Report*. For the address, see Appendix E.

dermatome A part of the mesoderm in the early embryo that forms the deeper layer of the skin (dermis). The entire surface of the body forms an interlocking web of dermatomes, the pattern of which is very similar from one person to another. Loss of sensation in a dermatome means that a particular nerve root has been damaged.

"Dermatome" also refers to a surgical instrument for cutting different thicknesses of skin for use in skin grafting.

dermatomyositis A rare (sometimes fatal) disease involving skin inflammation and a skin rash. One of a group of autoimmune disorders, dermatomyositis is sometimes associated with an underlying cancer of an internal organ. It is most often found in middle-aged women.

About half the patients recover fully within two years; in about 30 percent of cases the condition persists, and the remaining 20 percent experience a progressive and sometimes fatal form of the disease that affects lungs and organs.

Symptoms Red rash on nose and cheeks, followed by purple discoloration on eyelids, and a red rash on the knees, knuckles and elbows. Muscles begin to weaken, becoming stiff and painful, and the skin over the muscles of the shoulders and pelvis becomes thickened. Other symptoms include weight loss, nausea and fever. The role of sunlight in this disease has not been thoroughly examined, but in certain patients, exposure to sunlight may worsen skin symptoms and probably systemic symptoms as well.

Treatment Corticosteroid and immunosuppressant drugs are prescribed to control the skin inflammation and are used in combination with physical therapy to prevent muscles from scarring and shrinking.

dermatopathology The study of the microscopic appearance of diseased skin.

dermatophagy The practice (by amphibians and reptiles) of eating their own skin. While scientists originally believed this was a rare practice, a new survey of more than 100 zoos and aquariums around the world has documented the practice in 285 species of frogs, lizards, salamanders, snakes, turtles, tuatara and caecilians. Herpetologists believe the animals eat their skin for the extra protein, although some argue that the practice protects the vulnerable animals from predators by eliminating the evidence of their presence.

Because animals can eat their skin very quickly, there had been few reports of dermatophagy until researchers at the Smithsonian Institution sought help from animal caretakers for the new data. They note, however, that observations still need to be made in the wild, since captivity may affect the skin-eating behavior.

dermatophytes Superficial fungal infections that affect the skin, hair and nails, usually caused by the fungi *Microsporum, Epidermophyton* or *Trichophyton*. This type of infection can be spread by personal contact from person to person or from an animal to a person. It usually has a Latin name using the term "TINEA" (ringworm) with the part of the body affected (such as "tinea pedis" for ATHLETE'S FOOT). Although there are many different kinds of dermatophytes, seven species cause more than 90 percent of all infections.

dermatophytid A skin eruption caused by hypersensitivity to a DERMATOPHYTE (type of fungus) such as ringworm.

dermatophytosis A type of fungus infection (also called TINEA) caused by *Trichophyton, Epidermophyton* or *Microsporum sp.*

dermatosis cinecienta Another name for a progressive pigmented disorder called ERYTHEMA DYSCHROMICUM PERSTANS.

dermis The lower layer of the skin beneath the EPIDERMIS. The dermis is comprised of fibers called COLLAGEN and ELASTIN, complex proteins responsible for the support and elasticity of the skin. It is collagen and elastin that enable your skin to snap back into shape after being stretched or pulled.

Also found in the dermis are tiny twig-like sensory nerve endings that allow a person to sense touch, temperature, vibration and pain.

Each square of dermis contains 15 feet of small blood vessels that provide nutrients and oxygen; it is the constriction and dilation of these vessels in response to extremes of heat and cold that help regulate temperature throughout the body. It is also these vessels that are responsible for keeping your skin healthy and removing harmful metabolic wastes.

Interestingly, nutrients can *not* be easily supplied to the skin by applying substances to the skin surface. This means that slathering on fruits, vegetables, cream, lotion or vitamins on your skin in the hope of getting the substance into the skin may be unproductive. Certain substances, however, can penetrate into the skin where they are biologically active.

dermoid Resembling the skin.

desquamation The continuous process of shedding of the skin. This is an important factor that limits the bacterial population on the skin, since epithelial cells colonized with bacteria are always being shed. The entire external layer of the skin is almost completely replaced every three to four weeks. Dead cells contain large amounts of keratin (a fibrous portion that forms the outer barrier of the skin).

developers Oxidizing agents (usually containing HYDROGEN PEROXIDE) that supply oxygen to the molecules of hair dye so that a particular shade is achieved.

DHA See DIHYDROXYACETONE.

diaper rash Known medically as diaper dermatitis, this is a common condition of infancy caused by skin irritation from substances in feces or urine. It is probably worsened by friction from rough diapers and prolonged wetting of the skin.

While babies vary in their susceptibility to diaper rash, skin inflammation in some infants can be severe. In general, breastfed babies have a lower incidence of diaper rash than bottle-fed babies, and the resistance continues long after the baby has been weaned. In some infants, diaper rash is the first indication of sensitive skin heralding a long series of later skin problems, such as ECZEMA.

About half of all cases of diaper rash go away by themselves within a day. The other half of these rashes may last up to 10 days or more.

Symptoms The skin appears reddened at first and, as the rash becomes chronic, the skin becomes dry and scaly. In chronic severe cases, the skin is covered with papules, blisters and erosions that can be mistaken for bacterial infection or even burns. A long-term rash that won't clear may be caused by a candida (fungus) infection, PSORIASIS or atopic eczema.

Prevention Prevention of this skin condition is always better than trying to cure it once it appears. The aim in a preventive diaper rash program is to keep the baby's skin as dry as possible for as long as possible. Since a newborn breast-fed baby urinates about 20 times a day and has a bowel movement after each

feeding, this can be a major undertaking! Still, diapers should be changed as often as possible followed by a water-repellant emollient with each change. (If possible, leave the diaper off at least an hour a day).

Critics still disagree on the relative merits of cloth vs. disposable diapers and diaper rash, with each contingent asserting that only one type of diaper prevents diaper rash. Recent research has indicated that diapers containing absorbent gelling material significantly reduces skin wetness, leaving skin closer to the normal pH than either conventional disposable diapers or cloth products. Proponents of cloth diapers insist that the cloth allows for more air circulation to the skin and, because the cloth diapers do not hold as much water, these type of diapers tend to get changed more often than disposable diapers do.

While it's important to keep the diaper area clean, drying sensitive baby bottoms with a towel can be irritating to some infants. Experts suggest drying irritated bottoms with a hair dryer *set on low*; afterward, apply zinc oxide ointments (diaper rash ointments). Since a baby's urine is sterile and clean, the infant's bottom need not be cleaned after urination—only patted or air-dried.

If you *do* use cloth diapers, try adding one ounce of vinegar to one gallon of water during the final rinse water to help match the cloth's pH to baby's skin, and make sure the cloth diapers are well rinsed. Diaper rash enzymes are most active in an environment with high pH (often found in cloth diapers after washing). Cloth diapers provided by diaper services are usually very close to a baby's pH level, and are usually tested at regular intervals to ensure their products' pH level.

Treatment Some of the oldest advice is still the best in this case—expose the rash to air; take off the diaper and lay the baby face down (with face turned to one side) on towels over a waterproof sheet, as long as you are there to watch the infant. Protective ointment (zinc oxide or "diaper rash ointment") will help prevent and clear the problem. In severe cases, a mild corticosteroid drug is necessary to control inflammation, often given in combination with an antifungal drug to kill any organisms that might cause THRUSH.

diascope A glass or clear plastic plate (usually a microscopic slide) placed against the skin to observe the skin after the blood vessels been compressed. This diagnostic tool is used to blanch away any redness, which allows the underlying color of any lesion to be seen.

diet and skin Experts generally agree that a good healthy diet is beneficial to a good, healthy skin; they also stress that ACNE is *not* caused by a diet rich in oil, chocolate or seafood.

A wide variety of studies has shown links with certain vitamins and healthy skin. Vitamin A is important for healthy, normal growth of skin cells. Studies now being conducted with natural and synthetic derivatives of vitamin A may soon reveal that the vitamin holds the key to bolstering the skin's immune system, preventing acne and skin cancer. These derivatives, called retinoids, may someday be to skin diseases what antibiotics are to infections.

In addition, some B-complex vitamins and zinc deficiencies cause scaling and redness, especially around the mouth and nose.

Dietary deficiencies can also profoundly affect your skin. For example, vitamin C deficiency may result in SCURVY, causing bleeding gums, swelling skin and large black and blue bruises over the body. (In fact, the British sailors are nicknamed "limeys" because during the heyday of the great sailing vessels, they were fed limes and lemons to prevent scurvy). Vitamin C is also important in

the production of COLLAGEN, the main supportive protein of skin.

A deficiency of vitamin A can cause acne and other skin problems. Extremely low levels of vitamin B_2 (riboflavin), B_3 (niacin) and B_6 are linked to skin inflammations and mucous membrane sores.

Severe malnutrition (such as experienced in Third World countries) can cause changes in color and texture of hair and skin, and low iron levels result in yellowish, pallid skin.

At the other end of the spectrum, too *many* nutrients can also cause skin problems. Excessive intake of iodine (from too much iodized salt or shellfish) can cause breakouts of deep pustules and cysts on the face and back. Too much beta-carotene (from some vegetables or carrots or supplements) can turn skin yellow; high levels of vitamin A can cause dryness and cracking skin and mucous membranes.

dihydroxyacetone (DHA) The FDA-approved active ingredient in topical SELF-TANNING PRODUCTS (lotions and creams). This is a harmless skin dye that reacts with an amino acid in the skin or sweat to produce a temporary tan that flakes off as you shed skin.

Back in the 1960s, the pioneering self-tanning lotions used concentrations of DHA as high as 5 percent, which caused an unsightly orange tone. Since then, DHA concentration and formulations have been perfected, and companies can offer different shades of tans for different skin tones. Because DHA is a dye and not a bronzer, the color lasts longer and needs to be reapplied only every three or four days; however, this longer-lasting color could be a drawback if the consumer doesn't like the color of the tan. The "tan" is lost as the stained cells of the horny layer are shed or washed off. In general, several coats are needed to achieve the desired color.

Consumers should understand that unless these products contain a SUNBLOCK, they offer no real protection from the sun. Several of these products are now being combined with a sunscreen.

DIN The European equivalent of SPF (sun protection factor), the rating system for sunscreen products. DIN stands for Deutsches Institut fur Normung, the company that developed the European rating system. The DIN rating system uses lower numbers than the American SPF system for equivalent sun protection. For example, SPF 12 is equal to DIN 9; SPF 19 is equal to DIN 15.

diphenhydramine An antihistamine drug used to treat HIVES; it may be given as an injection to treat anaphylactic shock (a severe allergic reaction).
Adverse effects Possible side effects include drowsiness, dry mouth and blurred vision.

discoid lupus erythematosus (DLE) A chronic type of lupus erythematosus that usually affects exposed areas of the skin. The more serious and potentially fatal form (SYSTEMIC LUPUS ERYTHEMATOSUS, or SLE) affects many systems of the body, including the skin, joints, kidneys and nervous system.
Symptoms In DLE, a rash starts as one or more red, circular, thickened areas that later scar. The lesions are reddened with follicular plugs, atrophy, scaling and spidery veins. They may be found on the face, behind the ears and on the scalp, sometimes causing permanent hair loss. Lesions can also occur on other parts of the body. Individuals with DLE tend to be photosensitive.

Although one-fifth of SLE patients also experience these discoid lesions less than 5 percent of patients with DLE ever develop SLE.
Cause This is an autoimmune disorder in which the body's immune system attacks a variety of tissues as though they were foreign, causing inflammation.
Treatment There is no cure; treatment aims at reducing inflammation and alleviating

symptoms. It is essential to use sun screens, and avoid the sun whenever possible. The use of a potent topical corticosteroid or an injection into the lesion is appropriate, since these lesions often cause permanent scarring or hair loss if left untreated. Otherwise, antimalarial agents (such as hydroxychloroquine) may help. Quinacrine or DAPSONE may also be effective for DLE.

dishpan hands See CHAPPED HANDS.

DLE See DISCOID LUPUS ERYTHEMATOSUS.

dressings Protective bandages over wounds that may be used to control bleeding, prevent infection or absorb secretions. Dressings may be sterile or nonsterile. Sterile dressings are used to avoid infection, and should be absorbent enough so the skin around the wound doesn't become moist, which could encourage infection. Unless the wound must be cleaned often, the dressing should not be disturbed.

Skin dressings also are used to keep topical medications in place, and to relieve itching or pain. The *occlusive dressing* is a very effective means to increase the local skin temperature and hydration, enhancing the absorption of topical medication. Occlusive dressings also promote the retention of moisture, which stops the medication from evaporating. In an occlusive dressing, an airtight plastic film (such as plastic kitchen wrap) is placed over the medicated skin. Plastic surgical tape containing corticosteroid in the adhesive layer can be cut to size and applied to individual lesions. Occlusive dressings should be removed for 12 of every 24 hours in order to avoid local skin atrophy, bandlike streaks, telangiectasia (small red lesions caused by dilated blood vessels), inflamed hair follicles, nonhealing ulcers and systemic absorption of corticosteroids.

Wet dressings are compresses soaked in water or saline, used for oozing, weeping, crusted, eroded or ulcerated skin, that are usually applied for 10 to 30 minutes three or four times a day. Evaporation from the dressing soothes and dries by cooling the skin surface.

drug reactions Skin reactions are some of the most common side effects of a wide range of drugs, and may be the first sign of a generalized toxic reaction. And yet, while skin symptoms of a drug reaction are quite common, scientists don't really understand the mechanism underlying most of the effects.

Skin rash is the most common adverse skin reaction to a drug, occurring in 2 to 3 percent of patients. The rash is characterized by a fine, papular eruption that usually appears within the first seven to 10 days after the drug is begun. Antibiotics and allopurinol may induce rashes two or more weeks after they are started. Drug rashes often begin in areas of trauma or pressure, such as on the backs of bedridden patients or on the extremities of patients who are not bedridden. Drugs most frequently found to cause a rash are antimicrobial agents, blood products, nonsteroidal anti-inflammatory drugs (NSAIDs) and central nervous system drugs. According to one survey, drugs with reaction rates above 1 percent include trimethoprim-sulfamethoxazole, ampicillin, amoxicillin, semisynthetic penicillins, penicillin, red blood cells and cephalosporins.

The risk of a drug-related rash is higher in certain groups: 35 to 50 percent more women than men, 50 to 80 percent of patients with infectious mononucleosis who take ampicillin. The risk of a drug rash is much higher in patients taking ampicillin and allopurinol together than either drug alone. Reasons behind the development of this rash are unknown.

Most cutaneous drug eruptions will fade away within two weeks after the drug is stopped, leaving no permanent scars or dis-colorations. However, some skin reactions may be life threatening, including anaphylaxis, toxic epidermal necrolysis, vasculitis, severe ERYTHEMA MULTIFORME and exfoliative erythroderma. Usually the wider the area of affected skin, the longer it will take for side effects to fade.

Hives are the second most common allergic skin reaction to drugs, and are most often caused by antibiotics, blood products, radiocontrast agents, NSAIDs and opiates. The hives usually last for less than 24 hours and are replaced by new lesions in new places.

Allergic contact dermatitis to topical medications is common, with papules, blisters and vesicles. Patch testing may be used to demonstrate contact hypersensitivity to a suspected topical medication. Agents found in topical medications that are often associated with allergic contact dermatitis include neomycin, benzocaine, ethylenediamine, diphenhydramine (in Caladryl), and parabens (preservatives found in many topical preparations, including some corticosteroids). Neomycin is the most sensitizing of currently-used topical antibiotics; approximately 5 percent of people have a sensitivity to it.

Complications There is concern that if a patient develops a rash following use of a certain drug, then continued use of the medication may induce a life-threatening eruption or an exfoliative erythroderma. Patients who have developed rashes due to sulfonamides, penicillin or carbamazine have been desensitized by withdrawing the drug until the rash resolves, and then restarting the medication gradually, increasing doses until therapeutic doses are achieved.

dry skin Also known as "xerosis," dry skin usually begins in the 30s and worsens as a person ages. Dry skin may come and go depending on the weather: it's worse in the cold, and it is related to a decrease in the relative humidity and dry air from central heating. If the dryness worsens, the skin may seem irritated to the point of developing into DERMATITIS, with redness and skin fissures. One of the worst aspects of dry skin is the itch, which may increase during stressful periods.

Treatment Daily bathing in lukewarm water with an added bath oil will also help to add water to the skin. The most effective emollients are often those people find least acceptable—semisolid oils that work to prevent evaporation, instead of moisturizers, which immediately soften the skin but can't seal the water into the EPIDERMIS. Studies have indicated that petrolatum and lanolin are very effective at abolishing dry skin within two weeks. There are many excellent moisturizers that, used daily, can prevent progressive dry skin. Relatively new moisturizers containing lactic acid, which helps to draw moisture from the dermis into the epidermis, may be effective.

Drysol A prescription ANTIPERSPIRANT useful in patients with severe HYPERHIDROSIS (excessive sweating). Drysol is the brand name for aluminum chloride hexahydrate, 20 percent solution in absolute alcohol. It can be used under the arms, on palms or soles, and is applied under plastic film at bedtime. Frequent use may cause irritation. See also DEODORANTS.

duck bumps See GOOSEFLESH.

Duhring's disease See DERMATITIS, HERPETIFORMIS.

dyshydrotic eczema See POMPHOLYX.

dyskeratosis congenita Almost all cases of this rare inherited X-linked recessive disorder have been found in males. By age five or six,

the child experiences blistering of palms and nail beds, leading to a loss of nail plates and atrophy of the ends of the fingers and toes. There is a very high incidence of carcinomas and leukemias. In the teenage years, hyperpigmentation surrounding a central lack of pigment appears on the face and trunk and patients may be photosensitive.

Treatment There is no treatment other than relieving the skin symptoms. Patients should avoid known cancer-causing substances, including ultraviolet light and tobacco.

dysplastic nevus syndrome See NEVUS SYNDROME, DYSPLASTIC.

Dystrophic Epidermolysis Bullosa Research Association of America An association for people with EPIDERMOLYSIS BULLOSA (EB, a group of inherited disorders of the skin characterized by blisters caused by minimal trauma) and their families. The association raises funds to promote and support research into the cause, nature and treatment of epidermolysis bullosa in all its forms and to provide practical advice, guidance, support and other assistance.

The group distributes educational material to the public and to physicians, and campaigns for federal funding for biomedical research of EB and related disorders. It operates a library, offers children's services and conducts educational programs.

Founded in 1979, the group hosts a semiannual conference and maintains a computerized database.

Its publications include the semiannual *EB Currents* and a semiannual newsletter, *EB Reporter*, which covers research, treatment and legislation about EB, and also includes regional news and a pen pals section. For address, see Appendix D.

E

ear repair See OTOPLASTY.

eau-de-cologne A light, fresh scent that can be reapplied often. It is not as strong as pure perfume (parfum), because it is diluted with water. Eau-de-cologne has a 2–6 percent concentration of pure perfume, compared to eau-de-toilette (4–8 percent) and eau-de-parfum (8–15 percent). See also FRAGRANCE.

ecchymosis The medical term for a BRUISE, a blue or purple hemorrhage in the skin or mucous membrane.

eccrine gland See SWEAT GLANDS.

econazole (Ecostatin) An antifungal drug used to treat RINGWORM of the scalp, ATHLETE'S FOOT, JOCK ITCH, nail fungus, candidiasis and others. Available in powder, cream, lotion, ointment or vaginal tablet, the medication acts quickly (often within two days), killing fungi by damaging the fungal cell wall. The drug may take up to eight weeks to cure the infection. It is rare, but the drug may cause skin irritation.

ecthyma A deep ulcerative skin infection caused by bacteria (usually group A streptococci or *Streptococcus aureus*) that often results in scarring, usually found on legs and protected areas of the body. The condition begins with one lesion which enlarges and encrusts; beneath this crust is a pus-filled "punched ulcer."

Children are more commonly affected with ecthyma, which is usually associated with poor hygiene and malnutrition and minor skin injuries from trauma, insect bites or SCABIES. The condition commonly occurs during unfavorable conditions, such as war or captivity.

Treatment Erythromycin or dicloxacillin is administered. The lesions should also be soaked, and crusts removed.

ectoderm The outermost of the three primary germ (living substance capable of developing into an organ) layers of the embryo. From it are developed the EPIDERMIS and epidermal tissues (such as nails, hair and skin glands), as well as the nervous system, the external sense organs (eye, ear etc.) and the mucous membranes of mouth and anus.

ectodermal dysplasia A genetic birth defect usually causing an abnormal development in the outer layer of cells in the embryo. It is characterized by poorly functioning sweat glands, sparse hair follicles, abnormal hair texture, absence of hair and skin oils, disfigured finger and toe nails. Other symptoms include hearing or visual problems, mental retardation, cleft palate and urinary tract problems. With good care, patients can live normal lives. For address, see Appendix D; see also NATIONAL FOUNDATION FOR ECTODERMAL DYSPLASIAS.

ectoparasite A parasite that lives on the skin, getting nourishment either from the skin or by sucking the host's blood; various types of ticks, lice, mites and some types of fungi may occasionally be ectoparasites on humans. (Parasites living *inside* the body are called "endoparasites.") Diseases caused by these parasites include SCABIES and PEDICULOSIS (louse infestation).

ectothrix A fungus that grows outside the hair shaft. See also ENDOTHRIX.

eczema A superficial inflammation of the skin primarily affecting the epidermis (outer skin layer) that causes itching and a red rash often accompanied by blisters that weep and then crust. This may be followed by scaling, thickening or discoloration of the area.

Eczema has many forms with two main divisions—eczematous dermatitis, which is caused by external factors, and endogenous eczema, occurring without any obvious outside cause. Classification of endogenous eczema is based on its appearance and site. The five types are *atopic* (commonly found in childhood and sometimes associated with a family history of allergy, also called atopic dermatitis); *discoid* (small well-defined areas, also called nummular eczema or nummular dermatitis); POMPHOLYX (found on hands and feet, formerly called dyshidrotic pompholyx); *seborrheic* (scaly plaques in areas of the greatest sebum production, also called seborrheic dermatitis) and *varicose* (develops on the legs in association with poor circulation). Other types of eczematous diseases include asteatotic eczema (due to overdrying of the skin) and polymorphic light eruption. See also DERMATITIS, ATOPIC; DERMATITIS, NUMMULAR; DERMATITIS, HAND; DERMATITIS, STASIS; DERMATITIS, SEBORRHEIC.

Treatment Treatment of eczema depends on the cause, but it usually includes the use of locally applied corticosteroids. Creams, lotions and antihistamines may help stop itching. Coal-tar ointments are often used when the problem has persisted for months or years and the skin has become thickened and leathery. To reduce scratching and irritation, soothing ointments should be covered by a dressing and absorbent, nonirritating materials should be worn next to the skin. Avoid fabrics such as wool, silk and rough synthetics.

Children with atopic eczema should be bathed quickly with a mild neutral soap no more than three times weekly. Bath oil may prevent excess skin drying, and fingernails should be clipped to decrease damage from scratching.

eczema, atopic See DERMATITIS, ATOPIC.

eczema, herpeticum A rare skin condition caused by the herpes simplex virus infection in a patient with a preexisting skin condition, such as DERMATITIS. See also HERPES, ECZEMA. It is characterized by extensive blistering, oozing and crusting. The condition usually remains only on the skin.
Treatment Administration of acyclovir is effective. Treat symptoms by applying compresses and bathing.

egg Commercially produced skin care products containing egg do not help the skin, since the proteins in egg cannot be utilized by the skin in this way. However, a fresh egg mask can create a film on the face, locking in water and allowing the skin to build up a supply of water, which will temporarily soften dry skin.

Ehlers-Danlos syndrome A hereditary group of disorders in which there is a deficiency or defect of normal COLLAGEN (the most important protein in the body) that causes easily bruising, stretchy, thin skin. Known medically as "cutis hyperelastica," the disease is also characterized by paperthin scars from wounds that have failed to heal properly.

Contortionists in circus side shows are often victims of Ehlers-Danlos syndrome, since the disease allows the skin to be stretched far beyond its usual length; the skin can still resume its original shape after distention.
Symptoms Patients with this group of disorders do not become obviously distorted until late in life, when they may begin to experience significant cosmetic deformity caused by loose skin, joint changes and scars resulting from the skin's fragility. Gaping wounds may develop from the slightest injuries, and surgical sutures don't hold well. Often, prominent

scars appear on sites of frequent injury, such as the forehead, chin, knees and shins.

Repeated tearing and bruises may cause skin to "outbag" and form pseudotumors. Joints may be hyperextendable; the fingers may often be able to bend 90 degrees backwards, and the thumb can be bent back to the wrist. Other characteristics include soft handshakes, high-arched palate, long neck and sloping shoulders, with possible spine deformities. Common injuries include dislocations of the kneecap, hips and temporal mandibular joints; eventually these can lead to arthritis of the large joints and spine.

Cause The syndrome includes a family of 10 or more separate genetic disorders with varying inheritance patterns, some dominant, some recessive and some X-linked. Four have been linked to specific enzyme deficiencies.

Treatment There is no known treatment, but unnecessary injuries should be avoided. Surgery of various defects may be attempted, but there is a danger of bleeding and poor wound healing. Patients should protect fragile skin and joints, and avoid unnecessary injuries or extending skin, ligaments or joints. Female patients should understand that pregnancy carries a serious risk of hemorrhage.

Outlook Despite the lack of treatment, most patients have a normal life expectancy. Milder cases may correct themselves with aging, but other patients experience a progressive decline into severe arthritis and skin looseness over distorted joints. Death may result from a number of related internal organ problems.

elastic fibers Connective tissue fibers that help to give the skin elasticity so that it returns to its normal position after stretching.

elastin The protein which (together with COLLAGEN) is the primary substance in connective tissue. While collagen gives connective tissue strength, elastin gives skin its elastic properties, allowing the skin to stretch and spring back into place. Elastin becomes less elastic with age; as the skin and subcutaneous fat thins with age, the skin becomes looser. Elastin can be further damaged by extensive sun exposure, which can lead to wrinkling.

In cosmetic products, elastin cannot make your skin tighter. Used as a moisturizer it is thought to form a film on the skin that helps lock in moisture.

elastomas A rare type of CONNECTIVE TISSUE NEVI characterized by overgrowth and distortion of the elastic fibers of the skin. Also known as "NEVUS ELASTICUS OF LEWANDOWSKY," this type of nevus is usually found as a collection of smooth skin-colored papules forming patches and plaques, most often on the trunk. No treatment is necessary.

elastosis Degeneration of elastic tissue. It is most often seen as the result of long-standing sun exposure in photo-aged skin.

elastosis perforans serpiginosa A disorder in which the skin is perforated, as though the body were trying to push out defective elastin, causing a circular or wavy indented lesion. The syndrome is found in a variety of connective tissue disorders, such as EHLERS-DANLOS SYNDROME, Marfan's syndrome, Down's syndrome, ACROGERIA and Rothmund-Thomson syndrome, although it may also occur without any accompanying disorder.

The syndrome may be inherited and usually appears during the 20s or 30s; male patients outnumber women 4 to 1.

Causes In addition to the above associated syndromes, this disorder has been associated with the administration of penicillamine for Wilson's disease or SCLERODERMA. (Penicillamine chelates copper, which prevents normal cross-linking of elastin). The disorder has also been reported to be associated with kidney disease.

Symptoms Lesions usually appear on the back of the neck or arms, although they may also appear on the face and lower extremities.

Treatment There is no satisfactory treatment for this syndrome; surgery may be attempted.

electrical injury Damage to the skin caused by the passage of an electric current through the body (and associated release of heat). More than 1,000 people die from electrical accidents in the United States each year, and many more are seriously injured. Because the internal tissues of the body are moist and salty, they are good electric conductors. On the other hand, dry skin provides good resistance. For this reason, a shock to someone in a full bathtub will probably be fatal, whereas someone who is standing dry outside the tub, and wearing rubber-soled shoes (that don't conduct electricity) is far less likely to be hurt by the same shock.

All shocks except for the most mild are likely to cause unconsciousness, but the extent of tissue damage depends on the size and type of current. Skin tissues become charred when larger currents enter and exit the body.

First aid for electrical injury

1. *DO NOT attempt any type of first aid until contact with the energy source is broken, and don't touch the victim with anything wet.*
2. Pull the plug out of the socket, or stand on a dry object and push the victim away from the source with a dry stick.
3. If the victim is unconscious and not breathing, start CPR.
4. If the victim *is* breathing, follow first-aid advice for burns and shock until an ambulance arrives.

---

electrodesiccation A dermatologic treatment method that destroys tissue by heat from a high-frequency electric current. The technique is used to treat a variety of skin lesions from SKIN TAGS, WARTS and precancerous changes in the skin to skin cancers. It may also be used to destroy small tumors.

In the technique (which is usually performed with a local anesthetic), the physician applies an electric probe to the tissue for one or two seconds; the current flows to and through the lesion, destroying the tissue. While this may be enough to destroy a small tumor, larger growths may also require curettage (See also CURETTAGE AND ELECTRODESICCATION).

electrolysis Use of an electric current to permanently remove excess body hair by destroying the hair's root bulb from which it grows. Although unwanted hair can be removed in a variety of ways (such as waxing, plucking, etc.), electrolysis is the only *permanent* hair removal method.

To remove a hair, a fine needle is inserted into the follicle along the hair shaft, destroying the root with a small electric current; the hair is then pulled out. The procedure may be slightly painful, but it is harmless when performed by trained operators. A number of sessions may be required until treatment is successful. At this point, there should be no more hair growth from that follicle, and minimal scarring.

Electrolysis can be performed on almost any part of the body, although it should be avoided on the lower margins of the eyebrows because the skin in this area is delicate and easily damaged. Some experts also disapprove of electrolysis in the armpits because of the danger of bacterial infection. Electrolysis is rarely used to remove leg hair because treatment of such large areas requires so many sessions that it is too time-consuming and expensive for most people.

Before selecting an electrologist, it is important to make sure the operator is fully trained, since incompetent electrolysis can cause permanent disfigurement.

electroporation A series of short electrical pulses that rearrange fatty layers in the outer skin layer to create temporary pores through which drugs may be administered. While the skin's outer layer of dead, flattened cells is an effective barrier to microbes, chemicals and other toxic agents, temporarily increasing the skin's permeability would be of benefit when it comes to administering certain medications.

Recently, researchers at Massachusetts Institute of Technology successfully achieved a 1,000-fold increase in skin permeability using the technique, which delivers a series of millisecond electrical pulses every five seconds.

Before the technique can be used in drug delivery, researchers will need to answer questions about the technique's safety and effectiveness. The technique may also be used to transport fluids out of the body (such as a noninvasive way to take blood samples).

elephantiasis Massive swelling of the legs caused by obstruction of the lymph vessels that prevents drainage of lymph from the surrounding tissues, resulting in inflammation and thickening of the vessel walls, eventually blocking them. The syndrome gets its name from the appearance of the skin of the legs, which resembles elephant hide. While the legs are most commonly affected, the arms, breasts, scrotum or vulva may also be affected. Worldwide, the most common cause of this chronic swelling is the tropical disease FILARIASIS, caused by infestation with worms (*Wuchereria bancrofti* and *Brugia malayi*).
Treatment There is no treatment that can reverse elephantiasis, although the massive enlargement of the scrotum may be relieved with surgery. Elastic bandages applied to the affected parts and the elevation of limbs may

help. Larval forms of the worms in the blood that cause filariasis are killed with diethylcarbamazine.

emollients Substances that soften and smooth the skin, helping to replace oils and prevent moisture loss. Common emollients present in almost all skin creams include LANOLIN, petrolatum, mineral oil and squalane. See also AGING AND THE SKIN.

emotion and the skin Many experts believe that emotion plays a role in all skin diseases, whether or not the cause of the disorder is a physical one. Emotional factors sometimes cause skin disease, and often can either reduce or intensify itching and pain—even when the physical disease itself remains unchanged.

The psychological stress of illness or a variety of personal and family problems are often exhibited outwardly as skin problems. For example, even though SHINGLES or recurrent genital herpes (see HERPES SIMPLEX) are caused by a virus, and PSORIASIS is hereditary, negative emotions can trigger the onset of these diseases—or worsen a condition that already exists. Stress has also been linked with increased ACNE breakouts and worsening of hives.

One study evaluated more than 4,500 people to determine the link between emotional stress and skin disorders, as well as the time it took for the stressful event to trigger the disorder. Emotions were found to trigger itching almost 100 percent of the time; hives, 68 percent; and psoriasis, 62 percent.

endothrix A dermatophyte (superficial fungus) whose growth and spore production are confined primarily within the hair shaft, without forming conspicuous spores on the outside of the hair. See also ECTOTHRIX.

entoderm The innermost of the three primary germ layers of the embryo, from which are derived the epithelium of the pharynx, respiratory tract, digestive tract, bladder and urethra.

ephelis   Another name for FRECKLE.

epidermis   The surface layer of the skin. This layer covers the DERMIS and contains the basal cell layer, STRATUM SPINOSUM, STRATUM GRANULOSUM, STRATUM LUCIDUM and STRATUM CORNEUM.

There are two major zones of the epidermis—an inner region of moist cells and an outer layer of flattened dead cells known as the "stratum corneum" (or horny layer).

In the epidermis, there are three layers of living cells—the basal, spinous and granular layers. The basal cells at the bottom of the dermis constantly divide, giving birth to daughter cells that begin to move toward the skin's surface, where they become part of the horny layer. It is this horny layer that protects against external chemical and antigen damage and inhibits injury from microbes, fungi, parasites or insects.

epidermoid cysts   There are two types of epidermoid cysts—epidermal and pilar cysts. *Epidermal cysts* may be found alone or in groups, most often on the face, neck, upper chest and back. As they enlarge, the skin thins and begins to look yellow white; if the cysts become infected the skin becomes red and tender. Ultimately, these cysts may rupture and drain pus.

Pilar cysts involve hair follicles and are much less common than the epidermal variety. They are found most often on the scalp, although they may also crop up alone or in groups on the face, neck and trunk. They look identical to an epidermal cyst, but they can be differentiated under the microscope by the appearance of the epithelium (tissue that covers the external surface of the body). Pilar cysts tend to be multiple and run in families.

Treatment   Both types of cysts must be completely removed or the epithelial sac must be destroyed; otherwise, the lesion may recur. Some lesions are completely cut out in a wedge excision, while in other cases the sac may be removed through a small overlying incision after drainage of the cyst.

epidermolysis bullosa   A rare inherited condition that loosens the outer layers of the skin, allowing the cells to be easily separated into its various layers. As a result, blisters form either spontaneously or after minor injury. The disorder is found primarily in young children and may range in severity from mild foot blistering in hot weather to widespread and severe blistering and scarring all over the body. In mild cases, there may be gradual improvement, but more seriously affected children may experience progressive serious disease.

Cause   Epidermolysis bullosa is a group of inherited defects. Some are autosomal dominant (each child of an affected parent has a 50 percent chance of inheriting the defect); others are autosomal recessive (each of the children of two unaffected carrier parents has a one in four chance of inheriting the defect).

Treatment   Even the slightest injury to the skin should be avoided. Wound care is essential once blisters or open sores develop. There is no specific treatment for this disorder.

epidermotropism   The infiltration of the epidermis (top-most layer of the skin) by lymphocytes.

epiloia   An acronym for TUBEROUS SCLEROSIS that designates "epilepsy, low intelligence and ADENOMA SEBACEUM."

epithelioma   Any tumor derived from EPITHELIUM.

epithelium   The cells that cover the entire surface of the body. The epithelium varies in cell type and thickness, according to its function in any particular area. There are three basic cell shapes: squamous (thin and flat), cuboidal (resembling a cube) and columnar (resembling a column). The skin consists of many layers of epithelium. Because it is constantly subject to trauma, the outermost layer of cells are dead and constantly being shed.

epsom salts Magnesium sulfate crystals used in baths to sooth the skin. It is effective in drying an oozing, inflamed area of skin and is also very effective as a soak for tired, sore muscles. To use, follow directions on package.

erysipelas Formerly called St. Anthony's fire, this is a contagious infection of the facial skin and subcutaneous tissue usually caused by group A streptococci and marked by rapid-spreading redness and swelling which is believed to enter the skin through a small lesion. While this disease is contagious, it does not produce huge epidemics like those of SCARLET FEVER.

Before the advent of antibiotics, this disease could be fatal (especially for infants and the elderly). Today, it is quickly controlled with prompt treatment.

Symptoms After a 5–7 day incubation period, the patient's skin feels tight, uncomfortable, itchy and red, with patches appearing most often on the face, spreading across the cheeks and bridge of the nose. The patient also may notice sudden high fever (above 100°F) with headache, malaise and vomiting. It also occurs on the scalp, genitals, hands and legs. Within the inflammation, pimples appear, blister, burst and crust over.

Treatment Penicillin and antibiotic relatives of penicillin are the usual choice of treatment, and should cure the infection within seven days. Bed rest, hot packs and aspirin for pain and fever may also help.

See also NECROTIZING FASCIITIS.

erythema Redness of the skin that may be caused by inflammation that may occur for a variety of reasons. Reddening of the skin is caused by an increased amount of blood in dilated blood vessels in the skin. Unlike a hemorrhage, the red skin color of erythema fades when the skin is compressed, since the blood is pushed out of the skin's vessels. In a hemorrhage, the blood remains in the tissue outside the blood vessels so that compression does not remove the blood, and the red color does not disappear.

A range of external factors may cause erythema, such as heat, sun rays, cold and chemical irritants. Internal causes may include hot flashes, blushing, histamine release, fever, hot drinks, alcohol or spices. Erythema also may be caused by a range of inflammatory skin conditions such as ACNE, DERMATITIS, ECZEMA, ERYSIPELAS and ROSACEA.

In addition, erythema is a symptom of disorders including ERYTHEMA MULTIFORME, ERYTHEMA NODOSUM, LUPUS ERYTHEMATOSUS, and FIFTH DISEASE. Erythema often occurs with other primary skin lesions such as macules, papules, nodules or surrounding blisters.

erythema ab igne A condition of reddened skin that may be itchy and dry that is caused by long-term exposure to direct heat, such as by holding a hot water bottle against the abdominal skin for too long. In the past, it caused the typical telangiectasia (distended blood capillary vessels) and red-brown discoloration on the legs of those who sat in front of open fires or coal stoves in Great Britain and Europe. The condition became less common with the development of central heating. In the United States, the rising popularity of space heaters, wood-burning stoves and fireplaces saw a resurgence in this syndrome. Erythema ab igne is also seen on the skin of glassblowers, bakers and kitchen workers. Chronic use of heating pads may also lead to this problem.

Treatment The dryness and itching may be eased by applying an EMOLLIENT; the redness will fade, although the telangiestasia and discoloration does not usually disappear completely.

Complication Erythema ab igne rarely may lead to skin (usually squamous cell) cancer. Examples of this sort of heat-related damage have been reported throughout the world; "kangri cancer of India" is caused by holding pots of coal next to the skin; kange cancer of China is caused by sleeping on hot bricks; kairo cancer of Japan is associated with benzene-burning flasks next to the skin, and Turf or peat fire cancer in Irish women was caused by sitting too close to a peat fire. These aggressive types of squamous cell cancers may appear after a latency period of 30 years.

erythema annulare centrificum   This is one of a group of "annular erythemas" characterized by expanding ring-shaped plaques. The lesions, which are usually found on the trunk, enlarge slowly. While the disorder can occur at any age, most patients are young adults when stricken. Symptoms may last for only a short time, or they may persist for decades, depending on the cause.

Causes This type of erythema may be associated with a dermatophyte infection, yeast infection (*Candida albicans*), blue cheese, parasitic bowel disease or autoimmune disorders.

Treatment Eliminate the cause (that is, the fungus or parasite). Erythema annulare centrifugum caused by a yeast infection has been cured following treatment with oral and vaginal nystatin (an antibiotic effective against fungi).

erythema chronicum migrans   See LYME DISEASE.

erythema dyschromicum perstans   This is a progressive pigmented disorder of unknown cause that is one of the group of "reactive erythemas." It has also been called "ashy dermatosis" because of the characteristic slate-gray color of patients' skin.

Other than the ashy appearance of the skin, there are few symptoms; patients usually are dark-skinned individuals of Latin American heritage. Some researchers suspect that the pigment changes represent a post-inflammatory hyperpigmentation. The condition is chronic and tends to spread.

Symptoms Many slate-gray macules and patches develop over the trunk, arms and legs; the scalp, palms, soles and mucous membranes are usually not affected.

Treatment There is no effective treatment, but makeup can cover cosmetically unattractive areas. Deliberate suntanning can also mask the lesions.

erythema gyratum repens   One of a group of disorders called "annular erythemas" characterized by a red annula (ring-like rash). There are several different kinds of erythemas, caused by different things and resulting in different reactions.

Erythema gyratum repens causes an erythema (redness) in a wood-grain pattern that is usually (although not always) associated with cancer, most often of the breast, lung, uterus or upper gastrointestinal tract. This rare reactive erythema begins with an itchy rash, found mostly on the trunk, arms and legs, characterized by large lesions that flow together. The eruptions often look like coils of rope running parallel to each other, or growth rings on a tree. In about 60 percent of cases, the lesions occur before the cancer is diagnosed; in the other 40 percent of cases, erythema gyratum repens is diagnosed at the same time or shortly after the cancer diagnosis.

Treatment Treating the underlying cancer usually results in complete disappearance of the eruption. While topical therapy is of little benefit, emollients may help relieve the itch.

erythema infectiosum   See FIFTH DISEASE.

erythema marginatum   This type of reactive erythema is associated with rheumatic fever, a delayed complication of the upper respiratory tract caused by hemolytic streptococci, and characterized by rapidly changing ring-shaped red patches. The lesions tend to appear on the trunk, changing in size and shape, fading and reappearing over a matter of months. The syndrome is becoming less common with the decline in rheumatic fever cases.

In addition to the reddish lesions, patients usually have signs of active rheumatic fever including arthritis and fever, etc.

Treatment The skin symptoms do not itch and do not require topical treatment, but rheumatic fever requires immediate attention.

erythema multiforme An acute inflammation of the skin and mucous membranes characterized by a distinctive lesion called the "target lesion." Erythema multiforme literally means "skin redness of many varieties." Traditionally, the condition has been divided into major and minor forms (the latter is known as STEVENS-JOHNSON SYNDROME.)

Erythema multiforme is most common in women in their mid-20s; the characteristic rash, which consists of a number of target lesions, is self-limiting, but may recur in up to 37 percent of cases, especially when caused by the HERPES SIMPLEX virus.

Symptoms *Erythema multiforme minor* is usually preceded by malaise, fever, headache, sore throat and cough for seven to 10 days. Target lesions then appear on the skin of palms and soles for three to five days and last up to two weeks. The target lesion may appear abruptly or slowly develop over two days, beginning as a pale central area surrounded by one or more rings of erythema; the center may occasionally blister. Lesions usually heal without scarring. Occasionally, erythema multiforme minor does not cause a target lesion, but instead produces hive-like plaques.

Erythema multiforme major is a more severe condition, beginning with an initial illness of fever, malaise and prostration followed by an explosive eruption of target lesions over the body and mucous membranes, with severe ulceration, inflammation and bleeding in the eyes, mouth, nasal passages and genitals. Appearance of these symptoms is a dermatologic emergency. Secondary infection is common; 20 percent of patients experience significant pain, eye problems, breathing problems and difficulty maintaining oral fluid intake. Diagnosed most often among children, fluid and electrolyte imbalance or breathing problems can be fatal in 3 to 15 percent of patients. Involvement of the conjunctiva of the eyes may cause severe eye damage that can result in blindness. If the patient survives, there may be problems related to scarring in the eyes other mucous membranes.

Cause The etiology of erythema multiforme is not well understood, but it is believed to be a hypersensitivity reaction to a variety of substances. It may be caused by a drug reaction from penicillin, sulfonamides, salicylates or barbiturates. Drug-associated erythema multiforme may occur at any age, and is usually seen one to three weeks after first taking the offending drug.

Alternatively, it may be associated with a viral or bacterial infection, radiation therapy, internal disease, chemical exposure, vaccination or pregnancy. Herpes virus–associated erythema multiforme is found most often in teenagers and young adults; the minor form usually occurs 10 days after an acute eruption with either type 1 or type 2 herpes virus.

Half of all cases have no apparent cause.

Treatment In mild cases, no treatment may be required and the condition will fade away within two to three weeks. If no cause can be found, symptoms are treated and supportive care may include wet dressings or soaks and painkillers. If possible, however, the underlying cause of erythema multiforme should be diagnosed and treated. Erythema multiforme caused by a drug reaction is treated by stopping the medication. Antihistamines are not effective against this condition.

Short courses of topical corticosteroid drugs are given to relieve the inflammation of erythema's minor form, although there is little support in the literature for this treatment.

Herpes virus-associated erythema multiforme is treated with daily doses of oral acyclovir.

The severe (major) form of the condition is treated with painkillers, fluids and sedatives. Lesions may be treated with wet compresses; extensive erosions should be treated as a third-degree burn. Use of corticosteroid drugs in the severe form is controversial, although often given despite a lack of controlled studies proving their effectiveness. These patients usually respond to treatment, but they may become seriously ill if shock or systemic inflammation sets in. IV fluids and electrolyte replacement may be necessary; mouth lesions may be treated with a topical anesthetic, and petrolatum or other ointments may reduce cracking of dry lips.

erythema nodosum An inflammatory skin disease associated with reddish purple swellings typically on the lower legs that also may be a result of another illness, such as SARCOIDOSIS, inflammatory bowel disease, collagen disease, lymphoma, leukemia or from drug hypersensitivity or infectious agent. It occurs most often in women between ages 20 and 50, although the disease can appear in both sexes at any age.

Pain may be severe and disabling, but permanent problems from this disease are rare. Lesions usually disappear within one or two months, although recurrences are common. Even when the cause is not known, the prognosis for recovery is good.

Cause Streptococcal throat infection is the most common underlying cause in the United States, although erythema nodosum is also frequently associated with tuberculosis and SARCOIDOSIS elsewhere in the world. Frequent other associations include drug reactions from sulfonamides, penicillin, salicylates and the birth control pill. About 30 percent of the time no cause can be found. The exact mechanism behind the disease is not known, although it is believed to be some type of immune reaction around large blood vessels in the subcutaneous fat.

Symptoms Shiny, tender swellings up to 4 inches across appear suddenly on shins, thighs and sometimes arms. There is usually also fever and pain in muscles and joints, and there may be other symptoms, including chills, malaise, headache or sore throat.

Treatment Treat any underlying illness; alter medication if condition is a response to drugs. Bed rest with the legs raised is important; for ambulatory patients, support stockings may help. Warm water compresses may be soothing and tenting the bedcovers may relieve discomfort from rubbing against material. Otherwise, treatment may include painkillers or sometimes nonsteroidal anti-inflammatory drugs to reduce inflammation. Some experts find potassium iodide to be effective, although the reason is unknown.

erythema toxicum neonatorum A common, transient skin condition found in newborn infants during the first few days of life that usually disappears before the end of the first week and is characterized by papules, pustules and pink macules. The skin condition may consist of only a few lesions or may cover the entire body except for palms and soles.

Less common in premature infants, the condition has been attributed to allergies, although its true cause is unknown.

Symptoms The condition usually develops in the second to fifth day after birth, but it may appear as late as two weeks post-partum. While a few infants may be born with the condition, it may in fact represent a different but similar disorder called transient neonatal pustular melanosis.

The typical skin lesion of erythema toxicum neonatorum is a white pustule on a red base; if pustules do not appear, there may be papules or macules or a splotchy red mark. While the condition may appear anywhere, lesions are usually found on the trunk. There may be one or two lesions or a generalized eruption.

Treatment The condition does not require any treatment and has no effect on future health; there are no complications.

erythrasma A chronic bacterial infection of the toe web, groin and underarms that causes mild burning and itching. More common in warmer climates, it is caused by *Corynebacterium minutissimum,* which produces porphyrins that fluoresce a coral red color that is observable under Wood's light exam. Recurrences are common.

Symptoms Sharply outlined dry, brown, slightly scaly and slowly spreading patches.

Treatment C. minutissimum is very sensitive to a wide variety of antimicrobial drugs; extensive cases may also require oral administration of erythromycin, but topical treatment with antibiotics such as erythromycin or antifungals such as clotrimazole are usually effective.

erythroderma Redness over the entire body. See also DERMATITIS, EXFOLIATIVE.

erythromycin An antibiotic used to treat a variety of infections including some skin infections. It is often used as a systemic treatment for ACNE and in patients allergic to penicillin. In children under age 14 it is the alternative to tetracycline (an antibiotic that can permanently stain developing teeth and bones).

Because uncoated erythromycin is destroyed by acid in the stomach, the drug should be taken in enteric coated forms or as a compound. Otherwise, it could cause stomach distress.

Adverse effects Possible side effects include nausea and vomiting, abdominal pain, diarrhea and an itchy rash. To reduce side effects, certain brands of erythromycin may be taken with food to reduce the chance of irritating the stomach. Check with your physician or pharmacist regarding the proper method of taking this medication.

erythroplasia Red plaque on the mucous membranes of the mouth that may be benign or malignant. Two types of erythroplasia are often malignant—smooth macular plaques and velvety red patches dappled with white.

erythropoietic protoporphyria A profound photosensitivity disorder beginning in childhood, characterized by itching, burning and stinging skin almost immediately after exposure to sunlight. There may also be redness, swelling and fluid-filled blisters in the exposed area. Chronic exposure to the sun may cause thickened skin and fine scars, most often seen on the upper lip and the backs of the hands.

While the exact incidence of this disease is not known, it is not rare. It begins (often in infancy) when children are first exposed to sunlight; they cry and begin to develop swellings in the exposed areas of skin. The skin may erode and scar, especially on the hands, nose, eyes and ears. As the child ages, the skin over the knuckles appears thick and wrinkled.

Other internal findings include gallstones, mild hemolytic anemia, liver failure with jaundice, and cirrhosis of the liver.

Prevention/treatment Patients with this condition should avoid sunlight and wear protective clothing when outdoors. Oral administration of beta-carotene may reduce photosensitivity. Some patients have responded to treatment with iron or hematin, though this type of treatment has been found to worsen the condition of other patients.

eschar A scab produced on the surface of the skin by BURNS, corrosive agents, some skin diseases and infections or GANGRENE.

essential fatty acids Polyunsaturated fats necessary for healthy skin. Without them, dry scaly skin and hair loss will develop. However, deficiency is quite rare, since just one teaspoon per day of a polyunsaturated fat (such as corn oil) provides enough EFAs.

While these acids are recognized as important in the diet, there is no evidence that they can be absorbed from the skin. Most experts believe that EFAs are important in slowing the evaporation of water from the skin's surface. One EFA, gamma linolenic acid (otherwise known as EVENING PRIMROSE OIL), is thought to be helpful in the treatment of ATOPIC ECZEMA.

essential oils Oils extracted from real flowers and herbs. This term is often more loosely used to mean any perfumed oil that imitates a real scent.

estrogen A female sex hormone produced by the ovaries that can reduce the risk of dry skin and wrinkles. It is used in some facial creams designed for dry skin that enable the skin to retain water. Research shows estrogen may reduce some age-related skin deterioration, but smoking and sun exposure are more powerful causes of wrinkling.

etretinate (trade name: Tegison) A derivative of vitamin A used to treat PSORIASIS and some disorders of keratinization. Etretinate, like ISOTRETINOIN, is an analogue of vitamin A. It is more effective than isotretinoin for disorders of keratinization such as PSORIASIS and PITYRIASIS RUBRA PILARIS while isotretinoin is more effective for ACNE, especially in treating pustular and erythrodermic types of psoriasis. Unlike acne, psoriasis requires long-term treatment with etretinate.

Etretinate may be used alone, or together with more conventional psoriasis treatment (such as topical corticosteroids, tars, ANTHRALIN, PUVA or METHOTREXATE).

Combining etretinate with photochemotherapy using oral PSORALENS and PUVA (called RE-PUVA) is widely used in Europe to treat extensive psoriasis. It has the benefits of reducing the amount of UVA exposure and the dose and length of etretinate therapy.
Side effects Dry skin and eyes, nosebleeds, hair loss, bone and joint pain. Etretinate is a very potent cause of birth defects and should never be taken during pregnancy.

evening primrose oil A type of essential fatty acid (also known as gamma linolenic acid). Taken in capsule form, this oil (alone or in combination with fish oil) is believed by some to significantly improve cases of atopic ECZEMA when taken in high doses. One study, however, has not been able to confirm findings of earlier studies (according to a study published in the British medical journal *The Lancet*).

Those who support the use of evening primrose oil do admit it takes six to eight capsules per day for at least six months before any results may be observed in patients. Experts also report cases of fake capsules, so consumers should avoid evening primrose oil available in no-name brands.

exanthem subitum The medical name for ROSEOLA INFANTUM, a viral exanthem caused by human herpes viruses 6 and 7 (HHV 6 and HHV 7).

excoriation Injury to the skin's surface caused by abrasion (scratching) or chemical reaction that causes a raw area.

exercise and the skin Research suggests that exercise has especially important benefits for the skin. When comparing middle-aged athletes with a matched group of people who did not exercise, scientists found the athletes' skin denser, thicker, more elastic and stronger.

Researchers suspect that exercise flushes the skin, bringing oxygen-rich blood to the surface. It may also be that the production of COLLAGEN is enhanced by internally-generated heat (which is not the same as applying heat from the outside). Movement itself also seems to send messages to the cells in the body that manufacture the skin's elastic fibers.

When working out, never wear makeup because blocking the evaporation of sweat by sealing the skin with makeup interferes with the process of cooling the body by perspiring.

Before exercise, cleanse the face and neck where skin is most sensitive with a cleansing lotion and water; rinse well. If you have long hair or bangs, tie back your hair or use a sweat band; sweat that is trapped against skin by hair is thought to be a cause of after-exercise skin breakouts. Don't use a harsh astringent before you begin to remove skin oils, because these natural skin oils can protect your skin against the acid content of perspiration.

For outside exercise, always apply a moisturizing sunscreen whether or not you have oily or dry skin.

While some people joke that they have an "allergy to exercise," in fact as many as one million Americans are truly at risk for a potentially serious allergy linked to exercise. Symptoms include itching, hives, hoarseness, wheezing, breathing problems and a precipitous drop in blood pressure. While researchers aren't sure what triggers these symptoms, they suspect it could either be the activity itself or the heat generated by the exercise.

exfoliation Removal of dead cells on the surface of the skin with a cosmetic buffing sponge or a grainy cleanser.

As the skin matures, the turnover of epidermal (upper-layer) skin cells slows down. Because the dead skin cells cling together on the surface, the complexion may appear dull and rough.

By exfoliating properly, some dermatologists say, it's possible to increase the epidermal-cell turnover, making the skin look smoother and pinker again. Exfoliation also helps stimulate the production of young epidermal cells.

However, the subject of exfoliation generates strong and differing viewpoints among dermatologists. Some believe this procedure may help skin look newer, fresher, plumper and younger-looking, and encourage faster cell renewal. Others (including the American Academy of Dermatology) insist the skin does not need any help in sloughing off dead skin and rank overcleansing as the biggest skin care mistake because it can overdry and irritate the skin.

Exfoliation supporters say the technique works best for those with healthy, normal or dry complexions, and for those with dull, sun-damaged skin or skin with lots of blackheads. Even thin skin can be helped by milder exfoliants as long as there are no broken blood vessels. Patients who have had acne but whose complexions have improved may find that mild exfoliating keeps the pores unclogged and the complexion healthier.

Techniques There are two types of exfoliation—mechanical and nonmechanical. *Mechanical* exfoliants include a wide range of techniques ranging from very mild (washcloths and sea sponges) through exfoliation sponges, loofahs—to the severe exfoliation methods utilizing pumice stones, cleansing grains and scrubs.

Mechanical exfoliants stimulate the skin, and they may be too rough for sensitive skin or skin with broken blood vessels. People with this type of skin usually have fair, thin skin that reddens if touched. Dermatologists suggest that patients with acne not use mechanical exfoliation either, since the whiteheads or closed comedones may rupture beneath the skin when rubbed, leading to more inflammatory acne.

Nonmechanical exfoliants include cosmetic masks that work on the skin surface cells, RE-TIN-A, and chemical exfoliants (such as ALPHA-HYDROXY ACID). Masks never penetrate deeper than the dead superficial layer of the skin, and vary in strength according to the chemical used and its concentration. Depending on the concentration and the amount of time chemical exfoliants are kept on the skin, these can penetrate to living tissue, and **they should be used only under medical supervision.**

Generally, it's not possible to exfoliate the same way all year; the skin changes depending on the season and the temperature. In the summer, skin has more moisture and in the winter tends to dry out.

The mildest exfoliations are the sea sponge, the face cloth and cosmetic masks designed for sensitive or dry skin. A complexion brush moved in circular motions with some moisturizer can be a good exfoliator. For normal to thick skin, sea sponges or exfoliation sponges can be used effectively, but should be used no more than three times weekly in summer and no more than once a week in the winter.

Body exfoliation, on the other hand, is safe for all skin types, as long as any areas with inflammatory acne are avoided. It's especially beneficial for knees and elbows, especially when immediately followed by moisturizers. Self-tanning lotions also look best when applied after exfoliation.

exfoliative dermatitis See DERMATITIS, EXFOLIATIVE.

exudate Fluid containing PUS, cells and protein that has been discharged from blood vessels into a tissue (or tissue surface) and is usually a result of inflammation.

eyelid lift A cosmetic operation (blepharoplasty) that removes wrinkled, drooping skin from the upper and/or lower eyelids. The outpatient operation is usually performed with a local anesthestic, and takes about one and a half hours. As a person grows older, the skin loses its elasticity and fat stores, becomes redistributed, causing the skin to look creased and droopy. This aging process, which can be accentuated by weight loss and stress and is accelerated by sun exposure, makes the eyelids look baggy. Removing the excess skin and redistributed fat can greatly improve appearance.

During the operation, the surgeon removes a horizontal fold of skin from the center of the upper lids, so the scar will run in a natural crease line. Incisions in the lower lids are made either just below or just above the eyelashes to minimize the scar. Excess fat is removed from the lower lid but extra skin is not usually present and does not have to be removed.

After the operation, the patient can minimize swelling and bruising by applying ice packs to both eyes. Swelling usually subsides within three days, but bruising may last from two or three weeks.

Three to five days after the operation, the surgeon removes some of the stitches, and removes the remaining stitches within 7 to 10 days. The scars usually fade in time to unnoticeable marks within a year. Effects of the surgery can be expected to last between 10 and 20 years. Patients can go back to work within 5 to 14 days.

Actual cost may vary depending on the part of the country in which the surgery is performed.

F

Fabry's disease (Anderson-Fabry disease) The common name for angiokeratoma corporis diffusum. This is a hereditary disorder of lipid metabolism resulting from an enzyme deficiency that causes widespread lesions (especially in the umbilical and knee areas), extremely painful neuralgias in hands and feet during hot weather, hardening of the arteries and kidney disease. It is primarily characterized by the angiokeratoma, a 1- to 3-mm reddish purple raised skin lesion. Other skin symptoms include enlarged blood vessels, fingernail deformities and reddened skin. Sweating may be inhibited.

Kidney problems can lead to kidney failure and high blood pressure. Tissue death in the brain or heart due to decreased blood flow is common.

Fabry's disease is an X-linked recessive disease caused by a defect on the X chromosome, usually leading to problems in males only. Women can be carriers of the defect; their male children have a 50 percent chance of being affected by the disease.

Treatment There is no specific treatment. Kidney transplants can replace the missing enzyme and help ease pain and sweating. The angiokeratomas may be destroyed, but this does not often occur because they are small.

face-lift (rhydectomy) Cosmetic surgery to improve the appearance by smoothing out wrinkles and lifting sagging skin in the lower third of the face.

A face-lift is usually performed on an outpatient basis using a local anesthetic. Loose skin is separated from underlying muscle and pulled upward and backward all around the face, going back 3 to 4 inches from the side of the face. When the skin is lifted well away from the face, it is pulled up and draped over the face. The excess skin that overlaps the incision line is removed, and the skin is sewn at the incision line.

Cotton and gauze pads are placed over the face and eyes, and the whole face (except nostrils and mouth) is wrapped in an elastic bandage. Pads are kept in place for 24 to 48 hours, and then removed. After less than a week, the entire bandage is removed.

Bruising is expected and there may be some discomfort, which is usually controlled with minor painkillers; within a few weeks, however, these signs of surgery disappear and the face begins to show improvement. The stitches are removed three days after the operation, and the scars are usually hidden by natural crease lines and the hair, fading within a year.

Patients may be back to work in 10 to 14 days, although bruising can last up to three weeks. After a face-lift, the face must be cleaned twice a day with a mild, neutral soap and creams should not be used because the pushing and pulling of creaming the face puts strain on the newly sewn tissue, which can cause the skin to sag again. Facial massage should never be applied after cosmetic surgery, since it will spread the scars and make them seem broader and thicker, and puts strain on newly sutured skin.

Face-lifts cost an average of $4,000, although the exact amount will vary depending on the part of the country where the operation is performed. The operation lasts between two and four hours, and results last for two to 10 years. A face-lift can successfully be repeated several times in a lifetime. Although many people believe that repeated face-lifts will cause a mask-like expression, in fact a mask effect after a face-lift is an indication that the skin was tightened too much during the surgery.

Adverse effects The two most significant side effects are oozing and infection. Occasionally, bleeding under the skin causes a hematoma that interferes with successful healing. An infection may lead to severe scarring that may require a SKIN GRAFT.

See also PLASTIC SURGERY; PLASTIC SURGEON.

facial A skin treatment of the face designed to clean, tone and improve the skin's texture. Facials range from a simple mask applied at home to a sophisticated regimen in a beauty salon that may involve electrical currents, aromatic oils or specialized creams. While the facial may moisturize or stimulate circulation in the skin, it cannot remove or prevent wrinkles.

A full facial in a salon usually begins with an examination of the skin itself, followed by cleansing and toning. Steaming may follow so that skin impurities can then be removed (using extraction or exfoliation, for example). The face may be massaged to increase circulation and to relax muscles before a mask appropriate to skin type is applied.

factitial dermatitis See DERMATITIS ARTEFACTA.

Farber's lipogranulomatosis An inherited connective tissue disorder characterized by multiple subcutaneous nodules. Infants typically have a weak, hoarse cry and swollen joints. Most patients die by age two, and almost none live beyond age 10. There is no known treatment.

The disease is an autosomal recessive disorder, which means that a defective gene must be inherited from both parents to cause the abnormality. Generally, both parents of an affected person are unaffected carriers of the defective gene. Each of the children has a one in four chance of being affected, and a two in four chance of being a carrier.

The disease is caused by a deficiency in lysosomal acid ceramidase, which allows free ceramides to build up in tissues. This leads to the development of subcutaneous nodules.

fat atrophy The presence of fat in the subcutaneous tissue under the skin gives it its full, supple appearance. When fat cells are destroyed or removed, the surface of the skin appears to be depressed. The bony prominences of the body contribute to a gaunt appearance.

A group of rare disorders featuring localized or generalized fat atrophy are known as the lipodystrophies or lipoatrophies. They include partial lipodystrophy (Barraquer-Simmons disease), lipoatrophic diabetes (generalized lipodystrophy) and insulin lipoatrophy.

Barraquer-Simmons disease is characterized by the partial loss of subcutaneous fat over a large part of the body over a course of several years, and is often triggered by a fever. The depletion of fat cells usually begins on the face and proceeds downward, and occurs four times as often in women.

Generalized lipodystrophy can be either congenital or acquired (usually after a high fever). In both cases, the fat loss appears over the entire body. Symptoms also include a wide variety of other complaints, including insulin-resistant diabetes.

Insulin lipoatrophy is caused by repeated injections of insulin that reduce fat cells in a localized area. The depression appears about six months after injection, though rotating injection sites minimizes this problem. Spontaneous resolution of the depression may take up to 10 years.

Treatment New treatments have been developed using fat transfer, the technique of fat injection. Fat is removed from the patient's unaffected areas, cleansed, and then reinjected into the affected sites, where it appears to stay permanently.

See also FAT TRANSPLANTS.

fat transplants One of the newest methods in cosmetic surgery. By this procedure, fat removed from deposits in the hips, thighs, belly or buttocks is injected into deep wrinkles on the face, or into the breasts to enlarge them. Since the fat already belongs to the patient, it won't be rejected. However, results may be temporary because the body reabsorbs much of the fat. Therefore, physicians usually remove enough fat for several treatments (sometimes up to eight), and freeze it. After four or five injections (at four- to six-week intervals), the patient will see a marked improvement, with up to 80 percent of the furrows filled permanently.

The technique costs between $700 to $1,500, depending on the area of the country in which it is performed. See also FAT AT-ROPHY.
Side effects Temporary stinging, bruising, burning sensation, redness, swelling or excess fullness.
Risks Infection or contour irregularities.

fever blisters Another name for a "COLD SORE."

Fibrel A gelatin extracted from the patient's own plasma and, combined with gelatin and the clotting agent aminocaproic acid that stimulates the natural production of COLLA-GEN at the site of the injection. The material is injected until the scar or WRINKLE is elevated; the injections are given one or two weeks apart. As with collagen implants, overcorrection is necessary because there is some absorption by the body. Local redness, swelling, burning and bruising may occur at the site.

New collagen is then deposited at the site of the Fibrel injection; it usually takes three months for the newly formed collagen to replaced the injected substance. It is typically injected into wrinkles to smooth the skin. As with collagen injections, it's important to test

for allergy before treating, although a positive reaction occurs in less than 1 percent of all cases. Fibrel is less allergenic and longer-lasting than other liquid collagens (such as Zyderm). (See also SOFT TISSUE AUGMEN-TATION.)

fibroblasts Cells in the dermis (middle layer of skin) that produce COLLAGEN and elastin fibers.

fibrosis The deposition of fibrous tissue (scar) or connective tissue that may occur as a response to infection, inflammation or injury. Fibrosis may also be caused by a lack of oxygen in a tissue because of reduced blood flow.

fibrous hamartoma of infancy See FIBRO-MATOSES.

fibroxanthoma of skin A typically benign tumor of the skin found most often on the sun-exposed areas of older people's skin. The lesion usually appears first as a small nodule that slowly gets bigger, though seldom exceeds 3 cm. This type of lesion rarely becomes malignant and is cured by surgical excision.

Fifth disease Also known as "slapped cheeks" disease because of its dramatic herald symptom of a bright red rash across the cheeks, this is the least well known of the five common infectious childhood diseases—MEA-SLES, mumps, CHICKEN POX and RUBELLA (German measles).
Cause A parvovirus (B 19) usually occurs in small outbreaks among young children in the spring.
Symptoms Rash starts as rosy red spots on the cheeks that join into a red rash; within a few days, the rash has spread over the body, buttocks and arms and legs. There is often a mild fever in addition to the skin rash.

Treatment With bed rest, clear fluids and acetaminophen to lower fever, the rash usually clears within 10 days.

filariasis A group of tropical diseases caused by a range of parasitic worms and larvae that transmit disease to humans. About 200 million people are affected by filariasis, which occurs in tropic and subtropic areas of Southeast Asia, South America, Africa, Asia and the Pacific. When mosquitoes bite into the skin they inject the worm larvae, which migrate to the lymph nodes where they develop into mature worms in about a year.

Some of the species live in the lymphatic vessels, which become blocked, causing ELEPHANTIASIS (swelling of limbs with thickened, coarse skin). Another type of worm can be seen and felt just underneath the skin, which produces irritating and painful swellings called calabar swellings.

Symptoms Initial inflammatory symptoms occur between three months to a year after the mosquito bite, with swelling, redness and pain in arms, legs or scrotum. Abscesses may occur as a result of dying worms and secondary bacterial infection. Repeated episodes of inflammation lead to obstruction of the lymphatic system, especially in the genital and leg areas. Chronic swelling stimulates the growth of connective tissue in the skin, causing massive permanent enlargement and deforming (elephantiasis).

Treatment Three weeks of the antihelminthic drug diethylcarbamazine cures the infection. Large doses are not given initially because reactions to large numbers of dying parasites are severe—fever, malaise, nausea and vomiting—so doses are usually low at first. Oral antihistamines may help control hives and elastic stockings may help control swelling. No treatment, however, can reverse elephantiasis. Surgery may ease massive enlargement of the scrotum.

Prevention In infested areas, filariasis can be controlled by taking diethylcarbamazine preventively, and by using insecticides, repellents, nets and protective clothing.

filiform warts Slender fingerlike WARTS that are often found on the face (especially around the eyes and eyelids). They can be treated by cryotherapy, simple excision or ELECTRODESICCATION. See also PAPILLOMAVIRUS, HUMAN; PLANTAR WARTS; GENITAL WARTS; FLAT WARTS.

fingernails See NAILS.

fissure A crack or split in the skin.

flap A section of full-thickness skin that has been left attached at one end while the other end is surgically transferred to an adjacent part of the body. A flap differs from a graft in that a portion of tissue is attached to its original site and retains its blood supply. Flaps are used to cover wounds or repair defects caused by congenital deformity, accident or surgery.

Because a flap retains its color and texture, it is more apt to survive than a graft. However, several operations usually are needed to move a flap. The major complication is necrosis at the base because of failure of blood supply.

Free flaps, on the other hand, are completely severed from the body and transferred to another site, when it receives its blood supply. The procedure is usually completed in only one surgery.

flat warts Multiple WARTS commonly found on the face, neck, forearms, knees and the backs of the hands, especially among children. These flat, flesh-colored papules may appear in groups of up to 100. They are often found in lines or streaks, as a result of scratching and passing on the virus. On the face, they can resemble ACNE, melanocytic nevi or SEBORRHEIC KERATOSES. Flat warts on the arms or legs may resemble LICHEN PLANUS.

Treatment Treatment is by LIQUID NITROGEN cryotherapy or ELECTRODESICCATION with or without CURETTAGE. Flat warts are stubborn and require repeated treatments. Treatments applied once or twice daily have been reported to help. See also PAPILLOMAVIRUS, HUMAN; FILIFORM WARTS; PLANTAR WARTS; GENITAL WARTS.

fleas There are several types of fleas that cause skin problems: the human flea (*Pulex irritans*), the cat and dog flea (*Ctenocephalides felis* and *C. canis*) and others found on mammals and birds. Flea bites cause wheals and red papules, depending on how sensitive the person is to flea bites.

As a person is repeatedly bitten, he or she becomes gradually sensitized (for example, infants do not respond to flea bites); however, those who are continually exposed eventually may become desensitized.

Prevention Elimination of fleas and larvae can be accomplished by spraying insecticides in crevices of furniture, under rugs, in beds etc. Remove rubbish or sandpiles, and dust pets and pet bedding every two weeks with insecticides.

Treatment Itchy bites can be treated with topical steroid creams and systemic antihistamines.

flesh-eating bacteria See NECROTIZING FASCIITIS.

flucytosine (Ancobon) A synthetic fluorinated pyrimidine used to treat fungal infections. The drug is usually prescribed together with AMPHOTERICIN B OR KETOCONAZOLE for the treatment of chromoblastomycosis or CRYPTOCOCCOSIS. Newer antifungals are replacing the agent.

fluocinolone A medium-strength corticosteroid prescribed as a topical agent either as a cream, solution or ointment to relieve skin inflammation, itching and redness caused by disorders such as ECZEMA or PSORIASIS.

fluorescent lights and the skin While past studies have reached differing conclusions, a study in the 1992 issue of the *American Journal of Epidemiology* found that the more time men in the study spent under fluorescent lights, the higher their incidence of malignant melanoma. The link was not relevant for women in the study.

Fluorescent bulbs emit small amounts of ultraviolet radiation, the type of solar radiation that has been blamed for skin cancer.

In 1989, the National Institutes of Health said that the long-term effect of exposure to fluorescent bulbs is "an unresolved issue" and in 1990, the International Radiation Protection Association stated that ultraviolet radiation exposure from indoor fluorescent lighting should not be considered a malignant melanoma risk.

While the data remains inconclusive, those who are concerned can attach a plastic diffuser to their fluorescent lighting fixture (many lights come this way), which can eliminate or reduce the intensity of the ultraviolet emissions.

fluoroquinolones A group of antimicrobial drugs that are effective against many bacteria, including most *Pseudomonas* bacteria. Several of the fluoroquinolones are also active against *Mycoplasma, Chlamydia, Legionella* and a few other mycobacteria. Fluoroquinolones are not particularly effective against anaerobic organisms.

The drugs, which have fewer side effects than many other antibiotics, are used to treat many types of infections, including soft tissue infections and urethritis. However, these drugs are not recommended for children or adolescents, since they may have toxic effects on developing cartilage.

Fluoroquinolones include norfloxacin, ciprofloxacin, ofloxacin, enoxacin, pefloxacin, fleroxacin, lomefloxacin and several other compounds.

Side effects The most common side effect is loss of appetite and photosensitivity. Less common effects include nausea, abdominal pains, diarrhea, dizziness, rash etc.

fluorouracil An anticancer drug often used on the skin; also known as 5-fluorouracil or 5-FU. It is used to treat multiple ACTINIC KERATOSES and for flat, genital and intraurethral WARTS, BOWEN'S DISEASE, and superficial BASAL CELL CARCINOMA or KERATOACANTHOMAS. It is of particular benefit when surgical removal of several tumors located together is difficult. It is applied according to various schedules—from twice a day two consecutive days a week for nine weeks, to daily or twice daily for four to six weeks. It is also injected within the lesion for patients with KERATOACANTHOMAS.

Adverse effects As treatment progresses, patients develop intense inflammation and irritation that is worsened by exposure to ultraviolet light. For this reason, patients with many lesions are often not treated until winter. Irritation is significant and occurs with all patients. It can be soothed by using moisturizers; occasionally, topical steroids are necessary.

Other possible side effects include nausea and vomiting, diarrhea, hair loss and impaired blood cell production. The drug applied as a cream may cause skin inflammation.

flush Transient redness and warmth (primarily of the face and neck) associated with certain medications and pathologic conditions. See also ROSACEA; BLUSH.

Flynn-Aird syndrome A genetic disorder associated with skin ulceration in which subcutaneous tissue atrophies and forms ulcers similar to WERNER'S SYNDROME and SCLERODERMA. In addition, other symptoms include retardation, deafness, convulsions, baldness and stiff joints, which may appear during the first or second decade of life. This disorder is transmitted as an autosomal dominant disorder, which means that only one defective gene (from one parent) is needed to cause the syndrome. Each child of an affected person usually has a one in two chance of inheriting the defective gene and of being affected.

focal dermal hypoplasia See HAIR, DISORDERS OF.

follicle See HAIR FOLLICLE.

follicular hyperkeratoses Disorders of keratinization characterized by thickening of the skin around and/or on hair follicles. These disorders include KERATOSIS PILARIS, disseminated and recurrent INFUNDIBULOFOLLICULITIS and KYRLE'S DISEASE.

follicular mucinosa See MUCINOSES.

follicular orifice See PORE.

folliculitis Inflammation of at least one hair follicle. Folliculitis has many causes, including the bacteria *Staphylococcus aureus*, irritants and chemical exposure. While staphylococcal folliculitis can occur anywhere on the skin, it is most often found on hairy areas of the face, neck, armpits, thighs or buttocks. Staph folliculitis on the face is characterized by PUSTULES; in the armpits, it may lead to BOIL formation.

Treatment Antibiotics cure staphlococcal folliculitis. Depending on the cause, it may also be necessary to avoid irritants or chemical exposure.

Prevention Because the infection may be spread from one person to the next in the same household, each family member should use separate towels and washcloths, bathe often and wash underclothes in boiling water to kill the bacteria.

Food, Drug and Cosmetic [FDC] Act of 1938 The primary law governing the composition of cosmetics (including all skin care products). The act was passed in the wake of a serious cosmetics-related injury in 1933, when at least one woman was blinded and others were injured by using Lash Lure, a tint administered in beauty salons to color eyelashes and eyebrows.

In addition to the FDC Act of 1938, cosmetics packaging and labeling is governed by the Fair Packaging and Labeling Act; both of these are enforced by the U.S. Food and Drug Administration (FDA). Because the FDA is severely hampered by its budget (only about 1 percent of which is spent on cosmetics regulation), in an average year, the FDA makes only about 400 on-site inspections of cosmetics manufacturers.

In 1977, regulations on cosmetics labeling were added to the FDC act. According to this law, the outside wrapper or container must tell the consumer the manufacturer's name, address, maker or distributor, the product's weight, ingredients, and warn of any potential dangers. Ingredients listed must include any that are contained in the product in concentrations exceeding more than 1 percent in descending order of predominance. Ingredients should be listed only by their recognized names. If the cosmetic also qualifies as a drug, the drug ingredients must be listed as "active ingredients" at the top of the list. (For example, sunscreens are considered to be over-the-counter drugs, as are dandruff shampoos, acne medications etc.)

Fragrances can be listed only under the general heading "fragrance," and not under the specific ingredients from which the fragrance is derived—sometimes 10 or more substances.

Color ingredients can be listed in any order, no matter how much or little of the color they make up. Colors used in cosmetics are very strictly regulated, especially for products intended for use around the eye area. Many colors used in cosmetics are certified coal tar colors, which are prohibited for use around the eyes. Coal tar colors include any having the initials D&C or FD&C before the color name and number (such as D&C Yellow #10).

The FDA prohibits very few ingredients for cosmetics; those that are prohibited or restricted include bithionol, mercury compounds, vinyl chloride, halogenated salicylanilides, zirconium complexes, chloroform, chlorofluorocarbon propellants and hexachlorophene.

There are significant differences in how the FDA handles the approval of a cosmetic and a drug. If a cosmetic is promoted as a way to improve appearance, a company can place it on the market without any pre-market approval from the FDA—provided the manufacturer understands that it is safe. If the FDA later discovers there is a safety concern with the cosmetic, officials can take action to remove it from the market.

For the purposes of the FDA, a drug is considered to be any product that purports to cure, treat or mitigate a disease. Drug manufacturers must prove their medication is safe and effective before it is placed on the market.

Furthermore, a product that the FDA has considered to be a cosmetic may be relisted as a drug if the product subsequently is found to have a definite physiological effect on the body—even if the company did not market the product as a drug.

food reactions Allergies to certain foods can cause a wide range of reactions in up to 7 percent of the population, including specific skin symptoms such as itching, HIVES and swelling. However, a more serious response known as anaphylactic shock (ANAPHYLAXIS) can result in loss of consciousness or even death. If the reaction occurs immediately after the food allergen is eaten, the problem is not hard to trace. In cases where itching and redness do not occur until hours or even days after the food is eaten, the problem may be harder to track.

A range of common foods may bring on skin symptoms, including citrus fruits, eggs, fish, cola drinks, artificial coloring or milk. Infants prone to allergies may be particularly sensitive to milk and milk products, wheat, eggs and citrus fruits. Acute hives usually result from an allergic reaction to foods such as shellfish, nuts, berries, tomatoes, eggs, citrus fruits and pork.

Food *additives* may also cause problems. About 15 percent of people who are allergic to aspirin are sensitive to Yellow Dye #5 (tartrazine).

Allergic reactions can be caused by even very tiny (often undetectable) amounts of the food. For example, someone allergic to peanuts could go into anaphylactic shock if he or she eats food that only has been touched by peanuts.

Many food allergies disappear with time, especially in children. About a third of proven allergies disappear in one to two years if the patient carefully avoids the offending foods.

Diagnosis/treatment A food allergy is diagnosed following a detailed food history, physical exam and pertinent tests; skin testing may help identify cases of food allergy in cases of acute itching. However, skin testing is not usually helpful in diagnosing chronic itching due to food allergy. For these cases, a food diary and trial elimination of suspect foods may help.

Treatment involves eliminating or reducing the sensitive food, and drug therapy may be necessary for those with multiple food sensitivities not responsive to elimination measures. Drug therapy involves the use of antihistamines, adrenergic agents, corticosteroids and cromolyn sodium.

Treatment of an anaphylactic reaction to food depends on the severity of the reaction. If the person's heart has stopped, CPR should be initiated. Epinephrine is injected, and antihistamines and steroids may also be given to prevent recurrences of the reaction, and to control hives and swelling.

Prevention After a Johns Hopkins study found that fatal and near-fatal reactions to food allergies were more likely to be caused by foods prepared away from home, a new program initiated by the National Restaurant Association (NRA) and the Food Allergy Network will help restaurant workers understand food allergies. The NRA will provide free information to restaurants about the proper way to handle food allergy requests by calling (202) 331–5900.

formaldehyde, sensitivity to Many people can develop a sensitivity to formaldehyde, which is used in industry and in medicine as a preservative or antimicrobial and, in larger amounts, in nail care products. Household products often contain formaldehyde as a preservative. Substances that release formaldehyde contained in cosmetics or industrial products may be listed under a trade name and not under "formaldehyde" on the product label.

Formaldehyde can be irritating to some people, and because of its toxicity the Food and Drug Administration limits its concentration in nail products to 5 percent. See also ALLERGIES AND THE SKIN.

Fort Bragg fever See LEPTOSPIROSIS.

foundation Cosmetic product generally applied first to the skin to even out skin tone. Choosing the right foundation requires finding the product that most closely resembles your skin color and that is appropriate for your skin type. Because foundation is worn next to the skin, it should not be too oily nor contain too much alcohol.

Dry skin benefits from foundations containing mineral oil, cream-formula or oil-in-water emulsions. Products with a "matte finish" or those labeled "pore minimizing" are good choices for oily skin. Those with combination skin should choose an oil-free, pancake or matte foundation.

No matter what kind of skin you have, don't apply foundation directly to skin without first applying a layer of light-weight, skin-matched moisturizer that absorbs easily. Even women with oily skin or breakouts should use this buffer layer, and tone down the shine with a dusting of loose translucent powder. Skin that is at all sensitive needs this protective shield of moisturizer to reduce the chance of developing a reaction from something in the foundation.

Because a person's neck skin is often a different color than facial skin, experts suggest matching the color of the foundation with the jawline. Never test foundation color on the skin of your wrist or hand, because it won't match your facial skin. Never buy foundation with the intention of changing your skin color (to approximate a tan, for example) because the results will appear unnatural.

If you can't find a foundation that matches your skin perfectly, buy two (one lighter, one darker) from the same company and blend your own.

See also COSMETICS.

Foundation for Ichthyosis and Related Skin Types An educational foundation for persons suffering from ICHTHYOSIS, a group of rare hereditary diseases that cause the skin to be thick, dry, taut and scaly. Founded in 1981, its 3,000 members include dermatologists, scientists, and others interested in the disease.

Formerly known as the National Ichthyosis Foundation, the group acts as a support for persons with ichthyosis, helps link families with the disease and provides infor-

mation about the technical, social and psychological aspects of the disease.

Its publications include the quarterly *Ichthyosis Focus,* a newsletter featuring medical news, information on foundation activities, coping tips and correspondence column for members looking for penpals. The group also publishes booklets including *Overview, The Genetics of Inheritance, New Patient Booklet* and *Guide for Teachers and Healthcare Workers.* For address, see Appendix D.

Fox-Fordyce disease Also known as apocrine miliaria, this is an uncommon chronic disorder of the sweat glands causing itchy lesions of the skin under the arms, in the pubic area, around the nipple parts of the genitalia and sometimes on the chest and abdomen. It is characterized by retention of apocrine sweat leading to the formation of yellow papules. There may also be hair loss in the affected areas. The itching is often associated with emotional situations.

The disease appears after puberty, and is 10 times more common in women than men. Temporary improvement occurs during pregnancy. It is believed to be associated with an endocrinologic problem. Some women may find that the disease may regress after menopause.

Treatment This disease often causes no symptoms and requires no treatment. Topical application of corticosteroids or tretinoin may help relieve symptoms, and birth control pills or estrogen alone are often helpful. The only permanent cure is to excise and graft affected skin areas.

fragrance and the skin Modern fragrances usually contain about 50 different scent materials that may come from floral oils (flower petals), essential oils (such as citrus fruit peel) or animal perfumes (such as ambergris). By isolating the primary odor from a plant and combining it with chemicals, a new odor—or isolate—is formed. Fragrances may also contain man-made scents derived from petrolatum, coal tar etc.

Fragrance may be found in a variety of forms, including perfumes (alcohol solutions of 15–25 percent perfume concentrate) toilet water (3–5 percent perfume), or eau-de-cologne (about the same perfume concentration as toilet water, but whose scent blends the oils of lemon, bergamot and rosemary).

The odor of a fragrance depends on the chemistry of the wearer's skin, which is affected by genes, medication, diet, hormones and skin type (oily skin traps fragrance and dry skin tends to let fragrance evaporate). Therefore, to test a fragrance, it is better to dab a few drops on your skin and wait a few seconds before sniffing it, and also realize that the true "heart" of the scent will not be apparent for several hours. Fragrances are created with different top, middle and end "notes" that change the scent gradually as you wear it over a period of hours. The top notes are the way the fragrance smells right after you apply it to your skin, and last for approximately 15 minutes after application. The middle notes take over for the next few hours, and are the heart of the scent.

To test a fragrance, apply it to the inside of your wrist or ask the salesperson for a blotting-paper tester strip. You may want to wait 20 minutes before making a purchase. To prolong fragrance, try layering it, using several different preparations of the fragerance (oil or lotion, powder, and toilet water or perfume). Cologne lasts for approximately two hours. Eau de toilette lasts two to four hours, and perfume lasts four to six hours. Keep in mind that dry skin does not hold fragrance as well as oily skin, and if your skin is dry, soaking in bath oil before applying the same-scent fragrance or wearing body lotion can help the fragrance last. Remember that pulse points (behind the ear, backs of the knees, wrists) are the best places to apply fragrance, since they tend to be warmer than other skin areas. See also ALLERGIES AND THE SKIN; COSMETICS; MAKEUP.

fragrance, sensitivity to See ALLERGIES AND THE SKIN; FRAGRANCE AND THE SKIN.

frambesia See YAWS.

freckles Tiny round or oval patches of pigmented skin that are found on areas of the skin exposed to the sun. The tendency to freckling is inherited, and usually occurs in fair and red-haired individuals. Generally the more exposure to the sun, the more numerous the freckles. While freckles are harmless, those with highly freckled complexions should avoid excess sunlight and use SUNSCREENS. Freckles (also called ephelids) are temporary—they come and go with the sun. On the otherhand, liver spots (lentigines) come and stay forever.

Freckles are caused by the skin's efforts to tan in spots where there is an uneven distribution of melanin, resulting in an irregular tanning pattern. Some people find they can prevent freckles by applying a sunscreen with a high SPF (SUN PROTECTION FACTOR); once freckles appear, however, they may take an entire season to fade away.

free-flap surgery A procedure by which free flaps of skin are transplanted with blood vessels attached, thereby ensuring the health of the graft. In the past, when surgeons had to rely on simple skin grafts in areas that had little blood supply or in which the blood vessels were impaired, blood flow could not be restored and the transplanted tissue would often die. Attempts to transplant additional blood vessels to the site required multistage operations that caused long recovery delays.

With free-flap surgery, physicians can transplant skin and blood vessels, using microscopes that magnify the operating field up to 40 times. Sutures are only one-third the width of a human hair. Employing a team approach during the operation allows donor and recipient sites to be operated on simultaneously, connecting the transplanted blood vessels to other veins and arteries located outside the injury zone.

Common sites for the donor skin and blood supply include the groin, scalp, armpit, forearm, thigh or back.

When more than one of these tissues is needed in a special configuration unavailable naturally, the right kind of flap, called a prefabricated flap, can be pieced together gradually and then transplanted to its new home once the new structure is viable. For example, a new nose can be created on the forearm, where it is less conspicuous than on the face, and transplanted once it is complete.

Some uses for free flap surgery include breast reconstruction and movement restoration in fingers etc. See also SKIN GRAFT.

free radicals A highly charged, destructive form of oxygen generated by each cell in the body that destroys cellular membranes through the oxidation process, contributing to premature aging, loss of elasticity, discoloration and saggy skin. Rusting iron, crumbling stone and flaking paint on a canvas are all the result of oxidation, an environmentally triggered free radical reaction.

Because free radicals are essential to many reactions in the body (they are generated by the immune system to fend off microbes and help the digestive system break down food), they should not be destroyed entirely. It is only when the levels become excessive that skin damage can occur.

Free radical damage can be offset by molecules called antioxidants, which neutralize free radicals before they can damage skin cells. They include beta carotene, selenium, the synthetic antioxidant molecule BHT and Phloroglucinol, a natural antioxidant extracted from algae. Vitamins E and C are particularly potent antioxidants. While there is no guarantee regarding the effectiveness of

the dietary supplements of antioxidants in preventing cell damage, many physicians believe and recommend the benefits of the antioxidants beta carotene, vitamins C and E to their patients. Still, the Food and Drug Administration and the National Academy of Sciences believe it is premature to recommend increases in vitamin C, E and beta carotene intake. Other research groups and public health organizations are recommending daily doses of some vitamins and minerals that are four to 16 times higher than the current recommended daily allowances. No one is suggesting that vitamin supplements should take the place of a healthful diet and lifestyle, however.

While vitamins C and E are particularly good antioxidants, taking these vitamins orally may do a better job of protecting against free radicals in the body than on the skin. For this reason, some researchers are recommending that consumers apply these molecules directly to the skin. Some cosmetics are incorporating antioxidants into their ingredients as a way to make antioxidants more available to the skin.

frostbite Exposure to very cold temperatures for a long period of time can freeze the skin and underlying tissues, resulting in the condition known as frostbite. The areas most likely to be affected are the feet and hands, nose and ears. While anyone can become frostbitten, those with circulatory problems are at greatest risk.

Although it is theoretically possible for tissue to freeze in temperatures at about 32° F, the body's local internal temperature must fall to levels lower than that before freezing occurs at a specific area of the body. The danger of frostbite increases if the person is without adequate food, clothing or shelter; wind or wet skin also hastens the outward transfer of heat and increases the risk of frostbite.

Symptoms Frostbitten skin appears as firm, pale, cold white patches with a lack of sensitivity to touch, although there may be a sharp, aching pain on the affected area. As the skin thaws, it becomes raw and painful. Frostbite damage may be described as "superficial" (FROSTNIP), involving skin and subcutaneous tissues or "deep" (true frostbite), affecting muscle, nerve, vessels, cartilage and bone. In mild cases, damage can be reversed, but if frostbite is severe the flow of blood to the area stops. Unless immediate treatment is begun, the area will be irreversibly damaged and amputation of the extremity may be required.

Treatment Normal body temperature should be restored before thawing any frostbitten flesh. A small area of frostnipped skin can be rewarmed by placing fingers or the heel of the hand over the affected area. Rapid thawing of the affected part in warm water baths is the current preferred treatment method for more extensive frostnip and for frostbite. If immediate emergency assistance is unavailable, severely frostbitten hands or feet should be thawed in warm, *not hot,* water (between 100–105° F). Other heat sources (such as heating pads) should not be used because the frostbitten tissue can still be burned by temperatures that under normal conditions would not harm the skin. If the skin tingles and burns as it warms, circulation is returning. *If numbness remains as the area is warmed, professional help should be obtained immediately.* Never rub a frostbitten area as it thaws, and if feet are affected, the victim should not walk on them. In addition, frostbitten victims should not smoke cigarettes, since nicotine causes the blood vessels to constrict and may inhibit circulation. Neither bandages nor dressings should be used.

Thawing time is determined by the temperature of the water and the depth of freezing; it is complete when the extremity flushes pink or red. After rapid thawing, small blisters appear, spontaneously rupturing in four to 10 days, followed by a black scab. Normal tissue may have formed below. Constant dig-

ital exercises should be performed to preserve joint motion. Further treatment is designed to prevent infection and preserve function of the affected part.

In severe cases, antibiotics, bed rest and physical therapy may be necessary after the affected part has been warmed; cigarettes should be avoided during the entire recovery period.

The best chance of successful healing after frostbite occurs is when the affected part has not been frozen long, when thawing is rapid and when blisters develop early. The outlook is more uncertain when thawing is spontaneous at room temperature, when the part is frozen for a long time and if the frostbite occurred in an area of fracture or dislocation. A poor outlook is indicated if thawing is delayed or occurs due to excessive heat, if blisters are dark or if thawing is followed by refreezing. (Refreezing almost always ends in amputation).

Major complications include infection, tissue death, sensory loss, persistent deep pain and limited joint movement. Permanent effects may include fixed scars, small muscle wasting, deformed joints, arthritic bone changes and increased sensitivity to cold.

Prevention Frostbite is theoretically simple to prevent by wearing proper clothing in cold weather (dry and layered, warm and loose), especially on hands and feet. Nose and ears should be protected; tight apparel (boots, gloves or clothing) should never be worn. Conditions that increase the likelihood of frostbite include emaciation, fatigue, dehydration and previous frostbite.

To stay warm, wear cotton blend socks (such as Orlon and cotton), not pure cotton socks. Make sure clothes are loose, and dress in layers to help trap heat. The inner clothing layer should be made of a synthetic fabric, or a silk or wool blend that wicks away perspiration from the skin. The next layer should be something that insulates, like a wool shirt for example. Choose waterproof, breathable boots and outer jacket. Since the head is the source of greatest heat loss, be sure to wear a hat in cold weather; choose mittens, not gloves, because they trap heat from the whole hand.

Patients who must go outside in cold weather should eat warm food (oatmeal, hot soup etc.) to raise core body temperature, and drink plenty of fluids (hot cider or herbal tea, for example) to stave off dehydration. Dehydration can worsen chills and frostbite by reducing blood volume. Do NOT drink caffeinated beverages, which constrict blood vessels and interfere with circulation. While alcohol may temporarily warm up hands and feet, it has a cumulative negative effect by increasing blood flow to the skin, reducing the core body temperature.

In any situation where freezing has occurred, thawing must be prevented if refreezing is a possibility. While it is possible to survive local freezing of an extremity, the body's *internal* temperature must be maintained, since loss of vital temperature can cause hypothermia and death.

frostnip The earliest stage of FROSTBITE, this condition is reversible. In this stage, the skin suddenly turns white and frosty and becomes less sensitive. Frostnip is treated by drying and gently rewarming the injured skin by placing it against warm skin (such as under the armpits or on the abdomen). If exposure to the cold continues, frostnip quickly deteriorates into full-blown frostbite, which causes permanent skin damage.

fucosidosis A genetic metabolic disorder caused by a lack of a lysosomal enzyme (α-1-fucosidase), resulting in the accumulation of fucose between the cells. There are three types of fucosidosis, but it is type III disease that causes skin symptoms, including pigmentary retinopathy (disorder of the retina) and (occasionally) HYPOHIDROSIS and purple nail beds. In addition, these patients have various neurologic problems, including seizures and recurrent pulmonary infections.

The disorder is an autosomal recessive disease, meaning that a defective gene must be inherited from both parents to cause the abnormality. Generally, both parents of an affected person are unaffected carriers of the defective gene. Each of their children has a one in four chance of being affected, and a two in four chance of being a carrier. There is no effective treatment.

Fulvicin See GRISEOFULVIN.

fungal infections Diseases of the skin (also called mycoses) caused by the spread of fungal organisms that may range from a mild skin condition to disseminated disease with fatal symptoms. Fungal skin infections are either considered to be superficial (affecting skin, hair, nails) or subcutaneous (beneath the skin).

The *superficial* fungal infections include THRUSH (candidiasis) and TINEA (including RINGWORM and ATHLETE'S FOOT). *Subcutaneous infections* are rare; the most common is *sporotrichosis*, occurring after a contaminated scratch; most examples of this type of condition occur in tropical climates. (See also FUNGUS)

Causes Harmless fungi and yeasts are present all the time on the skin, but they do not multiply there because of competition among bacteria or because the body's immune system fights them off. Superficial fungal infections are extremely common, and occur in perfectly healthy individuals. Widespread or deep fungal infections of the skin are most common in those taking long-term antibiotics, corticosteroid or immunosuppressant drugs, or in patients with an immune system disorder (such as AIDS).

Fungizone See AMPHOTERICIN B.

fungus A phylum of plants (including yeasts, rusts, molds, smuts, mushrooms, etc.) characterized by the absence of chlorophyll and the presence of a rigid cell wall. There are more than 100,000 different species of fungi around the world, most of which are harmless or beneficial to human health (such as molds used to produce antibiotics, yeasts used in baking and brewing, edible mushrooms and truffles, yogurt cultures etc.).

However, some fungi can invade and form colonies in the skin or underneath the skin, leading to disorders ranging from a mild skin irritation and inflammation to severe or fatal systemic infections. See also FUNGAL INFECTIONS.

furuncle Another name for a BOIL.

furunculosis A bacterial infection characterized by tender, subcutaneous nodules usually capped with a small pustule, and infected with *Staphylococcus aureus*. Furuncles (BOILS) occur when a few neighboring hair follicles become infected with *S. aureus*. If more follicles are involved, the furuncle becomes a carbuncle. Furuncles most commonly affect the neck and upper back. Recurrent boils may also occur for years.

Treatment Surgical drainage of pus is followed by the application of warm compresses for 20 minutes four times a day. Bathing with antimicrobial soap decontaminates other areas. Systemic antibiotics are frequently required.

Prevention The recurrence of furunculosis may be prevented by improving hygiene, by taking systemic antibiotics and by ensuring that the source of infection is cleared.

Futcher's line See VOIGT'S LINE.

G

gangrene Death of tissue generally associated with loss of blood supply, followed by bacterial invasion and putrefaction. It may affect either a fairly small area of skin or an entire limb.

In *dry gangrene,* an area of the skin dies because of blocked blood supply, without bacterial infection; this type does not spread to other tissue. It may be caused by arteriosclerosis, diabetes mellitus, a stroke, blood clot or FROSTBITE. *Wet gangrene* follows bacterial infection of dry gangrene or a wound. *Gas gangrene* is a particularly virulent form of wet gangrene caused by a deadly type of bacteria (*Clostridium welchii*) that destroys muscle while producing a foul odor. Gas gangrene has been responsible for millions of deaths during war.
Symptoms Pain occurs in the dying skin tissue, which becomes numb and black once it dies. If bacterial infection occurs, the gangrene will spread, giving off a noxious odor with redness, swelling and oozing pus around the blackened area.
Treatment Dry *gangrene:* Improving circulation to the affected area can improve dry gangrene if it is begun early enough.

Wet gangrene: Once the tissue becomes infected, antibiotics are given to prevent wet gangrene from setting in. Once wet gangrene is diagnosed, amputation of the affected part, along with neighboring healthy tissue, is required, in order to save the patient.

Gardner-Diamond syndrome This psychogenic purpura (self-induced bruising) syndrome affects women almost exclusively, and is characterized by painful bruising of the skin after minor injury. These patients share a similar personality profile—masochistic tendencies, dependent relationships and intense anger toward those closest to them.

Patients may first complain of tenderness, burning or stabbing pain in the legs; skin lesions become bluish from within a few hours to three days later, and eventually come to resemble bruises. Recurrent lesions in groups are common. The condition is thought to be self-inflicted.

The prognosis for syndrome patients, even with extensive psychotherapy, is poor.

Gardner's syndrome A hereditary disorder featuring benign skin (and other tissue) growths that appear during the first 10 years of life. The skin growths include epidermal and sebaceous cysts, lipomas and fibromas. The disorder is an autosomal dominant disease, which means that only one defective gene (from one parent) is needed to cause the syndrome. Each child of an affected person usually has a one in two chance of inheriting the defective gene and of being affected.

gastrointestinal bleeding, skin symptoms of If enough bleeding in the gastrointestinal tract occurs, the skin may appear pale. Cirrhosis of the liver may include skin symptoms of redness, spidery VEINS or jaundice.

Gaucher's disease A hereditary disorder of lipid metabolism most often found among Ashkenazi Jews. A lack of the enzyme B-glucocerebrosidase, important to the metabolic process, leads to a buildup of fatty compounds (cerebrosides) in the liver, spleen, lymph nodes and nervous system. Gaucher's disease is an autosomal recessive disorder, which means that a defective gene must be inherited from both parents in order for the abnormality to occur. Generally, both parents of an affected person are unaffected carriers of the defective gene. Each of their children has a one in four chance of being affected and a two in four chance of being a carrier. The disease is fatal in infancy; a less-severe form may become apparent only in adulthood. A biochemical assay is now available to identify carriers.

Symptoms The most common skin symptom is a yellow-brown discoloration appearing over exposed areas, mimicking MELASMA when it occurs on the face. If bone marrow or liver are involved, symptoms may include blue/purple hemorrhagic patches, purple papules, pale skin or jaundice.

Treatment Researchers are studying the feasibility of replacing the deficient enzyme.

gel A clear, jelly-like, solid vehicle that becomes liquid when warmed or rubbed onto the skin. They usually contains volatile solvents that evaporate quickly when applied to the skin. Many gel products have been pared down to eliminate oils, fragrances, color or emulsifiers. Gel moisturizers and cleansers also have a higher water content than most creams and lotions, which makes them feel cool and soothing on the skin.

While most creams can leave the skin feeling greasy, gels are absorbed almost instantly, like water. Gels work well for women with normal to oily skin because they add moisture without adding oil. But for those with dry skin who may need more moisture, a better skin-care choice is an emollient-rich cream or lotion, because gels have a tendency to be drying.

genetic disorders of the skin There is a wide range of genetic diseases affecting the skin. Genetic hair defects that cause loss of hair include hidrotic ectodermal dysplasia, ANHIDROTIC ECTODERMAL DYSPLASIA, CARTILAGE-HAIR HYPOPLASIA, trichorhinophalangeal syndrome, biotin responsive carboxylase deficiency, marie-unbna hair dystrophy, congenital skin defect (APLASIA CUTIS), CONRADI'S DISEASE, incontinentia pigmenti, focal dermal hypoplasia, and Hallermann-Streiff syndrome. Other genetic hair disorders include low sulfur hair syndromes and hypertrichosis lanuginosa.

Genetic blistering disorders include EPIDERMOLYSIS BULLOSA; ACRODERMATITIS ENTEROPATHICA; Tyrosinemia type II (RICHNER-HANHART SYNDROME) PACHYONYCHIA.

Genetic diseases associated with photosensitivity include BLOOM SYNDROME, XERODERMA PIGMENTOSUM, DYSKERATOSIS CONGENITA. Genetic diseases associated with premature aging and hardening of the skin include WERNER'S SYNDROME and PROGERIA. Those associated with abnormal skin elasticity include EHLERS-DANLOS SYNDROME, CUTIS LAXA, BUSCHKE-OLLENDORFF SYNDROME, FARBER'S LIPOGRANULOMATOSIS PACHYDERMOPERIOSTOSIS.

Genetic skin disorders involving multiple new skin growths include epidermodysplasia verruciformis and GARDNER'S SYNDROME.

Other genetic diseases include: GENODERMATOSIS, ANGIOKERATOMA, arginosuccinicaciduria, lentigo simplex, MULTIPLE LENTIGINES SYNDROME and LENTIGINOSIS PROFUSA. See also CHROMOSOMAL DEFECTS AND SKIN DISEASE.

genital warts A type of wart found in the genital area, anorectal region and occasionally the urethra, bladder and ureters, caused by infection with human papillomavirus (HPV) (see PAPILLOMAVIRUS, HUMAN). The disorder is readily spread by sexual contact.

The warts primarily appear in the moist genital folds and creases. While just one wart may appear, they are commonly found in heaped-up bunches that form cauliflower-like masses. They are subject to injury and can bleed, and they are usually painless.

Women who are pregnant or take birth control pills are more likely to be affected by these warts.

This type of wart is not common in children, and their presence should raise a suspicion of sexual abuse.

Infants born to mothers who have vaginal genital warts may acquire HPV infection of the larynx and develop large, rapidly growing laryngeal warts that obstruct the airway. Medical attention should be sought in such cases.

Genital and anal warts may undergo malignant change to SQUAMOUS CELL CARCINOMA.

Treatment There is no known treatment that specifically eradicates HPV from the skin. Treatments are nonspecific and destructive and therefore only somewhat effective. Recurrence rates are high.

Most lesions in moist areas can be treated with podophyllum resin in tincture of benzoin, which is painted on the lesion and allowed to dry. It is then washed off several hours later. Extensive areas should not be treated at one time, since absorption of the resin can be toxic. For the same reason, pregnant women should not be treated. The active component of sodophylin podofilotoxin is now available in a colorless liquid that can be applied by the patient at home. It is slightly less irritating than the podophylin resin, and less toxic.

CRYOTHERAPY with liquid nitrogen is often effective: it is nontoxic, does not require anesthesia and, if done properly, does not scar. CURETTAGE AND ELECTRODESICCATION may also be successful.

While alpha interferon is available for treatment of resistant cases, it has a high likelihood of toxicity. It is also expensive and its effectiveness is marginal.

The CARBON DIOXIDE LASER may be helpful in cases of extensive growths, especially for those who have not responded to other treatments.

For pregnant patients, cryotherapy is most effective. Women taking birth control pills may have to stop taking the pill before the warts can be successfully treated. See also WARTS.

Certain HPV types are associated with SQUAMOUS CELL CACINOMA. In cases where the wart looks unusual, this possibility should be considered.

Prevention Transmission of the virus that causes genital warts can be prevented by avoiding contact with infected individuals or by the use of contraceptive barriers such as condoms.

genodermatosis Any genetically determined disorder of the skin, such as EPIDERMOLYSIS BULLOSA, PROGERIA, GARDNER'S SYNDROME ETC. See GENETIC DISORDERS OF THE SKIN.

gentamicin An injectable antibiotic sometimes given in combination with another antibiotic to treat serious grem negative bacterial infections. It cannot be given by mouth because it is inactivated during digestion.

Blood tests are taken during treatment to reduce the risk of toxic kidney damage.

German measles The common name for rubella, this is a viral infection like MEASLES that causes a rash on the face, trunk and limbs. Rubella, which causes a mild illness in children and a slightly more problematic one in adults, is serious only when contracted by pregnant women in the early months of gestation. During this time, there is a chance the virus will infect the fetus, which can lead to a range of serious birth defects known as rubella syndrome.

Although rubella was once found throughout the world, it is now much less common in most developed countries because of successful vaccination programs. The United

States has tried to eradicate the disease by vaccinating all school-age children. By 1986 there were only 551 reported cases of rubella, and only 14 cases of rubella syndrome.

Symptoms The infection usually affects youngsters between the ages of six and 12 with a rash that lasts for a few days, a slight fever and enlarged lymph nodes. Sometimes the symptoms are so mild, the entire infection comes and goes without notice. Adolescents and adults may have slightly more pronounced symptoms. The virus is contagious from a few days before the symptoms appear until a day after symptoms fade.

Rubella may be confused with other conditions characterized by rashes, such as SCAR-LET FEVER or drug allergy.

Treatment There is no specific treatment for rubella, although acetaminophen may reduce the fever.

Prevention Vaccination which can provide long-lasting immunity, is administered in the United States to all infants at about 15 months of age as part of measles and mumps immunization. There is not usually any reaction to the vaccine. Infection by rubella also provides immunity.

Gianotti-Crosti syndrome This condition (known as papular acrodermatitis) is characterized by skin-colored or slightly pink papules on the face, arms, legs and buttocks of children. The lesions do not usually itch. There is a frequent association with hepatitis B virus. Other viruses that have caused the eruption include hepatitis A virus, Epstein-Barr virus, coxsackievirus A16, parainfluenza virus, respiratory syncytial virus and polio-vaccine enterovirus.

The child usually feels fairly well, but has diarrhea or an upper respiratory infection when the skin suddenly breaks out in crops of papules lasting up to two months which then fade spontaneously.

Treatment There is no specific treatment, but itching may be relieved with an antipruritic lotion, weak topical corticosteroid lotion or systemic sedating antihistamines.

ginseng The dried root of the *Panax schinseng* plant that is reported to contain hormones and vitamins. Research has not found any evidence that ginseng can improve the appearance of the skin. Ginseng has been associated with allergic skin reactions.

glanders An infection found in Asia, Africa and South America that afflicts horses and donkeys and that may be occasionally transmitted to humans. The infection, which is caused by the bacterium *Pseudomonas mallei*, causes an ulcer or abscess where it enters a wound in the skin.

The infection causes a papule or vesicle at the site of infection that may become filled with pus. If the mucous membranes in the nose or mouth are involved, extensive tissue death and damage to the septum and palate may occur.

Glanders may appear as an acute disease, in which it may be rapidly fatal, or as a chronic condition that may persist for months or years. Death may occur as a result of liver disease or continuing infections.

Treatment There is no satisfactory treatment, although tetracyclines, streptomycin and chloramphenicol may be effective. Immediate surgical removal of lesions followed by treatment with sulfonamide is recommended.

glomus tumor A small, uncommon painful swelling usually found on the extremities, especially in the finger or toe near the nail. This benign tumor is more painful if the area is exposed to hot or cold. It appears as a soft or firm blue-red papule and is caused by an excess of "glomus bodies" (structures with many nerve endings that usually control blood flow and skin temperature). Lesions may be painful. Occasionally, the tendencies toward multiple glomus tumors may be inherited.

Treatment Glomus tumors may be surgically removed, especially if they are painful.

glutamic acid An amino acid included in some expensive cosmetics that purport to improve the appearance of the skin. All amino acids combine to form proteins under certain chemical conditions, but because more than two different amino acids are needed to form useful proteins, simply including glutamic acid in a skin cream will not provide much benefit. Further, is not possible to rebuild the proteins of your skin with amino acids, and they are not absorbed when applied to the skin.

glycerin A clear liquid made by combining water and fat that is used in many cosmetics and toiletries because it improves the consistency of creams and lotions, and helps them retain moisture. Glycerin, however, tends to draw water out of the skin, and can make skin drier. It has not been found to cause allergic reactions.

glycogen storage diseases Although there are at least 12 distinct disorders caused by defective glycogen metabolism, only one—Type 1, or von Gierke's disease—causes skin manifestations, which include yellow papules in association with hyperlipoproteinemia (the presence of abnormally high blood levels of lipoproteins due to faulty lipoprotein metabolism).

glycolic acid One of a number of ALPHA HYDROXY ACIDS available both as over-the-counter and prescription mild skin peels. This topical product improves the skin's appearance by accelerating the natural process of shedding dead skin cells. Used properly, the acids work gently, producing only a slight tingling or stinging sensation in some consumers.

Derived from sugar cane, glycolic acid can clear up ACNE-prone skin, soften tiny lines around the eyes and mouth, smooth dry skin and fade dark spots caused by sun or hormonal changes (such as in pregnancy). Fastest results are usually obtained in a doctor's office, since higher strength products are available to dermatologists.

By federal law, all alpha hydroxy acid products are considered to be cosmetics, not drugs, and are not regulated by the U.S. Food and Drug Administration.

Over-the-counter products manufactured by reputable companies are usually mild, containing less than 10 percent alpha hydroxy acid. Beauty salon operators use products up to 40 percent, and physicians use solutions of up to 70 percent for their in-office peels.

Reputable firms don't sell stronger products over the counter because of the danger to consumers and the accompanying liability threat. But the FDA is reviewing glycolic acid to see whether strength percentages should be established by law. Irritations and even burns have been reported by those who have used "bootleg" products. (See also CHEMICAL PEEL).

gnathostomiasis A form of larva migrans caused by a nematode (*Gnathostoma spinigerum*) found in Southeast Asia (especially Thailand). In humans, the parasite may live in body tissues—including subcutaneous tissue—for as long as 10 years. Symptoms include occasional palm-sized swellings with mild redness, itchiness and tenderness (usually on the chest and abdomen), with small hemorrhagic spots or abscesses. Swelling usually lasts for a few days and then suddenly fades.

Treatment Surgical removal is the preferred treatment.

Goeckerman regimen An intensive treatment regimen for patients suffering with PSO-

RIASIS combining ULTRAVIOLET B LIGHT and tar ointments. This regimen has been a standard in-patient treatment for 50 years. It involves applying 2 to 5 percent crude coal tar ointment to the entire body at bedtime, which is then left on the skin overnight. Application for two hours before exposure to ultraviolet light is an effective alternative. In the morning, the excess tar is removed with mineral oil and the patient is exposed to UV light; afterwards, the patient bathes away remaining tar. The amount of UV light is gradually increased over successive treatments. Hospitalization usually lasts for three or four weeks, and may result in remission for six to eight months.

A modified form of treatment involves applying topical corticosteroids at night instead of coal tar. In the morning the steroids are removed and the patient applies tar before UV treatment. Corticosteroids can't be used more than four or five days because of the danger of a rebound attack of psoriasis.

gold sodium thiomalate A water-soluble gold salt used in chrysotherapy (gold therapy) to treat rheumatoid arthritis. More recently, it has been used intramuscularly to treat PEMPHIGUS.

A few patients experience a specific reaction within minutes after treatment with gold sodium thiomalate, including flushing, redness, weakness, vertigo and low blood pressure. Other symptoms that appear within a day after treatment include arthralgia, joint stiffness, myalgia and malaise. See also GOLD THERAPY.

gold therapy The common term for chrysotherapy, this treatment is most often used to treat rheumatoid arthritis sometimes associated with PSORIASIS. PEMPHIGUS also has been treated with gold salts. Gold, which is administered orally, has an anti-inflammatory effect that can relieve pain and stiffness, and prevent further joint damage. Two different

gold preparations are used: the water-soluble GOLD SODIUM THIMALATE and the oil-based AUROTHIOGLUCOSE.

Side effects Possible side effects of gold therapy to the skin include exfoliative dermatitis (see DERMATITIS, EXFOLIATIVE), macules or papules, or lesions resembling LICHEN PLANUS or PITYRIASIS ROSEA. The drug is usually stopped if itching occurs. After gold therapy stops, the lesions typically fade away up to three or four months later. After that, most patients will tolerate further gold treatments without skin symptoms.

Other side effects of gold therapy may include the diffuse depositing of metallic gold within the skin (a condition known as chrysiasis). Patients who are going to be treated intramuscularly are usually given a test dose to gauge sensitivity, followed by gradually increasing doses. Patients with pemphigus may require a cumulative dose of 500 mg before noticing improvement.

Possible side effects unrelated to the skin include problems with the liver and kidney, liver and bone marrow changes, appetite loss, diarrhea, nausea and abdominal pain, and sometimes anaphylactic shock.

Because of the risk of side effects, patients are usually monitored with serial complete blood counts, platelet counts, urinalysis and liver function tests.

goose bumps See GOOSEFLESH.

gooseflesh Formation of temporary raised bumps of skin caused by the reaction of blood vessels to cold or to strong emotion.

In the presence of cold or of strong emotion, blood vessels contract, which also contracts the small muscle attached to the base of each hair follicle, causing the hairs to stand up. This makes the skin look like the skin of a plucked goose—hence, the name "goose flesh" or "goosebumps." The medical name for goosebumps is cutis anserina.

Gougerot-Blum syndrome Pigmented papular lesions that coalesce into itchy plaques known as "pigmented purpuric lichenoid dermatitis." The lesions are most often found on the lower legs, but may also appear on the lower trunk, abdomen and arms. The disorder is primarily a cosmetic problem, since the lesions don't usually itch and don't affect internal organs. The syndrome is caused by inflammation of the capillaries that causes blood to leak into tissues, causing the rust-colored pigment changes and lesions.

Treatment There is no specific treatment. Systemic corticosteroids may be effective, but their risk generally outweighs their usefulness. Topical corticosteroids may be helpful.

graft-versus-host disease (GVHD) The first symptom of this common complication to bone marrow transplantation is a skin rash. The condition is caused by cells present in the transplanted bone marrow (graft) that attack the transplant recipient's tissues (host). The disease may occur soon after any organ transplant (acute GVHD), or it may not appear until months later (chronic GVHD).

Symptoms In addition to the skin rash, there may be diarrhea, abdominal pain, jaundice, inflammation of eyes and mouth and breathlessness.

Prevention Giving immunosuppressant drugs (such as cyclosporine) may head off the reaction. Once the disease develops, it is treated with corticosteroid drugs and other immunosuppressants.

granular cell tumor A type of skin tumor that, like NEURILEMMOMA, is derived from SCHWANN CELLS. While people of all ages can get this type of tumor, they are most common in people between the ages of 40 and 60. The tumors can be found on almost any part of the body, but are most commonly located on the tongue. Though usually appearing alone, multiple outbreaks may occur. Only about 3 percent of all granular cell tumors are malignant.

Treatment Surgical excision.

granulation tissue Red, moist granular tissue on the surface of an open wound or ulcer during healing. It gets its name from the appearance of the skin surface, which has numerous granules. It is made up of healing tissue consisting of numerous blood vessels, white cells and fibroblasts.

granuloma Grouping of cells associated with chronic inflammation that can occur in any part of the body. They are usually a reaction to certain infectious agents, although they may occur with no known cause.

They are typical of certain infections such as tuberculosis and LEPROSY, of granulomatous disorders such as SARCOIDOSIS or Crohn's disease, and in reactions to foreign substances such as silicone, berylium, starch, talc and some tattoo pigments. See also GRANULOMA ANNULARE; GRANULOMA, LETHAL MIDLINE.

granuloma annulare A harmless skin condition characterized by a raised circular area found most often on children's knuckles or fingers, the upper part of the feet, the elbows or ears. The raised area spreads to form a ring up to 3 to 5 cm wide, with raised edges and a flat center, before slowly disappearing.

Although granuloma annulare is usually localized, it may become widespread (generalized granuloma annulare). This type is occasionally associated with diabetes. See also GRANULOMA; GRANULOMA FACIALE; GRANULOMA, LETHAL MIDLINE; GRANULOMATOUS DISEASES.

Cause Unknown.

Treatment In most cases, the skin eventually heals completely over a period of months or years. In cases where the appearance or itching is bothersome, topical corticosteroids are occasionally helpful.

granuloma faciale A fairly rare skin disorder characterized by a single persistent red-brown macule, plaque or nodule (usually on the face) with a smooth, intact surface. It usually appears in middle age. See also GRANULOMA; GRANULOMA ANNULARE; GRANULOMA, LETHAL MININE; GRANULOMATOUS DISEASES.

Treatment Usually not consistently successful, the drug DAPSONE is most commonly administered, although cryotherapy, topical or systemic corticosteroids and x-rays have sometimes been helpful.

granuloma, lethal midline A rare disorder characterized by an inflammation of the skin of the nose and facial structures, which are progressively destroyed. The condition primarily affects middle-aged women. It may be subclassified into midline malignant reticulosis, idiopathic midline granuloma and Wegener's granulomatosis. Recent research suggests that this disease is a manifestation of lymphoma.

Symptoms Ulcers and swelling within the nose spreads to tissue destruction in the facial sinuses, gums and eye orbits, leading to extensive destruction of the face, sinuses, hard palate and larynx. Death may result from infection or hemorrhage.

Treatment Radiation therapy usually stops the progression of the disease and may improve symptoms. Wegener's granulomatosis responds to corticosteroids and cyclophosphamide.

granulomatous disease A chronic disorder associated with an impaired immune system that is usually an X-linked hereditary disorder, which means that it is caused by a defect on the X chromosome and usually leads to problems in males only. Mothers and sisters of most male patients may be carriers, and half of their sons may be affected. Carriers of this disorder are not more susceptible to serious bacterial infections, but do have characteristic skin lesions that slowly become red and painful.

While infection gradually becomes less of a problem in adulthood, the possibility of severe, life-threatening bacterial infections exists throughout life for these patients.

Treatment All infections should be treated by broad-spectrum antibiotics after culturing lesions at the first sign of infection. Long-term treatment may be needed since these infections often do not respond well to antibiotics and recurrences are frequent. Human recombinant gamma interferon has helped some patients and is being studied as a possible prevention of infection.

Symptoms Patients with this disease have recurrent bacterial infections of the skin, with lesions of the scalp, mouth, nose and ears. Minor cuts and bruises often lead to furunculosis and abscesses. See also GRANULOMA; GRANULOMA ANNULARE; GRANULOMA, LETHAL MIDLINE; GRANULOMA FACIALE.

grenz zone A border of connective tissue separating the EPIDERMIS from a cellular infiltrate in the mid-dermis.

grenz ray therapy A now-abandoned treatment for inflammatory skin disease once used for ECZEMA, PSORIASIS, LICHEN PLANUS, TINEA CAPITIS and ACNE. While superficial MYCOSIS FUNGOIDES, SEZARY SYNDROME, KAPOSI'S SARCOMA and superficial BASAL CELL CARCINOMA also respond to grenz rays, soft x rays are preferred because of their better penetration.

Grisactin See GRISEOFULVIN.

griseofulvin (trade names: Griseofulvin, Fulvicin, Grisactin) One of the oldest antifungal drugs available in America, this antibiotic penicillin derivative is given orally to treat TINEA (ringworm) infections that haven't responded to creams or lotions. It is particularly effective against superficial DERMATO-PHYTE infections of the scalp, beard, palms, soles and nails, as well as ringworm of the scalp (TINEA CAPITIS), ringworm of the body (TINEA CORPORIS) and ATHLETE'S FOOT. Even with prolonged treatment, many nail infections do not respond completely, or they recur. Resistance may develop to this drug. It is not effective against bacteria, deep fungi, *Candida albicans* and TINEA VERSICOLOR. It is less effective against fungal infections of the nail.

When griseofulvin is taken with a high-fat meal, it is better absorbed and tolerated by the patient.

Griseofulvin should not be taken by patients suffering with acute intermittent POR-PHYRIA, since it may cause an acute abdominal attack. The drug may also interact with birth control pills, producing breakthrough bleeding or pregnancy.

Adverse effects The most common side effects are headache and gastrointestinal problems; others include loss of taste, dry mouth and increased sun sensitivity. Long-term treatment may cause liver or bone marrow damage.

group B streptococci infections, in infants The most common bacterial infection in newborns that may cause skin abscesses. A small number of infants with *Listeria* poisoning have skin lesions (including papules, pustules, and vesicles).

Treatment Antibiotic treatment should begin at once since blood poisoning is likely and prognosis is poor if the case is advanced and there are many lesions on the body.

Grover's disease The common name for transient acantholytic dermatosis, a keratinization disorder that is fairly common (especially in men over age 40). Despite its name, the lesions of this disease frequently persist. It is believed that sunlight may play a role in the development of this problem.

Symptoms Reddened crusted papules or vesicles appear on the upper trunk and extremities. Itching may or may not be a problem.

Treatment There is no definitive treatment. Topical corticosteroids and retinoids (such as Retin A).

gypsy moth caterpillar allergy See DERMATITIS, CATERPILLAR (GYPSY MOTH).

H

Hailey-Hailey disease The common name for familial benign chronic pemphigus, a rare genetic bullous disease characterized by the appearance of crusts with redness and blisters on the neck, under the arms, in the groin and sometimes on the scalp that may itch or cause pain. Lesions tend to get bigger, although they may spontaneously fade away without scarring; recurrences are common. The disease usually appears between ages 15 and 35.

The disease is an autosomal dominant trait, which means that only one defective gene (from one parent) is needed to cause the syndrome. Each child of an affected person usually has a one in two chance of inheriting the defective gene and of being affected. However, a positive family history can only be traced in 70 percent of patients; it is not hereditary in some cases.

While the disease is benign, it tends to last for a long time, with alternating periods of remission and active lesions. Some patients show improvement with age.

Cause The development of lesions can be set off by bacterial or candidal infections and may be exacerbated by exposure to sunlight. A hot, moist environment and sweating can contribute to the problem.

Prevention Patients with a family history are urged to avoid heat, moisture and friction, and to be careful to avoid bacterial or candidal infection when possible.

Treatment Treatment is aimed at controlling infection, relieving symptoms and avoiding heat, moisture and friction. Cold water compresses and antibacterial creams or ointments may be applied to the skin. Steroid creams may ease inflammation and discomfort; systemic steroids are not effective. Systemic antibiotic treatment (tetracycline or erythro-

mycin) may help. Surgical removal of chronic lesions followed by SKIN GRAFTS may be required.

hair, anatomy of Hair is composed of KERATIN, the protein that makes up NAILS and the outer skin layer (EPIDERMIS). Each hair shaft sits in a hair FOLLICLE, and each has a spongy semi-hollow core (the medulla) surrounded by long, thin fibers (the cortex) with several overlapping cell layers on the outside (the cuticle).

There are about 100,000 hairs on the average head, growing about 1/72 of an inch each day. At this rate, it takes about 75 days for scalp hair to grow an inch. (See also HAIR, CARE OF).

Growth stages Hair goes through distinct growing stages, growing for two to six years and then resting for three months. At any one time, about 85 percent of a person's hair is active, 1 percent is entering the resting phase, and about 14 percent is resting. In its growing phase, there is live tissue called the hair bulb at the tip of each hair that supplies keratin and melanin; this is the pale-colored swelling that may be seen if a hair is pulled out of the follicle. The upward growth of keratinocytes which become keratin-filled, forms the hair.

Hair that is in the resting phase separates from the bulb, and is shed. The rate of shedding of a normal adult scalp is about 100 hairs daily (usually after brushing or shampooing). The hair loss is continuous, but is always in the process of being replaced.

Types of hair The first kind of hair, developed in the uterus at the fourth month of gestation, is called LANUGO, a downy fuzz that is shed during the last month of pregnancy. After birth and until adolescence, fine,

Hair Anatomy

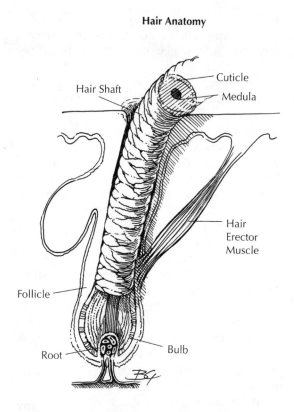

short and colorless hair (vellus hair) covers most of the child's body. "Terminal hair" is thicker, longer and often pigmented, and grows on the scalp, eyebrows and eyelashes. At puberty, it also begins to grow in the secondary sexual areas such as the pubic area and the armpits, in addition to the face, chest, legs etc.

Appearance The color of a person's hair is determined by the amount of pigment (MELANIN) in the hair shaft and its type. Melanin is produced by special cells (MELANOCYTES) in the base of the hair follicle. Red melanin causes red and auburn hair, and black melanin causes all other colors. White hair occurs when the cells receive no pigment.

Whether the hair is curly or straight depends on the shape of the hair's follicle. Straight hair grows from a straight follicle, whereas curly hair grows from a very curved follicle; wavy hair grows from a curved follicle.

Other types of hair Eyebrows and eyelashes have a different growth period from scalp hair. Both eyebrows and eyelashes grow for about 10 weeks and then rest for nine months. This is why it takes so long to grow the eyebrows back after shaving them. Plucking the eyebrows, however, stimulates the follicles and makes them grow back faster. (This is the exception to the rule that cutting hair doesn't make it grow in faster). See also HAIR, CARE OF; HAIR DYE; HAIR, DISORDERS OF.

hair, care of There are a host of old wives tales when it comes to hair, and caring for hair. For example, it's not true that shampooing too often will harm the hair follicles, that massaging the scalp will prevent hair loss, or that shaving will make hair grow back faster or thicker.

There are two types of hair—terminal hair, which grows on the scalp, eyelashes, eyebrows and areas of sexual development; and vellus hair, the fine hair that covers the body until puberty. The same follicles can produce different types of hair at different times in a person's life.

In general, it takes two and a half months for scalp hair to grow an inch; it tends to grow for up to six years, and then rest for three months. When a new hair begins to grow below the old hair, it loosens and sheds. At any time, about 85 percent of scalp hair is growing, 1 percent is beginning to rest, and 14 percent is resting. It's this hair in the resting phase that ends up in your comb, or in the bathtub drain.

As hair grows out, it is subject to weathering and injury to the overlapping cuticle scales that protect the inner cortical fiber of the hair. Once the hair is injured, it cannot be repaired because the shaft consists of dead cells. Cuticle scales near the scalp are smooth because they have not been injured; those near the ends of the hair have been repeatedly damaged and may be worn away, exposing the inner cortical fibers, and resulting in split ends.

Exposure to the sun or to chlorine from swimming pools can cause changes to the keratin, making the hair's texture change. While hair can tolerate changes such as permanents or dying if they are done carefully and not too often, these processes can cause alkaline oxidation damage.

Trauma In addition, combing and brushing may cause a great deal of injury to the cuticle scales. Hair and scalp should be washed as often as necessary with shampoos to remove oily buildup, dead cells, microorganisms, cosmetics and dirt. Because shampoos remove oil very well, those with oily scalps don't really need to choose a specially formulated shampoo. Most North Americans shampoo more often than is really necessary, but even daily shampooing is not really harmful nor is there evidence that frequent washing increases the production of sebum.

Dandruff shampoos While there is no cure for DANDRUFF, frequent shampooing is the most effective treatment and helps to alleviate symptoms in mild cases. Shampoos that are effective against dandruff contain selenium sulfide, zinc pyrithione, tar sulfur or salicylic acid. It may help to rotate different antidandruff shampoos to get the best results. When using such a product, apply the shampoo immediately and then leave on the scalp for five minutes to allow the ingredients time to work. Using a conditioner afterward won't help the dandruff, but many improve manageability. (See also DERMATITIS, SEBORRHEIC).

Acid-balanced shampoo Researchers say that using a shampoo with an acid pH on normal hair or scalp does not provide any additional benefits. However, hair damaged by sunlight or dyes, bleaches or straighteners may feel slimy when regular shampoo for damaged hair is used. An acid pH shampoo may make the hair feel more normal.

Baby shampoo These types of shampoos contain amphoteric detergents that irritate the eyes less, which make them useful for young children.

Conditioning shampoos While some products contain conditioners and shampoos, it is usually more effective to use a separate conditioner after shampooing.

Conditioners Cream rinses are made up of quaternary cationic polymers, which form a layer on the hair shaft and lubricate it. This reduces the damage caused by combing or brushing. Because anionic detergent shampoos remove oil, the hair develops a static electric charge; conditioners help to dispel the charge. Rinses also allow the strands to be aligned and reflect light. Blacks in particular may benefit from using cream rinses because very curly hair does not align well and does not reflect light uniformly, which causes the hair to appear dull. Some cream rinses also have oils to increase lubrication. While damaged or treated hair can be improved by using conditioners, fine hair can be overconditioned and appear dull and greasy.

Silicone One of the newest ingredients in hair care products is silicone (liquid plastic), which smooths the hair shaft and increases shine and manageability. Silicone works especially well for coarse or curly hair. However, regular use of silicone gels, shampoos and serums can leave hair feeling sticky, dull and hard to style.

Silicone works like clear nail polish, coating the hair so it reflects light and appears shiny. Since silicone doesn't dissolve in water, it helps prevent the hair from getting frizzy on damp days. However, because it doesn't easily rinse off, silicone tends to build up on the hair and when used too much, it causes the hair to look dirty and feel rubbery.

Fortunately, silicone will not permanently damage the hair, and it isn't absorbed into the scalp. Experts recommend using a build-up remover shampoo weekly if you use silicone products. Some salons also offer special treatments to remove silicone buildup from the hair.

Setting/permanent wave solutions These chemicals work by breaking the chemical bonds that result in the hair's normal consistency, giving it more curl or straightness (depending on their purpose), and then forming new bonds to keep the hair in place. Neither setting nor permanent wave solutions badly weaken normal hair, but if they are too strong or left on too long they can cause minor problems such as split ends or dullness, or can lead to profound structural damage and hair loss. If too strong or if used too long, they cause breakage. Only rarely, however, do the chemicals actually damage the hair follicle itself. Therefore, chemically damaged hair will be replaced by normal hair eventually.

Bleaching Bleaching products can damage the hair's protein if they are used for too long or too often, leaving the hair dull and almost colorless, and more susceptible to injury.

See also HAIR, ANATOMY OF; HAIR, DISORDERS OF; HAIR DYE.

hair, disorders of While many disorders of the hair may seem to be simply a cosmetic problem, in fact some may be evidence of an underlying disease. While brittle, unhealthy-looking hair may be caused by excessive blow-drying, combing or shampooing, it may also be a sign of a vitamin or mineral deficiency, or hypothyroidism. Very dry hair is probably caused by too much perming, tinting, bleaching or use of hot rollers—but it could also be a sign of malnutrition.

Ingrown hairs are another hair condition that can cause problems, especially in blacks or people with very curly hair. In this condition, the free-growing end of the hair penetrates the skin near the follicle and can cause severe inflammation.

hair dye Products used to alter the color of the hair that occur in two basic categories—permanent and semipermanent. Permanent dye can lift out the natural pigment and replace it with a different color. Each strand of hair is protected by an outer cuticle constructed of transparent overlapping scales much like shingles on a roof, and an inner cortex where the hair's natural pigment resides.

Permanent dyes contain ammonia, which opens the scales of the cuticle to allow the dye to penetrate the hair shaft, and peroxide, which removes the hair's natural pigment from the cortex so the new color can be layered on like paint on a canvas. The color doesn't just wash away because once it's deposited in the cortex, the dye produces a color molecule so big it gets trapped. The drawback to permanent dyes is that as the hair continues to grow, the natural color will begin to show up again in about 10 days.

Vegetable dyes Vegetable dyes deposit a coating of dye on the cuticle of the hair shaft; HENNA is an example of a vegetable dye. These dyes only keep their color with repeated applications.

Synthetic (aniline) dyes These dyes (including paraphenylenediamine) are the most popular, since they are easy to apply and their color is stable. Because they react chemically with hair, however, they can also react with skin protein and trigger an allergic reaction (see DERMATITIS, CONTACT). About 10 percent of the people who use these dyes will develop an allergy to them, and break out in red splotches. This is why a sensitivity test must be performed on every person each time an aniline product is used. While the hair can protect the scalp skin from damage, unprotected skin that touches the dye may react. In allergic individuals, these dyes used in areas around the eyes, on the eyebrows or the eyelashes can cause blindness as a result of the severe allergic reaction. This is why hair dye should never be used on eyelashes or eyebrows, and why eyelash and eyebrow dyes are forbidden by the U.S. Food and

Drug Administration to contain aniline dyes or derivatives.

Metallic dyes Metallic dyes (now only rarely used) can cause poisoning when the metal (silver, copper, iron or lead) reacts with the sulfur in the hair. Also called color restorers, they are a progressive type of dye that is combed through the hair and after several days, gradually covers gray hair. Hair dyes with metallic products will not react well to waving, straightening or to any other type of hair coloring.

Hair dye and cancer A large study by the American Cancer Society appears to put to rest the fears of a possible cancer risk for people who dye their hair. Most of the previous studies that raised concerns about hair dye were relatively small, and looked at the former habits of people who had already gotten cancer. The new study, which involved more than a half million women, looked forward—none of the women had been diagnosed with cancer when the study began. After six years, 9,500 women had died of cancer. In general, the results showed that women who dyed their hair—even those who had used hair color for more than 20 years—were at no greater risk than those who never colored their hair.

There was one exception to these findings: women who for many years use permanent black dye, the most concentrated form of hair dye. The few women who did use the black dye for at least 20 years did have a higher risk for two rare types of cancer.

Those who do use black hair dyes are advised to wear rubber gloves, avoid mixing different products, leave dye on as briefly as possible, rinse scalp completely and never dye eyebrows or eyelashes.

See also HAIR, ANATOMY OF; HAIR, CARE OF; HAIR, DISORDERS OF.

hair follicle A sheath of epidermal cells and connective tissue that surrounds the root of a hair.

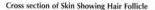

Cross section of Skin Showing Hair Follicle

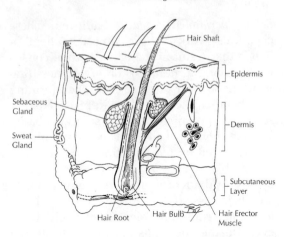

hair, gray In most people, what appears to be "gray" hair is actually a combination of pigmented and nonpigmented hair. Most people with some gray hair are not usually entirely gray, but have a mixture of white hairs among those of the normal shades of brown, blond, red or black.

As you age, your body's production of melanin decreases. New hair contains less pigment and the shaft eventually grows in without any pigment at all. The only color left in the hair is the color of the keratin itself: yellowish gray. Eventually, more and more hair continues to grow in the same way until the entire head is filled with gray hair.

White hair is due to a lack of melanin granules in the cortex of the hair shaft; usually occurring with advancing age, this lack of melanin granules means the body is losing its ability to synthesize the pigments from enzymes and proteins. True gray hairs are quite rare, and are caused by a decrease—not a total lack—of the pigment content in the hair shaft. In most people, what appears to be "gray" hair is actually a combination of pigmented and nonpigmented hair. Some hereditary diseases also predispose a person to premature grayness. See also HAIR, CARE OF.

Most people begin to develop a few gray hairs at about age 30, becoming progressively grayer over the next 20 years as more and more of their hair lacks pigment. By age 60 or 70, the hair often turns completely white, which means that all of the hairs on the head have lost their pigment granules.

Premature gray hair When hair turns gray prematurely (in the early 20s) this may often be the result of genetic factors, since the tendency seems to run in families. Severe stress, mental illness, serious physical ailments and traumatic experiences have been associated with premature gray hair and the acceleration of graying, although scientists don't know why. A few cases of premature graying are due to a deficiency of vitamin B12 (a disease known as pernicious anemia); this can be reversed by replacing the vitamin. Vitamin B is probably most effective for those whose grayness began after a severe strain, such as a long debilitating illness or severe stress.

Hair that begins to turn gray because of genetics and age is not reversible.

Throughout history, a number of famous individuals who experienced great stress were said to have turned gray overnight. Sir Thomas More in the 16th century and Queen Marie-Antoinette in the 18th both were said to have suddenly gone gray when they got the news that they were to be executed.

Although hair strands don't actually change color within hours, a person's hair can seem to turn gray in a matter of days. The phenomenon is caused by ALOPECIA AREATA, thought to be an autoimmune disorder in which the body's immune system attacks the hair follicles. While scientists don't know why the antibodies begin the attack, severe psychological stress may play a role. Alopecia areata can cause varying degrees of hair loss, from small bald patches to the loss of every bit of hair.

When the hair goes gray quickly, it is believed that the antibodies are selective and home in on just the pigment-producing cells in the follicles, causing only pigmented strands to fall out. If this occurs in someone whose hair is in the process of going white, the sudden loss of darker hair will make the person look as if he or she suddenly "went gray." Because alopecia can disappear, rapid graying isn't always permanent.

Treatment Once hair has started to gray, there is nothing that can be done to reverse the process. However, there are some hair dyes that are specifically used to color gray hair.

Some gray hair appears to have a yellowing tinge, apparently as a result of age-related changes in melanin production. This discoloration can be worsened by tobacco smoke, carbolic acid found in dry powder shampoos, setting lotions, and especially dandruff shampoos containing RESORCINOL. The easiest way to get rid of this tinge (from either external or internal factors) is to treat the hair with a bluing rinse. Do not use setting lotions or hair sprays, which have a tendency to turn gray hair yellow.

hairiness See HIRSUTISM.

hair loss The gradual loss of hair, either as a result of a disease, such as ALOPECIA AREATA or by hereditary and aging pattern baldness. In the United States, about 30 million men and 20 million women experience hair loss every year. About 40 percent of all men will show some degree of hair loss by age 35; 25 percent of all women experience some hair loss by age 40, but about 60 percent of all women experience hair loss by the time they reach menopause. Contrary to common belief, hereditary hair loss is not caused by a sudden stop in hair growth. Instead, it is the result of the gradual miniaturization of certain hair follicles; as this progresses, hairs become shorter and thinner, eventually ceasing to grow.

Every human follows a genetically programmed schedule for growing, resting and shedding hair. At any one time, as much as 85 percent of the scalp hair is growing up to an inch a month, and it may continue to grow for two to six years without stopping. When the growth phase ends, each hair begins a two-to-six month resting phase, and then begins a shedding phase. Only 10 to 15 percent of hair is in the resting phase at any one time; shedding occurs randomly. Eventually, a new hair begins to sprout from the root deep within the hair follicle, replacing the older hair above it as a new growth period begins.

It's normal to shed between 50 to 100 hairs daily—a loss that is not noticed, since most people have about 100,000 hairs on their head. Excessive shedding (more than 200 hairs) usually becomes noticeable within months, and can be caused in men and women by medical disorders (including malnutrition), medications or (most often) heredity.

Causes In most cases, hair loss is related to "androgenetic alopecia," or hereditary hair loss. Normal genes and androgens (especially testosterone) cause progressive shrinking of certain scalp follicles over time. The shrinking follicle produces a smaller, finer hair with each growth cycle. In addition to a smaller follicle, androgenetic alopecia is characterized by a shortened growth phase, which results in shorter hair.

The balding process is a gradual conversion of active, large follicles to less active, smaller follicles, resulting in short, thin hairs that are barely visible and eventually disappear completely. In men, hereditary baldness (also called "male pattern baldness") is characterized by a receding hairline above the forehead and loss of hair at the crown. If male pattern baldness progresses to its final stage, the person is left with hair only around the sides and back of the head. This is also known as pattern thinning in women. Hereditary hair loss is a general or diffuse thinning of the hair over the top of the head—women rarely lose all their hair.

The second most common cause of hair loss is ALOPECIA AREATA, which causes hair to fall out in clumps. This disorder often starts at a young age and may progress to the point where the person loses all scalp hair (alopecia totalis) or all body hair, including eyelashes and eyebrows (alopecia universalis). In some cases, alopecia areata follows a stressful event, such as divorce or death of a significant other. In most people, the hair will grow back, but the exact cause of the hair loss is not known. Most experts believe it may be caused by an immunological disorder in which antibodies are produced that attack the hair follicles.

Hair loss may be caused by medical disorders, such as a hyperactive or underactive thyroid gland, certain tumors, diabetes, severe infections, secondary syphilis, anemia and systemic LUPUS ERYTHEMATOSUS. It may be caused by medications for gout, arthritis, high blood pressure or depression, as well as high doses of vitamin A and anti-cancer drugs. Oral contraceptives may cause hair to fall out because of the increase of hormones. Hair loss due to medication is reversible once the medication is stopped.

Hair that is constantly damaged by excess bleaching, dyeing or permanent waving may begin to break and fall out; over-teasing hair or excessive straightening with hot irons can also cause hair loss. Metal combs can damage hair and scalp as well.

Traction alopecia is caused by ponytails, braids or cornrows that are pulled too tight, pulling the hair out by its roots. Friction alopecia is caused by constantly wearing snug-fitting wigs or hats.

Finally, poor diet low in protein or iron may cause abnormal hair loss.

Treatment Ever since ancient Egyptians anointed their bald spots with fats from ibex, lion, crocodile, serpent, goose and hippopotamus to encourage hair growth, humans have been trying to treat hair loss. In 420 B.C., Hippocrates tried to fend off his hair loss by whipping up typical potions of opium, horse-radish, pigeon droppings, beetroot and spices.

Today, there are several options for coping with hair loss, ranging from sophisticated styling and hair transplantation to medical treatment.

Concealing hair loss Concealing hair loss is easier for women. Women can work with their hairdressers to make their hair appear fuller through properly applied mousses, shampoos, perms and dyes. Shorter hair styles hold a curl more easily and can help hide thin hair. Both men and women find that powdered eye shadow applied to the scalp provides a darkened background that can disguise thinning hair; wigs and hairpieces may completely cover the problem.

Hairpieces Hair weaving and bonding are the most common methods of affixing a hairpiece to the head. Hair weaving ties the hairpiece with a tough nonshrinkable thread to clumps of existing natural hair that has been woven together to form anchoring places for the piece. Bonding uses a medical glue to anchor the piece to the natural hair. Both techniques must be performed by a trained hairdresser and require regular visits to have the piece washed and dyed. Periodic tightening is required.

Implants are another way to attach hairpieces, but they must be performed by a physician. By this method, the physician implants sutures or surgical threads into the scalp to which the hairpiece can be attached.

Surgical treatments Hair transplants, scalp reduction and transposition flaps are also available. In a transplant, surgeons move skin from areas of the scalp that grow hair, such as the back and sides, to areas of the scalp that are no longer growing hair. After a period of about three months, the transplanted hair begins to grow. Hair transplant techniques have been refined for a more natural look. Smaller grafts are now used for a more natural look.

Scalp reductions treat hair loss as too much scalp rather than too little hair. In this procedure, surgeons cut out areas of the scalp that no longer grow hair. The scalp is then pulled back together and help in place with sutures or surgical staples until it heals. Scalp reduction may also be successfully combined with hair replacement.

Transposition flaps are a variation of hair replacement, which involves transplanting an entire strip of hair-bearing skin instead of individual grafts. Used to cover a large area of hair loss, the flaps are a good choice for men. However, because they involve complicated multiple surgery and are expensive, the procedure is not often performed.

Medical treatment Minoxidil (trade name: Rogaine Topical Solution) is the only medically proven product that will regrow hair in men and women. Clinical tests conducted by dermatologists at 27 U.S. medical centers involving more than 2,300 men with male pattern baldness resulted in regrowth in about half (48 percent) of male patients. An additional 36 percent had minimal regrowth; the rest (16 percent) had no regrowth. In other studies, almost two out of every three women were evaluated by physicians to have regrown some hair; 13 percent had moderate regrowth and 50 percent had minimal regrowth. The rest (37 percent) had no regrowth. Among subjects who didn't use minoxidil, 39 percent also saw some regrowth.

Future research Scientists are studying the anti-androgens (drugs that would counteract the effect of the male hormone testosterone) that are responsible for signaling hair to fall out. Growth factors are also being studied to see if they can encourage growth in the tissue of the hair follicle.

hairpieces Also called toupees, these products provide fodder for jokes, but a high-quality, well-fitted piece can be successfully worn by some men. The key to a natural-looking toupee is to buy a good quality, custom-made hairpiece that is carefully matched to individual hair color and texture. Lifestyle and hobbies should also be considered when making this purchase.

A hairpiece consultant can recommend ways the hair can be attached to the head. Hairpieces should be handled carefully and washed or cleaned periodically. Hairpieces range in price from about $100 to well over $1,000, and last between two and three years.

hair removal Hair is usually removed from a part of the body for cosmetic reasons, although it may also be removed from a planned surgical site prior to an operation.

Shaving removes hair at the skin level on legs, armpits, pubic area, and facial beard area. However, hair quickly grows back from shaved areas and shaving can cause irritation.

Depilatory creams dissolve the hair just below the skin's surface, creating a smooth effect, but the cream may irritate sensitive skin areas and should be used only on the legs. *Waxing* is a technique used to remove hair from legs or face. Warm wax is applied to the skin and peeled off, pulling out the hair as it goes. *Plucking* with tweezers is a good technique for stray eyebrow hairs.

One type of *laser* has been approved for hair removal, eliminating 30 percent of hair in 70 percent of patients.

ELECTROLYSIS permanently removes hair through the use of an electric current to destroy the hair's root.

hair transplants A surgical operation in which a person's skin is moved from areas of the scalp genetically programmed to grow hair (such as the back and sides) to areas of the scalp that are no longer growing hair. After a period of about three months, the transplanted hair begins to grow.

Transplants are less often performed in women because women tend to experience diffuse hair thinning all over the scalp, which complicates the identification of hair that is not genetically coded to fall out.

Transplanation is best done before an area is completely bald. This way, the appearance of "new" hair is more subtle and the procedure less obvious. Further transplants may be needed periodically as natural hair continues to fall out, but the hair that is transplanted will remain. Results of this procedure may be enhanced by reducing the size of the scalp area or stretching scalp skin with temporary inflatable silicone bags, and then reducing the scalp area. Most physicians charge between $25 and $35 a plug; the average transplant includes about 500 plugs (totalling about $12,500 to $17,500).

Transposition flaps, a variation of hair replacement, involves transplanting an entire strip of hair-bearing skin instead of individual grafts. Used to cover a large area of hair loss, the flaps are a good choice for men who have large bald areas. But because this technique involves complicated multiple surgery, the flaps are expensive and the procedure is not often performed.

hair weaving This technique requires some natural hair to be present on the head. Hair weaves are made by tying a hairpiece with a tough nonshrinkable thread to clumps of existing natural hair which have been woven and braided together to form an anchoring for the piece. This technique must be performed by a trained hairdresser, and requires regular visits to have the piece washed and dyed. Results vary depending on hair style and texture; since the natural hair will continue to grow, regular sessions to tighten the braids will be needed. While the technique may be performed on both men and women, it is more commonly done for men. A weave generally lasts two to three years.

Implants are another way to attach hairpieces, but these must be performed by a physician. Implants are beneficial for those with little natural hair to anchor the wave. With this method, the physician implants sutures or surgical threads into the scalp to which the hairpiece can be attached.

haloderma Any skin eruption caused by the ingestion of halide.

haloprogin (trade name: Halotex) A topical treatment for fungal infections available as a 1 percent cream or solution that is usually applied two or three times a day. It is effective against DERMATOPHYTES and, to a lesser degree, against *Candida* and *Malassezia furfuri* (the cause of TINEA VERSICOLOR.)

Halotex See HALOPROGIN.

hand cream A cream designed to soften and moisturize the skin of the hands that may contain alcohol, stearic acid, lanolin and gum substances. Hand creams are usually not as greaseless as those designed to be used under makeup.

hand dermatitis See DERMATITIS, HAND.

hand, foot and mouth disease A common infectious disease of toddlers that produces blistering of palms, soles and the inside of the mouth, caused by the coxsackievirus. The condition often sweeps through day care centers in the summer. The mild illness usually lasts only a few days; there is no treatment other than painkillers to relieve blister discomfort. There is no connection to hoof-and-mouth disease, which affects cattle.

Toddlers sometimes exhibit no symptoms, but infants may develop flu-like symptoms which last several days.

hangnails Small torn pieces of skin on the sides or base of a nail that expose a raw, painful area. Hangnails may result after immersion in water, or from nailbiting. The raw

area may go on to become infected and develop into a PARONYCHIA.

Treatment Trim a hangnail with scissors and keep it covered with a Band-aid until it heals. Hangnails can be prevented by using a moisturizing cream.

Hansen's disease See LEPROSY.

harlequin color change A phenomenon caused by vascular autonomic imbalance most often seen in premature newborns during the first week of life. When the infant is lying on its side, the bottom half of the body becomes red, in sharp contrast to the top half of the body, which is quite pale. The condition may last briefly or up to 20 minutes.

harlequin fetus A rare genetic form of ICHTHYOSIS in which infants are born with very thick, hard skin with deep moist fissures that produce a grotesque appearance. The fissures appear most often over areas of movement, such as the joints, neck, underarms and groin. Ears may be underdeveloped and flat, and hair and nails may be absent. Most are born dead, or die shortly after birth from respiratory failure and the inability to eat. However, recent treatment of children born with the syndrome with etretinate, a derivative of vitamin A, has showed them to have shed the armor-like thick skin and live, albeit with severe remaining icthyosis.

The condition, which can be diagnosed before birth, may be linked with a defect in lipid metabolism or abnormal protein metabolism. More than one genetic defect may produce this syndrome.

Hartnup disease A rare hereditary metabolic disorder in which there is an eruption of lesions similar to PELLAGRA. Usually seen in children between age three and nine, the disease is an autosomal recessive trait, which means that a defective gene must be inherited from both parents to cause the abnormality. Generally, both parents of an affected person are unaffected carriers of the defective gene. Each of the children has a one in four chance of being affected, and a two in four chance of being a carrier.

Symptoms Other physical symptoms include progressive dementia, spasticity, short stature, abnormal hair and diarrhea.

Treatment Patients are treated with supplements of nicotinamide.

head lice See also LICE.

heat disorders The body maintains its optimum internal temperature through the hypothalamus. When the temperature of the blood rises, the hypothalamus sends nerve impulses that stimulate the SWEAT GLANDS and dilate the blood vessels in the skin. The act of sweating doesn't cool off the body. The cooling effect is caused by the evaporation of the sweat from the skin. Dilation of the blood vessels increases blood flow near the surface of the skin, increasing the amount of heat that is lost by convection and radiation.

When the hypothalamus does not function properly, the body may progressively overheat, leading to a fatal heat stroke if untreated. Any malfunction or overload of the body's mechanisms for keeping temperature on an even keel may result in a heat disorder. Poor adaptation to heat may cause heat cramps, heat exhaustion or heat stroke. High summer temperatures may cause PRICKLY HEAT, and an out-of-control infection can set off high fever, further damaging the body. Excessive sweating can cause an imbalance of salts and fluids in the body, which can lead to heat cramps or heat exhaustion throughout the day. To prevent heat disorders caused by excessive sweating, drink liquids (preferably water) throughout the day.

Prevention Most environmental heat disorders can be prevented by acclimation to hot conditions over a three-week period, eating a light diet, avoiding alcohol and wearing loose, lightweight clothes.

heat rash A rash that occurs at high tempertaures when sweat ducts are blocked by tight clothes made of fibers that do not breathe. Heat rash is most common on the chest and back, where perspiration is greatest, and is typified by widespread slightly raised red vesicles or even pustules. It settles down over a period of hours to days once the heat and sweating are eliminated. To protect against this rash, wear cotton clothing and use oil-free SUNSCREENS instead of heavier versions, which may trap perspiration.

helminthic infections An infestation by any species of parasitic worms. Several types of worms (or their larvae), ranging from microscopic in size to many feet long, can parasitize humans.

There are two main classes, the ROUNDWORMS and the platyhelminths, which include cestodes (tapeworms) and trematodes (flukes).

Worm disease with skin symptoms include FILARIASIS and SCHISTOSOMIASIS.

hemangioma A benign tumor or birthmark caused by an abnormal number of blood vessels in the skin as a result of proliferation. Hemangiomas may be either superficial, superficial and deep, or deep.

Superficial hemangiomas, known as STRAWBERRY MARKS or capillary hemangiomas, are bright red and protuberant. These marks develop shortly after birth; at about the age of 6 months, the tumor begins to subside and the redness slowly fades; by age 7 the hemangima completely disappears.

Deep (or cavernous) hemangiomas (see HEMANGIOMA, CAVERNOUS) are blue-purple growths that are often compressible. They do not spontaneously clear.

Treatment Superficial hemangiomas do not require treatment for any medical reason, unless they interfere with a vital function (such as those blocking the eyes, ears, mouth, nose or anus). If the marks appear on their face, there may be psychological reasons to remove these superficial tumors. A hemangioma that bleeds frequently also may require removal, especially if located on the lip or tongue, or on the vulva or anus, where it could be disturbed by constant pressure. Superficial hemangiomas may be removed by PULSED DYE LASERS, which is most successful in young patients, or by surgical excision. Deep hemangiomas are best treated surgically.

hemangioma, cavernous (or deep) A large tumor composed of large blood vessels in the subcutaneous fat and deep DERMIS that is deep, blue and never clears spontaneously. Like strawberry (capillary) hemangiomas, these most often occur in young children, usually on the head and neck. Cavernous hemangiomas, however, are composed of dilated veins rather than capillaries, and are distinguished by their slow growth and by the fact that they do not clear spontaneously.

A capillary (or strawberry) hemangioma, on the other hand, is a superficial, red growth that always disappears by age seven. *Treatment* Cavernous hemangiomas subject a patient to profound psychological stress and can permanently rob children of their sight or distort their facial features if present for too long. Systemic or intralesional corticosteroids may cause the lesions to shrink, and cryotherapy, electrodesiccation or carbon dioxide or argon laser treatments have proven successful. Selective vessel embolization followed by excision has also been used to treat patients.

hemangiosarcoma See SARCOMA.

hemochromatosis A disease also known as "bronze diabetes" in which too much dietary iron is absorbed, resulting in a bronzed skin color due to pigment deposited under the skin.
Cause This is an inherited disease primarily affecting men; women rarely are affected because they regularly lose iron during their menstrual periods each month. While the disease is known to be genetic, its exact mode of transmission is not known.
Symptoms During middle age, the first signs of the disease are a loss of sexual desire and shrinking testes; left untreated the iron overload causes chronic liver damage, impaired insulin production leading to diabetes mellitus, heart problems and liver cancer.
Treatment The disorder is treated by removing some of the patient's blood once or twice weekly; once the iron level is normal, the procedure is done only three or four times yearly. Early treatment can prevent complications; for those who have already developed the disease, regular blood removal (called "venesection") can head off problems. In some cases, chelation therapy (administration of chemicals that bind to iron and remove it from the body) may be used.

henna The most popular of the vegetable dyes, this powdered substance is made from the crushed leaves of the *Lawsonia* shrub and is used primarily to give red-orange highlights to the hair. The color can be built up to give the hair body and added shine that complements brown hair particularly but does not cover gray very well. Henna can be very messy to apply, staining anything it touches and drying and stiffening the hair (making it a good choice for oily hair). Because henna builds up on the hair, it shouldn't be used more than three times a year, and once it has been used, very little else can be done with the hair until it grows out. The color doesn't allow for permanent waving, straightening or coloring with semipermanent dyes. While henna has not been found to cause allergic reactions to the scalp, it can damage the hair.

Henoch-Schonlein purpura Inflamed blood vessels that leak blood into the skin, joints, kidneys and intestine. The disease is most common in childhood (especially among boys) after an infection such as a sore throat.

Cause Unknown, although it is suspected to be linked to an abnormal allergic reaction in resonse to infection.

Symptoms Purpuric rash on buttocks and backs of the legs and arms, with painful joints and swollen hands and feet. There may be abdominal pain and intestinal bleeding.

Treatment With bed rest and mild analgesics, most children recover within a month. In severe cases, corticosteroid drugs may be administered.

heparin necrosis Also known as anticoagulation syndrome, this condition is characterized by lesions at the subcutaneous injection site, and appears between four and 11 days after treatment with heparin (an anti blood-clotting drug) has begun. The lesions quickly enlarge into large necrotic areas. There is no successful treatment, but the disease is self-limiting. Amputation is recommended for severe cases involving the penis or breast; other areas require excision and grafting. See also COUMARIN NECROSIS.

herald patch The initial red, scaly eruption of PITYRIASIS ROSEA that occurs days before the disease spreads. It resembles a ringworm infection that is soon followed by multiple lesions, usually appearing first on the trunk.

hereditary disorders of the skin See GENETIC DISORDERS OF THE SKIN.

Hermansky-Pudlak syndrome A form of ALBINISM featuring white or pale yellow hair, many freckles, deeply-pigmented nevi, eye

problems and heavy bleeding. Sufferers also have problems with lipid storage, which may cause complications such as pulmonary fibrosis and pulmonary insufficiency. The condition is found in one of every 2,000 Puerto Ricans. On Lencois Island, Brazil, it is even more common—one in every 30 people there may be affected.

herpes gestationis A rare skin disorder occurring during pregnancy that is characterized by HERPES-like blisters on the legs and abdomen. Unrelated to the herpes simplex virus it is named because of the appearance of the eruption.

Cause Unrelated to any disorders caused by the herpes simplex virus, herpes gestationis is an autoimmune blistering condition somewhat similar to bullous PEMPHIGOID.

Treatment Systemic corticosteroids are used to treat the disease. Experts debate whether herpes gestationis is associated with an increased incidence in maternal or fetal death. The condition usually fades after delivery but tends to recur in subsequent pregnancies.

herpes progenitalis See HERPES SIMPLEX INFECTION.

herpes simplex infection A group of inflammatory skin diseases characterized by spreading or creeping small clustered BLISTERS caused by the herpes simplex virus. Forms of the virus result in COLD SORES and the sexually transmitted disease GENITAL HERPES characterized by blisters on the sex organs. More than 25 million people in America are affected by the herpes virus.

There are two forms of the herpes simplex virus—type 1 and type 2. Herpes simplex, type 1 (HSV1) is usually associated with infections of the lips, mouth and face, while herpes simplex, type 2 (HSV2) is usually associated with infections of the genitals and in babies, who acquire the disease at birth.

However, there is a certain amount of overlap between the two, and conditions usually caused by HSV2 may be caused by HSV1 and vice versa. Both types are highly infectious, spread by direct contact with the lesions or by the fluid inside the blisters. Most people have been infected with HSV1 by the time they reach adulthood.

A person suffering an immunodeficiency disorder (such as AIDS) or someone taking immunosuppressant drugs who is exposed to the virus may experience a severe generalized infection that can be fatal.

Symptoms Before a blister develops, it is often preceded by a "prodome"—burning, tingling sensation in the area where the blister subsequently appears. There may also be swollen and tender lymph glands. While the first infection by this virus may cause no symptoms at all, there may be a flu-like illness in addition to ulcers on the skin around and inside the mouth for type 1 (oral) herpes. The first outbreak for type 2 also involves a sore, appearing three to seven days after exposure, but with type 2, the infection may be so severe as to cover the penis or vagina with blistering. It may be accompanied by high fever, tender swollen glands in the groin and may last as long as two to six weeks before healing spontaneously. In women, the swelling from inflammation may be so severe as to impede urination. Exceptional pain, tenderness, high fever and extensive blister may require hospitalization.

Afterward, the virus remains in the nerve cells. Many people experience recurrent reactivations of the virus (both type 1 and 2), suffering with repeated attacks of sores, especially during a fever or after prolonged sun exposure.

The virus may infect any other part of the body, but often affects the finger, causing painful blisters called a herpetic whitlow. In patients with a preexisting skin condition (such as DERMATITIS), the virus may cause an extensive rash of blisters called ECZEMA HERPETICUM.

Treatment The antiviral drugs ACYCLOVIR, famciclovir and valacyclovir can ease the symptoms.

Prevention There is still no successful HSV vaccine. New antiviral drugs can lessen recurrences.

herpes zoster See SHINGLES.

heterograft Also known as a xenograft, this is a living tissue graft transferred from one animal species to another, such as a heart valve transplanted from a pig to a human.

hexachlorophene An antiseptic once widely used, effective against many gram-positive organisms such as *Staphylococcus*. However, it also has been associated with some unpleasant effects, including neurotoxicity in children and burn patients. It is not as safe as other antiseptics, such as chlorhexidine and iodine compounds.

See also ANTISEPTIC CLEANSERS.

HHT Foundation International Support group that promotes research into the treatment, causes and cure of hereditary hemorrhagic telangiectasia (HHT), also known as OSLER-WEBER-RENDU DISEASE. This rare genetic blood vessel disorder causes malformations of arteries and veins so that hemorrhaging from the nose occurs. Founded in 1991, the foundation has 300 members and sponsors an annual conference. It publishes the quarterly *HHT Newsletter*. For address, see Appendix D.

hidradenitis suppurativa Inflammation of an apocrine SWEAT GLAND, characterized by painful malodorous lesions in the armpits and groin area. The lesions, which are most common in those with dark skin, appear in late adolescence and are related to bacterial infection.

Treatment This condition is very difficult to treat, and scarring is a frequent complication. Good hygiene is critical; skin should be washed with a mild antibacterial soap and cleansed fastidiously. If obesity is a problem, losing weight is essential. Treatment with systemic antibiotics is guided depending on the results of the bacterial culture. In more severe problems, the dermatologist may consider administration of Accutane, steroids or surgery to remove affected tissue may help.

hidrocystoma An uncommon benign cystic tumor in the sweat gland that usually appears near the eye. The tumor usually appears alone, as a dome-shaped bluish growth. They also appear on the face, scalp, ears or chest. Treatment involves surgical excision or carbon dioxide laser vaporization.

hirsutism Excessive hairiness that occurs in females in a male pattern on face, trunk and limbs. The condition is often seen in Hispanics and women from the Mediterranean basin. However, hirsutism may be the sign of a hormonal imbalance or endocrine disease characterized by high levels of male hormones.

Treatment Several drugs can treat the problem: leuprolide, Proscar and Aldactazide, bromocriptine and Tagamet. However, none has been approved by the FDA for treating hirsutism. In cases where no medical cause is found, the unwanted hair can be bleached or removed in a variety of ways. See HAIR REMOVAL; ELECTROLYSIS.

histamine A chemical found in cells throughout the body which is released during an allergic reaction, resulting in inflammation. The effects of histamine can be offset by ANTIHISTAMINES. Histamine plays an important role in regulating the immune response. Its effects include the dilating of small venules and constriction of larger vessels, causing redness, swelling and HIVES, among other effects.

histiocytoma cutis See DERMATOFIBROMA.

hives A skin reaction also known as *urticaria* (from the Latin word *urtica* for "nettle"), these are raised, red, blotchy welts or wheals of various sizes that appear and disappear randomly on the surface of the skin. About one in five people experiences hives at one time in his or her life. Hives are physically uncomfortable but are generally harmless, leaving no lasting marks.

Cause While the cause of the reaction is often unknown, hives may result from the release of histamine and other chemicals into the skin and/or blood. A wide variety of things have been known to cause hives, including food, pollen, animal dander, drugs, insect bites, infections, illness, cold, heat, light or stress. Foods that have been linked with the development of hives include shellfish, fish, berries, nuts, eggs and milk. Penicillin and aspirin may also be related to hives in some susceptible patients.

There may also be a hereditary component in the tendency to develop hives. Termed HEREDITARY ANGIOEDEMA, this condition is characterized by diffuse nonitching swelling lasting three or four days, and may be triggered by trauma or may appear to occur spontaneously. Treatment is the same as for common hives.

Treatment The standard treatment for hives is antihistamines, but other drugs may also be used (including adrenaline or epinephrine, terbutaline, oral corticosteroids or cimetidine). In addition, sufferers should provide physicians with a detailed medical history, including a detailed diary of exposure to foods, chemicals, new products and possible irritants over a period of two weeks to a month. Because hives may be brought on by such a wide variety of agents, it may never be possible to document its exact cause.

hives, sun-induced See SOLAR URTICARIA.

homograft See ALLOGRAFT.

hookworms A small, round blood-sucking worm that penetrates the skin, causing a red, itchy rash on the feet called "ground itch" or cutaneous larva nigrans. The worms are of the species *Necator Americanus* or *Ancylostoma duodenale* (New and Old World hookworms respectively), and infest about 700 million people, in tropical Third World countries. There is very little risk of contracting hookworms in the United States. The worms are found in animal feces deposited on beaches all over the world. If an individual lies on such a beach, he or she risks becoming infested.
Symptoms In minor infestations, there may be no symptoms. In more severe cases, there is red linear rash caused by the worms crawling slowly through the skin, typically at the top of the sole of the foot or buttock. The worms also can become systemic, causing anemia, cough and pneumonia, in addition to the itchy rash.
Treatment Antihelmintic drugs (such as mebendazole applied as a topical cream) kill the worms. Improved diet and blood transfusions may also be necessary.
See also LARVA MIGRANS, CUTANEOUS.

hordeolum See STYE.

hormones and acne Hormonal activity is important in the development of ACNE, since it depends on the stimulation of the hair follicles by male sexual hormones (androgens) found both in men and women. Some women with acne may have excessive levels of androgens. This should be suspected if a woman has irregular periods or facial hair. The most frequent cause of androgen excess in females is polycystic ovarian disease.

horn, cutaneous A hard, benign pink, yellow-or-skin-colored growth most often seen in older persons. A slow-growing horn may develop on the former site of a wart a SEBACEOUS KERATOSIS, ACTINIC KERATOSIS or SQUAMOUS CELL CARCINOMA; left untreated, it may grow quite large and may protrude as much as ¾ of an inch. Surgery can remove the growth.

Horner's syndrome A group of symptoms that indicates damage to part of the sympathetic nervous system, including absence of sweating (ANHIDROSIS), narrowing of the pupil of the eye and drooping of the eyelid. The syndrome is caused by damage to the sympathetic nerve fibers (usually in the lower neck).

Howel-Evans syndrome A genetic disorder of keratinization characterized by keratosis of the palms and soles and cancer of the esophagus. It was first described by Howel and Evans in 1958, when two Liverpool families were reported to have a 70 percent incidence of esophageal cancer with the related keratosis. No cancer was found in family members without keratosis.

The disorder is inherited in an autosomal dominant pattern, which means that only one defective gene (from one parent) is needed to cause the syndrome. Each child of an affected person usually has a one in two chance of inheriting the defective gene and of being affected.

No one knows why the cancer and the keratosis appear together.

HPV See PAPILLOMA VIRUS, HUMAN.

human bites Human bites (particularly on the hand) are common, and because of the bacterial composition of the mouth, may often cause soft tissue infection. Septic arthritis or osteomyelitis may follow a bite. *Staphylococcus aureus* and *Streptococcus* are often found.

Treatment Thoroughly clean, soak and elevate the wound for 48 hours. It should be left open; oral antibiotics are often administered. Infected injuries may require local debridement, hospitalization and intravenous antibiotics.

humectant Substance that preserves the moisture or water content of the skin. Most dry skin lacks moisture rather than oil, and therefore humectants and moisturizers are needed instead of creams or oils. The most effective humectant is lactic acid, which, when applied to the skin, draws water from the dermis into the epidermis.

Hunter's syndrome A genetic metabolic disease with skin symptoms in 20 percent of cases, characterized by white or flesh-colored papules or nodules that are often found on the nape of the neck, the chest and the upper arms and legs. Lesions may appear in children before age 10, spontaneously disappearing later in life.

Hunter's syndrome is an X-linked recessive disorder, which means that it is caused by a defect on the X chromosome and usually leads to problems in males only. Women can be carriers of the defect, and half their sons may be affected.

The condition is one of seven major types of mucopolysaccharidoses, diseases characterized by a lack of certain enzymes. Other clinical findings that do not involve the skin may include deafness, dwarfism, mental retardation, clawlike hands and early mortality. There are also milder forms that allow the patient to live into adulthood.

Treatment There is no effective treatment for this disorder, although researchers hope one day the condition can be cured by replacing the missing enzymes.

Hutchinson's freckle The common name for lentigo maligna.

hyaluronic acid A substance in human skin cells that helps them to retain moisture. This acid is very effective in cosmetics but very expensive. It also helps bind and protect connective tissue.

hydrogen peroxide An antiseptic used to treat skin infections. The solution combines with catalase (an enzyme present in the skin) to release oxygen, which kills bacteria and cleanses the infected areas.

Adverse effects Hydrogen peroxide sometimes causes soreness and irritation.

hydropic degeneration Damage to the cells of the basal layer, which produces tiny spaces (vacuoles) in the cells.

hydroquinone (paradihydroxybenzene) A skin bleaching agent that can reduce the intensity of pigmentation of FRECKLES, MELASMA and senile LENTIGINES. It suppresses pigmentation by blocking the activity of tyrosinase, the enzyme involved in the synthesis of MELANIN.

When applied to the skin over a period of several months, the skin temporarily becomes somewhat lighter. For continued and increased effectiveness it must be used for a longer term. Sun exposure should be avoided because it reverses the effect of hydroquinone by increasing skin pigmentation. It is sometimes combined with tretinoin for better skin penetration, and with corticosteroids to reduce the irritation occasionally caused by tretinoin.

The medication was discovered when black workers who were handling rubber products containing hydroquinone noticed that the skin on their hands and other areas exposed to the chemical were getting lighter. Hydroquinone is prescribed in a 1 to 4 percent lotion, gel or salve.

Adverse effects Occasionally, at higher concentrations a patient will have an adverse reaction to the agent and experience *increased* pigmentation or development of MILIA. Other adverse effects could include mild skin irritation or allergic reaction.

hydroxyurea The generic name for Hydrea, an anticancer drug that inhibits DNA synthesis, that may be helpful for patients with extensive PSORIASIS.

Adverse symptoms Patients who have received prior radiation therapy may experience worsening of erythema. Other side effects include skin eruptions, gastrointestinal disturbances, bone marrow abnormalities and (rarely) neurologic symptoms. Because it causes birth defects in animals, it is not recommended for use during pregnancy. It may also cause temporary kidney problems.

hyperbilirubinemia A yellowish discoloration of the skin, sclerae, mucous membranes and eardrums caused by excessive levels of bilirubin in the blood.

hypergranulosis An increase in the number of keratin-producing cells in the granular layer of the skin, often associated with ORTHOKERATOSIS (normal keratinization).

hyperhidrosis This disorder causing excessive sweating begins at puberty, worsening in the summer and affecting the palms, soles and armpits. It may also be symptomatic of certain diseases, such as fevers, or the effect of using certain drugs. Excessively sweaty armpits and feet may cause unpleasant body odor. The condition often improves when the patient enters the middle 20s to 30s. See also SWEAT GLANDS; ANTIPERSPIRANTS; DEODORANTS.

Treatment Applications of aluminum chloride to the affected areas blocks sweat pores. Aluminum chloride is the active ingredient of most anti-perspirants. Patients should also wear clothing and shoes made of natural, absorbent material. The prescription deodorant DRYSOL (high concentration aluminum chloride) has been very effective in some patients who suffer from excessive sweating.

hyperkeratosis Thickening of the outer layer of the skin caused by an excess amount of KERATIN (a protein component of the outer skin layer). The most common types of hyperkeratosis are CORNS and CALLUSES (caused by pressure or friction).

Hyperkeratosis is often seen in scaly conditions such as WARTS, ECZEMA, and LICHEN PLANUS.

hyperpigmentation Greater pigmentation (and therefore darker) than usual skin. Darker skin (except for very black skin) often responds to trauma with hyperpigmentation, but the phenomenon occurs in all racial and ethnic groups.

Many chemicals can cause hyperpigmentation, but heavy metals can cause discoloration by being deposited within the skin. Arsenic, which some patients may ingest by drinking water from contaminated wells or by being exposed to insecticide sprays used in fruit orchards, can stimulate melanin formation within the EPIDERMIS, causing a brown hyperpigmentation. The hyperpigmentation is not caused by arsenic deposits within the dermis. Bismuth can also cause a brown hyperpigmentation; both bismuth and arsenic were once contained in medications.

hyperplasia An increase in the production and growth of normal cells in skin tissue. It can result in a thickened EPIDERMIS (outer layer of the skin). During pregnancy, the breasts grow in this fashion.

hypertrichosis Excessive hair growth in places not normally covered with hair. This excess hair growth is often caused by certain drugs (such as cyclosporine, MINOXIDIL and diazoxide). The condition is not the same as HIRSUTISM, which is excess hairiness in women.

hypertrophic scars An enlarged or thickened scar, remaining within the confines of the original wound in which excessive scar tissue rises above the skin during the healing process.

hypochondria, cutaneous See ACNE EXCORIEE.

hypohidrosis Lessened or inability to sweat. It is a symptom of HYPOHIDROTIC ECTODERMAL DYSPLASIA, a rare inherited condition characterized by the decreased ability to sweat, dry wrinkly skin, sparse dry hair, small brittle nails and cone-shaped teeth. Other causes of the hypohidrosis include exfoliative dermatitis and some anticholinergic drugs. See also DERMATITIS, EXFOLIATIVE.

hypohidrotic ectodermal dysplasia A rare, incurable genetic condition characterized by a decreased ability to sweat, dry wrinkly skin, sparse dry hair, small brittle nails and cone-shaped teeth.

hypomelanosis of Ito A congenital disorder of pigmentation also known as incontinentia pigmenti achromicans. It is characterized by bizarre hypopigmented macules in whorls, streaks and splashes on the skin of the trunk and extremities. The pigment changes are present at birth, and are often the first indication that the infant is not normal. In addition to skin symptoms, most patients also have other problems, including disorders of the central nervous system, eyes, hair, nails, teeth, musculoskeletal system or internal organs. Up to 40 percent of these patients are also mentally retarded and have seizures.

The disorder has an autosomal dominant mode of genetic transmission, which means that only one defective gene (from one parent) is needed to cause the syndrome. Each child of an affected person usually has a one in two chance of inheriting the defective gene and of being affected. Males are almost twice as likely to have the disorder as females.

Treatment As with other similar hypopigmentation disorders present at birth, there is no specific treatment for the skin problems with this disease. Topical application of methoxsalen and exposure to ultraviolet A radiation may lessen the hypopigmentation and minimize the skin disfigurement.

hypopigmentation Decreased pigmentation causing lightening of the skin. Pigment cells may be absent from an area of skin, may make too few melanosomes (melanin-producing cells) or may be incapable of synthesizing normal amounts of melanin.

Disorders of congenital hypopigmentation due to abnormal formation of melanosomes include TUBEROUS SCLEROSIS, HYPOMELANOSIS OF ITO, NEVUS DEPIGMENTOSUS and CHEDIAK-HIGASHI SYNDROME. Oculocutaneous albinism is a congenital hypopigmentation due to decreased or absent synthesis of melanin. TINEA VERSICOLOR is an example of an acquired case of hypopigmentation due to decreased synthesis of melanin. PITYRIASIS ALBA is an acquired type of hypopigmentation caused by the decreased transfer of melanosomes.

Finally, hypopigmentation may be caused by a post-inflammatory hypopigmentation. Many infectious and inflammatory skin disorders fade away while leaving hypopigmented macules and patches in the distribution and pattern of the original dermatosis. Dark skin responding to trauma often exhibits hypopigmentation, but the phenomenon occurs among all racial and ethnic groups—the more common disorders that produce post-inflammatory hypopigmentation include PSORIASIS, eczematous dermatitis, atopic dermatitis, seborrheic dermatitis, tinea versicolor, CHICKEN POX, SYPHILIS, LICHEN PLANUS, PITYRIASIS ROSEA, pityriasis lichenoides chronica and lichen striatus. Drugs also can cause hypopigmentation. Chloroquine may cause hypopigmentation of the skin or bleaching of the hair; cosmetics and skin bleaches often available without prescription may cause hypopigmentation.

hypopituitarism and skin color The lack of MELANOCYTE-STIMULATING HORMONES (MSH), which causes a generalized decrease in skin color. See also DEPIGMENTING DISORDERS; PIGMENTATION DISORDERS.

I

iatrogenic atrophy Thinning of the skin, often produced by CORTICOSTEROIDS taken either by mouth or administered on the skin, apparently because the steroids interfere with the formation of COLLAGEN. The more potent the topical steroid, the faster and more severe the atrophy. Thinning of the skin associated with systemic corticosteroids affects the skin everywhere on the body. ("Iatrogenic" describes conditions that result from treatment.)

ibuprofen (trade names Motrin, Advil, Nuprin) A nonsteroidal anti-inflammatory drug (NSAID) used to ease pain and reduce inflammation in a wide variety of skin disorders.
Adverse effects Ibuprofen may cause skin rash, abdominal pain, diarrhea, nausea, heartburn and, occasionally, dizziness. However, it is less likely to cause peptic ulcers than other NSAIDs.

ice packs A treatment to reduce inflammation, bruising and swelling of the skin by applying ice in a towel or other material. Cold causes the blood vessels in the skin to contract, reducing blood flow; it also numbs nerves and can reduce pain.

Ice wrapped in a wet cloth should be applied to the skin's surface. Chemical ice packs may also be used; these are struck or shaken, which mixes the chemicals and produces a liquid with a very low temperature.

If no ice is available in an emergency situation, a chilled soda can, frozen meat or other frozen food may be used as an ice pack (wrapped in material to avoid burning the skin).

ichthyosis Any of several generalized skin disorders characterized by dry, rough, scaling, darkened skin that occur because of an excess amount of KERATIN (the main protein component of the skin). The disorder's name is derived from the Greek word *ichthus* meaning "fish," the appearance and condition of the skin resembles scales. This group of genetic diseases ranges from mild generalized dry skin in ichthyosis vulgaris to severe widespread thickened scaly dry skin in LAMELLAR ICHTHYOSIS.

Ichthyosis vulgaris, which affects the thighs, arms and backs of the hands, usually appears at or shortly after birth and improves as the child grows older. However, in severe conditions, the infant is usually born dead, encased in skin as hard as armor plate.
Treatment There is no cure for any of the ichthyoses, but lubricants and ointments may help the dryness, and bath oils can moisten the skin. Ichthyosis improves in a warm, humid environment and worsens in cold weather. Washing with soap aggravates the condition.

icterus See JAUNDICE.

immersion foot Also known as "trench foot" during World War I, this condition causes the skin of the feet to turn pale, and then red, swollen and painful. It occurs among shipwreck survivors and soldiers whose feet have been wet and cold for a long time. It is caused by death of skin tissue after prolonged immersion in water.
Treatment At the initial stage (where the skin is pale and there is no detectable pulse), rewarm the skin gradually and carefully, since overheating may lead to GANGRENE (tissue death). If the condition has progressed to the latter stages, with red and swollen skin

and a strong pulse, the foot should be gradually *cooled.* Even so, the feet may subsequently be overly sensitive to cold for several years.

Untreated, the condition can lead to severe muscle weakness, skin ulcers or gangrene.

immunity and sunlight The sun has a detrimental effect on the body's immune system, decreasing its ability to recognize and destroy potentially lethal pathogens ranging from bacteria to cancer cells.

Ultraviolet-B light suppresses the function of T-lymphocytes, which are important in immune surveillance. There is evidence from animal research that this UV-B-induced supression may decrease the immune system's ability to recognize and destroy malignant cells which initiate skin cancer.

immunotherapy A preventive technique to combat allergy to substances such as pollen, dust mites, wasp or bee venom, etc. The treatment involves giving increasing doses of the allergen (irritating substance) to make the patient's immune system less sensitive to the irritant.

Before immunotherapy begins, the patient and physician try to determine, most often through skin and blood tests, the trigger factors for the allergy.

A purified extract of a small amount of the allergen is injected into the skin of the arm once a week for about 30 weeks, after which injections can be administered every two weeks. Eventually, the injections can be given once a month. The therapy must be given for three to four years before the patient can be considered immune. It increases a person's ability to tolerate the allergen.

Adverse effects Because there is a risk of a severe allergic reaction called anaphylactic shock shortly after an injection, the technique requires close medical supervision.

See also BEE AND WASPS.

impetigo See IMPETIGO, COMMON; IMPETIGO, BULLOUS.

impetigo, Bockhart's A superficial form of FOLLICULITIS.

impetigo, bullous Also called "staphylococcal impetigo," this is a superficial skin infection caused by *Staphylococcus aureus* bacteria that requires immediate attention. This disease has been more frequently diagnosed since the 1970s.

Symptoms Thin-walled, flaccid fluid-filled blisters that rupture easily; their fluid may be clear or full of pus. After rupture, the base quickly dries to a shiny veneer, which looks different than the thicker crust found in common impetigo. Lesions are usually found in groups, most often on the face or trunk instead of arms or legs.

Treatment As with common impetigo, bullous impetigo is treated orally/internally with dicloxacillin, cephalosporin or erythromycin. Blood poisoning complications are rare. It is important to wash the affected areas thoroughly twice a day with soap and water to keep the area as clean as possible.

impetigo, common A superficial skin infection most commonly found in children, caused by streptococcal or staphyloccal bacteria, or sometimes both, requires immediate attention. Impetigo should be treated as soon as possible to avoid the spread of the infection to other children and to prevent a rare complication: a form acute glomerulonephritis, a form of kidney disease.

Impetigo is spread through contact and usually is found on exposed body areas such as the legs, face and arms. Because impetigo is spread quickly through play groups and day-care centers, children with the infection should be kept away from playmates and out of school until the sores disappear.

Symptoms The condition starts as tiny, almost imperceptible blisters on a child's skin, usually at the site of skin abrasion, scratch or insect bite. Most lesions occur on exposed areas, such as the face, scalp and extremities. The red and itchy sores begin to ooze for the next few days, leaving a sticky golden crust. Untreated, the infection usually will last from two to three weeks but may continue indefinitely if not treated. It is most prevalent during hot, humid weather.

Treatment Parents should not let impetigo run its course. They should get treatment for children immediately to avoid spreading the infection to other children. Studies show nupirocin treatment alone is highly effective in simple uncomplicated impetigo and is now the treatment of choice. In widespread disease, systemic antibiotics also can be used. Oral dicloxacillin, cephalosporin or erythromycin for 10 days.

Complications Although rare, impetigo can lead to a form of kidney disease known as acute glomerulonephritis.

Prevention Cleanliness and prompt attention to skin injury can help prevent impetigo. Impetigo patients and their families should bathe regularly with antibacterial soaps, and apply topical antibiotics to insect bites, cuts, abrasions and infected lesions immediately. Impetigo in infants is especially contagious and serious. To prevent spreading, pillowcases, towels and washcloths shouldn't be shared, and should be boiled after each use.

impetigo contagiosa See IMPETIGO, COMMON; IMPETIGO, BULLOUS.

impetigo, staphylococcal See IMPETIGO, BULLOUS.

impetigo, streptococcal See IMPETIGO, COMMON.

impetigo, superficial See IMPETIGO, COMMON.

Imuran See AZANTHIOPRINE.

incontinentia pigmenti achromicans See HYPOMELANOSIS OF ITO.

incontinentia pigmenti See BLOCH-SULZBERGER SYNDROME.

infant acne See ACNE, INFANT.

infantile acropustulosis A newly discovered disease in black infants that causes severe itching, restlessness and fretfulness and is commonly diagnosed between two and 10 months of age. The disorder is characterized by pinpoint red macules evolving into papules and pustules on the hands and feet, with scattered lesions on other parts of the body. The disorder disappears spontaneously by the time the child is two or three years old.

Treatment Administration of diphenhydramine may help control itching. DAPSONE may also be helpful, but the risk of side effects usually outweighs need for treatment.

infant skin care See SKIN CARE FOR INFANTS.

infant skin diseases Infants are affected by a wide range of problems unique to their age group, and they may also show unusual symptoms of more common skin problems found in older patients. Because many skin problems of infants are related to systemic disorders, a complete physical exam is important to diagnosis. Treatment for infant skin problems is also difficult, complicated by the risks and toxicity of various medications that would be appropriate for an older patient.

Infant skin problems can include MILIA, SALMON PATCH, ERYTHEMA TOXICUM, PRICKLY HEAT, harlequin color changes, neonatal acne, hemangiomas, PORT WINE STAINS, lymphatic disorders, transient neonatal pustular melanosis acropustulosis, APLASIA CUTIS, EPIDERMOLYSIS BULLOSA, INCONTINENTIA PIGMENTI, ICHTHYOSIS, bacterial infections (such as IMPETIGO, SYPHILIS, SCALDED SKIN SYNDROME), and viral infections (such as HERPES SIMPLEX, cytomegalovirus, RUBELLA, AIDS, toxoplasmosis).

Other problems include histiocytosis X, juvenile xanthogranuloma, MASTOCYTOSIS, and subcutaneous fat necrosis of the newborn. There are pigmentary abnormalities, such as CAFE AU LAIT SPOTS, BLUE NEVUS, and CONGENITAL MELANOCYTIC NEVI. Infants may also be affected by seborrheic dermatitis of infancy, diaper rash and neonatal lupus erythematosus.

inflammation An essential part of the body's response to injury, inflammation results in redness, swelling, pain and heat in the skin tissue because of either a chemical or physical injury or an infection. Inflammation occurs when skin tissue is damaged. A chemical called HISTAMINE is released, which increases blood flow to the damaged tissue, causing redness and heat; white blood cells enter the tissue and attack the bacteria and other foreign particles. Similar cells from the tissues remove and consume the dead cells, sometimes producing pus. Histamine also makes blood capillaries leak, causing fluid to ooze out and create swelling.

Occasionally, inflammation is an inappropriate response (such as in autoimmune disorders) and results in disorders such as rheumatoid arthritis, causing joint inflammation.

Treatment Inflammation may be suppressed with corticosteroid drugs or nonsteroidal anti-inflammatory drugs. They work by reducing the production of prostaglandins (fatty acids that produce inflammation in injured tissue) and reduce the release and activity of white blood cells and normalize the size of blood vessels.

infrared light Light in the part of the electromagnetic spectrum immediately after the red end of the visible light. This invisible form of electromanetic radiation heats the skin and underlying tissues. Chronic exposure, such as in cases of bakers or furnace workers can produce photoaging, similar to that produced by longstanding sun exposure.

infundibulofoliculitis A disorder of keratinization characterized by flesh-colored follicular papules on the neck, trunk and extremities found almost exclusively in black patients. The cause of this recurrent dermatosis is unknown. It is treated with mild topical corticosteroids (such as 1 percent hydrocortisone cream) and emollients.

ingrown toenail A painful nail condition in which one or both edges of the nail has grown inward into the skin around the nail bed, causing inflammation and infection. The condition is usually caused by wearing ill-fitting shoes, poor personal hygiene or improperly cut toenails.

Prevention Toenails should be cut straight across, not angled down along the sides.

Treatment Antibiotics can relieve the infection; removal of the nail edge under local anesthetic may be necessary. Pain may be relieved by soaking the foot in strong, warm saline solution twice daily and covering the area with a dry gauze bandage.

insect bites Minute puncture wounds in the skin by any of a variety of arthropods such as insects, mites, mosquitoes, midges, gnats, sand flies, ticks, fleas and bedbugs. Most insect bites are not terribly painful, causing only a temporary itch for several days. They are extremely common, especially in children. Papular urticaria (HIVES) occurs most often in two- through seven-year-olds, usually in late spring or summer. Episodes last only two to three weeks, but can recur over a three- or four-year period.

Direct tissue injury may result from biting, stinging or burrowing. Local hives may occur by venoms introduced with a bite or sting, or by contact with various secretions. Necrosis (tissue death) has been produced by the bite of certain spiders (such as the BROWN RECLUSE). Secondary abrasions or infections may occur. Arthropods may bite either on exposed areas of the skin or parts of the body where clothing fits tightly (in these areas, the movement of the insect is halted and it bites to feed or as a defense).

Treatment Itch and redness can be reduced with topical corticosteroids; calamine lotions also helps the itch. Topical antihistamines or anestheics such as Benadryl and benzocaine should be avoided. Household insect control is important.

integument A medical name for the skin.

interface dermatitis See DERMATITIS.

internal malignancy, skin signs of See MALIGNANCY, SKIN SIGNS OF INTERNAL.

International Association of Trichologists A professional organization for individuals licensed to practice or perform manipulative, electrical, light or cosmetic therapy on the scalp that promotes the study, research and legitimate practice of the treatment and care of hair and scalp. The association prescribes and administers courses of study in trichology, conducts tests, grants certification and offers placement services. Founded in 1973, the association has 100 members and publishes the bimonthly newsletter *Guide to Hair Loss*. It sponsors an annual conference in January. For the address, see Appendix E; see also NATIONAL ALOPECIA AREATA FOUNDATION; ALOPECIA AREATA; HAIR, CARE OF.

International Guild of Professional Electrologists A professional organization for electrologists, electrology schools, and manufacturers and suppliers of electrolysis equipment. The group works to improve the image of electrolysis and promote it as an acceptable allied health profession. It establishes standards for practice and promotes licensing of electrologists. The group also compiles statistics, provides a referral service and conducts seminars and research programs.

It publishes brochures, a quarterly newsletter and biennial conference reports. Founded in 1978, the guild has 2,200 members and sponsors a biennial meeting. For address, see Appendix D; see also AMERICAN ELECTROLOGY ASSOCIATION; COUNCIL ON ELECTROLYSIS EDUCATION; NATIONAL COMMISSION FOR ELECTROLOGIST CERTIFICATION; SOCIETY OF CLINICAL AND MEDICAL ELECTROLOGISTS.

International Society for Burn Injuries A professional society for those who treat or research BURNS that seeks to disseminate knowledge and stimulate prevention in the field. The society promotes scientific, clinical and social research in burns, promotes first aid, nursing and other types of education in all phases of burn care and offers awards for research. Affiliated with the World Health Organization, the society was founded in 1965 and has 1,300 members. It publishes the monthly journal *Burns* and holds an annual conference and a quadrennial Congress on Burn Injuries, plus regional meetings and seminars. For address, see Appendix D; see also AMERICAN BURN ASSOCIATION, BURNS UNITED SUPPORT GROUPS, NATIONAL BURN VICTIM FOUNDATION, PHOENIX SOCIETY FOR BURN SURVIVORS, NATIONAL INSTITUTE FOR BURN MEDICINE.

International Society of Dermatology: Tropical, Geographic and Ecologic An international organization of dermatologists and general physicians that promotes interest, education and research in dermatology. Formerly known as the International Society of Tropical Dermatology, the group was founded in 1957 and has 3,000 members. It holds a quinquennial world congress and periodic seminars.

Publications include the biennial *Directory* and the monthly *International Journal of Dermatology*. For address, see Appendix E.

Interplast A professional group of medical professionals that sends volunteer teams into developing countries to perform free reconstructive surgery on patients with BURNS, birth defects or other deformities. An estimated 2,000 free surgeries are performed in Ecuador, Peru, Peru, Honduras, Nepal, Mexico, Brazil, China, Thailand, Vietnam and the Philippines. The group also conducts teaching programs during visits to these countries. Founded in 1969, the organization holds an annual meeting. For address, see Appendix E; see also NATIONAL FOUNDATION FOR FACIAL RECONSTRUCTION; AMERICAN ACADEMY OF COSMETIC SURGERY; AMERICAN ACADEMY OF FACIAL PLASTIC AND RECONSTRUCTIVE SURGERY; AMERICAN ASSOCIATION OF PLASTIC SURGEONS; AMERICAN BOARD OF PLASTIC SURGERY; AMERICAN SOCIETY OF PLASTIC AND RECONSTRUCTIVE SURGEONS; PLASTIC SURGERY RESEARCH COUNCIL.

intertrigo Skin inflammation occurring primarily in obese people on adjacent surfaces of the skin, such as the neck creases, groin, armpits, folds of the abdomen, between fingers and toes, and the area beneath the breasts.
Symptoms Red, moist skin, with scales or blisters and an unpleasant odor. The condition, which worsens with sweating, is sometimes accompanied by seborrheic DERMATITIS or THRUSH.
Treatment Weight reduction, good personal cleanliness, dry skin and corticosteroid or antifungal cream applied to dermatitis or thrush.

iododerma Any skin eruption caused by iodine or iodide ingestion.

isotretinoin (trade name: Accutane) A synthetic oral form of VITAMIN A that has been used since the late 1970s to treat severe cystic ACNE that has failed to respond to other treatments. Recent research has also found it is effective in the healing of oral LEUKOPLAKIA. It is also given to treat severe ICHTHYOSIS (disorders characterized by thickened, scaling skin).

Isotretinoin works by decreasing formation of oily plugs of SEBUM, reducing the formation of KERATIN (the tough outer layer of skin) and by shrinking SEBACEOUS GLANDS— so well that it can cause unpleasant side effects such as skin dryness and nosebleeds. Isotretinoin cures or greatly reduces severe disfiguring acne in up to 80 percent of patients. However, it can be dangerous to a fetus, causing severe birth defects (including fetal brain, heart and skeletal deformities); for this reason, pregnancy must be avoided during treatment and for at least two months after treatment has ended.

Currently, isotretinoin is given for four or five months for the first treatment; after treatment has ceased, the condition may continue to improve for at least two more months and sometimes for as long as one year, although the sebum production gradually returns to its original levels before treatment. However, only about one third of patients need a second course of the drug, which should be administered only after a six-month hiatus. This second course may require higher doses.
Adverse effects In addition to itching, thinning hair, dry and flaky skin, isotretinoin may occasionally cause aching muscles and bones, thinning hair, increased lipid levels in the blood and, rarely, liver damage. It carries a serious risk of birth defects. See also RETIN-A; RETINOIDS.

itching An intense tickling sensation on the skin that makes one want to scratch. The precise reason for this response is not fully understood. Itching is the most prominent symptom in many skin diseases.

Skin that is too dry and scaly commonly causes itching. Many drug reactions result in itching (especially reactions to codeine, cocaine and some antibiotics) and some types of rough clothing, soaps and detergents can trigger an itching response in some people.

In addition, a wide range of disorders produce itching, including HIVES, ECZEMA and FUNGUS INFECTIONS (tinea). PSORIASIS, LICHEN PLANUS and DERMATITIS HERPETIFORMIS may also experience bouts of itching. Itching around the anus may be caused by hemorrhoids, anal fissure or persistent diarrhea, or by too-rough cleaning after defecating. Worms are the most common cause of anal itching in children.

Itching around the vulva (pruritus vulvae) may be caused by *candidiasis* (a yeast infection), hormonal changes at puberty, pregnancy or menopause, or the use of spermicides or vaginal suppositories, ointments and deodorants.

Itchiness all over the body may be caused by diabetes mellitus, kidney failure, JAUNDICE, thyroid disorders, Hodgkin's disease or blood disorders.

Infestations of lice and scabies cause severe itching, as can insect bites.

Treatment Specific treatment depends on the underlying cause of the itching, but in general, cooling lotions (such as calamine) can relieve the itching and irritation. EMOLLIENTS can reduce skin drying and help ease itching.

Because soap can irritate itchy skin (especially if the skin is dry or has a rash), it should only be used when really necessary. Mild cleansing solutions or water alone may be enough to keep itchy skin clean.

While scratching can temporarily ease the itch, it can actually make itching worse over time by overstimulation. The urge to scratch can be suppressed by using lotions, salves or applying cool, wet compresses to the affected area, or systemic agents such as antihistamines.

J

Jarisch-Herxheimer reaction Also known as therapeutic shock, this reaction usually occurs within 12 hours of treatment with antitreponemal drugs (drugs used to kill *Treponema* bacteria, such as those that cause SYPHILIS).
Cause The reaction is caused by the widespread death of spirochetes.
Symptoms The reaction is characterized by a flu-like illness, including a rise in temperature (101–102° F) with chills, malaise and worsening of symptoms. Although the reaction is benign in secondary syphilis (it heralds a favorable response to treatment), in neurosyphilis this reaction, although rare, may be severe. In these cases, oral corticosteroids may minimize the reaction.

jaundice Yellow discoloration of the skin caused by the accumulation in the blood of the yellow-brown bile pigment called bilirubin. Jaundice is a primary symptom of many different disorders of the liver and biliary systems.

Bilirubin is formed from hemoglobin as old red blood cells break down. The pigment is absorbed from the blood by the liver, where it is dissolved in water and excreted in bile. The process can be disrupted in one of three ways, causing one of the three types of jaundice—hemolytic, hepatocellular and obstructive.

In *hemolytic jaundice*, the body breaks down too many red blood cells, producing too much bilirubin. A similar type of jaundice can develop in a newborn, whose liver has not yet developed the capacity to break down bilirubin. In adults, a type of jaundice much like hemolytic jaundice can develop as a symptom of mild liver disease.

In *hepatocellular jaundice*, the transfer of bilirubin from liver cells to bile is prevented, causing a buildup of bilirubin. This is usually the result of acute hepatitis or liver failure.

Obstructive jaundice is caused by a blockage of the bile ducts, which prevents the bile from flowing out of the liver. Obstructive jaundice can also occur if the bile ducts are missing or have been destroyed. As a result, bile can't pass out of the liver, and bilirubin is forced back into the blood.
Treatment In all cases treatment is for the underlying disorder.

jellyfish stings The true jellyfish family includes about 200 species that drift along the shoreline, dragging tentacles capable of stinging when touched. While most stings from jellyfish may cause little harm, some jellyfish (and Portuguese men-of-war) can inflict severe stings, causing a victim to panic and drown. In the water, the shock of the sting often causes the victim to jerk away, which only stimulates the tentacles to release more poison. If stung by a jellyfish on dry land, more poison is released if the victim tries to rip off the sticky threads of the tentacles.
Symptoms Stings can cause a severe, burning pain and a red welt or row of lesions at the site of the sting. There may also be generalized symptoms, including headache, nausea, vomiting, muscle cramps, diarrhea, convulsions and breathing problems. The wound site becomes red and blistered and can leave permanent scars. One or two weeks after a sting, the victim may experience a recurrence of the lesions at the site.

The sting of the Portuguese man-of-war (another type of jellyfish) is rarely fatal, but causes HIVES, numbness and severe chest, abdominal and extremity pain. Death is usually the result of panic and drowning.

Treatment Because tentacles continue to discharge their stinging cells as long as they remain on the skin, the most important first aid intervention is to remove all of the tentacles. Alcohol, ammonia or vinegar and salt water (*do not use fresh water*) can be poured over the sting site to deactivate the tentacles, which should then be scraped off with a towel, or with sand held by a towel. DO NOT REMOVE OR RIP OFF TENTACLES BY HAND. Pull, don't rub, the tentacles away. Baking soda in a paste can be applied to the sting to relieve pain; after an hour, moisten again and scrape off the baking soda with an object to remove any remaining stinging cells. Calamine lotion will ease the burning sensation, and painkillers may help with the stinging pain. (Other popular remedies for pain include meat tenderizer, sugar, ammonia and lemon juice. Some persons swear by the application of urine.)

If given early, the calcium blocker verapamil may be effective. Antivenin is effective against more dangerous species, but it must be given immediately.

Jellyfish stings may also cause an allergic reaction, which can be treated with Benadryl or corticosteroids. A severe reaction to the sting may require hospitalization.

jock itch The common term for tinea cruris, a common fungal infection of the genital area characterized by reddened, itchy areas spreading from the genitals outward to the inner thighs. It is uncommon in women.

Treatment Antifungal drugs in topical forms such as lotion, cream or ointment can ease the itchy rash. Treatment should be continued for some time after the symptoms have passed to make sure the fungi has been eliminated, to prevent recurrence. Mild infections on the skin surface may require treatment for up to six weeks.

K

Kaposi's sarcoma A condition characterized by skin tumors that is the most common malignant manifestation of acquired immunodeficiency syndrome (AIDS). Before the advent of the AIDS epidemic, Kaposi's sarcoma was a fairly rare skin condition that developed slowly and was seen almost exclusively in elderly Italian and Jewish men. Today, it is at least 20,000 times more common in the general population and 300 times more common among immunosuppressed groups in the United States. About 95 percent of the epidemic Kaposi's sarcoma in the United States is found in homosexual and bisexual men, whereas other risk groups have an incidence of 3 percent. In patients with AIDS, Kaposi's sarcoma is highly aggressive and causes widespread tumors.

Cause The cause of this disorder is unknown, although there is some evidence that it may be the result of a sexually transmitted infectious agent other than HIV, the virus that causes AIDS.

Symptoms Epidemic Kaposi's sarcoma may appear early in HIV infection, or late in its course. Purple macules first appear on any body site. In time, they may thicken into plaques or nodules and are often seen in the mouth, on the hard palate and the gums. In those with AIDS, tumors also often affect the gastrointestinal and respiratory tracts, where they may cause severe internal bleeding.

Prognosis The outcome in adult patients with AIDS and Kaposi's sarcoma depends on the activity of the HIV disease, and the degree to which the person's immune system is suppressed.

Treatment Treatment should include an antiretroviral agent such as zidovudine, which will not affect the tumors but will diminish the degree to which the immune system is suppressed. Antiretroviral agents may also boost the effectiveness of other drugs that do affect Kaposi's. Localized lesions respond well to radiotherapy, cryotherapy, surgical excision or injection with vinblastine, bleomycin or interferon alfa. Oral administration of interferon alpha is effective in about half of patients with mild Kaposi's sarcoma. In more severe cases, chemotherapy is often required.

Kawasaki disease An acute childhood disease of unknown cause featuring a measles-like rash over the body that usually occurs during the first years of life. Also called mucocutaneous lymph node syndrome, it was first observed in Japan during the 1960s.

Symptoms The first symptom is a persistent fever, coupled with conjunctivitis, dry and cracked lips, swollen lymph nodes, red swollen palms and feet, and a measles-like rash. By the end of the second week, the skin at the tips of the fingers and toes peels and the other symptoms subside. The disease can last for more than three months and can recur.

Complications/Treatment While most children recover completely, sudden death occurs in 1 or 2 percent of cases, usually due to coronary thrombosis during the acute phase of the illness. Aspirin and intravenous immune globulin may help prevent heart complications.

keloids Large permanent and sometimes disfiguring scars that may develop after surgery or other injury to the skin or occasionally spontaneously. Similar in appearance to hypertrophic scars, keloids tend to grow indefinitely, (although they generally run in families). They are particularly apt to occur in blacks or Asians, and are less common in whites.

Keloids are often found on the upper shoulders, the earlobes (after ear piercing), and the face, chest and neck. Rare in infancy and old age, they appear more often throughout childhood, reaching a maximum outbreak between puberty and age 30. They slowly improve as patients get older. This relationship to age (and the fact that they sometimes appear during pregnancy) suggests a possible hormonal influence.

Treatment Treatment is usually not satisfactory, since keloids tend to recur after excision, at which point they can become even larger and more unsightly.

Small keloids may be treated by corticosteroids injected into the lesions. Large keloids can be debrided surgically but must be injected with corticosteroids immediately after surgery and four weeks later.

keratin A protein containing high amounts of sulfur that is the primary component of the outermost layer of the skin, nails, horny tissue and hair. Keratin is a tough substance that resists damage from a wide range of chemical and physical agents. See also KERATINIZATION, DISORDERS OF; KERATINOCYTES.

keratinization, disorders of These disorders are usually characterized by obvious skin problems such as fissures, scales or thickening of the stratum corneum (top layer of the epidermis). These disorders of keratinization include DARIER'S DISEASE, a variety of ICHTHYOSES (see ICTHYOSIS), epidermolytic hyperkeratosis, KID SYNDROME, NETHERTON'S SYNDROME, REFSUM'S DISEASE, CONRADI'S DISEASE, HARLEQUIN FETUS, lipid storage disease, FOLLICULAR HYPERKERATOSES, GROVER'S DISEASE, ACANTHOSIS NIGRICANS, POROKERATOSIS, PALMAR-PLANTAR KERATOSIS.

keratinocytes Responsible for maintaining the skin's barrier, these cells make up about

80 percent of the body's epidermal cells. The keratinocytes are made of the protein keratin; soft keratin is found in the epidermal cells and hard keratin is found in hair and nails.

The lowest layer of the epidermis is called the basal layer, where the cells of the epidermis are born; these cells reproduce rapidly and rise gradually toward the surface. These cells lie right next to the dermis, with its rich supply of blood vessels and glandular secretions. Their health and growth is dependent on the food and oxygen that the tiny capillaries of the dermis carry. As the cells in the basal layer are pushed up into the other layers, they undergo many changes, including the increase in the amount of keratin they produce. By the time the cells of the basal layer reach the top layer of the epidermis, they are no longer alive and they are entirely formed of keratin. This process of growth, maturation and death is called KERATINIZATION. Problems in the speed and mount of keratin formation, as well as its disposal, lead to many different skin problems, such as thickened, cracked and infected skin.

If the cells contain too little keratin, the appearance begins to look cracked and flaky as cells slough off. This can leave the lower layers exposed to infection and irritation. Keratin needs water to keep it pliable and healthy; when there is not enough water, the keratin crumbles and the cells can't stay together. This is what happens when the skin becomes dry.

keratitis-ichthyosis-deafness syndrome See KID SYNDROME.

keratoacanthoma A skin nodule that usually appears on the face or arm of elderly people, it is often very difficult to distinguish from invasive SQUAMOUS CELL CARCINOMA. A biopsy may be necessary to tell the difference.

Initially small it grows rapidly for two to three months, reaching a maximum size of about 2 cm across. The mature nodule has the slope of a volcano with bulging sides and a crater-like center.

Cause Unknown, but it tends to be more common in those who have had years of exposure to strong sunlight and in those taking long-term immunosuppressant drugs.

Treatment Left alone, keratoacanthoma regress completely, often leaving unpleasant scarring. They are best excised.

keratoderma A group of skin disorders characterized by thickening of the STRATUM CORNEUM on the palms and soles.

keratohyaline granules Deep, irregular grains in the outermost layer of the skin.

keratolysis Dissolution of the STRATUM CORNEUM.

keratolytic drugs Drugs that soften and loosen KERATIN (the tough outer layer of the skin) and remove scales. They include preparations of SULFUR, SALICYLIC ACID and lactic acid, which are used in the treatment of skin and scalp disorders such as WARTS, calluses, ACNE, DANDRUFF and PSORIASIS.

For example, salicylic acid works by softening the intracellular cement and decreases cell-to-cell adhesion, encouraging the shedding of cells in the stratum corneum layer of the skin (the most superficial layer of the epidermis, consisting of dead cells).

keratosis follicularis See DARIER'S DISEASE.

keratosis, seborrheic These skin lesions of unknown cause range from flat, dark brown rough patches to small, warty protrusions that are covered with a greasy, removable crust. Completely harmless but unsightly, they usually appear on light-skinned people after age 40. Their occurrence increases with age. While the lesions may appear alone, they are usually found in groups on the face, chest, back, abdomen and extremities. As time goes on, the lesions become more deeply pigmented, become increasingly raised from the skin and develop a rougher contour. They are not caused by exposure to sunlight or by a virus.

Treatment When large, irritated or inflamed, they can be treated with a variety of techniques including CRYOTHERAPY, ELECTRODISSICATION or CURRETAGE. See also KERATOSIS PILARIS; DARIER'S DISEASE.

keratosis, solar Also known as actinic keratosis, small, these rough pink or flesh-colored growths appear on exposed parts of the body as a result of overexposure to sun over a period of years. Rarely they may develop into skin cancer, usually becoming a SQUAMOUS CELL CARCINOMA.

Treatment They should be removed because of the risk of skin cancer, which can be on an outpatient basis using CRYOSURGERY (destruction of tissue with extreme cold) or curretage.

keratosis pilaris A type of follicular hyperkeratosis characterized by sandpaper-like skin with skin plugs that typically occurs on the upper outer arms. It may first begin in childhood or during adolescence, and is more severe in winter. An associated form of the condition is associated with a red halo around each plugged follicle. Less frequently, it may affect the thighs or the cheeks.

This disorder is chronic, but it improves during the summer months. While it is a nuisance, it is of no medical significance.

Treatment Emollients (such as Eucerin cream), agents containing lactic acid (Eucerin Plus), lachydrin or tretinoin (RETIN-A) may be effective, but they must be used continuously for continuous effect. Most patients improve after being exposed to ultraviolet radiation. See also KERATOSIS; DARIER'S DISEASE.

kerion An inflammatory fungal infection of the scalp characterized by a red, pustular swelling. The swelling lasts for up to two months, but may leave a scar and permanent loss of hair from the affected area. See also TINEA.

Treatment Aggressive treatment with a systemic antifungal such as GRISEOFULVIN with systemic steroids is usually recommended.

ketoconazole (Trade name: Nizoral) An antifungal drug used to treat TINEA VERSICOLOR or candidiasis (THRUSH), superficial dermatophytoses and some systemic fungal infections.

Adverse effects Ketoconazole may cause nausea, but this may be avoided by taking the drug with food. It should not be taken at the same time as antacids, however, because ketoconazole requires an acidic stomach for absorption. Other side effects include itching, headache, dizziness, abdominal pian, constipation, diarrhea, nervousness, rash and liver damage. Occasionally, patients may experience hives and allergic reactions with the first dose.

Drug interactions with ketoconazole can be serious; this drug should not be taken with rifampin, isoniazid, warfarin, cyclosporine or phenytoin.

kidney disease and skin symptoms While symptoms in the skin are not often associated with kidney disease, both organs can be affected by immune complex disease. However, glomerulonephritis with kidney insufficiency can complicate the course of LUPUS ERYTHEMATOSUS and SYSTEMIC VASCULITIS and have prominent skin features. In addition, patients with progressive SYSTEMIC SCLEROSIS can also develop kidney failure.

Other skin symptoms associated with kidney disease include NAIL-PATELLA SYNDROME, with nail plate abnormalities and progressive renal disease; FABRY'S DISEASE, featuring small blue-black papules around the navel and kidney failure; pruritus (itching) of hemodialysis, characterized by generalized itching during hemodialysis; bullous dermatosis

of renal failure, characterized by tense blisters while on hemodialysis and sometimes on those with chronic kidney failure; skin lesions (WARTS, chronic HERPES, SQUAMOUS CELL CARCINOMA, ALOPECIA, bacterial and fungal infections) in kidney transplant patients.

KID syndrome The common name for keratitis-ichthyosis-deafness, this rare keratinization disorder leads to blindness and is associated with deafness and an unusual skin scaling. Patients with this condition have leathery skin texture, thickened palms and soles, and sparse hair.

Other associated health problems may include mental retardation, tight heel cords, tooth problems and recurrent skin infections. The biochemical basis for this disease is unknown.

kissing bug bites Kissing bugs (members of the family Reduviidae), are also known as assassin bugs, cone-nose bugs, Walapai tigers or Mexican bedbugs, and cause hive-like nodules or plaques with severe itching lasting up to a week. Sensitive individuals may experience hemorrhagic, giant hives or anaphylactic shock. The bugs bite at night in small clusters on uncovered body parts such as the face or arms.

While most are found in South America, about 15 species are found in the southwestern United States. They usually live near rodents, armadillos and opossums, but they can also be found in houses, living off humans.

Klippel-Trenaunay Support Group A support group for individuals affected by KLIPPEL-TRENAUNAY SYNDROME and their families. The support group acts as a clearinghouse of information and correspondence between members. Founded in 1986, the group has 180 members, publishes the quarterly *K-T Newsletter,* and holds a biennial conference.

Klippel-Trenaunay syndrome A congenital malformation of the extremities characterized by port wine birthmarks, varicose veins, and other symptoms. The cause is presently unknown, but is believed to be either genetic or the result of an intrauterine trauma between the third and sixth week of gestation. See Appendix D; see also KLIPPEL-TRENAUNAY SUPPORT GROUP; STURGE-WEBER FOUNDATION.

Koebner's phenomenon Lesions found in skin diseases induced by trauma such as PSORIASIS or LICHEN PLANUS.

koilonychia Also called "spoon nails," this is a condition in which nails are thin, dry, brittle and concave (spoon shaped), with raised edges. In nail-patella syndrome, the nail may be split into two spoon-shaped parts.
Cause Injury to the nail, iron-deficiency anemia and LICHEN PLANUS are the main causes; the condition may be inherited.
Treatment None.

kwashiorkor A severe type of malnutrition in young children occurring mainly in poor rural areas in the Third World, in which the child's skin flakes off, leaving a raw, weeping area beneath. Hair may lose its curliness, become sparse and brittle and turn from dark to fair. The nails tend to be soft and thin.

Derived from the Ghanaian word meaning "disease suffered by a child displaced from the breast," kwashiorkor usually affects only those children between ages one and three. Most children treated for the condition recover, but those younger than age two are likely to suffer permanent stunted growth.

Severe untreated cases can be fatal; blood poisoning kills about 30 percent of patients with kwashiorkor.

Kwashiorkor may also be found among elderly people and in some patients with systemic diseases characterized by problems in absorbing or digesting protein.
Cause The illness begins when the child is suddenly weaned on a poor diet low in calories, protein and essential micronutrients (such as ZINC, selenium and vitamins A and E).
Symptoms In addition to the skin and hair symptoms, growth is stunted, and there may be swelling. Behavioral symptoms in children include apathy, weakness, irritability and inactivity. The liver becomes enlarged, and the child loses resistance to disease.
Treatment Continually replace fluids, keep child warm and treat any infection. The child should first be fed milk and vitamin/mineral tablets, with the administration of ZINC to prevent further skin flaking. When the child's appetite returns, a high-calorie, protein-rich diet should be given.

Kyrle's disease A disorder of keratinization known medically as hyperkeratosis follicularis et parafollicularis or en cutem penetrans.
Symptoms It is characterized by horny plugs surrounded by a red rim that may enlarge to form plaques. The lesions are found most often on the extremities, although they may occur anywhere on the body. A similar condition may appear in patients undergoing kidney dialysis.
Treatment Administration of a keratolytic agent or liquid nitrogen may be effective, but the disease is difficult to treat.

L

laceration A torn ragged wound.

LAMB syndrome See MULTIPLE LENTIGINES SYNDROME.

lamellar dystrophy of nails The splitting of nails into layers, also called onychoschyzia, often found in those who must immerse their hands in water. Scientists believe the condition is caused by the constant absorption and evaporation of water from the nail plate. It is usually found in those whose hands are continually in and out of water, such as dish washers or launderers.

lamellar ichthyosis A disorder of keratinization characterized by redness and scaling at birth with large, dark scales and scaling of face, palms and soles of the feet. This is usually a severe form of ichthyosis that can produce considerable disability and deformity throughout life.

This condition is a rare autosomal recessive trait, which means that a defective gene must be inherited in a double dose to cause the abnormality. Generally, both parents of an affected person are unaffected carriers of the defective gene. Each of the children has a one in four chance of being affected, and a two in four chance of being a carrier.

Symptoms The condition is always noticeable at birth, often as a condition of prematurity. Babies may be born encased in a membrane that is eventually shed. There is generalized severe dryness and scaling; in some patients, large platelike dark scales predominate over all body surfaces. Redness is noticeable in infancy and usually remains throughout life; hair loss occurs in some patients.

Treatment Infants should be kept in a continuous humid environment and the membrane encasing the child should not be debrided. Moisturizing the skin is essential, moisturizers containing lactic acid are especially helpful. Systemic therapy with etretinate or isotretinoin is extremely helpful, but results only last as long as treatment continues. The side effects of high dose therapy are significant.

Langerhans cells A type of cell that makes up only about 4 percent of all epidermal cells, they are an extremely important part of the body's immune system. It is believed that the Langerhans cells play an important part in protecting the body against invading foreign substances.

Langer's lines Lines of cleavage of the skin determined by the position and orientation of COLLAGEN bundles and elastic fibers.

lanolin A mixture of a yellow, oily substance obtained from sheep's wool and purified water that is used as an EMOLLIENT to treat dry skin. Lanolin is a common ingredient of bath oils and hand creams. It is also used to treat mild DERMATITIS. Occasionally lanolin can irritate the skin and in some individuals an allergic reaction develops.

lanugo The fine, downy hair on the body of a fetus that first appears in the fourth or fifth month and usually disappears by the end of the pregnancy. It can still be seen in some premature babies.

Lanugo hair (hypertrichosis lanugiosa) sometimes reappears on the skin of adults with cancer (especially of the breast, bladder, lung or large intestine), in patients with anorexia nervosa, or as a side effect of some drugs (especially cyclosporine).

larva migrans, cutaneous Also known as creeping eruption, this disease is caused by hookworm larvae that normally parasitize dogs, cats or other animals. It is contracted by walking barefoot on soil or beaches contaminated with animal feces. The larvae penetrate the skin of the feet and move randomly, leaving intensely itchy red lines (sometimes accompanied by BLISTERS).

Because several different parasites produce similar symptoms, there may be difficulty in diagnosing specific disease such as many fall under the umbrella of "cutaneous larva migrans." Usually the term refers to disorders caused by cat or dog hookworm larvae.

Larva migrans is caused when human skin is in contact with soil contaminated with cat or dog feces. Shaded, moist and sandy areas—such as beaches, children's sandboxes and areas underneath houses—are the most likely spots to harbor larvae. The eggs passed in the feces hatch into infective larvae that can penetrate human skin (even through beach towels).

Skin lesions usually appear in areas that are in contact with soil, such as feet, hands and buttocks. A red papule appears within a few hours after the larvae penetrates the skin. After a latency period of a few days to a few months, the larvae migrate, causing a red, raised intensely itchy red line that may loop and meander all over the skin. Complications include bacterial infections, which can result from excessive scratching.

About half of the larvae die within three months, even without treatment.
Treatment Thiabendazole is the drug of choice; its topical form is best for mild infections, applied to the tracks and normal skin around the traces. Systemic thiabendazole is also effective, but causes many side effects (dizziness, nausea and vomiting).

laser resurfacing One of the newest techniques for removing medium to fine wrinkles with the use of a pulsed or scanned CO_2 laser. It can also resurface edges of ACNE and chicken pox scars.

The pulsed CO_2 laser works by emitting a very brief pulse of high-intensity light that's fast enough to limit heat damage in the skin, yet strong enough to vaporize tissue cleanly. Since the heat penetrates the skin no deeper than half the thickness of a human hair, it can remove the wrinkled skin layer by layer without scarring. The procedure can be done in an outpatient basis, and takes on average about *30 minutes to an hour.*

Another version of the laser—the scanned CO_2 laser—does not produce a pulse of laser light, but utilizes mirrors to rapidly scan the laser spot in a spiral pattern. While experts don't yet have enough information to make direct comparisons between the two versions, they say both appear to achieve impressive results.

Less expensive than a facelift, laser resurfacing doesn't cause bleeding and doesn't require general anesthesia. And while facelifts are good for sagging skin, they aren't ideal for lots of sagging skin. While laser resurfacing does not *replace* a facelift, it can improve the appearance after a facelift has been performed by removing the fine lines that may remain.

Unlike other cosmetic techniques, most patients report little or no pain *during* with the pulsed CO_2 laser treatment, and areas of the skin that can be completely anesthetized (such as the skin around the mouth) are usually pain free. After the technique, the skin may ooze and become puffy, crusting and red; while the skin remains reddened for about six weeks, it can be covered completely by makeup after the first few days. Full healing takes place within about three months.

Many dermatologists today believe the pulsed CO_2 laser is a better way to treat wrinkles than either dermabrasion and chemical peels because it allows for better control and safety, and sharply decreases the risk of scarring.

laser treatment The acronym for "Light Amplification by Stimulated Emission of Radiation," lasers produce light of specific wavelengths in a nondivergent beam of monochromatic radiation that can mobilize immense heat and power when focused at close range. They can be used as a tool in both diagnosis and surgical procedures. A laser is a device that contains an active medium made up of either a gas, such as carbon dioxide or argon; a solid, such as ruby or neodymium: yttrium aluminum garnet (Nd:YAG); or a liquid, such as a dye that is powered by a source (such as electricity) to produce a beam of single-colored light up to 10 million times more powerful than the sun.

Laser light is absorbed by different types of substances in tissue, depending on its wavelength, and it is the absorbed light which produces the effect on tissue. In a matter of seconds, this intense beam of light can hit a target and remove a skin problem, leaving little or no scarring. Most laser surgery can be done in the dermatologist's office, causes little or no blood loss and poses less risk of infection and faster healing than other conventional treatments.

Physicians wielding lasers can treat all sorts of skin problems, from precancerous growths to port-wine stains. The color of the light a laser emits determines what kind of skin problem it can be used to treat.

Ruby lasers, which produce red light (694 nm), remove some tattoos and pigmented lesions such as cafe au lait macules and a LENTIGO or liver spot. The *Nd:YAG laser* at 1064 nm (in the infrared spectrum) is also effective for tattoos and pigmented disorders. The CARBON DIOXIDE LASER also produces invisible infrared radiation (10,600 nm) and is used to remove benign skin growths, warts, and to resurface the skin. The PULSED DYE LASER is the best treatment for birthmarks such as the PORT-WINE STAIN, while ARGON LASERS have been used to treat port-wine stains, but they are best for TELANGIECTASES, SPIDER ANGIOMAS and venous lakes.

Not all skin problems respond to laser treatment, however. While several laser devices are being studied for the treatment of spider veins in the legs, for example, they are still best treated by sclerotherapy, which involves injections of a saline solution or an agent called aethoxysclerol.

Dermatologists don't usually use lasers to remove malignant skin growths, unless the patient is taking blood-thinners that could heighten the risk of hemorrhage during conventional surgery. Lasers can be extremely dangerous when used around the eyes. A stray beam can hit the cornea or be absorbed by the retina and blind the patient. Protective goggles and eye shields are used to prevent eye damage.

Before consenting to laser surgery, make sure your physician has had formal training and hands-on experience.

For a list of dermatologists in your area qualified to perform laser surgery, call the American Society for Dermatologic Surgery at (800) 441-2737 or the American Society for Lasers in Medicine and Surgery.

latex allergy Natural rubber latex, the stretchy material used in everything from balloons and baby bottle nipples to surgical gloves and condoms, is causing an outbreak of widespread allergic skin reactions ranging from mild irritation to life-threatening anaphylactic shock. Those most at risk are health-care workers, rubber plant workers and children with birth defects requiring multiple surgeries early in life.

One recent study found that in the general population, the risk for latex allergy was much higher than earlier suspected—6.5 percent. The study was conducted by researchers in the pediatric allergy and immunology department at Henry Ford Hospital in Detroit, in connection with the American Red Cross.

Hives and other allergic responses are being reported by users of latex products, especially medical workers. One study found that 7 percent of surgeons and 5 percent of operating room nurses are now allergic to the latex in their surgical gloves. Some health care workers develop generalized reactions to the rubber product.

In addition, the Food and Drug Administration has traced 17 deaths to a violent allergic reaction to an inflatable latex cuff used when administering barium enemas; the enema apparatus was later recalled by the manufacturer.

Symptoms About a third of patients who develop hives from contact with latex also develop other symptoms, including hay fever, asthma and even anaphylactic shock. (In anaphylactic shock, a victim can develop shortness of breath, swollen lips, and throat, heart and breathing difficulties within minutes). Death can result from anaphylactic shock without prompt treatment.

Reactions to latex were rarely reported before 1970, but since the late 1980s many reactions began to be reported each year. Scientists are not sure why, but allergic responses often develop with increased exposure to a product. It could be that because the AIDS epidemic has required the increased use of latex gloves and condoms, more and more people are being sensitized. Most health care workers now use a new set of gloves for each patient they treat. Patients at highest risk are those who undergo repeated surgical procedures such as urologic surgery in which latex exposure is heightened. (See also ALLERGIES AND THE SKIN:)

Lawrence-Seip syndrome A skin manifestation of insulin-resistant diabetes of both congenital and acquired types, this condition is characterized by the wasting away of subcutaneous fat, thickened skin, enlarged genitalia, excessive hairiness, excessive pigmentation, central nervous system disease and liver or spleen problems. There is no treatment.

leg ulcers An open sore on the leg that does not heal, usually caused by an inadequate blood supply from the area. Leg ulcers are most often found among the elderly.

BEDSORES (also called decubitus ulcers) develop on pressure spots on the legs as a result of poor circulation, pressure and immobility over a period of time. Leg ulcers may also be due to peripheral vascular disease (restricted blood supply to the extremities caused by thickening of the artery walls). Diabetes mellitus, which increases susceptibility to blood vessel disease and skin infection, may also lead to leg ulcers.

Treatment Prevention is preferable to undergoing treatment. Anyone susceptible to leg ulcers should avoid obesity, leg injury and immobility. Treatment should be sought as early as possible. If an ulcer is filled with pus, apply a wet dressing under a bandage. This should be changed only every three to seven days to avoid removing new skin from the area.

leishmaniasis A variety of diseases that affect the skin and mucous membranes caused by infection with single-celled parasites (called leishmania). The parasites are found in dogs and rodents in many parts of the world except Australia, Antarctica, the United States (with the exception of Texas) and large areas of Africa. Parasites are transmitted from the animals to humans via the bites of sand flies, which live on the fur of the animals. There are at least three types of the disease that affect the skin, one of which is common in the Middle East, North Africa and the Mediterranean; the others are found in Central and South America.

No effective vaccine currently exists.

Symptoms A persistent ulcer that may eventually heal but can leave an ugly scar forms at the sand-fly bite. In the South American form, there is more extensive tissue damage (often on the face), often causing severe disfigurement.

Treatment It is essential to understand the different geographic strains of the different parasites in order to properly treat the disease. All forms of this disease are treated effectively with drugs (such as sodium stibogluconate or glucantime) given by injection into a muscle or vein. All types of this disorder with secondary bacterial infection should also be treated with antibiotics.

lemon A fruit that contains both citric acid and vitamin C, lemon is good at cutting grease and is one of the few natural ingredients that can retain its properties after chemical extraction. For best results, however, cosmetics should contain concentrated lemon juice and not just the essence for a lemony fragrance. Fresh-squeezed and diluted lemon juice is an excellent rinse for oily hair. See also OIL OF BERGAMOT.

lentiginosis profusa Also known as generalized lentiginosis, this disorder is characterized by the appearance of many lentigines (small dark brown spots). It is different from MULTIPLE LENTIGINES SYNDROME, which involves multiple lentigines and many other developmental problems, such as deafness and short stature. See also LENTIGO; LENTIGO, ACTINIC; LENTIGO, MALIGNA.

lentigo A harmless flat, pigmented area of skin similar to a FRECKLE, lentigines (the plural of lentigo) are usually brown and may be found alone or in groups in either exposed or unexposed areas of skin. They are more common in middle-aged and elderly people,

and in those who have been exposed to the sun.

Treatment No treatment necessary, but if cosmetically unacceptable they are best treated with cryotherapy or laser therapy. Irregular brown flat lesions may suggest the presence of a potentially malignant pigmented lesion, such as a MELANOMA. These should be shown to a dermatologist.

lentigo, actinic Also known as a solar lentigo or liver spot, this harmless small brown macule differs from a LENTIGO simplex by its larger size and by its appearance later in life on sun-exposed areas of skin, especially the face and the backs of the hands. Similar in appearance to a FRECKLE, lentigines do not clear once sun exposure is stopped. They may be found alone or in groups and are more common in middle-aged and elderly people and in those who have been exposed to the sun. See also LENTIGO, MALIGNA; LENTIGINOSIS PROFUSA.

Treatment No treatment is necessary, but if raised, darker brown areas appear inside the lentigines, a physician should be consulted since these areas could develop into MALIGNANT MELANOMA. Lentigines can be relatively easily treated with liquid nitrogen or by laser treatment with either the Q-switched Nd:YAG laser, the Q-switched Alexandrite laser or the Q-switched ruby laser.

lentigo maligna Also known as a melanotic freckle of Hutchinson, and more common in women, this is considered to be a precancerous lesion that may transform itself into a malignant melanoma. It is different from an ordinary LENTIGO, which is benign.

A lentigo maligna may start out as small fawn-colored macule—usually on the face—very similar to a benign seborrheic keratosis; as the patient ages, it becomes larger and irregularly shaped and colored. It gradually gets bigger until it forms an irregular patch with jagged or notched borders, irregularly colored from tan to dark brown or black. It may also be red or white. Scientists now believe that about 5 percent of these lesions turn into lentigo maligna melanoma.

The lesions are always seen on sun-exposed skin, as opposed to melanoma, and they are seen in patients older than those who are seen with melanoma. See also MELANOMA, MALIGNANT.

Treatment Surgical removal, or cryotherapy or radiation.

LEOPARD syndrome Another name for MULTIPLE LENTIGINES SYNDROME. The acronym stands for the range of developmental symptoms that characterize the disorder: Lentigines, Electrocardiographic abnormalities, Ocular hypertelorism, Pulmonary stenosis, Abnormalities of the genitals, Retarded growth and Deafness. See also LENTIGO SIMPLEX; LENTIGO, MALIGNANT; LENTIGO ACTINIC.

leprosy A chronic bacterial infection (also called Hansen's disease) that damages nerves in the skin, limbs, face and mucous membranes. Untreated leprosy can lead to severe complications, which can include blindness and disfigurement. Contrary to popular belief, it is not highly contagious. While the disease still carries a significant stigma, patient care has become integrated with routine health care, and anti-leprosy organizations have fought to repeal stigmatizing laws and practices. Patients are no longer referred to as "lepers."

Although leprosy is one of the oldest diseases in human history, it was not until 1873, when Armauer Hansen first saw the bacillus causing leprosy under a microscope, that the disease was discovered to be infectious instead of hereditary.

There are currently about 20 million leprosy patients in 87 countries, primarily in Asia, Central and South America and Africa; but probably fewer than 20 percent have access to treatment. India has the highest prevalence of leprosy, followed by Brazil. There are more than 6,000 known cases in the United States. Most cases occur in California, Florida, Hawaii, Louisiana, New York and Texas. There are about 200 new cases of leprosy each year in the United States, and 12,000 new cases each week around the world. Children represent approximately 16 percent of the new cases of leprosy.

History Ancient religious traditions associated with leprosy continued to influence social policy well into the 20th century. Leprosy was first mentioned as a curse in Shinto prayers of 1250 B.C.; it was also mentioned in some Egyptian legends to explain the exodus of the Hebrews. For hundreds of years, those with leprosy were taken to a priest, not a doctor, and were found "guilty," not sick.

These customs led to the forcible confinement of patients in "leprosaria," or leper colonies; their children, whether infected or not, were denied education in community schools. In eighth-century France, leprosy was considered grounds for divorce, and under the Roman Empire, was cause for banishment. Some countries passed legislation providing for the compulsory sterilization of leprosy patients, and others would not permit patients to handle the nation's currency. Others "steam treated" letters before allowing them in the mail, and some countries did not allow patients to vote. In medieval Europe, leprosy patients had to carry a "clapper" to warn others that a person with leprosy was approaching. Even as late as 1913, state Senator G.E. Willett of Montana was forced to give up his seat after he was diagnosed with leprosy.

Religious customs also affected many treatments for leprosy. In 250 B.C., Chinese patients pricked their swollen limbs to let out the "foul air." Ramses II of Egypt believed that people with leprosy who used his water wells would be cured. And in medieval Europe, it was believed that leprosy could be cured by the touch of a king.

Historically, topical treatments ranged from turtle soup, whiskey and various poultices (onion, sea salt and urine in Egypt; arsenic and powdered snake bones in China; water mixed with blood of dogs and infants under age two in Scotland; elephants' teeth; the flesh of crocodiles, snakes, lions and bears.) Other ingredients ranged from carbolic acid, creosote, phosphorus, mercury and iodine, and plant extracts, including madar, cashew-nut oil, gurjum oil or chaulmoogra.

The idea of caring for patients with leprosy became popular among missionaries following biblical directives and the teachings of Jesus; this service became fashionable about A.D. 1100 in Europe, after Crusaders (including a king) returned with the disease. Special hospitals were built, operated and supported by cathedrals, but with the outbreak in the 1300s of bubonic plague, which wiped out populations, patients with leprosy began to be segregated again. Some countries seized the property of those with leprosy before burning them alive.

Leprosy is erroneously associated with the Old Testament, where references to "tsara'-ath," a term which most closely translates to "leprosy," actually refers to a broad spectrum of problems that affected cloth, leather, linen and house walls as well as humans. Most medical historians doubt, and archaeologists have not found evidence to support, the idea that leprosy existed among the Hebrews in Moses' time. Biblical scholars also have problems with the translation of the Greek term *lepra* partly because the Greeks had a specific term for leprosy. The Greek word *lepra* was most likely used to refer to a variety of severe skin diseases. Greek medical writings later than the third century B.C. provide the earliest clinical references to modern leprosy. No mention of leprosy occurs in the New Testament after the Gospels.

Cause Leprosy is caused by a rod-shaped bacterium, *Mycobacterium leprae*, that is spread in droplets of nasal mucus. A person is infectious only during the first phase of the disease, and only those living in prolonged close contact with an infected person are at risk. Leprosy is probably spread by droplet infection through sneezing and coughing. In those with untreated leprosy, large amounts of bacteria are found in nasal discharge; the bacteria travel through the air in these droplets. They can survive three weeks or longer outside the human body, in dust or on clothing.

Although relatively infectious, leprosy is still one of the least contagious of all diseases. This—together with the fact that only 3 percent of the population is susceptible to leprosy—means that there is no justification for the practice (still prevalent in some countries) of isolating patients. Only a few people are susceptible because most people acquire a natural immunity when exposed to the disease.

Most of the body's destruction is caused not by bacterial growth but by a reaction of the body's immune system to the organisms as they die. In *lepromatous leprosy*, damage is widespread, progressive and severe. *Tuberculoid leprosy* is a milder form of the disease.

Symptoms Damage is first confined to the nerves supplying the skin and muscles, destroying nerve endings, sweat glands, hair follicles and pigment-producing cells. It first causes a lightening (or darkening) of the skin, with a loss of feeling and sweating. Some types of the disease produce a rash of bumps or nodules on the skin. As the disease progresses, bacilli also attack peripheral nerves; at first patients may feel an occasional "pins and needles" sensation, or have a numb patch on the skin. Next, patients become unable to feel sensations such as a light touch or temperature. Gradually, even hands, feet and facial skin eventually become numb as muscles become paralyzed. Delicate connections between nerve cells and nerve endings are severed, and whole sections of the body become totally numb. For example, if the nerve above the elbow is affected, part of the hand becomes numb and small muscles become paralyzed, leading to curled fingers.

When a patient can no longer sense pain, the body loses the automatic withdrawal reflex that protects against trauma from sharp or hot objects, leading to extensive scarring or even loss of fingers and toes. Muscle paralysis can lead to further deformity, and damage to the facial nerve means eyelids can't close, leading to ulceration and blindness. Direct invasion of bacteria may also lead to inflammation of the eyeball, also leading to blindness.

Treatment Several antibiotic agents are effective against leprosy and are best used in combinations of two or three. This multidrug therapy (MDT) is the current preferred treatment: it combines DAPSONE, clofazimine and rifampin. The MDT was developed as leprosy bacilli became resistant to dapsone alone after decades of constant use. (Dapsone, a sulfone drug, was introduced during the 1940s). The most powerful of these is rifampicin, a drug first used against tuberculosis and found to be effective against leprosy in 1968. Particular combinations of these drugs were recommended in 1984 by the World Health Organization as standard treatment for mass campaigns against leprosy.

MDT is often distributed in blister packs containing a month's supply of pills; dapsone is taken daily; clofazimine is taken every other day; and rifampin is taken monthly. There are now more than 1 million people receiving these drugs worldwide, and more than 1 million others have already completed treatment.

While the medication usually can cure leprosy within six months to two years, patients are no longer contagious within a few days after treatment begins. To prevent a relapse, treatment needs to be administered for at least two years after the last signs of the disease have disappeared. In the United States, patients are eligible for treatment by the Public Health Service at special clinics and hospitals, or at the Gillis W. Long Hansen's Disease Center in Louisiana, the only institution in the United States devoted primarily to treatment, research, training and education related to leprosy. Eleven regional centers, located primarily in major urban areas, treat those with leprosy on an outpatient basis.

No vaccine for leprosy is available because scientists have not been able to grow cultures in lab environments. However, about 95 percent of the population is immune to leprosy, which occurs naturally in armadillos.

Post-treatment care After leprosy is cured, patients must learn to watch for wounds and injuries they don't feel, and must learn to wear special shoes to protect insensitive feet.

leptospirosis A rare disease characterized by a skin rash and flu-like symptoms caused by a spirochete bacterium excreted by rodents. Also known as Weil's disease, there are about 100 cases and a few deaths reported in the United States each year.

Symptoms After an incubation period of up to three weeks, an acute illness characterized by headache, fever and chills, severe muscle aches and minute red spots and purple papules appears. The kidneys are often affected, and liver damage and JAUNDICE are also common.

Treatment Antibiotics are effective, and in about one-third of cases the patients improve rapidly. Some patients go on to suffer a more persistent illness with slow recovery of kidney and liver function. The nervous system may also be affected, often producing signs of meningitis.

L.E. Support Club A patient support group designed to aid people with LUPUS ERYTHEMATOSUS and other autoimmune diseases. The club offers support and self-help education via newsletters and personal interchange, and also provides information on nutrition and medication. Founded in 1984, the club has 2,500 members and contributes to lupus research. It publishes the bimonthly newsletter *LE Beacon*. For address, see Appendix D; see also AMERICAN LUPUS SOCIETY; LUPUS FOUNDATION OF AMERICA; LUPUS NETWORK.

leukonychia A whitish discoloration of the nails that may involve the entire nail, a portion of it, or a discolored band. Some patients inherit the condition; it may also result from certain treatments for leukemia (arsenic and antimetabolites). Patients with liver disease may also have complete discoloration. No treatment is available.

leukoplakia A smooth, opaque white patch found mostly on the mucus membranes of the lips and inside the mouth, primarily among the elderly. Some patches are benign, some are premalignant conditions and others are malignant. Therefore, patients must see a dermatologist or oral surgeon to confirm a diagnosis.

Cause Leukoplakia in the mouth may be caused by to tobacco smoke (especially pipe smoking), trauma from rubbing of dentures or a rough tooth. In some cases, it is genetic.

Treatment The patches develop slowly and are, of themselves, harmless. Once the cause has been treated, the patches may clear up of themselves.

lice Small wingless insects about the size of a sesame seed, with six legs and claws for grasping the hair. Lice feed on human blood. They are crawling insects that cannot jump or fly. Lice are divided into three species: *Pediculus humanus capitis* (head louse); *pediculus humanus corporis* (body louse) and *Phthirus pubis* (the crab, or pubic, louse). All three have flat bodies that measure up to 3 mm across.

Head lice live on and suck blood from the scalp, leaving red spots that itch intensely and can lead to DERMATITIS and IMPETIGO. The females lay a daily batch of pale eggs called "NITS" that attach themselves to hairs close to the scalp. The nits hatch in about a week, and the adults can live for several weeks.

Head lice can be found among people of all walks of life. About 6 million cases of head lice occur each year among U.S. schoolchildren between ages 3 and 12, even among those who shampoo daily. Children most often contract lice through direct contact, usually at school by sharing hats, brushes, combs or headrests. Pets cannot contact head lice.

Because lice move so quickly, it is the nits that will be seen on the hair shaft. Head lice and their nits can also be found on eyebrows and eyelashes. If one person in a family has head lice, all family members should be checked. Only those who are infested should be treated with lice pesticide.

Body lice live and lay eggs on clothing next to the skin, visiting the body only to feed. Body lice affect people who rarely change their clothes.

Crab lice live in pubic hair or (rarely) armpits and beards. Pubic lice are commonly known as "crabs" because under the microscope they resemble a crab. Crab lice cause incessant itching. They are visible to the naked eye and are easily transmitted during sex. It is also possible to pick them up from sheets or towels. They can live away from the host's body for up to one day, and the eggs can survive on their own for several days. Affected patients who don't wash underwear, sheets and towels in hot enough water may be reinfected.

Treatment For *head lice*, lotions containing malathion or carbaryl kill lice and nits quickly. The lotion should be washed off 12 hours after application, followed by combing the hair with a fine-toothed comb to remove dead lice and nits. Shampoos containing malathion, lindane or carbaryl are also effective if used repeatedly over several days. Combs and brushes should be plunged into very hot water to kill any attached eggs.

The National Pediculosis Association discourages the use of LINDANE products (such as Kwell), because they consider them to be potentially more toxic and no more effective than other treatments. There is no national consensus in this regard, however. Still, no product kills 100 percent of nits, and a fine-toothed comb should be used to remove the remaining nits. Lice medications are not intended to be used on a routine or preventive basis.

All lice-killing medications are pesticides, and therefore should be used with caution. A pharmacist or physician should be consulted before using or applying pesticides when the person is pregnant, nursing, has lice or nits in the eyebrows or eyelashes, or has other health problems (such as allergies). Because the head lice pesticides can be absorbed into the bloodstream, they should not be used on open wounds on the scalp, or on the hands of the person applying the medication. These pesticides should not be used on infants, and should be used with caution on children under age two. In these cases, lice and nits should be removed manually or mechanically.

Pesticides should be used over a sink (not a tub or shower) to minimize pesticide absorption and exposure to the rest of the body. Eyes of the affected individual must be kept covered while administering any pesticide.

All nits must be removed from the hair shaft. Bedding and recently worn clothing should be washed in hot water and dried in a hot dryer. Combs and brushes should be cleaned and then soaked in hot (not boiling) water for 10 minutes. Lice sprays should not be used, according to the National Pediculosis Association. Vacuuming is the best way to remove lice and attached nits from furniture, mattresses, rugs, stuffed toys and car seats.

Neighborhood parents and the school, camp or child care providers should be notified of any infestation. Children should be checked once a week for head lice.

Body lice can be killed by placing infested clothing in a hot dryer for five minutes, by washing clothes in very hot water or by burning.

Pubic lice can be treated with an over-the-counter treatment, including A-200 Pyrinate, RID or Nix.

For more information about *lice,* contact the National Pediculosis Association, P.O. Box 149, Newton, MA 02161, or call (800) 446-4NPA. For more information about *head lice treatment,* write for a free brochure to the Office of Public Affairs, Nonprescription Drug Manufacturers Association, 1150 Connecticut Avenue NW, Washington, DC 20036.

lichenification Thickening of the skin caused by repeated scratching, often by trying to relieve the intense itching of ECZEMA.

lichenoid drug eruptions A type of drug reaction causing an itchy eruption of papules most often appearing on the forearms, less often on the lower legs, genitalia, and mucous membranes. While the rash resembles LICHEN PLANUS, the histology and cause is different. Substances most often associated with this condition include gold, antimalarials, thiazides and tetracyclines.

lichen myxedematosus A condition of metabolic dysfunction characterized by skin symptoms, including lichenoid papules of the ears, neck, scrotum and perianal area. Facial features are exaggerated with deep furrows, which are sometimes very thickened. Other patients have groups of pink wheals and red or flesh-colored small papules. Still others have lichenoid plaques resembling LICHEN PLANUS. Occasionally patients with this condition develop multiple myeloma.

The condition is a proliferative process related to an abnormal immunoglobulin that stimulates production of mucinous material that deposits in the skin. See also LICHEN SIMPLEX.

Treatment Cyclophosphamide, radiotherapy, dermabrasion or systemic corticosteroids may eradicate the cells producing the immunoglobulins so that the disease can go into full remission.

lichen planus A common skin disease of unknown origin causing small, shiny, flat-topped, itchy pink or purple raised spots on the skin of the wrists, forearms or lower legs, particularly in middle-aged patients. The inside lining of the cheek may be covered by a lacy white network of spots. Most cases resolve spontaneously within two years.

Treatment Potent topical steroids and antihistamines are the mainstay of therapy. For extensive cases, PUVA and GRISEOFULVIN or systemic steroids have been used.

lichen simplex Patches of thickened itchy and sometimes discolored skin caused by repeated scratching, usually found on neck, wrists, arms and ankles. It is most prevalent among women and is believed to be caused by extended scratching caused by a psychological condition. Patients often rub patches unconsciously when agitated or during stressful situations. This contributes to a cycle of skin thickening and scratching. The skin thickens in reaction to the itching which in turn causes the skin to thicken.

Treatment Corticosteroid creams applied twice daily and whenever the patient has an urge to scratch are the treatment of choice to relieve the itching, which allows the scratching to subside. Psychological counseling may help.

light treatment See PHOTOTHERAPY.

limes and the skin See OIL OF BERGAMOT.

lindane A drug (gamma benzene hexachloride, included in such products as "Kwell") that is used to treat infestation by SCABIES or LICE. It is no longer recommended by the NATIONAL PEDICULOSIS ASSOCIATION (NPA) because of its potential toxicity. Other products, such as permethrin (Elimite), according to the NPA, work equally well with less risk.

Lindane may irritate the scalp and skin, or cause itching. It is thought by some to be toxic to the nervous system. In at least one case, a child was allegedly permanently brain damaged after being treated with a lindane–based pediculicide. Critics feel that this and other reports are inaccurate.

lipoid   proteinosis See   URBACH-WIETHE DISEASE.

lipoma A common benign tumor composed of mature fat cells. It is doubtful whether malignant changes ever occur. Women are affected much more often, usually in early-to-middle adult life. The tumors appear on the neck, trunk, abdomen, forearms, buttocks and thighs.

Treatment Most require no treatment, although liposuction or surgical excision are both effective means of their removal.

liposuction The removal of unwanted fat deposits in certain areas of the body, most commonly the thighs, buttocks, abdomen, "handlebar" areas, chin and knees. It has become the most popular cosmetic surgical procedure in the United States—even more popular than face-lifts. The procedure is effective because fat cells do not regenerate after they are destroyed or removed; for example, people who gain weight after liposuction do not regain significant amounts of weight in areas where fat has been removed.

Best candidates for the surgery are those who are healthy, at near-normal weight, with good skin turgor. Provided the patient maintains a stable weight pattern, the results will be permanent. The best candidates are people in their 30s and 40s whose skin still retains some elasticity, which helps the skin drape properly after the fat is removed.

Technique While some surgeons perform liposuction under general anesthesia, it is most frequently done under local anesthesia. Sometimes, the removed fat can be transferred into other areas where the fat has wasted away as a way to augment soft tissue. (See FAT TRANSPLANTS).

The surgeon inserts a tube (called a canula) through a small skin incision. The tube is attached to a suction pump and is moved through fat, removing the cells. As the canula moves through the fat, it creates tunnels that scar, resulting in a permanent flattening of the area. With newer anesthesia techniques (tumescence anesthesia), the risk of blood loss is very low and the procedure is easier to perform.

The surgery lasts between 30 minutes and three hours, and patients can be back to work in one day to a week, depending on the extent of the procedure. Bruising and swelling will last between one to six months. The final improved appearance is not apparent until the healing process is completed.

The cost of this procedure averages about $2,000 per site, although the exact cost will vary depending on the part of the country where the surgery is performed.

Side effects Temporary bruising, swelling, numbness and soreness result. The most frequent side effect is a ridging of the skin's surface—this is an external reflection of the tunneling created by the procedure. Ridging may be unattractive, but it is not apparent when the patient is fully dressed.

Risks Infection, local irregularity of contour or blood loss.

liquid nitrogen Freezing with liquid nitrogen, otherwise known as cryotherapy, destroys tissue by means of extremely low temperatures of -125 degress to $-130°$ C ($-195°$ to $-200°$ F). The liquid nitrogen is delivered with either a Q-tip, a spray thermos device or a contact probe.

It is used for the treatment of LENTIGINES, seborrheic keratoses, actinic keratoses, WARTS, benign tumors, some basal cell and squamous cell carcinomas, and occasionally LENTIGO MALIGNA. Liquid nitrogen on plantar or palmar warts may cause painful blood-filled blisters, however. See also KERATOSIS, SEBORRHEIC; KERATOSIS, ACTINIC; BASAL CELL CARCINOMA; SQUAMOUS CELL CARCINOMA.

livedo reticularis A condition characterized by a reddish blue net-like mottling of the skin, usually on the lower legs. The condition, may be intermittent, appearing simply as a normal response to the cold. The permanent form of livedo reticularis may be caused by an underlying sytemic disease, such as arteriosclerosis, diseases of COLLAGEN, cerebrovascular disease etc.

Cause Enlargement of blood vessels underneath the skin.

Treatment Treatment of the underlying condition.

liver spots Also called "age spots" or LENTIGINES, these spots are the result of the skin's defensive mechanism against long-standing sun exposure in which pooling pigment in some spots to protect the skin leaves uneven brown patches that don't fade away—most commonly on the back of the hands. Those with fair skins are at greatest risk for developing the spots.

Treatment While skin bleaching creams may provide some relief, they can't prevent new spots from forming, nor are they effective at completely lightening most lesions. Dermatologists may permanently remove brown spots from hands by a technique called CRYOSURGERY (removal with acids similar to those used in chemical peels). Retin-A is an effective, albeit very slow, treatment. Treatment with lasers (Q-switched Ng:YAG, ruby or alexandrite, or 510 nm pulsed dye) are very effective.

loiasis A form of the tropical parasitic disease FILARIASIS caused by an infestation of the *Loa loa* worm, which travels beneath the skin and causes an inflammation known as a calabar swelling.

loofahs A type of natural fibrous sponge harvested from the luffa plant, which grows like a gourd and is then dried and made into sponges, mitts or woven cloths. Loofahs are a good alternative to a body brush or washcloth, since they help remove dead skin cells. They should not be used on the face, neck, or on broken skin.

Because loofahs are a nutrient source for bacteria and cellular debris from the skin and are usually kept in a damp environment, these products are liable to become contaminated.

To keep a loofah clean, thoroughly wash with mild soap, rinse and then dry after each use. Since this process will not kill some organisms, soak the loofah twice a week in a solution of one part bleach and nine parts water to sterilize.

Loofahs may not *look* contaminated (such as a color change or odor), so be sure to buy new ones regularly—about every two months. A loofah needs to be replaced if it gets soft, or if pieces start to fall off.

Synthetic products are less likely to become contaminated, but they should still be washed and rinsed after each use and replaced after two months of use.

Loofahs, sponges and brushes should not be shared and if used on an infected part of the skin, they should be thrown away.

Look Good . . . Feel Better program A free public-service program of classes taught by makeup, hair and nail aestheticians to help cancer patients cope with the cosmetic crises that may accompany chemotherapy or other treatments, such as loss of hair, eyelashes and eyebrows; uneven skin tone and texture; fragile fingernails.

The program was founded by the Cosmetics, Toiletry and Fragrance Association Foundation in partnership with the American Cancer Society.

To find a local program, call (800) 395-LOOK or contact the nearest American Cancer Society office.

Loprox See CYCLOPIROXOLAMINE.

lotion A liquid drug preparation that can be applied to the skin. Lotions have a soothing effect and can be used to cover large areas.

Louis-Bar syndrome (ataxia telangiectasia) This genetic disorder causes, among other symptoms, telangiectases on sun-exposed areas, the butterfly areas of the face, the back of the neck, tops of the ears etc. Other skin symptoms include GRAY HAIR, loss of skin elasticity and subcutaneous fat. Researchers suspect the problem may be caused by a defect in DNA repair. Lymphomas are common, and death usually occurs by the fifth decade of life. There is no treatment.

lubricants Topical preparations containing fats or oils used to help hydrate and protect the skin by trapping water within the stratum corneum (top layer of the EPIDERMIS), making the skin more pliable.

Lubricants work better if the skin is first soaked for 5 to 10 minutes in water. They may contain animal fats (such as LANOLIN), vegetable oils (such as olive oil), mineral oil, paraffin, petrolatum, or waxes.

Different brands or types of lubricants may have quite different consistency, and choice of preparation should depend on its use.

lunula The white crescent area at the base of the nail.

lupus erythematosus A chronic autoimmune disease that causes inflammation of connective tissue, which affects the skin and internal organs. When wolves roamed Europe, it was said that the victim of a wolf attack bore the sign of the wolf (*lupus*)—a red mark on his or her face. Others who had never been attacked yet bore similar marks, were believed to have the disease of the *lupus*—lupus erythematosus.

Lupus involves the body's immune system, which launches an attack against itself. In one form (discoid lupus erythematosus, or DLE), the disease affects only the skin; in the second form (systemic lupus erythematosus, or SLE), the disease affects the skin and organs throughout the body.

Lupus strikes nine times as many women as men, usually those of childbearing age, and is found throughout the world. However, its incidence is higher among certain ethnic groups (such as blacks in the United States). In high risk groups, the incidence may be as high as one in every 250 women.

Although this disease may be life threatening if the kidney is involved, the outlook for patients has improved a great deal over the past 20 years. Today many patients can survive for at least 10 years after diagnosis.

Cause An autoimmune disorder, lupus causes the body's immune system to attack its own connective tissue, causing inflammation. Attacks can be triggered by sunlight and by certain drugs (hydralazine, procainamide and isoniazid). It is believed that the disease is inherited, and that hormonal factors play a part. Sometimes, a viral infection may set off the disorder.

Symptoms In both forms of the disease symptoms wax and wane with varying severity.

In DLE, the rash presents itself as one or more red, circular, thickened areas of skin on the face, behind the ears and on the scalp. The rash may cause permanent hair loss in affected areas and result in facial scars.

SLE causes a red, blotchy butterfly-shaped rash over the face that does not scar. Most patients feel sick and are tired, experiencing fever, appetite loss, nausea, painful joints and weight loss. Complications include kidney failure, pleurisy, arthritis seizures and psychiatric problems.

Less than 5% of patients with DLE progress to SLE; patients with SLE may also have skin lesions of DLE.

Treatment Although there is no cure, treatment aims at reducing inflammation and alleviating symptoms with nonsteroidal anti-inflammatory drugs, antimalterials and corticosteroid drugs. Those whose condition is worsened by sunlight should avoid exposure wear protective clothing and use sunscreens.

Lupus Foundation of America A nonprofit voluntary health foundation serving patients with LUPUS ERYTHEMATOSUS by providing patient education, services and support, and education to the medical community and the public about the disease. The foundation offers a fellowship grant for lupus research and publishes the *Lupus News* three times a year, together with other publications. Founded in 1977, the foundation has 45,500 members and holds an annual meeting in July. For address, see Appendix D; see also AMERICAN LUPUS SOCIETY; L.E. SUPPORT CLUB; LUPUS NETWORK.

Lupus Network An informational group for educators, medical professionals and individuals suffering from systemic LUPUS ERYTHEMATOSUS to better understand the disease. Established in 1985, the group publishes the quarterly newsletter *Heliogram,* pamphlets and reprints. For address, see Appendix B; see also AMERICAN LUPUS SOCIETY; L.E. SUPPORT CLUB; LUPUS FOUNDATION OF AMERICA.

lupus pernio See SARCOIDOSIS.

lupus vulgaris A type of skin lesion that appears in skin tuberculosis in immune (or par-

tially immune) patients. Beginning early in life, the condition is characterized by scaly red plaques, which over time will spread, ulcerate and produce extensive scarring and tissue loss.
Treatment Administration of antituberculosis drugs.

lycopenia A condition characterized by an orange-yellow skin tint caused by eating foods (tomatoes or berries) high in lycopene, an isomer of carotene. In lycopenia, the skin discoloration may resemble that of hypercarotenemia. High blood levels of lycopene may be raised and mild liver dysfunction may also occur.

Lyme disease A tick-borne illness whose hallmark symptom is a red rash that forms an irregular ring shape surrounding the tick bite. Untreated, Lyme disease can cause a host of problems, including arthritis and disorders of the heart and central nervous system. It is most commonly found in the northeast coastal states from Maine to Maryland, in the upper Midwest and on the Pacific Coast. It is most often contracted in the late spring or early summer when ticks are abundant.
Cause The disease is caused by *Borrelia burgdorferi,* a spirochete form of bacteria. It is transmitted primarily by the deer tick, the tiniest of the ticks about the size of the period at the end of this sentence, which is found on deer, birds, field mice and rodents.
Symptoms Red raised irregular ring-shaped rash with a clear center at the site of the bite. There may be multiple individual rings in spite of only one bite. Flu-like symptoms, arthritic complications, abnormal skin sensations and sensitivities, insomnia, hearing loss, heart complications, fainting, dizziness, shortness of breath, depression and dementia. Pregnant women who contract the dis-

ease run the risk of miscarriage, stillbirth or birth defects.
Diagnosis and treatment Lyme disease is diagnosed on the basis of symptoms and a blood test and is treated with antibiotics (tetracycline or penicillin). Pregnant women may require hospitalization.

lymphangiosarcoma See STEWART-TREVES TUMOR.

lymphangitis Inflammation of the lymphatic vessels that cause tender red streaks to appear on the skin caused by a spread of bacteria (usually STREPTOCOCCI) from an infected wound. The streaks extend from the site of infection toward the nearest lymph nodes, and is usually accompanied by a fever and a general feeling of illness.
Treatment This condition is a clear indication of serious infection, and requires immediate treatment with antibiotics. Antibiotic treatment usually clears up the infection without complication.

lymphocytoma cutis One of a group of benign inflammatory skin conditions that resemble malignant lymphomas. This variant, (also known as cutaneous lymphoid hyperplasia), seen primarily in women, is usually characterized by a single firm, red-brown or purple nodule or plaque on sun-exposed areas such as the face and extremities. In most cases, the cause of this disorder is unknown, although it may be induced by bites or stings, injected drugs, vaccinations or acupuncture. If the lesion persists or spreads, a biopsy must be performed to rule out the possibility that the condition is malignant lymphoma and not a benign condition.
Treatment Although the lesions may be excised, they do respond to injections of corticosteroids directly into the affected area. Superficial, low-dose X-rays may also be administered.

M

macular amyloidosis See AMYLOIDOSIS.

macule A flat spot on the skin, visible only by differing color that is less than 1–2 cm in diameter.

maduromycosis See MYCETOMA.

Maffucci's syndrome A rare genetic syndrome characterized by raised cavernous hemangiomas on the skin and pathologic fractures early in the first 10 years of life.

magnesium aluminum silicate An oil-absorbing chemical that is included in some skin care products, such as oil-free foundations. It is not considered to be part of an effective treatment for ACNE.

Majocchi's granuloma A variant of TINEA CORPORIS (ringworm of the body), in which there is an infection in the hair follicules resulting in a granulomatous inflammation.

Majocchi's disease A disorder involving inflammation of blood vessels with particular skin symptoms. Known medically as purpura annularis telangiectoides, this condition is one of a group of diseases that are all characterized by rust-colored macules and papules on the lower legs. In this condition, early lesions may be redder, forming rings, but there is no itching involved.
Treatment All forms of these capillary diseases are chronic and tend to resist treatment, although topical steroids and UVB phototherapy may help.

makeup A group of COSMETICS including face powder, lipstick, mascara, eyebrow pencil, eye shadow and eye liner that are used to enhance a person's appearance.

Face powder covers up the outer greasy layer of the skin, creating a velvety finish on the face. This product usually contains titanium dioxide or zinc oxide, with talc, kaolin, zinc or magnesium stearate, color and perfume. Powdered silk, sometimes included in face powder, is a powerful marketing tool but contributes very little to the product's function.

Compact powder is compressed face powder with a binding component (such as gum arabic). *Translucent powder* offers an extra opaque quality through the addition of titanium dioxide.

Lipstick is made up of a number of components, including carnauba wax, beeswax, castor oil, lanolin, preservatives, perfumes and indelible dyes (such as D&C Red #21, D&C Orange #5, etc.).

Mascara is a soap that emulsifies when moistened; liquid mascara is emulsified with alcohol. *Eyebrow pencil* is made with the same pigments as in mascara and is basically a crayon. *Cream eye shadow* is a mixture of a petrolatum and pigment, whereas *stick eye shadow* contains most of the same ingredients as lipstick.

Eyeliner contains pigments in a resin solution that may often be irritating to the eyes. It also contains a small amount of mercury, which has been prohibited in all other cosmetics. However, the amount in eyeliner is not believed to be harmful.
Side effects Sensitivity can appear in response to any cosmetic, but the eyes are especially vulnerable. Too frequent or too harsh cleansing of the eyelid can also cause irritation.

mal del pinto See PINTA.

malar flush Often a sign of mitral stenosis (narrowing of a heart valve), malar flush is characterized by heightened color and a slight blue tinge, due to a lack of oxygen in the blood, over the cheekbones. It usually appears after a bout of rheumatic fever.

It is possible, however, to have a malar flush without any heart irregularities: Many people with this high coloring do not have cardiac disease.

mal de Meleda An extremely rare hereditary skin disease of the epidermis inherited by autosomal recessive transmission, which means that a defective gene must be inherited from both parents in order to cause the abnormality. Generally, the parents of an affected person are unaffected carriers of the defective gene. Each of the children of such parents has a one in four chance of being affected, and a two in four chance of being a carrier. This disease is progressive and persistent.

The condition was first described in 1826 on the island of Meleda off the coast of Bosnia Herzegovina, and most cases of this disease have been reported in Bosnia, Germany and France.

Symptoms During the first few weeks of life, the disease is characterized by yellow-brown, waxy, rough palms and soles of the feet. Other associated abnormalities include poor physical development, short nails and fingers, high palate, and abnormalities of the EEG.

Treatment Administration of keratolytics and lactic acid–based creams.

malignancy, skin signs of internal There are a range of signs that can appear on the skin in connection with cancer. Some of these signs include multiple sebaceous cysts, increased hairiness, dryness and scaling. Five percent of cancer patients may get metastatic nodules (lumps), usually in connection with cancers of the breast, lung or colon—but usually only after the cancer is well advanced. Up to 25 percent of lymphomas appear first as an skin rash, with small plaques, nodules or ulcers.

Other examples of cancerous diseases with skin symptoms include ACANTHOSIS NIGRICANS (darkening in body folds, underarms, neck and groin, with velvety brown eruptions), COWDEN'S DISEASE (small oral nodules), dermatomyositis (red, swollen thickened skin especially of the eyelids), GARDNER'S SYNDROME (disfiguring cysts on skin), Paget's disease (weeping, crusting or scaly skin inflammation in anal or groin region, vulva, armpits or breasts), PEUTZ-JEGHERS SYNDROME (dark pigmented oral spots), PYODERMA GANGRENOSUM (ulcer with bluish borders, covering large areas of skin), BOWEN'S DISEASE, BULLOUS PEMPHIGOID, DERMATOMYOSITIS, ERYTHEMA ANNULARE CENTRIFUGUM, ERYTHEMA GYRATUM REPENS, acquired ICHTHYOSIS (Hodgkin's disease or lymphoma), BAZEX SYNDROME, DERMATITIS HERPETIFORMIS, Paget's disease, PEMPHIGUS, PORPHYRIA cutanea tarda and leukocytoclastic vasculitis.

malignant melanoma See MELANOMA, MALIGNANT.

mammoplasty Plastic surgery of the breasts either to increase (breast augmentation) or decrease (breast reduction) their size.

Breast augmentation is the most popular of all operations to reshape soft tissue. In the past, fluids were directly injected into the breast, with some dreadful results. Today, a prosthesis is implanted into a pocket either directly under the breast tissue or underneath the major chest muscle (pectoralis). In the past the most common implants were silicone gel (see SILICONE IMPLANTS). After numerous medical reports questioning their safety and linking them to connective tissue disorders, saline inflatables have now become more popular. A third type, the double-lumen prosthesis, features a gel-filled inner portion surrounded by a saline inflatable outer jacket.

In breast augmentation, the incision through which the implant is inserted can be made either above the crease under the breast, near the nipple or high in the armpit. The first method is the most popular: The armpit incision leaves no scar on the breast itself, but it is more risky since the incision is so far from the area on which the surgeon is working.

After the procedure, the breast should look and feel natural: Scars are usually not noticeable.

Risks Problems with breast hardness, caused by scar tissue that forms around the implant, may occur in up to 30 percent of patients. This hardness may appear soon after surgery or years after the procedure. Other risks are rare and include loss of nipple sensitivity (5 to 10 percent), infection or poor healing of scars.

Because breasts that are too large may cause back pain, discomfort during sports, chronic back strain, rashes in the creases, or a psychological burden, some women choose *breast reduction* to solve their health problems. In this surgical technique, excess breast tissue is removed, the nipple position is raised and the skin is trimmed to fit the new shape. The operation usually requires a hospital stay and general anesthesia. Activities must be restricted for several weeks post-surgery. Some scarring occurs, usually around the nipple, under the breasts and between the nipple and the second scar. It is also possible that the nipple will be less sensitive, and that breast-feeding may become impossible. There is no evidence of an increase in breast cancer. Because breast reduction is not always sim-ply cosmetic, some insurance companies will pay for at least part of the operation.

See also MASTOPEXY.

manicures See NAILS, CARE OF.

Mantoux test See TUBERCULIN TEST.

mask of pregnancy See CHLOASMA.

mask A type of skin product that can either be rinsed or peeled off that helps the skin to exfoliate (shed its dead outer cells) in order for it to look fresh and vital. Masks also stimulate the skin's circulation, and some help the skin hold moisture better (at least temporarily).

Newer products have been developed for a wide range of tasks (such as improving puffy eyes) in addition to imparting a healthy glow to the skin and removing dead skin cells. Masks are designed to work quickly—most of them dry in 10 minutes or less and are then removed.

Today's masks are more effective because they include better ingredients designed to clean, tighten, refresh and moisturize the face. Mixed into these products are substances previously found only in moisturizers (such as talc and nylon, to cut down shine), buttermilk (a moisturizing ingredient), caffeine extract and grapefruit seed (to soothe and lessen redness).

Before choosing a mask, consumers should read the label carefully; it's important to know what active ingredients to look for to best treat a specific SKIN TYPE.

Oily skin The best masks for this skin type are made of kaolin (oil-absorbing clay), bentonite (white clay), aluminum magnesium silicate (talc), witch hazel, alcohol or zinc oxide. These masks work by cleaning the skin, absorbing excess oil (which cuts down on shine) and preventing bacterial growth. Kaolin and bentonite also cause the skin to perspire, which opens up the pores, allowing the ingredients in the mask to deep-clean the skin. Most oily-skin masks start as a thick paste and dry to a hard crust that is removed by water. Afterward, the skin feels temporarily tightened.

Dry skin The best masks for dry skin include those having collagen, buttermilk and protein as moisturizers; panthenol (a B vitamin), to help retain moisture; amino acids, to help water penetrate the skin, plumping up skin cells and temporarily filling in fine lines; and oils or lanolin, to help keep moisture close to the skin. Masks for dry skin are usually gel- or cream-based and do not dry and harden on the skin.

Blotchy skin The types of masks to help this skin problem include those made with kaolin, caffeine, grapefruit seed and plant extracts such as azulene, chamomile and aloe. All skin types can benefit from products with these ingredients, which can soothe and even out the complexion. Caffeine and grapefruit seeds diminish redness; chamomile extract cuts down inflammation and has a cooling effect on the skin.

Dull skin Masks made of menthol, peppermint or eucalyptus can help stimulate the skin, leaving it with a tingling feeling. These masks are sometimes made to dry into a stretchy film that is peeled off; others are cream-based and are rinsed off. Both types remove dead skin cells, which create a dull appearance.

mast cell diseases Diseases of the mast cell, a large cell in connective tissue with many coarse granules containing the chemicals heparin, histamine and serotonin, which are released during inflammation and allergic responses. Mast cell diseases (known collectively as mastocytosis) include a wide variety of different conditions characterized by tissue invaded by mast cells. These conditions include crops of benign hyperpigmented macules or papules (URTICARIA PIGMENTOSA), small nodules common in young children (MASTOCYTOMA) and malignant mast cell leukemia. Urticaria pigmentosa is the most common of these diseases. MASTOCYTOMAS represent 10 percent of all cases of mast cell diseases.

Most patients with mast cell diseases can expect an excellent prognosis with an uncomplicated recovery. In children, the skin lesions often clear up on their own, but in adulthood the lesions don't usually disappear. Occasionally, patients may experience systemic involvement with collections of mast cells in internal organs and a progressively more serious decline into a lymphoma-like illness, but this is uncommon. A few cases become malignant.

Symptoms Symptoms may include flushing, nausea, vomiting, upper stomach pain and shock, or "mastocytosis syndrome."

mastocytomas One of the more common MAST CELL DISEASES that is found almost exclusively in children, characterized by a solitary brown-tan plaque rather like an orange peel (PEAU D'ORANGE) that itches when stroked. Adults do not develop exterior symptoms from mastocytomas.

Symptoms Mastocytomas usually are diagnosed at birth or within the first few weeks of life. Usually solitary, they may occur in groups of up to four, and they are most often found on the body, neck and arm (especially near the wrist). The brown/tan plaques may swell or itch, usually the result of gentle rubbing or scratching. Blisters may also develop from the plaques. Attacks of flushing (either on the face or all over the body) may occur, sometimes related to bumping the lesion.

Treatment While isolated mastocytomas may be excised, especially with severe flushing, it may be best to leave them alone since they almost always spontaneously disappear.

mastocytosis The most common variety, also known as urticaria pigmentosa, is an unusual condition characterized by many itchy, yellow or orange-brown macules on the skin (most often found on the trunk and seldom the face, although they can appear anywhere on the body). They range in size from a few millimeters to several centimeters. The skin condition generally worsens after bathing or scratching the skin. The most common of all the MAST CELL DISEASES, mastocytosis usually appears during the first 12 months of infancy and fades away by adolescence.

Treatment There is not really any effective treatment, although antihistamine drugs may provide some relief.

mastopexy The medical term for reshaping the breasts by trimming excess skin and raising the nipple. Drooping breasts usually follow significant weight loss or frequent childbirth.

In mild cases, the breast appearance can be improved simply by placing an implant underneath the breast tissue in a procedure similar to breast augmentation (see MAMMOPLASTY). In this procedure, the implant fills out the extra skin and raises the nipple, giving the entire breast a more youthful appearance. This process also makes the breast larger; in patients who don't want larger breasts—just more youthful-looking ones—the surgeon can preform a mastopexy. This does leave the same scars as a breast reduction. With this technique, however, nipple sensations are usually left undisturbed and there may be no loss of the ability to breastfeed.

measles (rubeola, morbilli) A childhood viral illness causing a widespread blotchy, slightly elevated pink rash, which develops first behind the ears and then elsewhere. The rash lasts from three to five days. Although a commonplace disease, complications (including pneumonia) can lead to death. In the United States, widespread vaccines have decreased the occurrence of this disease. One attack usually confers lifelong immunity. The patient is infectious while the rash lasts; complete recovery may take two to four weeks.

Once common throughout the world, a few thousand cases of measles are still reported in the U.S. despite strict vaccination requirements for school-age children.

Measles is still a killer in developing countries, where more than 1 million deaths a year are recorded from the disease—especially among malnourished children with impaired immunity.

Cause The measles virus is very contagious, and is spread by airborne droplets from nasal secretions. Symptoms appear after an incubation period of between nine to 11 days, and the patient is infectious from shortly after the beginning of this period until up to a week after symptoms have developed. Infants under eight months of age rarely contract measles, because they still harbor some immunity from their mothers.

Symptoms The disease begins with a fever, runny nose, sore eyes and cough; the rash appears after three or four days, beginning on the head and neck and spreading down to cover the entire body. The spots may be so numerous that they appear together as a large red area. The rash begins to fade within three days.

Complications The most common complications include ear and chest infections, usually occurring as the fever returns a few days after the rash appears. There may also be diarrhea, vomiting and abdominal pain. About one in every 1,000 patients goes on to develop encephalitis (brain inflammation), with headache, drowsiness and vomiting beginning seven to 10 days after the rash begins. This may be followed by seizures and coma, sometimes leading to mental retardation or death. (Note: seizures are common with measles and don't necessarily indicate the presence of encephalitis). Very rarely (one in a million cases) a progressive brain disorder called subacute sclerosing panencephalitis develops many years after the illness.

Measles during pregnancy causes fetal death in about one-fifth of cases, but there is no evidence that measles causes birth defects. German measles during pregnancy can cause birth defects if the mother contracts the disease during early pregnancy. Girls should be immunized before puberty.

Treatment Give fluids and acetaminophen for fever. Antibiotics will not help the virus, but may be needed to treat a secondary infection.

Prevention In the United States, children are routinely vaccinated early in the second year by an injection usually combined with mumps and rubella that produces immunity in 97 percent of patients. Side effects are reported to be mild, including low fever, slight cold and a rash about a week after the shot.

The vaccine should not be given to infants under age one, to those with a history of epilepsy in the family, or to those who have had seizures before. In these cases, simultaneous injection of measles-specific immunoglobulin, which contains antibodies against the virus, should be given.

mechlorethamine A nitrogen mustard used for the past 30 years as a topical treatment for early stages of MYCOSIS FUNGOIDES (a disease featuring chronic irritating eruptions), which can result in a long-term remission. It is administered either as a liquid or ointment, usually over the entire body on a daily basis. Lesions clear up in between 50 and 75 percent of cases within two to six months, although prolonged treatment may be required for more stubborn cases. Some experts recommend daily treatments for six months even after active lesions have disappeared, in order to prevent recurrence, but the value of maintenance therapy has not been established.

Mechlorethamine is not effective in those with advanced tumor-stage mycosis fungoides.

Side effects This medication is relatively less toxic than other anti-tumor agents, although more than half of all patients develop an irritant or contact dermatitis. In fact, its most common side effect is contact hypersensitivity. Nitrogen mustard causes fewer problems when applied as an ointment in lower concentrations, gradually increasing the concentration over time. The drug should be stopped if diffuse hyperpigmentation occurs. See also SQUAMOUS CELL CARCINOMA; BASAL CELL CARCINOMA.

Mees' lines Single or multiple white horizontal bands on the nails that are a sign of arsenic poisoning.

Meissner's touch corpuscles One of three specialized nerve endings found in the skin. Meissner's touch corpuscles are oval structures composed of coiled terminal axons within a basal lamina and collagen fibers. They are primarily found in the palms and soles, and appear to assist in the sensory function of touch.

melanin The pigment that gives skin, hair and the iris of the eyes their color; the more melanin present, the darker the color. Its level depends on race, heredity and sun exposure.

Melanin is produced by cells called melanocytes (see PIGMENT CELLS), special cells of the epidermis that are controlled in part by the pituitary gland and by a hormone secreted from the hypothalamus, called melanocyte-stimulating hormone (MSH). Melanocytes produce two types of melanin, eumelanin and phaeomelanin; eumelanin is black or brown, and phaeomelanin is red. The ratio of these two types of pigment largely determines the tint of hair and skin.

Exposure to sunlight stimulates a protection reaction by the melanocytes that darkens the skin color by increasing the amount of melanin. Ultraviolet light B (UVB) causes an increase in the production of melanin; UVA oxidizes already-existing melanin to produce immediate darkening, which is what you see after several hours of sun exposure. UVB tanning is the slow darkening that develops one to seven days after the beach. Localized excess melanin production causes pigmented spots such as freckles and lentigines. Many physical and chemical agents stimulate the production of melanin.

Other agents that boost melanin production include prostaglandin E2, estrogens and other hormones, as well as some chemotherapy drugs (such as bleomycin). Ingested metals such as arsenic can darken skin by depositing melanin in the dermis.

PSORALENS are organic compounds found in many plants such as limes and celery that—in combination with UVA—stimulate the formation of melanin. See also PIGMENTATION DISORDERS; DEPIGMENTATION DISORDERS; PIGMENTATION.

melanocytes See PIGMENT CELLS.

melanocyte-stimulating hormone (MSH) A hormone that stimulates the production of MELANIN. Four different MSH peptides have been identified, all of which are formed in the pituitary gland. Lack of MSH (such as in HYPOPITUITARISM) may cause a decrease of skin color all over the body. See also PIGMENTATION; PIGMENTATION, DISORDERS OF; PIGMENT CELLS.

melanocyte system, tumors of These tumors include MOLES, congenital nevus, spitz nevus (see NEVUS, SPITZ), dysplastic nevus syndrome, halo nevus (see NEVUS, HALO); blue nevus (see NEVUS, BLUE), lentigines (see LENTIGO; LENTIGO MALIGNA), malignant melanoma (see MELANOMA, MALIGNANT). See also PIGMENT CELLS; PIGMENTATION.

melanoma See MELANOMA, MALIGNANT.

melanoma, acral lentiginous The second least common of four types of malignant melanoma (see MELANOMA, MALIGNANT), accounting for only 10 percent of all melanomas. It is, however, the most common malignant melanoma in blacks and Asians. The diagnosis of this form of melanoma is often delayed, which is unfortunate since a late diagnosis can be fatal.

Lesions are found on the palms, soles, fingers and toes, or on the mucosal surfaces. The first signs of acral lentiginous melanoma may appear as a darker streak in the nail, sometimes appearing with a brown discolored cuticle (Hutchinson's sign). Not all darker streaks in the nail are the result of malignant lesions. As the lesion develops it produces variations in color (brown, black, pink or blue) and it grows, occasionally becoming a nodule, which may ulcerate.

Treatment Treatment of acral lentiginous melanoma is described under malignant melanoma (see MELANOMA, MALIGNANT; MELANOMA, JUVENILE; MELANOMA, LENTIGO MALIGNA).

melanoma, juvenile Historic name for SPITZ NEVUS.

melanoma, lentigo maligna This type of malignant lesion develops from a preexisting lesion of LENTIGO MALIGNA (melanotic Hutchinson's freckle) and makes up about 5 percent of all primary skin melanomas. These lesions, which tend to occur in older patients and more often among women, always are found in sun-exposed areas (especially the face).

This type of malignancy tends to grow over a long period of time; the original pigmented lesion appears 10 to 15 years before it becomes malignant. This transformation takes place in up to 5 percent of all patients with lentigo maligna.

Melanoma first appears within the lesion as a slow-growing, deeply colored nodule. Once the malignant cells have invaded the dermis, they may spread as any other type of melanoma.

Treatment Treatment for lentigo maligna melanoma is the same as for malignant melanoma (see MELANOMA, MALIGNANT; MELANOMA, ACRAL LENTIGINOUS; MELANOMA, JUVENILE; MELANOSIS).

melanoma, malignant The most deadly form of the three major types of SKIN CANCER, melanomas are brown, black or multicolored patches, plaques or nodules with an irregular outline. Malignant melanoma is much more dangerous than other forms of skin cancer because of its tendency to spread rapidly to vital internal organs such as the lungs, liver and brain. One in five patients afflicted with malignant melanoma dies of this cancer. It is the most frequently diagnosed cancer among women between 25 and 29, and it ranks second in frequency of occurrence only to breast cancer among those aged 30 to 34.

Symptoms Melanoma usually begins as a pigmented growth on the skin, displaying many shades of color (including brown, black, pink, white, blue or gray). It often has irregular outlines and may be larger than ordinary moles. The spots may crust, bleed or itch, and at times they may develop within preexisting MOLES. It is therefore important that any moles that change in any way be examined by a dermatologist. Congenital moles (present at birth) seem to have an increased risk of becoming malignant, and therefore should be examined early in life by a dermatologist.

Causes In 1935 when few people habitually baked at the beach, melanoma was a rare disease, affecting only one in 1,500 Americans. Although malignant melanoma is still a fairly uncommon cancer, its incidence is growing at a faster rate than any other cancer except lung cancer in women. Today, the rate has climbed to one in 100; about 32,000 new cases are predicted each year, and 7,000 people will die.

Those at highest risk have a family history of skin cancer, an abundance of moles (more than 100), fair skin, light hair and blue-green or grey eyes. Recently, scientists have identified a defective gene that appears to cause an inherited tendency to this type of deadly skin cancer, and that may also play a role in non-inherited melanoma. About 10 percent of melanoma occurs in people with an inherited tendency, and it is unclear what percentage of inherited cases are due to this gene.

Normally, the gene acts as a brake on cancer, but those who inherit a defective version lose part of their protection, making them unusually susceptible to melanoma. The normal gene tells the body how to make a protein called p16, which helps regulate cell division. Earlier studies suggested that the p16 gene is a "tumor-suppressor" cell that discourages development of tumors. These earlier studies also indicated that defective versions play a role in cancer.

Defective versions of the gene also may be involved in many or even most cases of non-inherited melanoma, according to research. In those cases, the gene would be inherited in normal form but would mutate following exposure to sunlight or other causes. Researchers hope that studying this gene may someday lead to a screening test for those at risk, and for better treatments for the non-inherited disease. The genetic research was presented by the National Center for Human Genome Research (part of the National Institutes of Health) and at Myriad Genetics, Inc. in Salt Lake City in cooperation with the University of Utah.

In one study, nine of 18 melanoma-prone families screened showed defects in the p16; in another study, p16 gene defects appeared in two of 13 families known to have a melanoma-related abnormality in the neighborhood of the p16 gene.

Other risk factors for developing melanoma are severe sunburns in childhood; even one severe burn during childhood or adolescence is a potent precursor of melanoma later in life. Anyone with multiple moles may also suffer from dysplastic nevus syndrome (see NEVUS SYNDROME, DYSPLASTIC) and may be at increased risk for the development of melanoma.

Finally, new research suggests that alcohol use can contribute to the development of melanoma, according to Australian researchers. In one study, women who drank two or more drinks per day had two and a half times the chance of developing melanoma. A Harvard University study found that drinking more than one beer, glass of wine or cocktail daily led to an 80 percent higher melanoma risk.

Diagnosis Because the skin is so easily seen, malignant melanoma can be easier to spot than internal malignancies. To make sure that people notice skin cancer, dermatologists recommend that everyone examine their skin twice a year, using a full-length and a hand-held mirror. Any suspicious growths should be reported immediately to a dermatologist. (For a free brochure illustrating how to do the skin surface exam, send a stamped, self-addressed business-sized envelope to the Skin Cancer Foundation, Box 561, New York, NY 10156)

Treatment Most skin cancers—even malignant melanomas—can be cured if discovered early enough, which is why attention to symptoms and regular self-examination is highly recommended. When cancers of the skin are discovered early, there are a variety of treatment possibilities, depending on the type of tumor, size, location and other factors affecting the patient's general health. A biopsy is often needed before a treatment option is selected.

Recent research has suggested the possibility of using fat-like molecules to deliver DNA with cancer-killing potential into the tumors of people with skin cancer—one step closer to the dream of developing gene therapy for cancer treatment. Scientists at the University of Michigan Medical Center in Ann Arbor used liposomes (artificially produced fat particles) to transfer DNA into tumor cells in five patients with malignant melanoma. The five had an advanced form of the disease that would not respond to conventional anticancer treatment. There was evidence of an immune response in two patients; scientists hope that once the gene is deposited into the tumor cell, production of an alien protein will alert the immune system, which should then recognize the tumor cell as foreign and mount an attack. Unfortunately, only a fraction of tumor cells take up the gene, but researchers hope that once immune cells travel to the tumor site they may kick off a broad-based attack that will eventually seek out all malignant cells.

Although the study was not designed to prove the therapy's usefulness, one patient showed a dramatic, positive response—the skin tumor that had been injected completely disappeared, as did several other tumors that were not treated. This same patient also had one tumor that did not respond to treatment. The injections appeared to have no toxic effects.

Even newer research isolating a gene defect that appears to cause some types of inherited melanoma may eventually lead to better treatment for the non-inherited disease.

Melanoma and psychotherapy Recent studies at Stanford Medical School found that patients with malignant melanoma appear to live longer after a course of group therapy. In the study, 68 patients were divided into two groups after surgery. Once a week for six weeks, 34 of them met in small groups to express their feelings, give one another support and encouragement, and receive information and advice about the disease. The other 34 had only standard treatment. Five to six years later, 13 of the 34 patients in the control group had suffered a recurrence of the cancer, and 10 had died (numbers that were about average, given the patients' physical condition when the study began). Although the two groups were otherwise similar, only seven patients in group therapy had a recurrence, and only three died.

Prevention In addition to avoiding excess sun exposure, new research isolating a gene defect that may lead to some cases of malignant melanoma may be used as a screen for people at risk for the disease. These patients could then be counseled to take steps like avoiding too much sun, keeping track of possible pre-cancerous moles and using sunscreen, although sunscreen may not prevent all skin cancer.

Some foods and nutrients may offset the development of melanoma: fish with omega-3 fat and antioxidants (including vitamins E and C and beta carotene). In one Australian study, those who ate a half-ounce of fish daily were less likely to have melanoma than those who ate only one-fifth of an ounce of fish daily.

melasma See CHLOASMA.

meliodiosis See WHITMORE'S DISEASE.

Mendes da Costa syndrome A disorder of keratinization also known as erythrokeratoderma variabilis, this is a rare autosomal dominant disorder characterized by two types of lesions—fixed plaques and shifting red rings or arcs frequently caused to change by temperature change. The plaques are most often found on the face, extremities and buttocks; the red rings may last up to hours or days.

This genetic disorder is carried by only one defective gene (from one parent). Each child of an affected person usually has a one in two chance of inheriting the defective gene and of being affected.

meningococcal infections These infections caused by the bacteria *Neisseria meningitidis* may cause a rash ranging from masses of tiny pinhead-sized red dots to large blue-purple hemorrhagic areas or extensive gangrene. In the few who lack immunity, the meningiococcus bacteria infects the lining of the brain as a form of MENINGITIS, or the bloodstream as either acute or chronic meningococcemia.

Cause The disease is transmitted most often through the air in winter or by nasal droplets in spring. If the infection is introduced to people in closed quarters, it can become epidemic. Spread by a cough, a sneeze, a kiss or a shared drink, it can kill a healthy teenager within hours.

Symptoms In addition to the rash, other symptoms include fever, headache, vomiting, delirium, convulsions, stiff neck and back. Acute meningococcemia is rapidly progressive and often fatal, and needs early and aggressive diagnosis and treatment.

Treatment Aqueous penicillin G must be administered every 24 hours for 7 to 10 days by IV (or until the patient's fever subsides for five days). There is a vaccine for group A and group C meningococci. Treatment should also include symptom control, such as reducing fever, maintaining fluid and electrolyte balance, and administering heparin when necessary.

Menkes' kinky-hair syndrome A hereditary syndrome characterized by twisted, beaded (monilethrix) or fragile (trichorrhexis nodosa) hair shafts, usually associated with mental retardation seizures and problems in walking or balance.

The syndrome is caused by a problem with copper metabolism, resulting in poor absorption, low blood and tissue copper levels. Most untreated patients die by the age of four; many survive less than two years.

The condition is an X-linked recessive disorder, which means that it is caused by a defect on the X chromosome, usually leading to problems in males only. Women can be carriers of the defect, and half of their sons may be affected.

Treatment Supplements of intravenous copper are not effective.

metabolic disorders, skin signs of Disorders of metabolism often include symptoms of skin abnormalities. In some disorders, skin changes are the first signal of an underlying metabolic problem.

Metabolic diseases with skin symptoms include disorders of amino acid metabolism (phenylketonuria, homocystinuria, ochronosis, HARTNUP DISEASE, arginosuccinicaciduria and tyrosinemia type II). Diseases of lipid metabolism include xanthomatoses, REFSUM'S DISEASE, XANTHELASMA, GAUCHER'S DISEASE, and FABRY'S DISEASE. Diseases of metal metabolism include problems with the metabolism of zinc (acrodermatitis enteropathica), iron (HEMOCHROMATOSIS) or copper (WILSON'S DISEASE) and may result in numerous skin signs.

Other metabolic disorders include AMYLOIDOSIS, MUCINOSES, LICHEN MYXEDEMATOSUS, URBACH-WIETHE DISEASE, MUCOPOLYSACCHARIDOSES, FUCOSIDOSIS, gout and Lesch-Nyhan syndrome.

menthol A soothing white substance derived from oil of peppermint that is included in many skin-care products because it feels cool to the touch and may help relieve itching.

methotrexate Sometimes used to treat PSORIASIS, this powerful anticancer drug can cause many unpleasant side effects. (It can also make the skin increasingly sensitive to sunlight). *It should never be given to anyone else for any purpose, since patients require close medical supervision.*

Adverse effects Possible effects include severe nausea and vomiting, diarrhea and mouth ulcers, black stools, sore throat, fever, chills, unusual bleeding and bruising, abdominal pain, anemia, increased susceptibility to infections, abnormal bleeding, and liver damage with long term use. Extra fluid intake mitigates methotrexate toxicity. Infrequently, side effects can include hair loss, dizziness, seizures, shortness of breath and rash.

Physicians perform routine follow-up medical evaluations in all patients taking methotrexate, including tests to check liver and kidney functions and complete blood counts.

Methotrexate may negatively interact with a range of other drugs. Possible toxicity could occur when taken with anticonvulsants, anti-gout drugs, diclofenac, nonsteroidal anti-inflammatory drugs, oxyphenbutazone, phenylbutazone, phenytoin, probenecid, pyrimethamine, salicylates (including aspirin), sulfadoxine and pyrimethamine, sulfa drugs, and tetracyclines.

methoxsalen A PSORALEN drug used to treat PSORIASIS, MYCOSIS FUNGOIDES and VITILIGO. This drug belongs to the class of repigmenting agents. It is taken as a tablet or capsule two to four hours before exposure to sunlight or a sunlamp. In the treatment of vitiligo, it may take between six to nine months before results are apparent; results may be seen in 10 weeks or more for psoriasis. See PUVA.

Precautions Methoxsalen should not be taken with any other medication that causes skin sensitivity to the sun. Patients should avoid alcohol in any form from 12 hours before taking the drug to at least 24 hours afterward. Combining alcohol with methoxsalen may result in a reaction causing flushed face, severe headache, chest pains, shortness of breath, nausea and vomiting, sweating and weakness; severe reactions may be fatal.

Side effects In addition to the above, common side effects include increased skin and eye sensitivity to the sun, and nausea. Other possible side effects include red and sore skin, dizziness, headache, depression, leg cramps or insomnia.

methyl paraben A preservative used in eyeliners, hair care products and cold creams that is the frequent cause of allergic reaction to cosmetics.

metronidazole (trade names: Flagyl, Metryl, Protostat, Satric) An antibiotic particularly useful in fighting infections of the urinary, genital and digestive systems such as trichomoniasis, amebiasis and giardiasis, and for the treatment of ROSACEA. It is administered by mouth or by suppository.

Side effects Rare, but may include nausea and vomiting, appetite loss, abdominal pain, metallic taste, and dark-colored urine. Drinking alcohol during treatment with this drug can trigger particularly unpleasant reactions, such as nausea, vomiting, hot flashes, headache, etc.

miconazole Antifungal agent used for topical treatment of dermatophytes.

milia Also known as epidermal cysts, these are small, firm white papules usually found in clusters on upper cheeks and around the eyes. They are commonly (but wrongly) called "sebaceous cysts."

Painless and harmless, milia may appear following injury, chronic ultraviolet light exposure or blistering. More often they are caused by blocked pores as a result of moisturizer use.

Milia are also found in about 40 percent of full-term infants on the forehead, cheeks and nose.

Treatment Epidermal cysts and milia may be removed for cosmetic reasons or to prevent rupture using a fine-guage needle and a cotton-tipped swab or a comedone extractor. Inflamed lesions respond well to incision and drainage. Antibiotics are not normally required, unless pathogenic bacteria are present. In infants, no treatment is necessary.

miliaria See PRICKLY HEAT.

miliaria apocrine See FOX-FORDYCE DISORDER.

miliaria crystallina Transparent superficial blisters on uninflamed skin, often found in creased-skin areas (such as the groin or under the breasts). See also PRICKLY HEAT.

miliaria profunda White or red papules that usually aren't itchy. They are commonly associated with heat stress and may appear together with chronic MILIARIA RUBRA. See also PRICKLY HEAT.

miliaria rubra See PRICKLY HEAT.

miliaria tuberculosis See TUBERCULOSIS, SKIN.

milker's nodule A viral infection by a poxvirus that causes tricolored, sometimes-painful, black, red and white nodules on the fingers of people who milk cows. The poxvirus (paravaccinia) is found widely among cattle and can cause lesions called pseudocowpox in the animals. Cross-species infection can occur when human skin touches these lesions.

Symptoms Generally, a single red macule appears on the finger (although multiple lesions may occur) between four and seven days after infection. It progresses into a three-colored papule with a crusted center surrounded by a whitish area, in turn surrounded by a red base.

Prevention/treatment Infected cows should be isolated, and protective gloves should be worn when coming in contact with infected animals. There is no specific treatment, and the lesion usually heals on its own, although it may leave a scar. Topical antibiotics may help to minimize the risk of secondary bacterial infection.

mineral oil A clear, odorless oil derived from petroleum that is widely used in cosmetics because it is inexpensive and rarely causes allergic reactions. It can, however, sometimes induce ACNE lesions.

minocycline (trade name: Minocin) A tetracycline antibiotic used to treat ACNE.

minoxidil The brand name for Rogaine, this vasodilator (a drug that widens blood vessels) is used in a topical solution on the scalp to treat androgenetic alopecia (also known as pattern baldness) in men and diffuse hair loss or thinning of the front and top of the scalp in women. It was approved by the FDA in 1988 as a lotion treatment for male pattern baldness, and in 1991 for women with hair loss.

Research has found that after four months, about 25 percent of 2,300 men with male pattern baldness reported moderate to dense hair regrowth, compared with 11 percent using placebo. No regrowth was reported by 41 percent (60 percent using placebo). After one year, 48 percent of those who continued to use minoxidil rated their new hair growth as moderate or better.

Studies have shown that the response to the drug varies a great deal from one person to the next, but patients should not expect to see regrowth before four months of use. Minoxidil is a hair loss treatment, not a cure, and patients must continue to use the drug in order to maintain regrowth. New hair growth is shed after minoxidil use is discontinued.

In general, clinical studies have found that minoxidil works best for those patients who are younger, who have been losing their hair for a short period of time and who have less initial hair loss. The medication's effectiveness appears to be related to the activity level of hair follicles.

Side effects include itching and other skin irritations on the scalp.

mites Tiny eight-legged parasites belonging to the group (Acarina) that includes ticks. Much like tiny spiders, many of these mites have piercing mouth parts that suck blood from animals and humans. A mite has no antenna or wings. Medically important mites include the many species causing dermatitis (*Dermatophogoedes*). The SCABIES mite lives in human skin, and the CHIGGER's bite can cause a rash. Mites in grain or fruit can cause a variety of skin irritations (commonly called "grocer's itch" or "bakers' itch").
Prevention Mite infestations can be avoided by using insect repellents such as dimethyl phthalate when walking through infested areas.

Mohs' microscopically controlled excisions A type of dermatologic treatment in which thin layers of tissue are removed and immediately examined for malignant cells in a specially equipped lab in the doctor's office. Layers are removed until all tissue is cancer-free. The technique is used to remove basal cell and squamous cell carcinomas and a variety of other more rare skin cancers.

Developed by Dr. Frederic E. Mohs about 44 years ago, this method is now used to treat one out of every four or five skin-cancer patients. Mohs surgery offers the highest cure rate and sacrifices the least amount of healthy tissue because it almost always removes the entire cancer without removing too much surrounding normal skin. In this technique, using local anesthesia, the tumor may first be reduced by curettage and then excised; blood flow is usually controlled by electrodesiccation. The excised tissue is then mapped, flattened, frozen and then cut in horizontal sections and the entire undersurface checked for the presence of tumor. Repeated slices are performed until the margins are clear.

This technique is indicated for patients with recurrent tumors, primary tumors known to have high recurrence rates and primary lesions where tissue must be preserved (such as on the eyelids, nose, finger, genitalia and areas around facial nerves).

moisturizer While moisturizing can help dry skin (much like a raisin plumps up in water), no moisturizer can prevent wrinkling. (The only possible exception is a moisturizer containing ALPHA HYDROXY ACID, which may help keep skin young-looking by thinning out dried up cells on the surface). The right moisturizer should prevent dryness without causing the skin to break out. Consumers who experience problems with one moisturizer should switch moisturizers rather than discontinue their use. The problems may have resulted from reaction to a specific chemical in that brand.

It's important to test a moisturizer in the store, especially if you've had problems with other moisturizing products. Apply to an area (such as your neck) that you won't be washing immediately. Walk around for a while and assess the fragrance and feel of the product.

While moisturizers don't have "use by" dates, they can lose effectiveness if stored for too long. Shopping at a store with good turnover will ensure freshness. At most department and chain stores, the cosmetics company automatically changes the stock, but this may not be the case at off-price or discount stores that don't buy directly from a manufacturer.

Moisturizers may cost between $5 and $250. Some of the newest (and most expensive) products contain humectants (ingredients that help the water stay with the skin longer to keep it supple) and some of these substances are expensive. Some experts believe that two humectants—hyaluronic acid and ceramides—are excellent moisturizing ingredients, but they can add significantly to the price of a product. Whether hyaluronic acid is a good moisturizer remains to be proven.

The best humectants include lactic acid and urea, which is not expensive and is very effective. Over-the-counter products containing these compounds are available singly or together.

When shopping for moisturizers, experts suggest that consumers compare ingredients and try the lower-priced product first. While people with dry skin and no acne can use oil-based moisturizers, consumers who tend to break out need to be more careful. Those with acne-prone skin should choose water-based products while avoiding products that could aggravate the condition. However, recent information suggests that oil-based products are acceptable as long as they are not comodogenic. Acne-aggravating products include ingredients such as cocoa butter, heavy mineral oil, acetylated lanolin alcohols, isopropyl esters, isopropyl myristate, lanolin, lanolin fatty acid, linseed oil, oleic acid, olive oil, petrolatum and stearic acid. Moisturizer ingredients that are good for oily skin include beeswax, corn oil, isostearyl neopentate, light mineral oil, octyl palmitate, propylene glycol, safflower oil, sodium lauryl sulfate and spermacetti.

moles A type of pigmented NEVUS composed of NEVUS CELLS. The average young adult has at least 25 moles. However, a change in a mole may be the first sign of an early malignant melanoma.

Malignant melanoma is a serious skin cancer that begins in benign moles about a third of the time. In early stages it can be treated, but in later stages it spreads to other parts of the body and becomes very difficult to treat.

Regular self-examination is the best way to notice when a mole begins to change shape or size. It is important to realize that common moles and malignant melanoma *do not look alike.* A handy way to remember what features to look for is to remember "A-B-C-D" (asymmetry, border, color, diameter).

A mole that is asymmetrical, that has uneven borders, that changes color or is made up of more than one color, or that has a diameter larger than 6 mm. could be a malignant lesion and should be checked immediately by a physician.

molluscum contagiosum A harmless viral infection that causes clusters of pearly white tiny lumps on the skin's surface. Each papule is a small circle with a central depression that produces a cheesy fluid when squeezed.
Symptoms The papules appear primarily in children on the genitals, thighs and the face and in adults in the genital region and on the lower abdomen. They are also frequently seen in patients with advancing AIDS. Molluscum in patients with AIDS are most frequently seen on the face, in flexural areas and on the genitals.
Cause Infection is easily transmitted by direct skin contact or during sexual contact.
Treatment The infection may clear up within a few months without treatment, although it usually requires treatment with keratolytics, liquid nitrogen or by curettage.

Mongolian spot A congenital blue-black pigmented NEVUS found on the lower back or buttocks. The spot, which may appear alone or in a group, may be mistaken for a bruise. It is most common in Asian or black children, and is caused by a concentration of pigment-producing cells (MELANOCYTES) deep within the skin. The spots usually disappear by age three or four.

moniliasis See CANDIDA INFECTION.

monilethrix A rare condition of the hair shaft featuring multiple constrictions, causing the hairs to look like a string of beads. The disease is caused by a defect in the production of keratin. It is an autosomal dominant disorder that is characterized by hair that is normal at birth but which changes in the first months of life. The hair breaks off at the thinned area between the beads.

monobenzone A permanent depigmenting agent that causes permanent skin bleaching. It is used only in severe cases of VITILIGO to remove residual areas of normal pigmentation.

monochloroacetic acid Together with di- and trichloroacetic acid, these are caustic treatments used for WART removal, to treat XANTHELASMA and to perform moderate-depth facial peels.

morbilli See MEASLES.

Morgan's lines (Denny-Morgan) A crease often seen on the lower eyelids of patients with atopic dermatitis (inflammation of the skin). See also DERMATITIS, ATOPIC.

morphea A localized form of SCLERODERMA (hardening of the body's connective tissue) in which one or more well-defined, hard, flat, round or oval patches appear on the skin. The white or purplish patches may be up to several inches in diameter, usually appearing on the trunk, neck, hands or feet. There also may be hair loss or ulceration at the affected site. The condition is most often found in middle-aged women, although it can occur at any age. The condition may spontaneously regress over several years.
Treatment Treatment includes systemic antibiotics and potent topical steroids, colchicine and immunosuppressive drugs may have

limited benefit. New treatments being studied include gamma interferon (which may inhibit synthesis of collagen) and extra-corporeal photophoresis (which may alter immune response).

mosquito bites Female mosquitoes bite in order to obtain blood to produce their eggs. Because their eggs are laid and hatched in stagnant water, throughout the world they are most commonly found near marshes, ponds, reservoirs and water tanks.

Mosquito bites may cause swelling and itching for several days; the main problem of these bites is the infections that may be transmitted. In the United States, mosquitoes carry a variety of strains of viral encephalitis. *Treatment* Because mosquitoes can spread disease, wash the bite area with soap and water and then apply an antiseptic. To control itching, try a nonprescription antihistamine, calamine lotion, gels with mild anesthetic, or ice packs. Or try making a paste to put over the bite: salt moistened with water; 1 tsp. baking soda in a glass of water for 20 minutes; 1 Tbs. epsom salts in 1 quart of hot water that is then chilled.
Prevention Use insect repellents, such as:

DEET (N1N-diethyl-m-toluamide): By far the best repellant, it should be applied to all exposed skin. It comes in various strengths, but the more concentrated is more effective; children should use milder versions because there have been a few cases of toxicity involving small children.

chlorine bleach: Bathe in a tubful of warm water and two capfuls of bleach, but do not get the solution near eyes.

bath oil: Although many consumers swear by Avon's Skin-so-Soft, recent research by the military (and Avon) demonstrate that it is not nearly as effective as DEET.

zinc: Some experts recommend daily doses (at least 60 milligrams) of zinc, although they warn it can take up to four weeks to become effective; extra supplements should be taken only with approval of a physician.

thiamine chloride: A B vitamin that may repel insects when taken orally; however, it may also cause itching, hives and a rash in sensitive individuals.

Moynahan's syndrome See MULTIPLE LENTIGINES SYNDROME.

mucinoses A group of metabolic disorders involving mucin (the primary component of mucus). These disorders include LICHEN MYXEDEMATOSUS, URBACH-WIETHE DISEASE, and MUCOPOLYSACCHARIDOSES.

mucocutaneous lymph node syndrome See KAWASAKI DISEASE.

mucomycosis An uncommon invasive fungal infection of the lung and central nervous system usually associated with diabetics, kidney transplant patients or patients with cancers of the lymph or bone marrow. While primary skin infection is rare with this type of fungus, it may be commonly associated with burn wound infections:
Treatment Administration of intravenous amphotericin B plus treatment of underlying disease.

mucopolysaccharidoses A group of metabolic disorders comprising at least seven major types and 14 subtypes, each with an enzyme deficiency in the metabolism of mucopolysaccharides (a group of complex carbohydrates that help make up the connective tissue). None of these disorders can yet be treated, but someday it may be possible to replace the missing enzyme.

Hunter's syndrome is the only disease in this group with skin symptoms, which are white or flesh-colored papules or nodules that may merge to form ridges. They may appear before age 10 and may fade away later. In severe forms of this syndrome, patients are mentally retarded and die young. Milder forms may not be fatal, or affect intelligence.

multiple lentigines syndrome A genetic syndrome characterized by multiple lentigines (numerous lentigo lesions), heart irregularities, abnormal distance between the eyes, pulmonary stenosis, abnormal genitals, short stature and deafness. The syndrome is also known as LEOPARD or Moynahan's syndrome; variants include NAME syndrome centrofacial lentiginosis and LAMB syndrome. Multiple lentigines syndrome was originally described as progressive cardiomyopathic lentiginosis syndrome by Moynahan; the acronym LEOPARD was applied later to describe the unusual appearance of the numerous lentigines together with the major developmental defects. The acronym stands for the range of developmental symptoms that characterize the disorder:

Lentigines

Electrocardiographic abnormalities

Ocular hypertelorism

Pulmonary stenosis

Abnormalities of the genitals

Retarded growth

Deafness

At birth, patients have only a few lentigines (brown spots similar to freckles), but the number increases rapidly with age until there are hundreds of lesions by adulthood, including on the palms, soles, lips and genitalia. Patients with centrofacial lentiginosis have lentigines in a "butterfly" pattern over the nose and cheeks.

While freckles are flat tan or brown spots found only on areas of the skin exposed to the sun that darken with sun exposure, lentigines are medium to dark brown spots that appear on all areas of the skin and that do not clear in the absence of sun exposure.

Many patients with multiple lentigines syndrome are also mentally retarded, with abnormal EEGs. The NAME syndrome includes: *n*evi (moles), *a*trial myxoma (tumor in the heart), *m*yxoid neurofibromas and *e*phelides (freckles). The LAMB syndrome includes: *l*entigines (brown flat spots), *a*trial myxoma, *m*ucocutaneous myxomas (tumor of connective tissue) and *b*lue nevi. Both are believed to be a variant of multiple lentigines syndromes.

Generalized lentiginosis (LENTIGINOSIS PROFUSA) is a different genetic disorder characterized by numerous lentigines without other developmental problems.

Treatment Most of the symptoms and developmental problems associated with this syndrome are not treatable. Shortly after birth, the infant should be examined by pediatric cardiologists, endocrinologists and otolaryngologists aimed at early detecting of atrial myxomas or deafness. It is possible to improve the appearance of the facial skin by superficial DERMABRASION. The patient's family should understand that all forms of the multiple lentigines syndrome are transmitted as autosomal dominant disorders. This means that the defective gene must be present in only a single parent to cause the syndrome. Each child of an affected person usually has a one in two chance of inheriting the defective gene and of being affected.

mupirocin A fairly new topical antibacterial that is very effective in treating superficial streptococcal and staphylococcal infections of the skin. Many use mupirocin instead of systemic antibiotics to treat primary and secondary types of IMPETIGO.

mycetoma A rare tropical infection also known as Madura foot affecting skin and bone of the foot. It can be highly disfiguring, producing a hard swelling covered by the openings of multiple drainage channels that discharge pus. It most commonly affects farm workers, and can cause severe skin damage.

Cause Mycetoma is caused by usually harmless deep fungi or actinomycetes (a type of bacteria).

Treatment Treatment depends on the organism, but includes six to 12 months of drug therapy. Antibiotics used include ketoconazole, griseofulvin, sulfonamides, penicillin or tetracycline. Fungal disease may be hard to treat with drugs and it may be necessary to surgically remove affected skin.

mycobacterial skin infections Infections caused by a genus of rod-like gram-positive aerobic bacteria that cause disease in humans. MYCOBACTERIUM LEPRAE (or Hansen's bacillus) cause LEPROSY; *M. tuberculosis* (or Koch's bacillus) causes tuberculosis. *M. bovis* causes tuberculosis in cattle, but the mycobacterium can also infect the lungs, joints and intestines of humans.

Infection by atypical mycobacteria are caused by acid-fast organisms like *M. tuberculosis*, but their cultural characteristics are distinctive. Group I, the photochromogens, develop pigment only when growing cultures are exposed to light. They include *M. marinum*, *M. ulcerans* and *M. kansasii*. Many cases of infection with *M. marinum* occur in children and teenagers who swim or clean fish tanks; lesions most often appear on fingers, knees, elbows and the bridge of the nose. There is usually just one lesion, and the tuberculin test is positive. Most cases can be left to resolve spontaneously, although hot compresses may help relieve symptoms. Rifampin or sulfone drugs or minocycline may be effective.

In some tropical areas, *M. ulcerans* infections are common. Single, painless lesions usually appear on arms or legs, but may be found in other places (except on the palms and soles of the feet). The organism is sensitive to a number of drugs in the laboratory, although experiments with patients in a clinical setting have not been encouraging. Excisions and grafting are often necessary; tetracyclines such as minocycline are often helpful.

Group II, the scotochromogens, develop pigment in the absence of light; they do not usually cause human disease.

Group III, the nonchromogens, include *M. avium* and *M. intracellulare*.

Group IV are rapid growers and thrive at temperatures of 37° C and below; there is no pigment production. They include the *M. fortuitum* and *M. smegmatis*.

Mycobacterium leprae The organism that causes LEPROSY, it cannot be cultivated on artificial media or in cell culture. Instead, the organism has been grown in the footpads of mice and armadillos. Humans are its only natural host. See also MYCOBACTERIAL SKIN INFECTIONS.

mycosis Any disease caused by a fungus.

mycosis fungoides Also known as cutaneous T-cell lymphoma, this is a type of lymphoma primarily affecting the skin of the back, shoulders or buttocks. It starts in the skin and may remain there for years before eventually spreading internally.

Symptoms A red, scaly rash that does not itch and that may spread slowly or remain dormant for years. More severe forms of the disease may cause thick patches of skin followed by the development of ulcers.

Treatment For mild cases, nitrogen mustard, UV-B or PUVA (PSORALEN drugs and long-wave ultraviolet-A treatment) is effective. For more serious cases, anticancer chemotherapeutic drugs may be required.

Mycostatin (generic name: nystatin) An anti-fungal treatment available in cream, ointment, powder or suspension, and in combination with topical steroids. Nystatin is a good choice for the treatment of skin infections caused only by *Candida albicans* and other *Candida* species. It is not effective in the treatment of DERMATOPHYTOSIS or TINEA VERSICOLOR.

myiasis, cutaneous A fly larvae infestation of the skin usually found only in the tropics. When the African tumbu fly lays eggs on clothing, the larvae from the eggs penetrate the skin, eventually causing a swelling that resembles a boil. Various other types of flies may lay eggs in open wounds, on the skin or in the ears or nose.
Prevention Infestation can be avoided by covering open wounds and (in Africa) by thoroughly ironing clothes that have been drying outside.
Treatment Apply oil drops over the swellings. The oil suffocates the larvae, which then come to the surface, where they can be removed with a needle.

myxedema A condition characterized by dry, waxy swelling with abnormal mucin deposits (the principal constituent of mucus) in the skin. Often associated with thyroid disease, it is one of the results of hypothyroidism, causing thickened, coarse skin (especially on the lips and nose). It is also the clinical syndrome due to hypothyroidism in adult life, including coarse skin, weight gain, hair loss, sensitivity to cold and mental slowness. A separate condition known as pretibialmyxedema is characterized by a thick, pink-colored plaques on the shins.
Treatment Thyroid hormone replacement will reverse symptoms.

myxoma A soft, jelly-like tumor usually found in the skin of the limbs or neck, made up of mucous material that may grow very large. A myxoma is usually surgically removed.

N

Naftin See NAFTIFINE.

naftifine (trade name: Naftin) A new anti-fungal agent that, when applied to the skin, is effective against the DERMATOPHYTES and *Candida* species. It is used to treat ATHLETE'S FOOT, JOCK ITCH and RINGWORM of the body, among other diseases.
Side effects Burning or stinging feeling on treated areas is a common side effect. Less common are dry skin, itching and redness.

nail biting A common habit that is not related to any underlying medical problem. While many children bite their nails in their early school years, most grow out of the habit, although it can continue as a nervous mannerism into adulthood.

Nail biting is one of the causes of recurrent acute PARONYCHIA (inflammation of nail tissues), and viral warts around bitten nails are not uncommon. Because persistent nail biting can cause pain and bleeding, painting on bitter-tasting preparations may help end the habit.

nail discoloration The most common cause of nail discoloration is nail polish. The deeper the shade of polish, the more likely the pigment will stain the nail. Using a clear base coat before applying color seems to help a bit. Usually, externally induced discoloration involves the whole nail, while discoloration of just a portion usually means there is a problem underneath the nail.

Other causes of externally induced nail discoloration include the use of nail hardeners and synthetic nails, as well as contact with some chemicals (such as photo developer or gardening fertilizers), applying HENNA with your bare hands, and smoking.

The stain, which appears on the nail surface, usually ranges from yellow to brown to red, and could take from three to six months to fully grow out.

If the nail continues to be discolored, you should see a dermatologist because it could be a symptom of an underlying disease. Discoloration can also be caused by health problems such as yeast and bacterial infections, inflammatory syndromes (such as PSORIASIS), benign tumors and even certain cancers (such as melanoma). But in these cases, stains are located *under* the nail and cannot be removed.

Dark-skinned individuals may notice linear longitudinal brown streaks in their nails. Some antimalarial drugs may cause nail discoloration.

For best results in lightening or removing a stain, consumers should skip commercial stain-removing products, since many of them don't work well on nails. Instead, lightly buff the nail with a white emery block. Buffing will sand off the pigments in the top layers of the nail. (However, this should not be done on a regular basis, since too much buffing thins and weakens the nail.)

nail fungus These hard-to-cure infections also known as ONYCHOMYCOSIS can develop in warm, moist areas of the body and are more common as a person ages. The fungus can affect the end of the nail on fingers or toes, causing the nail to crumble and turn yellow, thickening and lifting up. Sometimes, white crumbly patches or white or yellow spots on the surface.
Treatment For mild infections, topical treatment, including cutting the nail back and applying an antifungal medication, may help, but recurrence is common. More severe cases

may require oral medication. Using conventional antifungals (griseofulvin), cure rates are about 30 percent. It takes up to a year for medication to cure a nail infection on smaller toes and up to two years for infections involving the big toe. Newer systemic antifungals are becoming available that are much more effective (cure rates are around 80 percent) in a much shorter period of time.

nail hardeners These are fingernail enamels, actually nail polishes, that form a particularly thick coat or that contain nylon fibers to protect or shield the nail. In the past, nail hardeners caused actual physical changes in the keratin through the action of formaldehyde; because these formaldehyde-containing products caused adverse reactions they are limited to concentrations of 5 percent by the Food and Drug Administration. See also FINGERNAILS, CARE OF; FORMALDEHYDE, SENSITIVITY TO.

nail-patella syndrome An hereditary disorder characterized by nail abnormalities (especially of the index finger and thumb), kidney dysplasia, mental retardation and lack of kneecaps (patella). The prognosis is poor for infants whose kidneys are involved.

The condition is an autosomal dominant disorder, which means that only one defective gene (from one parent) is needed to cause the syndrome. Each child of an affected person usually has a one in two chance of inheriting the defective gene and of being affected.

nail polish A lacquer used to apply color to the fingernails to enhance their appearance. Nail polish is comprised of solvents, plasticizers (to provide flexibility), resins (for body and adhesiveness), color and cellulose nitrate (to create a film for the nail).

Resins are responsible for most of the nail polish dermatitis, but the more severe aller-

gic reactions are often caused by the monomers contained in nail polish extenders.

A new, solvent-free water-based polish has been developed that peels off without polish removal. It can be worn by most people with nail polish allergies, children and pregnant women.

nails The horny plate at the top of the end of fingers and toes. It is made up of KERATIN (a tough protein that forms the basis of skin and hair), and takes up to six months to grow from base to tip on the finger; toenails take twice as long to grow. Nail growth is also affected by seasonal variations. While very tough, the nails may still be damaged by crush or pressure injuries.

Nails can be affected by bacterial and fungal disorders, especially TINEA (ringworm) and candidiasis (thrush). The nail folds can also become infected (PARONYCHIA).

Illness can cause nail symptoms, such as pitting seen in ALOPECIA AREATA, pitting and separation from the nail bed in PSORIASIS, or scarring and nail bed separation in LICHEN PLANUS.

More generally, some nail symptoms may be indications of a generalized disease. Concave, ridged and brittle nails can indicate the presence of iron-deficiency anemia, and fibromus nails can be a sign of TUBEROUS SCLEROSIS. Bleeding into the nail beds, causing

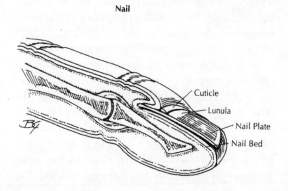

Nail

Cuticle
Lunula
Nail Plate
Nail Bed

vertical black lines on the nail bed, can be an indication of infection of heart valves.

Unusual nail color can also be an indication of disease; bluish nails may indicate heart or breathing problems; greenish black nails might be caused by a bacterial yeast infection, and hard, curved yellow nails may indicate breathing problems.

nails, care of Despite a wide variety of old wives tales, there is actually little that can be done—even by consuming calcium or gelatin—to strengthen a healthy fingernail. Preventive care can include avoiding injuries. Never pry open objects with your nails or file down rough splits with a diamond dust file (a type of file finer than an emery board). Wear cotton gloves when doing chores, and heavier gloves for gardening and outside jobs.

Because repeated drenching of nails in detergents and water can make nails brittle, this problem can be prevented by wearing cotton-lined rubber gloves. However, the rubber gloves should be removed before your hands begin to sweat. Constantly immersing hands in water can also lead to inflammation of the cuticle (PARONYCHIA). Dry nails tht split easily can be treated by applying Vaseline to the nail, cuticle and fingertips nightly.

Care of the cuticle When hands are damp, gently push back the cuticle with a soft towel and massage in hand cream. Cuticle removers contain substances that dissolve and soften the keratin, and because of the potential hazards of caustic products containing potassium hydroxide, many dermatologists recommend that they be avoided. People with inflamed cuticles should never use cuticle removers to achieve a smooth appearance. Although many manicurists do trim or clip the cuticle, this process can cause inflammation and should not be performed.

Hangnails These partly detached dried parts of the cuticle should be cut close to the base, and not be picked or torn (which can lead to infection). To head off hangnails, wear emollients and gloves in dry, cold weather or while using detergents.

Manicures Manicures may improve the appearance of fingernails. Carefully done, manicures can be beneficial. Be careful when removing dirt from underneath the free nail edge, which can cause infection. Overenthusiastic buffing of nails with abrasive powders may injure the nail matrix. Repeatedly applying and removing nail polish can dry out the nail. Allergic reactions to nail polish usually do not appear on the fingers but instead may be manifested on the eyelids or neck.

Sculptured nails Molded fake nails are created by applying an acrylic monomer on the nail plate. While this procedure is popular because it enhances the length of the nail, it can often induce inflammation and cause a painful separation of the nail plate from the bed.

nails, disorders of Although the fingernails are quite hard, they are susceptible to traumatic damage, usually caused by crushing or pressure. This can cause splitting, ridging, breaking or bleeding under the nail.

The nails may become abnormally thick and curved (ONYCHOGRYPHOSIS), a finding that usually occurs among the elderly. Fungal or bacterial infection may also damage the nails, especially TINEA and CANDIDA INFECTIONS, or the nails may also be affected by skin diseases or more general illnesses. For example, in ALOPECIA AREATA (hair loss) the nails may be pitted. In PSORIASIS, the nails may be pitted and separate from the nail bed (ONYCHOLYSIS). In LICHEN PLANUS, the nails may be scarred and separate from the nail bed. Brittle, ridged, concave nails suggest iron-deficiency anemia. Separation of the nail from its bed is seen in thyrotoxicosis, and fibrous growths on the sides of the nails are a sign of TUBEROUS SCLEROSIS. In endocarditis and bleeding disorders, the nails develop splinterlike black marks.

The color of the nails may also be indicative of possible diseases of the body. Blue nails may be a sign of respiratory or cardiac distress. Hard, curved yellow nails are seen in people with bronchiectasis and lymphedema.

Nail disorders are usually diagnosed by visual inspection. Treatment of nail disorders is not easy, since creams and lotions do not usually penetrate into the nail deeply enough, and oral medications may take months to be effective.

nails, pitted Small depressions in the nail plates, typically found in PSORIASIS.

NAME See MULTIPLE LENTIGINES SYNDROME.

National Alopecia Areata Foundation A support group for individuals concerned with ALOPECIA AREATA, a disease causing partial or total scalp hair loss, or total loss of body hair (alopecia universalis). Objectives of the foundation are to develop public awareness of the disease, provide a support network, raise funds for research and keep patients medically informed. The foundation maintains a medical advisory board, operates information booths at meetings of the AMERICAN ACADEMY OF DERMATOLOGY and offers research grants into alopecia areata.

Founded in 1981, the group has 5,000 members and publishes a bimonthly newsletter covering treatment, research and development (including wig and cosmetic tips). The foundation also sponsors an annual conference. For address, see Appendix D; see also the INTERNATIONAL ASSOCIATION OF TRICHOLOGISTS.

National Arthritis and Musculoskeletal and Skin Diseases Information Clearinghouse A clearinghouse that collects, publishes and disseminates professional and public educational materials for people concerned with skin diseases and maintains a Combined Health Information Database.

Its publications include the biannual *National Arthritis and Musculoskeletal and Skin Diseases Information Clearinghouse Memo* that provides information on clearinghouse resources and services and lists new materials. The clearinghouse also issues bibliographies and catalog of publications. For address, see Appendix D.

National Burn Victim Foundation A professional group for anyone interested in burns, fire prevention and burn care that maintains a 24-hour emergency burn referral service and crisis intervention team of professionals to provide counseling to burn victims and their families, addressing psychological problems and physical handicaps remaining after treatment. The group provides free blood services to burn victims, sponsors Burns Recovered, a self-help group, and conducts medical emergency burn care seminars and workshops for physicians, nurses, emergency medical technicians, and emergency rescue personnel.

The group also operates the Medical Disaster Response System, which utilizes private helicopters for transporting medical teams to disaster sites where large numbers of survivors have been burned.

The foundation collects burn data from New Jersey hospitals daily, and currently provides direct professional services in New Jersey and information and referral services nationally. It offers consultation and evaluation services regarding suspected child abuse or neglect to the Division of Youth and Family Services and to law enforcement agencies, and presents burn awareness and prevention programs to schools, civic organizations and day care centers. It also maintains speakers' bureaus, compiles statistics and conducts specialized education, children's services and research programs.

The foundation offers videos on disaster medical response, general burn awareness, training professionals in child abuse/neglect investigation and publishes the quarterly newsletter *Update* and other pamphlets. For address, see Appendix D; see also AMERICAN BURN ASSOCIATION, BURNS UNITED SUPPORT GROUPS, INTERNATIONAL SOCIETY FOR BURN INJURIES, PHOENIX SOCIETY FOR BURN SURVIVORS, NATIONAL INSTITUTE FOR BURN MEDICINE.

National Commission for Electrologist Certification A professional group that conducts a certification program for individuals practicing ELECTROLYSIS, a method of permanent hair removal. The commission establishes and promotes safety and proficiency in the practice of permanent hair removal, conducts research in occupational credentialing and develops and administers credentialing exams. Founded in 1983 with 1,200 members, the group seeks to enhance public confidence in electrolysis and compiles statistics. See also AMERICAN ELECTROLOGY ASSOCIATION; COUNCIL ON ELECTROLYSIS EDUCATION; INTERNATIONAL GUILD OF PROFESSIONAL ELECTROLOGISTS; SOCIETY OF CLINICAL AND MEDICAL ELECTROLOGISTS.

National Foundation for Ectodermal Dysplasias A support group for families of ECTODERMAL DYSPLASIA patients and the medical community that provides information. The group helps physicians acquire information, locates treatment facilities and makes referrals. The group also provides funds to qualified applicants for necessary care, conducts educational meetings, assists with research projects, establishes regional centers for diagnosis and treatment. The group also provides children's services, compiles statistics and publishes a number of brochures and newsletters. For address, see Appendix D.

National Foundation for Facial Reconstruction A foundation that sponsors surgical and rehabilitation service programs for patients suffering facial disfigurements from severe burns, accidents, birth defects and diseases such as cancer. The group maintains a patient referral service; its former name was the Society for the Rehabilitation of the Facially Disfigured.

Founded in 1951, the group publishes an annual newsletter and offers brochures. For address, see Appendix D; see also AMERICAN ACADEMY OF COSMETIC SURGERY, AMERICAN ACADEMY OF FACIAL PLASTIC AND RECONSTRUCTIVE SURGERY, AMERICAN ASSOCIATION OF PLASTIC SURGEONS, AMERICAN BOARD OF PLASTIC SURGERY, AMERICAN SOCIETY FOR AESTHETIC PLASTIC SURGERY, AMERICAN SOCIETY OF PLASTIC AND RECONSTRUCTIVE SURGEONS, INTERPLAST, PLASTIC SURGERY RESEARCH COUNCIL.

National Institute of Arthritis and Musculoskeletal and Skin Diseases One of the U.S. National Institutes of Health, this federal research group sponsors research on skin diseases and a variety of other related musculoskeletal diseases. The institute provides information and publishes a range of materials. For address, see Appendix D.

National Institute for Burn Medicine A professional group for those dedicated to preventing burn injuries and improving the survival rate of and developing the quality of life for burn victims. The institute provides consultation for the development of specialized burn care facilities, prevention programs and materials, education, information and statistics in burn treatment and care. The institute also maintains an international burn library of more than 35,000 citations. Founded in 1968 as the American Burn Research Corporation and later known as the Institute for Burn Medicine, the national institute publishes books, brochures, posters and films. See also AMERICAN BURN ASSOCIA-TION, BURNS UNITED SUPPORT GROUPS, INTER-NATIONAL SOCIETY FOR BURN INJURIES, PHOENIX SOCIETY FOR BURN SURVIVORS, NA-TIONAL BURN VICTIM FOUNDATION.

National Neurofibromatosis Foundation A support group for people with NEU-ROFIBROMATOSIS, their families, health care workers, teachers and other concerned individuals. Also known as von Reckling-hausen's disease, neurofibromatosis is char-acterized by changes in the skin and marked by spots and tumors on the skin, in addition to other symptoms. The foundation provides patients and their families with information about the disorder and how to find medical, social and genetic counseling; provides infor-mation to physicians and health workers; promotes scientific research; and holds work-shops and compiles statistics. Publications include the quarterly *National Neurofibro-matosis Foundation Newsletter* and *Neurofibro-matosis Research Newsletter*. Founded in 1978, the group has 5,500 members and sponsors an annual meeting. For address, see Appen-dix D.

National Pediculosis Association A non-profit organization established to build awareness about head LICE and to standard-ize head lice control policies nationwide. The NPA seeks to dispel myths about pediculosis while encouraging research and development for safer and more effective management procedures.

The NPA's program of education, preven-tion and early detection work is an effort to raise pediculosis as a public health priority for the protection of American children and their families.

Members represent a broad spectrum of individuals, organizations, health care sys-tems and medical professionals. The associa-tion offers broad corporation membership to businesses interested in demonstrating a joint

effort to improve public health policy and serve the best interests of children and their families.

The organization offers a number of infor-mational brochures, including *Child Care Pro-vider's Guide to Controlling Head Lice; Pharmacist's Guide to Controlling Head Lice, Keep Your Wits Not Your Nits,* and the NPA's *Progress*. It also offers a catalog, *Not Just An-other Lousy Catalog* with products including a wide variety of teeshirts, "check a head" sticks, laminated cards showing what nits look like, coloring books, screening packets, and a variety of handouts and mailers.

For address, see Appendix D.

National Psoriasis Foundation A profes-sional organization for people suffering from PSORIASIS, their families and friends, physi-cians and nurses, and representatives of drug companies. The foundation supports research at various university research centers; makes physician referrals; offers a pen pal program for teens and adults; and sponsors group ses-sions and other activities. The group testifies annually to Congress for funds for research; provides information to schools, libraries and the media; and supplies members with sam-ples of new nonprescription products.

Founded in 1968, the foundation today has 20,000 members and sponsors regional edu-cation symposia. It maintains a library of ma-jor medical journals and personal histories of psoriasis patients.

Publications include an annual report, a bimonthly *National Psoriasis Foundation—Bul-letin,* a newsletter covering psoriasis treat-ment and research with a doctor's question and answer column; a periodic *National Psori-asis Foundation—Pharmacy News;* plus pam-phlets, brochures and flyers.
For address, see Appendix D.

National Rosacea Society An educational organization that provides information on ROSACEA to physicians, patients and the public. For more information, contact the society at 220 South Cork St. Suite 201, Barrington, IL 60010.

National Sjogren's Syndrome Association The association promotes public awareness of Sjogren's Syndrome, an autoimmune disorder characterized by dryness of mucous membranes. The group also encourages research into the cause and cure of the disorder, sponsors support groups, offers information to the medical community, conducts educational and research programs, and maintains a speakers' bureau. The association is also associated with the National Organization for Rare Disorders.

Its publications include the quarterly *Patient Education Series*, the quarterly *Sjogren's Digest* and the guide *Learning to Live with Sjogren's Syndrome*. For address, see Appendix D.

National Tuberous Sclerosis Association A support group for families affected by TUBEROUS SCLEROSIS through a nationwide network of volunteer state representatives and informational packets. The association conducts educational programs for health professionals and provides grants for research into the diagnosis, cause, management and cure TUBEROUS SCLEROSIS. Founded in 1975, the group has 750 members and sponsors an annual meeting in June. For address, see Appendix D.

National Vitiligo Foundation A professional group for physicians and patients, contributors, and supporters that provides information and counseling to VITILIGO patients and their families. (Vitiligo is a disease that destroys pigment cells, causing smooth, white patches of skin).

Founded in 1985, the group has 9,500 members and seeks to increase awareness and concern for vitiligo patients. It raises funds for scientific and clinical research on the cause, treatment and care of vitiligo.

Publications include the semiannual *Newsletter* and brochures. For address, see Appendix D.

necrobiosis Gradual process by which cells lose their function and die. In necrobiosis lipoidica, there is patchy degeneration of the skin, resulting in white scars. It is most often seen in diabetics (about one in 300), although others can contract this disease.

The lesions usually appear as red papules or plaques, followed by a yellowish depressed plaque. Treatment with steroids injected into the lesions may be effective during early stages.

necrolysis, toxic epidermal A severe blistering skin rash in which the surface layer of the skin peels off, exposing large areas of raw skin over the entire body. The condition is similar to a third degree burn; both conditions carry serious risk of infection and fluid loss because of widespread skin damage. See also SCALDED SKIN SYNDROME, STAPHYLOCOCCAL.
Cause Adverse drug reaction (especially to barbiturates, sulfonamides, penicillins, nonsteroidal anti-inflammatory drugs and antiseizure medications).
Treatment The mortality rate of the disease approaches 30 percent. The offending agent must be identified and stopped immediately. Aggressive skin care is required, preferably in a burn center, where physicians can control fluids and temperature, and prevent infection.

necrotizing fasciitis A potentially fatal illness caused by the *Streptococcus* bacteria, the cause of strep throat, that is characterized by an infection with warm, red, tender subcutaneous plaque that becomes necrotic and spreads. In the spring of 1994, the so-called "flesh eating bacteria" illness attracted worldwide attention when numerous cases of the disease occurred in one community north of London. Although virulent forms of strep occur occasionally, it is very rare to see so many cases break out in one area. At least 12 people in Britain reported possible cases of the disease in a four-month period; normally about 10 cases are diagnosed in Britain in one year.

In these cases, more virulent strains of the strep bacteria destroy the body's protein, affecting the lungs, skin and bloodstream. The bacteria releases a toxin that can dissolve fat and muscle tissue, causing the skin above to die and leading to deadly gangrene. Between 2,000 and 3,000 people die from strep infections each year out of 10,000 to 15,000 cases of *serious* strep infections in the United States, according to the Centers for Disease Control. Of these 15,000 cases, between 500 to 1,500 involve necrotizing fasciitis; of these, between 150 to 450 people die.
Treatment The disease requires aggressive treatment with debridement and broad-spectrum parenteral antibiotics, including anaerobic coverage. See also BACTERIAL SKIN INFECTIONS.

neomycin (trade names: Mycifradin [oral]; Myciguent [topical]) An antibiotic rarely used to treat skin infections (often together with other drugs); possible adverse effects include nausea and vomiting, rash, itching, diarrhea, hearing loss, dizziness and tinnitus (ringing in the ears).

neonatal acne See ACNE, INFANT.

Netherton's syndrome A hereditary condition characterized by three primary defects: abnormality in the hair shaft (especially trichorrhexis invaginata, or "bamboo hair"), ICHTHYOSIS linearis circumflexa (a scaling skin disorder) and atopic dermatitis (see DERMATITIS, ATOPIC).

This disorder of unknown cause is inherited in an autosomal recessive pattern, which means that a defective gene must be inherited from both parents to cause the abnormality. Generally, both parents of an affected person are unaffected carriers of the defective gene. Each of the affected children has a one in four chance of being affected, and a two in four chance of being a carrier.

neurilemmoma (neurofibroma) A slow-growing, benign tumor of the nerve sheath derived from Schwann cells lying along a cranial, peripheral or sympathetic nerve. Usually about half of the lesions are found on the head and neck.
Treatment Surgical separation of the tumor from its nerve.

neurocutaneous disorders A group of conditions featuring abnormalities of the skin, nerves or the nervous system. The most familiar of these diseases are NEUROFIBROMATOSIS, a disorder causing brown patches and nodules on the skin, and TUBEROUS SCLEROSIS, characterized by small skin-colored swellings over the cheeks and nose, mental retardation and epilepsy.

neurodermatitis See LICHEN SIMPLEX.

neurofibroma A skin tumor that may occur alone or in groups, ranging in color from pale cream to lightly pigmented. See NEUROFIBROMATOSIS.
Treatment Single neurofibromas may be surgically removed.

neurofibromatosis Also known as von Recklinghausen's disease, this disorder is characterized by many soft, fibrous swellings (called NEUROFIBROMAS) growing from nerves in the skin and elsewhere in the body. There may also be CAFÉ AU LAIT MACULES (coffee-colored spots) on the skin. The disease occurs in one in every 3,000 infants, affecting males and females equally. Although it may be hereditary, half have no family history of the disorder and contract the disease as a spontaneous mutation.

Symptoms and complications Usually, this disease affects only the skin, causing discolored spots and large nodules and swellings. The number of colored spots increases as the patient gets older, and cosmetic disfigurement can range from mild to severe. Eventually, some of the neurofibromas may become malignant and can spread. Neurofibromas in the central nervous system can also cause epilepsy and other problems, including visual or auditory disturbances. Bone deformities may also occur, as well as spinal deformities.

Treatment Surgical removal of the neurofibromas is attempted if they are causing complications or for cosmetic purposes.

neurotic excoriations A psychogenic skin disease characterized by repeated picking of the skin. This condition should be suspected if the lesions, which are present in all stages of development, are distributed solely in accessible areas. Ulcers often appear in parallel or arranged in lines. There are no primary lesions.

Generally, patients pick at their skin because they feel restless; the root of the tension is sometimes related to a specific cause, such as family problems. Picking their skin is another outlet for these patients' emotional tension.

Symptoms Lesions are gouged in the skin, leaving white, round papery scars when they heal against a hyperpigmented background. Lesions are noticeable in all stages of healing, and the small ulcers are usually angular, the tip-off that they are self-induced and not primary. They are most often found on the tops of the forearms and over the shoulders.

Treatment Usually patients with these necrotic urges to pick at their skin do it compulsively and find it very difficult to stop. Therefore, treatment should center on efforts to identify the source of stress in the patient's life, although psychiatric help is not usually very effective. Attempts to physically prevent the patient from picking may result either in panic or depression. See also ACNE EXCORIEE.

nevus (plural: nevi) A birthmark or skin malformation characterized by too much (or not enough) normal epidermal, connective, adnexal, nervous or vascular tissue. There are many different types of nevi, with different appearances: colored or uncolored, with or without hair, lying flat, slightly raised or on a stalk above the skin. Some nevi may be congenital, but they may develop at any time.

A MOLE is still another common type of colored nevus, not usually present at birth. Some nevi have a bluish color, and are known as "blue nevi" often found on the backs of hands in young girls. Most black and Asian infants are born with one or more blue-black spots on their lower backs, called MONGOLIAN SPOTS.

The above examples are all forms of *melanocytic* (or pigmented) *nevi,* caused by an overactivity or abnormality of skin cells that produce MELANIN.

The other primary type of nevi are the *vascular nevi* (or HEMANGIOMA), caused by an abnormal collection of blood vessels. They include PORT-WINE STAIN, which does not fade but can be treated with lasers, and strawberry mark, which usually does disappear in early life.

Treatment Most nevi are completely harmless and do not require treatment. Some types of vascular nevi do require treatment for psychological reasons. Any nevus that suddenly appears, grows, bleeds, or changes color should be brought to the attention of a dermatologist to rule out the possibility of cancer.

See also NEVUS ARANEUS; NEVUS, BLUE; NEVUS, COMPOUND; NEVUS, CONGENITAL; NEVUS DEPIGMENTOSUS; NEVUS ELASTICUS OF LEWAN-

DOWSKY; NEVUS, HALO; NEVUS SPILUS; NEVUS, SPITZ; NEVUS SYNDROME, DYSPLASTIC.

nevus araneus The medical name for spider angiomas, which look like bright red vessels with branches radiating out from the center, much like a spider. This condition is common in pregnancy; it is suspected that estrogen plays a role in the development of these nevi, which are caused by the expansion of superficial arterioles in the skin. They are found most often over the face, the front of the neck and chest and the upper arms. They are also often seen in patients with chronic liver disease.

Treatment Those nevi associated with pregnancy normally fade after delivery, so generally they do not require treatment. If not, the lesions may be removed by laser surgery with the pulsed dye laser or a variety of continuous wave lasers, or they may be electrocoagulated with a fine needle.

See also NEVUS, BLUE; NEVUS, COMPOUND; NEVUS, CONGENITAL; NEVUS PIGMENTOSUS; NEVUS ELASTICUS OF LEWANDOWSKY; NEVUS, HALO; NEVUS, SPITZ; NEVUS SPILUS; NEVUS SYNDROME, DYSPLASTIC.

nevus, blue A type of melanocytic (or pigmented) NEVUS caused by an abnormality or overactivity of skin cells producing the pigment MELANIN, which is deep blue in color. The brown melanin pigment is placed in a specific pattern, deep enough in the skin for it to take on a blue color. See also NEVUS ARANEUS; NEVUS, COMPOUND; NEVUS, CONGENITAL; NEVUS ELASTICUS OF LEWANDOWSKY; NEVUS, HALO; NEVUS PIGMENTOSUS; NEVUS, SPITZ; NEVUS SPILUS; NEVUS SYNDROME, DYSPLASTIC.

nevus, compound One of three main types of benign NEVI, these are located within the dermal-epidermal junction and in the underlying dermis. Compound nevi are often raised and may have a flat area surrounding the elevated area.

See also NEVUS ARANEUS; NEVUS, BLUE; NEVUS, CONGENITAL; NEVUS ELASTICUS OF LEWANDOWSKY; NEVUS PIGMENTOSUS; NEVUS, HALO; NEVUS SPILUS; NEVUS, SPITZ; NEVUS SYNDROME, DYSPLASTIC.

nevus, congenital Unlike the common acquired nevi (skin malformation) (see NEVI, COMMON) that appear after birth, this type of nevus appears at birth or shortly thereafter, and remains throughout life. Most are small and look very much like acquired nevi. Rarely, congenital nevi may be large (giant congenital nevi), involving major areas of the body. These nevi are usually found on the trunk, upper back and shoulders. Most have a rough surface and hair.

There is debate over whether small congenital nevi can become cancerous (melanoma). If there is a risk, it is quite low. The lifetime risk of melanoma arising from giant congenital nevi is higher—approximately 6 percent. See also BIRTHMARK; MOLE; NEVI, COMMON; NEVUS, BLUE; NEVUS, HALO; NEVUS, SPITZ; NEVUS SYNDROME, DYSPLASTIC.

nevus depigmentosus A fairly uncommon disorder of pigmentation that may be either congenital or acquired, characterized by white macules and patches on the trunk or extremities. As the child grows, the macule enlarges. It represents a patchy irregular area without melanocytes.

Treatment There is no way to repigment the skin, though cosmetic concealment may be helpful in masking the problem.

See also BIRTHMARK; MOLE; NEVUS ARANEUS; NEVI, COMMON; NEVUS, BLUE; NEVUS, COMPOUND; NEVUS ELASTICUS OF LEWANDOWSKY; NEVUS, EPIDERMAL; NEVUS, HALO; NEVUS PIGMENTOSUS; NEVUS, SEBACEOUS; NEVUS, SPITZ; NEVUS SYNDROME, DYSPLASTIC; PORT-WINE STAIN.

nevus elasticus of Lewandowsky A type of connective tissue nevi that is characterized by an excess growth and distortion of the elastic fibers of the DERMIS (middle skin layer). The condition includes a group of smooth skin-colored papules that form patches or plaques, usually on the trunk.

Treatment No treatment is necessary for most of these connective tissue nevi, since they aren't unsightly. On rare occasions, surgical excision may be performed.

See also BIRTHMARK; MOLE; NEVUS ARANEUS; NEVUS, BLUE; NEVUS, COMMON; NEVUS, COMPOUND; NEVUS, EPIDERMAL; NEVUS DEPIGMENTOSUS; NEVUS, HALO; NEVUS PIGMENTOSUS; NEVUS SEBACEOUS; NEVUS, SPITZ; NEVUS SYNDROME, DYPLASTIC; PORT-WINE STAIN.

nevus, epidermal An uncommon congenital developmental abnormality causing errors in the production of mature epidermal structures. The tan-to-dark brown lesion may either appear small and singly or as large groups which are usually either linear or sworled. While they usually are present at birth, they may appear during the first few years of life up to puberty, and rarely later in life.

Treatment No treatment is normally required, unless they are cosmetically distressing. In that case, small lesions may be excised, but removal of larger epidermal nevi may be difficult or cosmetically unappealing, as the scar may look worse than the nevi. Superficial removal by laser or by chemical destruction are possible treatment options. See also BIRTHMARK; MOLE; NEVUS DEPIGMENTOSUS; NEVUS PIGMENTOSUS, NEVUS, SEBACEOUS.

nevus, epithelioid See NEVUS, SPITZ.

nevus flammeus See PORT-WINE STAIN.

nevus, halo A nevus in which the skin surrounding the lesion whitens in color, giving a characteristic "halo" appearance.

See also BIRTHMARK; NEVUS; NEVI, COMMON; NEVUS, COMPOUND; NEVUS, EPIDERMAL; NEVUS DEPIGMENTOSUS; NEVUS, HALO; NEVUS PIGMENTOSUS; NEVUS, SEBACEOUS; NEVUS, SPITZ; NEVUS SYNDROME, DYSPLASTIC; NEVUS ARANEUS; NEVUS, BLUE; PORT-WINE STAIN.

nevus of Ito and nevus of Ota Disorders of pigmentation characterized by benign blue-gray-brown pigmented patches of skin located on the face (nevus of Ota) and on the shoulder (nevus of Ito). About 50 percent of these lesions are congenital or appear soon after birth; most of the rest appear at puberty, although a few may not surface until the third decade of life. The two lesions are similar to the Mongolian spot with the melanin pigment found deep in the dermis, accounting for the typical blue-gray color.

Nevus of Ota is usually found over the cheek and temple, and is more commonly found in dark-skinned people and Asians; it affects 0.5 percent of all Japanese. Neither type fades with age; while both are benign, they have rarely been associated with melanoma (usually in Caucasians).

Treatment Highly effective treatment includes the use of short pulsed lasers. Most experience in the United States has been with the Q-switched ruby laser. This provides excellent results without textural change in most lesions.

See also BIRTHMARK; MOLE; NEVUS ARANEUS; NEVUS, BLUE; NEVI, COMMON; NEVUS, COMPOUND; NEVUS DEPIGMENTOSUS; NEVUS ELASTICUS OF LEWANDOWSKY; NEVUS, EPIDERMAL; NEVUS, HALO; NEVUS, PIGMENTOSUS; NEVUS, SEBACEOUS; NEVUS SPILUS; NEVUS, SPITZ; NEVUS SYNDROME, DYSPLASTIC; PORT-WINE STAIN.

nevus pigmentosus A benign tumor composed of MELANOCYTES. See also BIRTHMARK; MOLE; NEVUS ARANEUS; NEVUS, BLUE; NEVUS, COMPOUND; NEVUS DEPIGMENTOSUS; NEVUS, EPIDERMAL; NEVUS, HALO; NEVUS PIGMENTOSUS; NEVUS, SEBACEOUS; NEVUS, SPITZ; NEVUS SYNDROME, DYSPLASTIC; PORT-WINE STAIN.

nevus, sebaceous A nevus present at birth or shortly thereafter that usually appears as a hairless, yellowish orange plaque on the scalp that sometimes may be mistaken for a melanocytic nevus. These lesions should be removed during childhood because they have a tendency to become cancerous, usually at puberty (basal cell carcinoma or other benign or malignant adnexal tumor). See also MOLE; NEVUS DEPIGMENTOSUS; NEVUS, EPIDERMAL; NEVUS PIGMENTOSUS.

nevus spilus A light-brown patch (CAFE AU LAIT MACULE) sprinkled with dark brown macules that is present at birth or early infancy. While the overall size of the spot may vary, it is usually several centimeters in diameter and may be found on the trunk or extremities. No treatment is necessary, although short pulsed lasers such as the Q-switched ruby and O-switched Y:AG lasers can lighten the lesions. See also BIRTHMARK; MOLE; NEVUS; NEVUS ARANEUS; NEVUS, BLUE; NEVUS, EPIDERMAL; NEVUS DEPIGMENTOSUS; NEVUS, HALO; NEVUS PIGMENTOSUS; NEVUS, SEBACEOUS; NEVUS, SPITZ; NEVUS SYNDROME, DYSPLASTIC; PORT-WINE STAIN.

nevus, spindle and epithelioid cell Another name for a spitz nevus (See NEVUS, SPITZ).

nevus, spitz A solitary pink, purple or red papule or nodule that usually appears in childhood. While it resembles malignant melanoma (See MELANOMA, MALIGNANT) under the microscope, this lesion is benign. It usually appears on the face in young patients, but among adults is more common on the legs and trunk.
Treatment Simple excision.
See also BIRTHMARK; MOLE; NEVUS; NEVUS ARANEUS; NEVUS, BLUE; NEVUS, COMPOUND; NEVUS, HALO; NEVUS, EPIDERMAL; NEVUS DEPIGMENTOSUS; NEVUS PIGMENTOSUS; NEVUS, SEBACEOUS; NEVUS, SPITZ; NEVUS SYNDROME, DYSPLASTIC; PORT-WINE STAIN.

nevus syndrome, dysplastic An often-hereditary condition characterized by groups of melanocytic nevi, which in some patients may indicate a predisposition to malignant melanoma (see MELANOMA, MALIGNANT). Such cancerous melanomas may grow from the nevi themselves, or elsewhere on the body.

The trait usually has an autosomal dominant mode of transmission, which means that only one defective gene (from one parent) is needed to cause the syndrome. Each child of an affected person usually has a one in two chance of inheriting the defective gene and of being affected. A patient with dysplastic nevi with two or more primary family members with malignant melanoma has a very strong chance—almost 100 percent—of developing the cancer as well.

If a patient's parent has dysplastic nevi *without* melanoma, the chance of the patient developing melanoma is less definite; however, the patient still is at higher risk than the general population.

Patients with dysplastic nevi but no family history of melanoma have "sporadic" dysplastic nevus syndrome. If these patients have high numbers of nevi, they are still at a higher risk for developing malignant melanoma than the general population, but less than for those in the familial dysplastic nevus group.

Dysplastic nevi are different from ordinary nevi in that they are bigger and usually more prevalent (often more than 100). And while ordinary nevi don't usually appear in adulthood, dysplastic nevi continue to develop throughout life. When researchers followed the evolution of dysplastic nevi in 153 patients aged 12 to 73 for seven years, they found new nevi common—even among adults—continuing to appear in 20 percent of adults over age 50. The moles also changed appearance, or disappeared in people of all ages.
Prevention Patients with multiple dysplastic nevi and a family history of malignant mela-

noma should avoid the sun and use sunscreen, practice skin self-examination and see a dermatologist every six months. To spot signs of dysplastic nevi that may be turning malignant, check for the "ABCs": the blemish is *asymmetrical,* the *border* is notched or blurred (not smooth and distinct) and the *color* includes mixtures of shades.

Treatment Suspect nevi should be seen by a doctor and removed.

See also BIRTHMARK; MOLE; NEVUS; NEVUS ARANEUS; NEVUS, BLUE; NEVUS, COMPOUND; NEVUS, HALO; NEVUS, EPIDERMAL; NEVUS DEPIGMENTOSUS; NEVUS PIGMENTOSUS; NEVUS, SEBACEOUS; NEVUS, SPITZ; NEVUS SYNDROME, DYSPLASTIC, PORT-WINE STAIN.

niacin deficiency See PELLAGRA.

nickel dermatitis See DERMATITIS, NICKEL.

nifedipine A drug commonly used to treat angina that is also used in the treatment of circulation disorders such as RAYNAUD'S DISEASE.

Side effects Possible effects include fluid retention and swelling, flushing, headache and dizziness.

Nikolsky's sign A diagnostic technique in which the skin sloughs off with slight lateral pressure. Nikolsky's sign is seen in superficial blistering disorders such as in SCALDED SKIN SYNDROME, toxic epidermal necrolysis and in PEMPHIGUS, but it is not usually seen in deeper blistering diseases such as bullous pemphigoid.

nitrobenzenes Hair dyes used in semipermanent shampoo-in hair color. The color is formulated to last up to a month, but this depends on how often hair is washed.

nits The tiny eggs of a louse that are yellow when newly laid, turning to white once they hatch. Nits are small, oval-shaped eggs that are "glued" at an angle to the side of the hair shaft. Nits hatch within eight days, and the empty eggshells are carried outward as the hair grows. Both head and pubic lice lay eggs at the base of hairs growing on the head or pubic area. Nits can be seen anywhere on the hair, especially behind the ears and at the back of the neck.

Nits should not be confused with hair debris, such as fat plugs or hair casts. Fat plugs are bright white irregularly shaped clumps of fat cells stuck to the hair shaft. Hair casts are thin, long, cylinder-shaped segments of dandruff encircling the hair shaft; they are easily dislodged.

Lice infestations are diagnosed by the presence of nits; by calculating the distance from the base of the hair to the furthest nits, it's possible to estimate the duration of the infestation.

All nits must be removed, according to the National Pediculosis Association. Since no lice pesticide kills all nits, thorough nit removal will reduce or eliminate the need for more treatments.

Nits can be removed with a special nit removal comb, with baby safety scissors or with the fingernails.

Noah Worcester Dermatological Society A professional association for dermatologists and allied medical scientists that sponsors programs to exchange scientific information on diseases of the skin. The society is named for the author of the first American textbook of dermatology, published in 1845. The society maintains the Noah Worcester Library at the University of Cincinnati, supports research and offers yearly support to the DERMATOLOGY FOUNDATION.

Founded in 1958, the group has 170 members and holds an annual convention. It also publishes an annual membership roster.

nocardiosis An infection by a fungus-like bacterium (*Nocardia asteroides*) found throughout the world that starts in the lungs and spreads to tissues under the skin where fistulas develop. This infection is not normally found in healthy patients, and usually occurs in those with a compromised immune system. The prognosis is good with early diagnosis, before the infection spreads to the brain.

Symptoms Fever and cough similar to pneumonia that does not respond to normal short-term antibiotics, with lung damage and brain abscesses.

Treatment Sulfonamide drugs (sulfadiazine) or a combination of trimethoprim-sulfamethoxazole (TMP-SMX). Drainage or resection of abcesses may be necessary.

nodule A solid mass of tissue larger than 1 cm. in diameter that may protrude from the skin or occur deep underneath the surface.

non-Hodgkin's cutaneous lymphomas Non-Hodgkin's lymphomas are tumors of the lymphatic system. The skin findings in non-Hodgkins lymphoma are uncommon. They may appear in patients with systemic disease or may be the first sign of lymphoma. The skin lesions in this condition are red, blue or plum-colored and can be found on any part of the body. The lesions are firm and smooth.

Because most patients have (or will develop) widespread lymphoma throughout their body, their prognosis may not be promising.

Treatment The lesions generally respond to ionizing radiation or to systemic chemotherapy.

non-invasive cutaneous infections See TINEA.

Norwegian scabies A type of exfoliative erythroderma (mild to severe redness and scaling of the skin) characterized by thick crusted lesions on hands, nails and feet associated with a widespread infestation of scabies and mites. Mites are easily seen among the scales. Unlike ordinary SCABIES, there is little or no itching. It may be seen in retarded patients, patients with AIDS and other individuals suffering from debilitating medical conditions.

Treatment The same as for scabies.

nose repair An operation (also called rhinoplasty) that alters the nose structure to either correct a deformity caused by injury or disease, or to repair its appearance. In the technique, incisions are made within the nose to avoid visible scars, using a local or general anesthetic. Sometimes, a bone or cartilage graft is used, and the nose is splinted in position for about 10 days.

These operations usually cause considerable bruising and swelling. Final results may not be noticeable until weeks or months later. Rarely, complications may include recurrent nosebleeds because of persistent crusting at the site of the incision, or breathing problems because of narrowed nasal passages.

NSAIDS See NONSTEROIDAL ANTI-INFLAMMATORY DRUGS.

nucleic acids The building blocks of protein, these specific chemicals act on the nucleus of cells. They cannot stimulate growth when applied to the skin's surface or to the hair. However, like all proteins, nucleic acids in cosmetics can form a film on the skin or hair shaft to help retain moisture.

nummular dermatitis See DERMATITIS, NUMMULAR.

nutrition and the skin See DIET AND THE SKIN.

Nystatin See MYCOSTATIN.

O

oatmeal A colloid-containing grain that soothes the skin and can be very helpful for itchy skin conditions. Preparations containing oatmeal can soothe skin irritated by sunburn or allergic reaction. Oatmeal is also included in face masks and soaps because it absorbs oil from the skin's surface and lessens redness of irritating ACNE-prone skin. Non-irritating oatmeal soaps are a good choice for people with sensitive skin.

occupational skin disorders Because the skin has such a large surface area accessible to the environment, it is particularly vulnerable to problems related to occupational trauma and disease. In fact, after traumatic injuries, skin problems represent almost half of all remaining occupational illnesses. And, as new industrial chemicals and production processes are developed, new skin diseases and problems continue to appear.

Occupational skin diseases include systemic diseases (caused by absorption through the skin), contact dermatitis (see DERMATITIS, CONTACT), PHOTOSENSITIVITY DISORDERS, disorders of pigmentation, skin cancer, connective tissue diseases, hair and nail disorders, occupational infections and infestations, and disorders caused by physical and mechanical agents.

Skin absorption is one way that many toxic substances (such as agricultural pesticides) enter the body. Some of the major industrial chemicals that cause toxic systemic diseases by being absorbed in the skin include aniline dyes, arsenic, benzene, cyanide salts, mercury, methyl-*n*-butyl ketone, polyhalogenated aromatic hydrocarbons, organic solvents and neuromuscular insecticides.

About 90 percent of all skin diseases acquired via occupations are *contact dermatitis.*

Most cases are due to skin irritation, not allergy, through skin contact with an irritating substance. Some common industrial irritants include solvents, acids and alkalies, industrial detergents, cleaning compounds, abrasive soaps, waterless hand cleaners, poison ivy or oak, metallic salts, rubber antioxidants, epoxy resins and hardeners, acrylic resins, biocidal agents, and organic dyes.

Other substances encountered in the workplace may include fragrances, cosmetic preservatives and topical medications included in soaps, hand creams or first-aid products.

Certain industrial chemicals, when present on the skin and exposed to sunlight, can cause an acute sunburn or eczema on sun-exposed surfaces. The resulting *photosensitivity* may cause redness and swelling, with vesicles or blisters that later weep, crust or scale. Chemicals such as creosote and tar may cause burning and stinging after sun exposure. Severe blistering may occur in celery harvesters caused by toxins released by celery fungus, and certain new acrylic resins may produce both phototoxic and photoallergic reactions.

Acne may be induced or aggravated by experiences in the workplace as well. Tight-fitting masks may cause ACNE MECHANICA; lubricating oils or grease may irritate the follicles and cause oil acne (see ACNE, OIL). Finally, CHLORACNE is caused by exposure to specific aromatic hydrocarbons such as in the workplace.

The synthesis of melanin may be slowed down or speeded up by a variety of occupational substances, leading to *disorders of pigmentation.* Such changes in skin color may follow any contact dermatitis, and certain photosensitizers (especially tar, pitch and furocoumarins) may also alter skin pigmentation. Similarly, the loss of pigment may be caused by exposure to a variety of industrial substances such as phenol. Skin discoloration has been associated with heavy metal contact (especially silver and mercury), and from dyes.

Skin cancer was the first type of *tumor* to be associated with occupational risks back in 1775, when Percivall Potts discovered that soot caused SQUAMOUS CELL CARCINOMA in the scrotums of London's chimney sweeps. People who work outdoors in natural sunlight, or who are exposed to ionizing radiation, are at greatest risk for the development of skin cancer. While coal tar and its derivatives (such as pitch and creosote) may contribute to the development of premalignant skin warts and keratoses that eventually are transformed into squamous cell carcinoma, researchers have not yet proved that any chemical carcinogen causes malignant melanoma.

Connective tissue diseases such as SCLERODERMA may be caused by on-the-job exposure to silica in mining operations, and acrosteolysis has been linked to the manufacture of certain polyvinylchloride plastics.

Hair loss may be caused by a variety of toxic exposures in the workplace or by mechanical accidents. A wide variety of infections may be picked up on the job, often linked to poor hygiene or minor abrasions and lacerations. Finally, heat, electricity, cold, wind, vibration and radiation may cause a wide variety of skin problems.

Prevention Workers should wear protective clothing, use barrier creams (see CONTACT DERMATITIS) and practice good hygiene. Depending on the job description, gloves, boots, sleeves, aprons, coveralls and different types of face protection must be worn to keep out toxic substances.

oil of bergamot A phototoxic type of oil contained in the skin of lemons and limes that, when applied to the skin, can cause burns and blisters after exposure to sunlight.

Although lemons and limes are most notorious for their phototoxic reactions, many other plants and foods also contain the oil in lesser amounts—carrots, celery, figs, parsley, parsnips, coriander, caraway, fennel and anise. Even perfumes that contain the oil can cause burns when oil-soaked skin is exposed to the sun.

Young children who suck on limes or lemons in the hot sun are particularly prone to skin burns and blisters, since juice of the fruit dribbles onto the face or drops onto the chest, which then causes burns from the ultraviolet rays of the sun.

The chemical in oil of bergamot responsible for the phototoxic reaction is PSORALEN, ironically now used for its therapeutic benefits. Many years ago, a Cairo dermatologist found out that indigenous people along the Nile used plants containing psoralen as a folk remedy to treat VITILIGO, a skin disorder in which the immune system attacks and destroys the skin's pigment. While researchers aren't sure why it works, they believe that psoralens, when combined with sunlight, may suppress the immune system and stop the attack on the skin's pigment, or simply that the psoralen augments the sun's ability to produce pigmentation. Psoralens plus sunlight also decreases cells from making DNA, thus decreasing cell turnover, so it is also being used to treat PSORIASIS (a disease featuring excessive cell turnover).

ointment A greasy, semi-solid substance that is placed on the skin either to apply drugs or to provide a protective barrier. Most ointments contain petrolatum or wax with an EMOLLIENT for a moisturizing effect.

onychodystrophy Malformation of a nail.

onychogryphosis A curved overgrowth and thickening of the nail. The cause is unknown.

onycholysis Separation of part or all of a nail from its bed; the lifted nail becomes yellow. It is a common symptom that may be associated with thyroid disorders (including hypo- and hyperthyroidism), an injury to the nail, exposure to chemicals or use of nail cosmetics combined with a fungi, yeast or bacterial infection.

Treatment Regular clipping and application of a topical antifungal such as imidazole derivative is recommended. Patients with *Candida* infection should avoid water. Antibiotics may help if bacteria is present.

onychomalacia Softening of the nails.

onychomycosis A fungal disease of the nails that often occurs on the feet, where it may be associated with ATHLETE'S FOOT. It is much less common on the fingernails. The infection is usually caused by *Trichophyton rubrum* or *T. mentagrophytes.*

Symptoms The infection first causes a discolored nail edge, spreading until the entire plate is discolored, ragged, thickened and rough. Sometimes, however, there is only a slight infection of the upper surface of the nail, which has a chalky color.

Treatment Most topical antifungals aren't effective in treating fungal nail infections. Fingernail fungal infections may be treated with oral doses of GRISEOFULVIN until the nail grows out (usually as long as six months). The effectiveness of treatment depends on how faithfully the patient takes the medication. However, if the fungal infection returns, treatment is far less successful because the DERMATOPHYTE may develop resistance to the griseofulvin.

While infections of the toenail are less serious than the fingernail, they are more difficult to treat and are only about 30 percent effective (in part because it can take up to 18 months for a toenail to grow out). Except for young patients, griseofulvin is usually not prescribed for toenail infection unless the fingernails are also involved. Ketoconazole is a wide-spectrum antibiotic that is 50 percent effective against dermatophytes and *Candida* that may be used for patients who can't take, or haven't responded, to griseofulvin, but risk of toxicity restricts its long-term use.

Side effects A few patients don't tolerate griseofulvin because of nausea and vomiting, and develop headaches or PHOTOSENSITIVITY.

onychotillomania Manipulation (pulling, poking, tearing) of the nails that is a manifestation of DELUSIONS OF PARASITOSIS, in which the patient cuts down the nails in search of parasites. It may also occur as a nervous habit.

open wet dressings A type of topical preparation useful in conditions characterized by vesicles, pustules, exudates and crusts, such as in acute dermatitis (as in poison ivy). These dressings cool and dry the skin by evaporation, and as they are removed they help remove the crusts and exudate from the surface. Appropriate use of open wet dressings can control exudation and inflammation.

The solutions usually consist of room-temperature water or saline. Other agents include silver nitrate, BUROW'S SOLUTION, potassium permanganate, 5 percent acetic acid and sodium hypochlorite.

orf A viral infection caused by a subgroup of poxviruses found around the world in sheep and goats. Human infection is usually caused by direct contact with infected material from animals or animal products. Veterinarians, farmers, shepherds and butchers are especially at risk.

The infection is characterized by large crusting purple pustules with a white center and a red edge appearing on the hands. The infection will heal spontaneously within three to six weeks; primary infection confers lifelong immunity.

Symptoms Following an incubation period of up to a week, a firm red papule appears and enlarges into a large crusted hemorrhagic pustule. The lesions usually appear alone on the fingers, hands, forearms or (occasionally) the face. There is sometimes an accompanying low fever.

Prevention Those working with animals should watch for lesions around the mouths of sheep or goats. There have been no reports of infection spreading from one human to another.

Treatment No treatment (other than prevention of secondary infection) is required.

orthokeratosis Normal keratinization. See KERATINIZATION, DISORDERS OF.

Osler-Weber-Rendu disease An hereditary disease characterized by telangiectases (dilatation of small blood vessels) of the skin and mucous membranes. Also known as hereditary hemorrhagic telangiectasia, the lesions in this condition may be congenital, but more commonly they appear after puberty and progress with age. The lesions are usually found on the lips, mouth and ears, face, fingers, toes and nail beds, and in the gastrointestinal tract. Hemorrhage is common and often serious, especially from the nose and gut.

Treatment Treatment is difficult; surgical grafts may be necessary to replace mucous membranes with dilated vessels with normal skin. Laser destruction of blood vessels and administration of estrogen or amino aproic acid have been helpful.

osteopoikilosis with connective tissue nevus See BUSCHKE-OLLENDORFF SYNDROME.

otitis externa An inflammation of the outer ear caused by infection or the result of an inflammatory skin disorder (such as atopic ECZEMA or seborrheic dermatitis). It is also known as "swimmer's ear" because it can oc-cur after swimming in dirty or heavily chlorinated water. The risk of getting swimmer's ear rises with the frequency of swimming, the longer the person stays in the water and the longer the head is submerged.

Swimmer's ear usually causes redness and swelling in the ear canal, a discharge and sometimes eczema around the ear opening. Itching may become painful and deafness can occur if pus blocks the ear.

Swimmer's ear can also be caused by excessive washing, perspiration, irritation of the ear canal after removing a foreign object, allergies or a generalized skin disease such as ATOPIC ECZEMA.

Cause A generalized infection may be caused by bacteria or fungi, and may affect the ear canal and sometimes also the external ear.

Malignant otitis externa is a rare (and sometimes fatal) form of the disease caused by the bacterium *Pseudomonas aeruginosa*. This type of otitis sometimes spreads into surrounding bones and soft tissue, and usually affects elderly diabetics with a lowered resistance to disease.

Treatment Usually the only required treatment is a thorough cleaning and drying of the ear together with antibiotic, antifungal or anti-inflammatory drugs. Patients should avoid getting the ear wet until the condition is completely healed. A wick should be used to instill drops into the ear in ear canals that are badly swollen.

otoplasty A cosmetic operation to correct oversized or malformed ears. By the age of six, most children's ears have reached adult size and an operation to repair them may be considered. In the operation, an incision is made behind the ear, and excess skin is removed; at this time, the ear itself can be reshaped, recurled etc. The day after surgery, bandages are removed, and smaller, lighter bandages are applied until the sixth day, when stitches are removed. A ski headband can be worn at night for a month after the operation to prevent distortions of the ear as it heals.

oxytetracycline One of the tetracyclines, this is a type of antibiotic used to treat a wide variety of infections, including chlamydia, syphilis, Rocky Mountain spotted fever, cholera, the plague, etc.

Adverse effects Possible side effects include rash, increased skin sensitivity to the sun, nausea and vomiting. Because oxytetracycline may discolor developing teeth and bones, it is not prescribed during pregnancy or for youngsters under the age of 12.

P

PABA The abbreviation for the active ingredient in sunscreen—PARA-AMINOBENZOIC ACID—which is very effective in blocking ultraviolet B (UVB) rays of the sun.

Some people are allergic to PABA and its esters, especially if they are allergic to the "-caine" group of anesthetics (lidocaine, benzocaine etc.) or to certain hair dyes. Allergic reactions to PABA resemble sunburn.

pachydermoperiostosis A rare hereditary disease characterized by thickened furrows on the face (especially on the forehead), with large, active sebaceous glands and oily skin. In addition, there is often a marked folding of the scalp skin (cutis verticis gyrata).

It is an autosomal dominant disease, which means that only one defective gene (from one parent) is needed to cause the syndrome. Each child of an affected person usually has a one in two chance of inheriting the defective gene and of being affected, and a one in two chance of being unaffected.

pachyonychia Thickened nails that may occur as an inherited disease.

padimate O A derivative of PABA that can block the damaging effects of the sun.

pallor Abnormally pale skin (especially of the face) that may be a symptom of a disease or a simple deficiency of the skin pigment MELANIN or a constriction of blood vessels in the skin.

Melanin deficiency can be caused by a lack of exposure to the sun, or it can be the hereditary condition albinism.

Constricted blood vessels in the skin may be caused by severe pain, injury, fainting, extreme cold or excessive blood loss, leading to shock. Constriction of blood flow to the skin is a reaction of the body in an effort to shunt blood to the vital organs and the brain. Pallor may also be a symptom of anemia, caused by the lack of hemoglobin pigment in blood vessels in the skin.

Pallor as a symptom of disease may be caused by kidney disorders such as pyelonephritis or renal failure, or from hypothyroidism. Other diseases that might cause pallor include lead poisoning or scurvy.

palmar-plantar keratosis A descriptive term for the thickening of the horny layer of palms and soles as seen in a wide variety of acquired and hereditary disorders. These include CORNS, CALLUSES, WARTS, hand eczemas, HOWEL-EVANS SYNDROME, MAL DE MELEDA etc.

panniculitis A general term for a group of inflammatory diseases of the subcutaneous layer of fat tissue. It is caused by a wide variety of diseases. These diseases are characterized by pain, tenderness, reddened nodules and sometimes ulcers in the overlying skin.

panthenol A vitamin B complex that can add strength and body to hair by filling in cracks on the shaft, thereby firming up the fiber.

panthothenic acid A B vitamin found in liver, eggs and dried brewer's yeast (and the royal jelly of bees) that some people erroneously believe can prevent gray hair.

papilloma A generic term usually referring to a nonmalignant tumor resembling a wart with a broad base, that arises from the EPITHELIUM (cell layer that forms the skin and mucous membranes)—most commonly on the skin, tongue or larynx and in the urinary tract, digestive tract or breasts.

papillomavirus, human (HPV) This member of the papovavirus family is the cause of WARTS—common warts, PLANTAR WARTS, FLAT WARTS, FILIFORM WARTS, PARONYCHIAL WARTS, GENITAL WARTS (condylomata acuminata) and oral and laryngeal papillomas. Different lesions are caused by different HPV types (of which there are more than 50).

The viral infection is spread directly by person-to-person contact, or indirectly by contact on public shower floors, in swimming pools, etc. The virus may also be spread from one area of the body to another on the same patient.

papovaviruses One of a group of viruses producing nonmalignant tumors in humans (subgroup papilloma viruses).

papular acrodermatitis See GIANOTTI-CROSTI SYNDROME.

papular dermatitis of pregnancy Also known as Spangler's dermatitis of pregnancy, this condition is a rare, severely itchy disease that can occur at any time during pregnancy. Associated with 30 percent of stillbirth or spontaneous abortion cases, it recurs with subsequent pregnancies.

Symptoms The condition is characterized by uniform crusted, excoriated red papules that appear in groups of wheals. As the lesions fade, the skin may become hyperpigmented but these will fade after pregnancy.

Treatment Administration of systemic corticosteroids: Diethylstilbestrol (DES) is no longer used because of its established link with vaginal carcinoma.

papular mucinosis See LICHEN MYXEDEMATOSUS.

papular urticaria A condition caused by a hypersensitive reaction to insect bites (espe-

cially fleas, bedbugs, mosquitoes and dog lice). The condition appears primarily in children aged two to seven; the disease is rare in infancy and uncommon in adulthood. The lesions, which appear as a solid lesion instead of a swelling, are sometimes indistinguishable from an insect bite. They are generally found on exposed areas of the skin, especially the face and arms and legs. In some cases, they represent overreaction to insect bites, while in others papular urticaria lesions appear in sites distant to insect bites as a hypersensitivity or allergic reaction to the bite.

The lesions transform into an inflammatory, firm, red-brown persistent papule. Extremely sensitive people may also experience vesicles and blisters. Bacterial infection and excoriations may appear.

In the eastern United States, the problem appears almost exclusively in the summer when fleas are numerous; on the West Coast the problem is found throughout the year.

papules Small, solid slightly raised areas of the skin less than half an inch in diameter. They may have a varied appearance: either rounded, smooth or rough, skin-colored or red, pink or brown. The characteristic lesion in skin conditions such as ACNE or LICHEN PLANUS is a papule.

papulosquamous diseases These conditions are characterized by scaling papules or plaques, with sharply defined margins. Crusts, excoriation or weeping are rarely seen. PSORIASIS is the most typical of the papulosquamous diseases; others include PARAPSORIASIS, LICHEN PLANUS, SEBORRHEIC DERMATITIS, FUNGAL INFECTIONS and SYPHILIS.

para-aminobenzoic acid See PABA.

parabens, sensitivity to Some people are sensitive to parabens, the most widely used preservatives in foods, drugs and cosmetics. The parabens (esters of *p*-hydroxybenzoic acid) are included in one-third of all cosmetics registered in the United States. However, considering how widespread the use of parabens is, sensitivity to this preservative is low. See also PARA-AMINOBENZOIC ACID; ALLERGIES AND THE SKIN.

parapsoriasis A group of diseases characterized by different-sized superficial scaling plaques that don't usually itch and resist treatment. Resembling PSORIASIS, parapsoriasis is not related at all to that disease.

There are three main types of parapsoriasis: Parapsoriasis guttata (small plaque parapsoriasis), parapsoriasis lichenoides chronica and parapsoriasis en plaques (large-plaque parapsoriasis). PARAPSORIASIS VARIOLIFORMIS ACUTA is a completely different entity, and should not be classified amongst these diseases.

Symptoms Some forms of parapsoriasis are chronic and cause no serious complications, but parapsoriasis en plaques is serious and may progress to MYCOSIS FUNGOIDES. All forms of the disease usually begin with one lesion covered with a fine spreading scale, appearing first on the trunk, arms or legs.

In *parapsoriasis guttata*, the lesions are fine macules and papules resembling guttate psoriasis, dusted with a fine silvery scale. This condition does not respond to antipsoriasis treatment. The lesions appear on the trunk at any age in both men and women, and may persist for years. Itching does not usually occur.

Parapsoriasis lichenoides (or retiform parapsoriasis) is characterized by raised, dull red, lichenoid scaly papules that appears on the neck, trunk, arms and legs. The patient's general health is not affected, and itching is not a problem.

In *parapsoriasis en plaques*, lesions are larger than those of either lichenoides or guttata,

and they are flatter than those lesions in psoriasis. Lesions range from yellow-red to brown with a fine scale, found primarily on the trunk, thighs and buttocks. Unlike the other two types of parapsoriasis, these lesions may itch and in many cases this type of parapsoriasis may progress to MYCOSIS FUNGOIDES.

Treatment Treatment for both parapsoriasis guttata and lichenoides may not be necessary, since the lesions cause no problems, although sunlight (UVB and PUVA) or topical corticosteroids may be helpful in clearing them up. *Parapsoriasis en plaques* may respond to topical steroids, sunlight (ultraviolet B) or PUVA. Patients with parapsoriasis en plaques should be carefully followed by a dermatologist.

parapsoriasis varioliformis acuta A papulosquamous disease (disease that features a papular, scaly rash) unrelated to other forms of PARAPSORIASIS, also known as acute parapsoriasis, pityriasis lichenoides et varioliformis acuta, or Mucha-Habermann syndrome.

Acute onset appears much like CHICKEN POX with groups of papules vesicles, and pustular crusted lesions that progress to a necrotic stage, leaving chicken pox–like scars. They typically form on the insides of the forearms and back of the legs.

This condition primarily occurs in patients in their 20s and 30s and lasts from a few weeks to years. Often, it simply disappears without treatment.

Treatment Large doses of tetracycline, penicillin G or erythromycin are administered for a month; for chronic cases this treatment may not help. While small doses of oral methotrexate will control the disease, when the drug is stopped the lesions return.

parasitic infections A wide range of skin symptoms may occur with parasitic infections, which are endemic in many developing countries throughout the world where poverty, poor hygiene and poor sanitary facilities are prevalent. Infections from parasites are divided into those caused by protozoa (single-celled animals), by helminths (worms) and by arthropods (mites or ticks).

Protozoal infections that cause skin symptoms include LEISHMANIASIS, African and South American trypanosomiasis, amebiasis, trichomoniasis and TOXOPLASMOSIS.

Parasitic worm infestations with skin symptoms are divided into roundworms (class Nematoda) and flatworms (class Trematoda, or flukes, and Cestoidea, or tapeworms).

Arthropod infestations include mites, ticks and insects.

Treatment for parasitic infections depends on the particular parasite involved.

paresthesia See PINS AND NEEDLES SENSATION.

paronychia Swelling and inflammation of infected skin at the base of the nail usually caused by the yeast *Candida albicans.* Acute paronychia is the result of bacteria. The condition, which presents as a tender red area that may draw pus, is most often found among women with poor circulation or those who must wash their hands often.
Treatment Antifungal or antibiotic drugs will cure this problem. The hands must be kept dry. Any abscesses must be surgically drained.

patch A flat area of skin larger than 1 cm in diameter that differs in color from the skin around it.

patch test A test to discover the cause of an allergic reaction by reproducing allergic contact dermatitis. (See DERMATITIS, CONTACT). In the test, the physician places a suspected ALLERGEN in contact with the patient's unbroken skin under occlusion for 48 hours. Posi-

tive reactions show redness, swelling and/or blisters.

The physician can select suspected allergens from a screening tray of chemicals often found in commercial products or with the products that are suspected. The chemical is placed on an adhesive-backed gauze pad, taped in place on the back or inner arm for 48 hours. The reaction is influenced by the skin condition, the concentration and the volume of the testing substance and the vehicle used, the length of time of the test and the number of readings. The standard tray of allergens is frequently updated by the International Contact Dermatitis Research Group and the North American Contact Dermatitis Research Group.

The standard patch test covers the most common skin allergies, about 80 percent of contact sensitivities. To test for other allergies, supplementary patch testing must be carried out. The type of patch test is determined by the kind of dermatitis, the history of exposure and the experience of the dermatologist.

If a reaction occurs, the physician can then describe the substance, what common products contain that substance, and what substitutions are available.

Pautrier's micro abscess A characteristic small collection of leukocytes (or white blood cells—lymphocytes) found in the epidermis (top layer of skin) of MYCOSIS FUNGOIDES (a kind of tumor).

pearly penile papules See ANGIOFIBROMA.

peau d'orange French for "skin of an orange," this is a skin finding caused by fluid retention in nearby lymph glands, dimpling the skin like an orange peel. The fluid retention may be caused by breast cancer in the area around the nipple, in lichen myxedematosus or in some types of skin lymphoma.

pediculi See LICE.

pediculosis Any type of louse infestation. See LICE.

pellagra A nutritional disorder affecting the skin caused by a deficiency of niacin (found in meat, yeast extracts and some cereals), pellagra is found primarily in parts of India and southern Africa where people live primarily on corn.

Symptoms First signs of pellagra include itching and inflammation of the skin, especially in sun-exposed sites, weakness, weight loss, lethargy, depression and irritability. Severe attacks include bright red weeping blisters, a swollen tongue, DERMATITIS, diarrhea and, in severe cases, dementia and memory loss.

Causes While corn has as much niacin as other cereals, the niacin in corn is not absorbed by the body unless first treated with an alkali such as lime water. Corn is also low in tryptophan, an amino acid that the body converts to niacin. This is why other diseases that increase the breakdown of tryptophan, such as inflammatory bowel disease, can also cause pellagra.

Treatment Several weeks' supplementation with niacin and a varied diet rich in protein and calories is needed to reverse pellagra.

pemphigus A serious but uncommon skin disorder featuring skin blisters most often found in patients usually between ages 40 and 60. Pemphigus is a more serious disorder than another similar condition, bullous PEMPHIGOID, which features itchy blisters that are not normally fatal, and appears more commonly among Jews and other ethnic groups of Mediterranean and Indian descent.

Pemphigus may be associated with other autoimmune diseases, such as myasthenia gravis and LUPUS ERYTHEMATOSUS. Various forms of pemphigus include pemphigus vulgaris, pemphigus vegetans, pemphigus foli-

aceus, pemphigus erythematosus and fogo selvagem.

Cause In pemphigus, antibodies circulate in the blood that react against the intercellular substance of the epidermis. These antibodies cause separation of epidermal cells leading to blister formation.

Symptoms Blisters first break out in the mouth and nose, then on the skin; the precise location and type of lesions vary depending on the variety of pemphigus. The easily ruptured skin lesions often form raw, painful areas that may become infected and then form a crust. If the blisters appear over a large area, the skin condition can lead to secondary skin infections that may be fatal.

Treatment Corticosteroid drugs given over a long period of time together with immunosuppressant drugs can control the disease. Antibiotics may be given for any resulting skin infections.

pemphigus, familial benign chronic See HAILEY-HAILEY DISEASE.

pemphigoid, bullous This is a fairly rare skin disease characterized by large tense blisters on the skin that are extremely itchy, unlike the blisters in PEMPHIGUS, a similar but less serious disorder. Bullous pemphigoid is an autoimmune disorder that is usually found among older patients in their 60s or beyond. Antibodies form against the junction between the epidermis and dermis and cause separation of the two layers, leading to blister formation.

Symptoms The disease usually begins with itchy red plaques, followed by tense blisters over several weeks to months. The condition is progressive at first, spreading across the body, with oozing erosions that may be itchy or painful. Infection may lead to fluid or electrolyte imbalance.

Treatment A long-term course of corticosteroids or immunosuppressant drugs can effectively treat this disease, which is much easier to control than pemphigus. Warm baths, water compresses, topical steroids and anti-itching shake lotions won't affect the course of the disease but may provide some relief for itching and pain and may prevent infection.

penicillin and derivatives The first group of antibiotic drugs to be discovered (the sulfas are considered to be antibacterials); natural penicillins are derived from the *Penicillium* mold, but can also be produced synthetically. Penicillins are used to treat a wide variety of infections, and include amoxicillin, ampicillin, penicillin G, penicillin V and penicillin.
Side effects Allergic reactions include skin rash, hives and anaphylaxis. Any patient who has had an allergic reaction to one type of penicillin should not be given any other. Other side effects include vomiting and diarrhea. See also PENICILLIN RASH.

penicillin rash An allergic skin rash in response to the administration of PENICILLIN and derivatives. The red rash usually appears as hives or as a fine macular or papular rash; it can be widespread. These allergic reactions are not uncommon and range from immediate hypersensitivity (including potentially fatal anaphylaxis) to serum sickness reactions. Hypersensitivity of one type or another to penicillin is believed to occur in about 1 or 2 percent of the general population.

Anyone who develops such a rash should immediately stop taking the medication and contact a physician. Anaphylaxis should be handled as a medical emergency.

penile warts See WARTS.

peptides A combination of two or more AMINO ACIDS that are used in shampoos, conditioners and moisturizers because of their ability to retain moisture and strengthen the hair shaft. Peptides form a film on the hair shaft, making the hair seem thicker—they can also fill in cracks on the shaft and make hair shinier. On the skin, peptides form a film that retains moisture.

Physiologically, peptides are found throughout the body's endocrine and nervous systems. Many hormones are peptides; in the nervous system peptides are found in nerve cells throughout the brain and spinal cord.

percutaneous A medical term meaning "performed through the skin." Percutaneous procedures include injections into veins, muscles or other body tissues, and biopsies in which tissue or fluid is removed with a needle.

perforating disorders A family of several disorders characterized by perforation of elements of the dermis through the overlying epidermis. The perforating disorders include ELASTOSIS PERFORANS SERPIGINOSA, perforating collagenosis, perforating FOLLICULITIS, KYRLE'S DISEASE. Perforation has also been reported to occur in dermal diseases, including GRANULOMA ANNULARE, necrobiosis lipoidica diabeticorum and PSEUDOXANTHOMA ELASTICUM.

perfume sensitivity See FRAGRANCE, SENSITIVITY TO.

periarteritis nodosa An uncommon disease of small and medium-sized arteries also called polyarteritis nodosa. It causes the arterial wall to become inflamed and weakened and tends to form aneurysms. Many different groups of blood vessels may be involved, including the coronary arteries supplying blood to the heart, and the arteries of the kidneys, intestine, skeletal muscles and nervous system.
Causes This disorder has been linked to a poorly functioning immune system triggered by exposure to the hepatitis B virus. While it

may develop at any age, it is most common among adult men.

Symptoms Initial symptoms include fever and aching muscles, with a general malaise, appetite and weight loss and sometimes nerve pain. High blood pressure, muscle weakness, skin ulcers and gangrene are often associated with the disease.

Treatment Large doses of corticosteroid drugs are given together with immunosuppressant drugs. Without treatment, the condition is almost always fatal within five years by heart attack, kidney failure, intestinal bleeding or complications of high blood pressure. With treatment, about half of all patients survive for five years.

periderm The outer two layers of fetal epithelium (tissue that covers the external surface of the body) that generally disappear before birth, persisting only as the cuticle.

perifollicular fibromas Small lesions on the face made up of fibrous tissue around hair follicles. See also ANGIOFIBROMA.

periodic acid-Schiff (PAS) stain One of the most common tests for the presence of fungi and certain microorganisms in tissue sections.

perioral dermatitis See DERMATITIS, PERIORAL.

perleche Inflammation, dryness and cracking of the corners of the mouth, sometimes with infection. It may be caused by persistent lip-licking or by a vitamin-deficient diet.

permanent makeup Also known as "dermapigmentation," this is a technique in which pigment is implanted in the skin to simulate the lines drawn with makeup pencils on eyelids, brows or lips. Like tattooing, dermapigmentation involves dipping a needle into pigment that is injected into the bottom layer of the skin. Each injection leaves behind a tiny dot of pigment. The dots when placed closely enough together look like an unbroken line.

While the procedure is fairly straightforward, it is painful, it carries some risks and it is permanent.

The technique is most frequently performed by an aesthetician working in a skin-care salon. While a medical professional is better qualified to handle complications, many physicians do not perform the procedure.

Dermapigmentation (like tattooing) is not well regulated: anyone may perform the procedure, and any state or local ordinances are usually not well enforced. Consumers interested in the procedure should find out how the practitioner was trained; ask to see before-and-after photos; and call past clients to see how pleased they were with the work. Clients must also understand what the end result will look like; dermapigmentation does *not* look like real eyebrow hairs, for example—it looks like makeup. Consumers should realize that once placed in the skin, the pigment cannot be removed.

To some people, dermapigmentation on the sensitive eye or lip area is extremely painful, while others dismiss it as merely uncomfortable. Physicians may use injectable anesthetics (like those used by dentists) to numb the area, but these may cause swelling and bruising that would otherwise not occur.

It is very important that the procedure be performed in a sterilized environment. In a skin-care salon, the dermapigmentation area should be separate from other rooms to protect against contamination from fumes or hair. All parts of the machine that come in contact with the skin and the pigment must be disposable or removable for sterilization *after each use.*

Autoclave sterilization (steam under pressure) is acceptable; dry heat sterilization is not. Because blood is drawn during the procedure, the technician should wear goggles, a face shield and double gloves.

Pigments should be gamma-irradiated for sterility and approved by the Food and Drug Administration. Common tattooing dyes, India ink and vegetable dyes should never be used. Pigment used around the eyes must be an ophthalmologist-tested blend of iron oxide suspended in glycerine and alcohol.

While there have been no irritating reactions to eye pigments, lip lining requires an allergy test before the operation because the ingredients used to produce reddish tones often cause an allergic reaction.

To help decide on colors, bring in eye pencils and lipsticks. The pigment shades won't match the pencils exactly because the colors change in contact with skin tone. Custom-mixing colors is not a good idea, because if they are improperly blended they can separate and result in the absence of one of the desired hues.

Placement of the pigment is critical; if placed only on the top layer of skin it will soon be sloughed off. Special needle guns used in the procedure are designed to penetrate skin only as deep as is necessary. This is particularly important around the eyes, where contact must never be made with the eyeball. Occasionally eyebrow pigment is placed too high or with too much of a curve, but once applied, the color cannot be changed.

For more information or for a recommendation of dermatologists in your area, contact the American Academy of Dermatology, Box 681069, Schaumburg, IL 60168; for a trained anesthetician, call the Aestheticians International Association at (504) 469–1016.

permethrin   Permethrin 5 percent cream is a synthetic substance that is approved by the Food and Drug Administration for the treatment of SCABIES. Because of its low toxicity, it is widely prescribed, especially for children with scabies. In treating scabies, a single ap-

plication of permethrin is applied to the entire skin surface and washed off eight to 14 hours later.

pernio   See CHILBLAIN.

pet-borne illnesses   A wide range of pet-borne illnesses can cause skin symptoms. These include allergies to pet dandruff (See PET DANDER ALLERGY), HOOKWORM, infections from bites, CAT-SCRATCH FEVER, MITES fleas, RINGWORM and TOXOPLASMOSIS.

pet dander allergy   Allergies to pet dander can cause itching and skin rash in sensitive people. In the case of an allergy, the immune system identifies a normally harmless substance (called an "allergen") as dangerous, and produces antibodies to fight it.

Those allergic to cats experience an allergic reaction, which can cause itching, puffy eyes, wheezing, rash, or shortness of breath. The allergen stems from substances in the pet's oil-producing glands, in its skin or from its saliva. Some experts also believe that cat dander may also contribute to the problem.
Prevention   Not surprisingly, the best way to handle pet allergies is to avoid pets. But even if you rid your home of animals, it may take weeks or months for the allergens to be completely removed from carpeting and furniture. If you keep your cat or dog, washing the pet once a week for several weeks will reduce the amount of the airborne allergens by 90 percent. Get rid of carpeting and upholstered furniture, mop your floors often and vacuum with a high-efficiency filter. An effective air cleaner can remove up to 99 percent of the dust, including pet allergens. Keep your pet outside as much as possible, and don't let the pet on the bed or in other rooms where you spend a great deal of time. Because super-insulated homes have higher allergen levels, be sure to get lots of fresh-air circulation.

Treatment Antihistamines are the primary treatment for most allergies. Repeated allergy shots may allow you to build up immunity over a period of several months. However, because people may react adversely to the shots, and because repeated shots are inconvenient, a severe cat or dog allergy is best managed by removing the pet. See also PET-BORNE ILLNESSES.

petechiae Flat pinhead-sized spots of red or purple appearing in the skin or mucous membranes caused by a localized hemorrhage from small blood vessels. Petechiae are seen in individuals with bleeding disorders and sometimes appear with bacterial endocarditis (inflammation of the heart's lining).

petroleum jelly An inexpensive oily substance also known as petrolatum used in products to treat chapped, dry or raw skin. Derived from petroleum, it is commonly used as an ointment base, a protective dressing or an emollient to soften the skin. An excellent protectant against water evaporation, it is very mild and has not been associated with allergies or irritation. It can, however, trigger ACNE in people with oily or acne-prone skin.

Peutz-Jeghers syndrome An inherited autosomal dominant disorder featuring small brown or blue-brown spots on the lips and in the mouth. It is associated with many polyps in the small intestine. While there are often no other symptoms, the polyps may occasionally produce pain or bleeding.

Lesions appear early in childhood and may fade during adolescence. About one-third of affected individuals exhibit symptoms in the first 10 years of life.
Symptoms In addition to skin lesions, symptoms include abdominal pain, vomiting and gastrointestinal bleeding. There appears to be a 2 to 3 percent chance for the eventual de-

velopment of gastrointestinal cancer. Because the polyps are usually numerous and widespread, removal is not often possible.
Treatment Bleeding polyps may be removed, but generally treatment aims at symptom management.

Peyronie's disease A disorder in which part of the sheath of connective tissue within the penis thickens, causing it to bend at an angle during erection, often making intercourse painful and difficult. The disorder usually affects men over age 40; the cause is unknown.

The thickened area can be felt as a NODULE when the penis is not erect. If the condition progresses, the tissue may thicken to the point where the penis cannot maintain an erection.
Treatment The disorder may improve without treatment; otherwise, local injections of corticosteroid drugs may help in thinning the tissue. If the condition persists, the thickened area may be surgically removed and replaced with a graft of normal tissue, although this sometimes causes additional scarring that can make the problem worse.

pH A measure of acidity or alkalinity using a scale from 0–14 (the lower the number, the more acidic and the higher the number, the more alkaline). Vinegar has a pH of 2.3; the skin has a slightly acid pH (between 5.5 and 6.8); most soaps are pH 8–10. Plain water and blood are either neutral (pH 7) or very close to neutral.

phenytoin hypersensitivity syndrome A type of drug reaction to the anticonvulsant drug used to treat epilepsy that, while fairly rare, can be severe; it usually occurs during the first week of phenytoin use. Phenytoin (Dilantin) is also used occasionally to treat migraines and to control certain types of arrhythmia (irregular heart beat). Cross reaction with other anticonvulsants is common;

therefore, physicians should treat with caution.

Symptoms The syndrome is characterized by fever, a widespread eruption consisting of red papules and plaques with facial swelling, generalized tender swollen lymph nodes, leukocytosis, and liver dysfunction.

phlegmon Intense inflammation of connective tissue, often causing ulcers or abscesses.

Phoenix Society for Burn Survivors A self-help service organization for burn survivors and their families that works to ease the psychosocial adjustment of severely burned and disfigured persons during and after hospitalization so that they may return to normal and satisfactory lives within their communities. Former burn survivors work as volunteers on a one-to-one basis with other burn survivors and their families. The group offers a training program for volunteers, seeks to educate the public about the nature and problems of disfigurement, discourages concealment of disfigurement, conducts research on psychological ramifications of burn disfigurement and disseminates information on burns and trauma and their treatment. The society conducts school programs for burned children returning to class, and presents the Heroism Award to burn rescuers. It maintains a speakers' bureau and contains books on burn recovery, films and videocassettes.

The society publishes an annual list of audiovisual materials on burns, disfigurement and related subjects; an annual bibliographic references on burns in children; *Coping Strategies for Burn Survivors and Their Families* and *Guidelines for Burn Volunteers*; and the quarterly newsletter *Icarus file*.

Founded in 1977, the group has 6,500 members and sponsors an annual World Burn Congress. For address, see Appendix D; see also AMERICAN BURN ASSOCIATION, BURNS UNITED SUPPORT GROUPS, INTERNATIONAL SOCIETY FOR BURN INJURIES, NATIONAL INSTITUTE FOR BURN MEDICINE, NATIONAL BURN VICTIM FOUNDATION.

photoallergy (and phototoxicity) A condition in which a person experiences an adverse reaction after ingesting or applying a substance (called a photosensitizer) and subsequently exposing the skin to sunlight (usually ULTRAVIOLET RADIATION). The reaction is characterized by an itchy papular, eczematous lesions resembling contact dermatitis due to poison ivy or blistering, that may extend beyond the area of exposure. Immediate HIVES occur rarely.

Photosensitizers can be either exogenous (they penetrate the skin through topical application or systemic dissemination through the blood) or endogenous (occurring within the body). The only endogenous photosensitizers synthesized by the human body are porphyrin molecules; when produced in excess, they cause the PORPHYRIAS.

Topical photosensitizers are common ingredients of cosmetics, face creams, perfumes, after-shave lotions and soaps. Others include medications such as coal tars and PSORALENS that are deliberately used to induce photosensitivity to help treat various skin disorders, or phenothiazines and sulfonamides, which may produce unintended photosensitivity when applied to the skin. Antibacterial agents (such as the halogenated salicylanilides and related compounds) were once used in deodorant soaps; first-aid creams were responsible for an epidemic of photosensitivity reactions in the 1960s.

Plants such as celery, wild carrots, gas plant, limes and meadow grass contain photosensitizing psoralens. Industrial contaminants and air pollutants such as tars and polycyclic aromatic hydrocarbons are also potent photosensitizers.

Commonly used photosensitizers include sulfonamides, thiazide diuretics, sulfonylureas, phenothiazines and certain tetracycline derivatives (such as doxycycline). While some of these are more potent, thiazide diuretics produce the most reactions because they are used most frequently.

Treatment Prevention is the best option; patients using a known photosensitizer should avoid exposure to sunlight and those who develop a reaction should avoid the photosensitizer. Treatment of lesions depends on the type, extent and severity of response. Cool tap water compresses can be applied continually or intermittently; topical application of corticosteroid cream or lotion can reduce inflammation. Systemic antihistamines may lessen the itch. If the process is severe and extensive, systemic corticosteroids (such as those used in extensive poison ivy cases) may be needed.

photochemotherapy Treatments involving the interaction between chemicals and the sun, also called PUVA therapy (*Psoralens* molecules combined with *UVA* energy). The PSORALENS (a group of photosensitizing chemical compounds) are taken either orally or topically followed by irradiation with long-wave ultraviolet light A (UVA) rays one to two hours later, for five to 10 minutes two or three times per week until remission. The most common psoralen used in the United States is 8-methoxy psoralen.

Photochemotherapy in the treatment of VITILIGO has been practiced since 1400 B.C. in India, using plant-derived psoralens. Today, physicians use synthetic psoralens that become activated after they absorb UVA radiation.

This treatment has been successful in the treatment of a variety of conditions including PSORIASIS, vitiligo and MYCOSIS FUNGOIDES; other diseases such as solar HIVES may also respond.

Side effects Patients who receive too much drug or UV light can develop severe sunburn with blisters and swelling. The psoralen may produce nausea, vomiting or lightheadedness. Prolonged use of PUVA may cause cataracts, solar keratoses and skin cancer.

photodermatitis Skin inflammation caused by light or ULTRAVIOLET RADIATION.

photophytodermatitis Skin inflammation caused by plant products on the skin, activated by light or ULTRAVIOLET RADIATION. See OIL OF BERGAMOT.

photosensitivity Also known as sun sensitivity, this is a toxic skin reaction to the sun that can be caused by a variety of substances, such as some prescription medications and consumer products—as well as some physical disorders. It often occurs because a substance (called a photosensitizer) has been ingested or applied to the skin. Examples of photosensitizers include certain drugs, dyes, chemicals in perfumes and soaps; plants such as buttercups, parsnips and mustard; and fruits such as limes and lemons.

Any abnormal reaction to the sun causing exaggerated sunburn, painful swelling, hives or blistering should be considered to be a sign of photosensitivity. A photosensitive reaction can occur in less than half an hour or it can take until 48 to 72 hours after exposure.

Drugs are the primary cause of photosensitivity; those that are known to cause sun sensitivity include tetracyclines, furosemide (Lasix), griseofulvin, sulfonamides and nalidixic acid, phenothiazine, piroxicam and naproxen, tretinoin (Retin-A), diphendramine and birth control pills. Other medications that may cause a problem include anticancer and photochemotherapy drugs, antidepressants and antipsychotics, antihistamines, antiparasitic drugs, diuretics and hypoglycemics.

Sun sensitivity can also be triggered by the coal tars in some medicated soaps and shampoos, or the OIL OF BERGAMOT in certain perfumes, toilet soaps, lemons and limes.

Photosensitivity can also be caused by some disorders, including LUPUS ERYTHEMATOSUS and the porphyria group of blood disorders.

Fortunately, relatively few people ever become photosensitive; the risk is higher for those who only have intermittent exposure to the sun, those who have light skin and who tend to burn instead of tan.

About 10 percent of individuals have an adverse reaction to sunlight in the absence of photosensitizing medications. These individuals suffer from POLYMORPHIC (or polymorphous) LIGHT ERUPTION, an itchy eruption characterized by red papules 24 to 72 hours after sun exposure that last several days after the affected person avoids the sun. Frequently known as "sun poisoning," this reaction often develops on the first sunny outing in the spring or during a winter holiday to a sunny destination. It is usually mild, but the itch, swelling and rash can be so severe that it can ruin a holiday. It can be prevented by getting small amounts of sun before going on holiday, or with pretreatment (PUVA or PUVB).

Treatment Known photosensitizers should be avoided; susceptible people who report skin reactions without using any photosensitizing agents should also avoid exposure to the sun and should use a SUNSCREEN. Polymorphic (-ous) eruptions may be treated with systemic corticosteroids or antihistamines.

phototherapy Treatment with light, including sunlight, nonvisible ultraviolet light (UVA or UVB), or visible blue light. Moderate exposure to sunlight is the most common form of phototherapy and is effective in treating up to 75 percent of PSORIASIS patients.

The most recent form of phototherapy is called PUVA, which combines long-wave ultraviolet light (UVA) with a PSORALEN drug (such as METHOXSALEN) to sensitize the skin to UVA. It is especially effective in the treatment of psoriasis and some other skin diseases, such as VITILIGO and MYCOSIS FUNGOIDES.

Short-wave ultraviolet light (UVB) is effective in the treatment of PSORIASIS.

Visible blue light is the treatment of choice for infant JAUNDICE, caused by the accumulation of bilirubin (bile pigment) as the result of a poorly developed liver. Experts believe the light breaks down the bilirubin in the skin, allowing it to be excreted.

phototoxic Pertaining to injury by ULTRAVIOLET RADIATION or light.

COMMON PHOTOSENSITIZING DRUGS

Antibiotics
aureomycin (Chlortetracycline)
griseofulvin (Fulvicin)
minocycline (Minocin, Dynacin)
quinolone (Aprofloxacin, naladoxic acid)
sulfa drugs
tetracycline (Tetracycline)

Antiarrythmics
quinidine (Cin-Quin, Duraquin, etc.)

Antidepressants
amitriptyline (Elavil)
desipramine (Norpramin)

Tranquilizers
chlordiazepoxide (Librium)
chlorpromazine (Thorazine)

Diuretics
hydrochlorothiazide (Esidrix)
chlorothiazide (Diuril)
chlorathalidone (Hygroton)
furosemide (Lasix)
triamterene (Dyrenium)

Non-steroidal   Anti-inflammatory   drugs (NSAIDs)
Seldane

phrynoderma Also called "toad skin," this is an eruption of solid, elevated palpable lesions seen in patients with severe VITAMIN A deficiency.

pian See YAWS.

piebald skin A condition of two-toned skin, either white and black, or white and brown. It is an inherited autosomal dominant condition characterized by a white forlock and stable white flat discolorations with hyper-pigmented centers. The discolorations are usually found on the trunk, face, forearms and mid-leg (hands and feet are not affected).

Some patients are deaf (Waardenburg's syndrome).

Treatment It is difficult to repigment white areas, and the lack of melanin-producing cells in hair follicles next to affected skin means that PSORALEN and UVA (PUVA) therapy will not be very effective. Full thickness grafts of normal skin may result in successful repigmentation.

piedra See TRICHOSPOROSIS.

pigmentation Color of skin, hair and eyes determined by MELANIN (pigment) produced by special cells called melanocytes (PIGMENT CELLS). The more melanin in the body, the darker the color. The amount of melanin any person produces is the result of heredity and exposure to sunlight. Three other pigments that contribute to normal skin color are oxygenated hemoglobin, reduced hemoglobin and carotenoids. Skin color can range from a pale white to deep black, and hair color ranges from white, blond, light to dark brown, black, red or gray. Eyes can be any shade from the bluest sky-blue to the very blackest black.

In humans, pigmented skin and hair protects against the harmful effects of sunlight; in other animals, color may provide camouflage against predators (as in chameleons) or act as a sexual attractant (as in peacocks).

Some experts believe that the human pigmentation system may have developed as a skin protectant for animals with very little hair covering.

All pigment cells are produced from the neural crest (except those of the retina, which come from the primitive forebrain). A person's neural crest is formed by the sixth week of gestation, although the precursors of pigment cells probably begin their migration to the skin, ears, eyes and other organs before the neural crest is completely formed. By the eighth week of gestation, pigment cells can be identified in the DERMIS. See PIGMENTATION, DISORDERS OF.

pigmentation, disorders of Skin color is determined by the MELANIN—its amount, its distribution, its character and its chemistry—which together determine the color and hue of the skin's pigmentation.

Lightened skin Pigment cells that are absent from an area of skin, produce too few melanosomes or are unable to produce enough melanin, result in skin that is very light in color. An absence of pigment cells may cause PIEBALD SKIN, WAARDENBURG'S SYNDROME or VITILIGO. Lack of skin color may also be caused by trauma, exposure to cold or chemicals. Hypopigmentation (too little pigmentation), due to abnormal formation of melanosomes, may indicate TUBEROUS SCLEROSIS, HYPOMELANOSIS OF ITO, NEVUS DEPIGMENTOSUS or CHEDIAK-HIGASHI SYNDROME. Loss of pigment due to a drop in the production of melanin may be caused by ALBINISM and TINEA VERSICOLOR. PITYRIASIS ALBA is caused by a decrease in the transfer of melanosomes. Finally, there are many infections and inflammatory skin disorders that leave behind hypopigmented skin, including drug reactions, LEUKONYCHIA and post-inflammatory hypopigmentation. Patches of pale skin are also a symptom of a range of disorders, including PSORIASIS and PITYRIASIS ALBA and PHENYLKETONURIA.

Darker skin Hyperpigmentation is a common problem, especially among patients with dark skin. Among those with darker skin, most skin irritations cause heightened skin color. Hyperpigmentation may also be a sign of a serious metabolic or nutritional problem. Most lesions that are hyperpigmented are benign, although some (such as MELANOMAS) are cancerous.

Patients may notice patches of dark and light skin after an episode of ECZEMA, psoriasis or tinea versicolor. Those with CHLOASMA experience dark areas on the face caused by hormonal changes while taking birth control pills, or during pregnancy or menopause. Dark skin patches on the face may also be caused by some perfumes or cosmetics, especially when they contain photosensitizing chemicals. These chemically induced patches usually fade with time. Other types of skin darkening unrelated to sun exposure may occur with ADDISON'S DISEASE or Cushing's Syndrome.

Permanent areas of dark pigmented skin are usually caused by an abnormality in the melanocytes, such as with a FRECKLE or MOLE. The disease ACANTHOSIS NIGRICANS is characterized by dark patches of velvety thick skin usually found in the skin creases.

Other disorders involving hyperpigmentation include LENTIGO SIMPLEX, MULTIPLE LENTIGINES SYNDROME, NEVUS SPILUS, MONGOLIAN SPOT, NEVUS OF ITO AND NEVUS OF OTA, RECKLINGHAUSEN'S DISEASE, hereditary cases of hyperpigmentation and ADDISON'S DISEASE.

Other changes Still other pigment changes occur with an excess of bilirubin, which turns the skin yellow, or too much iron, HEMOCHROMATOSIS, which turns the skin bronze.

pigment cells Also called melanocytes, these pigment-producing cells are located in the BASAL CELL layer of the EPIDERMIS (top skin layer). They are controlled by a hormone secreted by the pituitary gland in the brain and produce MELANIN (pigment color) by oxidizing tyrosine. Pigment cells are also found in the hair bulb and are a normal part of cells in the mucous membranes. In dark-skinned people, these pigment cells normally produce large amounts of melanin, and oral mucous membranes are very dark. In Caucasians, pigmentation may not be normally visible in mucous membranes.

Large amounts of melanin indicate an efficient effective protection against many chemical and physical toxins. Short wave ultraviolet light, chemical carcinogens and phenols produce free oxygen radicals within the epidermis and dermis. It may be that a primary function of melanocytes is to remove FREE RADICALS formed in the skin during inflammatory conditions. Melanocytes protect other cells of the epidermis from damage by release of radical oxygens.

Human pigment cells produce two types of melanin: eumelanin (black and brown) and phaeomelanin (red). The ratio between the two types determines a person's skin and hair color. See also PIGMENTATION; PIGMENTATION, DISORDERS OF.

pigmented nevi See NEVUS.

pilar Pertaining to the hair.

pilosebaceous Relating to the hair follicles and their sebaceous glands.

pimples The common name for a small PUSTULE or PAPULE, pimples are usually found on the face, neck and back, especially in adolescents with ACNE. See also ACNE, ADULT; ACNE, TREATMENT OF.

pinch graft A small type of SKIN GRAFT used to cover leg ulcers. Only 4 to 10 mm thick, this graft is taken from anesthetized skin from the upper thigh by pinching up a small amount of skin with the tip of a small needle and slicing with a scalpel or razor blade. The grafts are kept in sterile saline and transferred to the wound area, leaving a 2–mm space between grafts. An adhesive spray is then applied, followed by a semipermeable dressing with edges extended beyond the margin of the ulcer. Gauze and an elastic dressing are used to cover the wound, which is left untouched for up to four days. Strict bed rest is required. The wound can be checked through the semipermeable dressing and accumulating fluid can be drained. Dressings are removed in five to six days. Wiping the wound with alcohol allows it to form a scab that will come off in two or three weeks. As the grafts take, the grafted sites grow together and cover the entire wound site. See also ALLOGRAFT, ARTIFICIAL SKIN; HETEROGRAFT.

pins and needles sensation The common term for PARESTHESIA, a tingly or prickly sensation in the skin that is usually associated with numbness or loss of sensation and sometimes with a burning feeling.

A temporary pins and needles feeling is caused by a disturbance in the nerve impulses along the pathway from skin to brain, such as when an arm is bent under the body during sleep. Persistent pins and needles sensations may be caused by a group of nerve disorders called neuropathy. For example, this is frequently seen in diabetes.

pinta A skin infection found in some remote tropical American villages caused by the microorganism *Treponema carateum,* a close relative of the bacterium that causes syphilis. It seems to affect only dark-skinned people and is thought to be transmitted either by direct contact or by flies that carry the infective spirochetes.
Symptoms Symptoms include thickening and loss of pigment of the skin, particularly on the face, neck, buttocks, hands or feet. Up to a year later red skin patches appear that turn blue, brown and then white.

Treatment Rarely disabling or fatal, penicillin or tetracycline will cure the disease, but patients may be permanently disfigured.

pitted nails See NAILS, PITTED.

pityriasis alba A common childhood skin condition featuring irregular, fine, pale scalp patches on the cheeks caused by a mild ECZEMA. The skin condition often worsens after exposure to the sun because inflamed skin in the patches doesn't tan well. The disease may persist into adulthood.
Treatment The condition usually responds well to EMOLLIENTS or mild topical steroids.

pityriasis rosea A common mild skin disorder of childhood and young adulthood characterized by a single large round spot (called a herald patch) on the trunk, followed days to a week later by slightly raised, scaly-edged, round or oval pink-to-copper colored spots on the trunk and upper arms. The condition is thought not to be contagious.
Cause The cause of the disease is unknown, although many speculate that it is due to a virus.
Symptoms In addition to the above symptoms that last for about six to eight weeks, pityriasis rosea may cause itching.
Treatment The rash usually clears up without treatment, but a physician should rule out other conditions that may cause a similar rash. Mild itching may be relieved by applying CALAMINE LOTION or ZINC OXIDE shake lotion; more severe itching may be treated with ANTIHISTAMINE DRUGS, topical steroids or phototherapy.

pityriasis rubra pilaris A chronic disease of keratinization that can be inherited or acquired and is characterized by follicular papules with greasy plugs, generalized skin redness, and yellow thickening of the palms and soles.

In the inherited form, the lesions, which may resemble PSORIASIS, may begin in infancy and last throughout life, with occasional periods of remission. The acquired type of pityriasis rubra pilaris usually appears in adulthood. The lesions disappear within three years in 80 percent of cases. Treatment may shorten that time.

Cause Unknown.

Symptoms Firm, pink, red or orange follicular papules may form groups of lesions that remain localized to the extensor surfaces of the skin or that eventually cover the entire body. There may be scaling on the scalp. When the lesions spread over the entire body, a few small clear areas of normal skin ("skip areas") may be seen on the trunk.

Treatment Etretinate, ISOTRETINOIN and methotrexate are the most effective treatments. Etretinate and isotretinoin produce remission within several months. Combining the retinoids with ultraviolet B (UVB) phototherapy may also help. Topical creams are not usually effective.

plague A serious infectious disease transmitted by the bites of rats or fleas that was the scourge of early history. It was nicknamed the Black Death during the pandemic of the 14th century because its primary symptom is the black patches on the skin caused by bleeding around the buboes (swollen lymph glands). Recent outbreaks among humans have occurred in Africa, South America and Southeast Asia. Plague is also found among ground squirrels, prairie dogs and marmots in parts of Arizona, New Mexico, California, Colorado and Nevada. Between 10 and 50 Americans contract plague during the spring and summer months each year.

Causes Fleas found on rodents throughout the world may carry the bacterium *Yersinia pestis.* The great pandemics of the past occurred when wild rodents spread the disease to rats in cities and then to humans when the fleas jumped off dying rats. A bite from an infected flea leads to bubonic plague, a form of the disease characterized by buboes. Pneumonic plague affects the lungs, and is a complication of bubonic plague; it is also spread via infected droplets during coughing.

Symptoms Two to five days after infection, patients experience fever, shivering, seizures and severe headaches followed by buboes—smooth, oval, reddened and very painful swellings in the armpits, groin or neck. Left untreated, half of plague patients will die. If blood poisoning occurs as an early complication, a patient may die before the buboes appear.

Treatment Administration of streptomycin, chloramphenicol or tetracycline reduces the risk of death to less than 5 percent. Those in contact with anyone who has pneumonic plague are given antibiotics as a preventive measure at the first sign of disease.

plantar warts A firm, rough-surfaced WART found on the sole of the foot that may appear alone or in clusters. It is usually contracted through contact with swimming pool or communal shower floors contaminated with the human papillomavirus that causes the wart. Because of the constant pressure from the body, the wart is compressed, flattened and forced into the sole of the foot.

Treatment Like many warts, plantar warts may disappear without treatment; others may persist for years or may recur. A foam shoe pad may relieve discomfort. Alternatively, the warts may be removed by CRYOSURGERY, using salicylic acid plasters, CURETTAGE and ELECTRODESICCATION and LASER treatment.

plastic and reconstructive surgery The specialty of plastic surgery includes two branches—reconstructive and cosmetic surgery. Plastic and reconstructive surgeons use special techniques to repair visible skin defects and problems in underlying tissue, caused by heredity, burns, injuries, operations, aging or disease.

The word plastic, from the Greek *plastikos,* means to fit for molding or to give form—it does not refer to the synthetic materials that are sometimes used in plastic surgery.

Reconstructive surgery is performed on abnormal structures of the body, caused by congenital defects, developmental abnormalities, trauma, infection, tumors or disease. It is generally performed to improve function, but may also be done to approximate a normal appearance. This includes procedures done to repair birth defects, such as cleft lip and palate repair, and deformities caused by accidents or disease, such as facial reconstruction following cancer surgery, burn care, re-attachment of limbs, and breast reconstruction following mastectomy. The average plastic surgeon spends 60 percent of his or her time performing reconstructive surgery.

Cosmetic surgery is performed to reshape normal structures of the body in order to improve the patient's appearance. This includes procedures such as facelifts, nose reshaping and other procedures done to improve appearance and enhance the quality of life for patients who choose to have this type of surgery.

Patients who have aesthetic surgery are from all segments of American society. A recent survey showed that 65 percent of patients undergoing aesthetic surgery are middle class; that is, they have household incomes of less than $50,000.

A variety of techniques are used to provide skin cover for damaged areas, including SKIN GRAFTS, skin and muscle flaps, Z-PLASTY and TISSUE EXPANSION. These techniques may be performed in addition to grafts or implants.

Over the past 10 years, the practice of plastic surgery has broadened through the use of microsurgical techniques to join blood vessels, allowing the transfer of blocks of skin and muscle from one part of the body to the other.

More than 1 million plastic and reconstructive surgeries are performed in hospitals each year, according to the National Center for Health Statistics. See also PLASTIC SURGERY, COSMETIC SURGERY.

Plastic Surgery Educational Foundation A professional group for plastic and reconstructive surgeons that sponsors demonstrations, lectures, educational seminars, symposia and workshops focusing on plastic surgery techniques and procedures. Founded in 1948, the group has 4,500 members and sponsors an annual scientific meeting. It publishes the *Plastic and Reconstructive Surgery* journal, booklets and *Plastic Surgery News.* For address, see Appendix E; see also AMERICAN ACADEMY OF COSMETIC SURGERY, AMERICAN ACADEMY OF FACIAL PLASTIC AND RECONSTRUCTIVE SURGERY, AMERICAN ASSOCIATION OF PLASTIC SURGEONS, AMERICAN BOARD OF PLASTIC SURGERY, AMERICAN SOCIETY FOR AESTHETIC PLASTIC SURGERY, AMERICAN SOCIETY OF PLASTIC AND RECONSTRUCTIVE SURGEONS, INTERPLAST, NATIONAL FOUNDATION FOR FACIAL RECONSTRUCTION, PLASTIC SURGERY RESEARCH COUNCIL.

Plastic Surgery Research Council A professional group designed to foster fundamental research in the fields of plastic and reconstructive surgery. Founded in 1955, the council has 232 members and sponsors an annual conference. For address, see Appendix E. See also AMERICAN ACADEMY OF COSMETIC SURGERY, AMERICAN ACADEMY OF FACIAL PLASTIC AND RECONSTRUCTIVE SURGERY, AMERICAN ASSOCIATION OF PLASTIC SURGEONS, AMERICAN BOARD OF PLASTIC SURGERY, AMERICAN SOCIETY FOR AESTHETIC PLASTIC SURGERY, AMERICAN SOCIETY OF PLASTIC AND RECONSTRUCTIVE SURGEONS, INTERPLAST, NATIONAL FOUNDATION FOR FACIAL RECON-

STRUCTION, PLASTIC SURGERY EDUCATIONAL FOUNDATION.

plethora A florid, bright red flushed complexion that may be caused by dilation of blood vessels near the skin's surface due to alcohol, heat, spicy food etc. More rarely, it can be caused by an excess number of red blood cells, as in polycythema rubra vera.

pockmark A term referring to the deep, pitted scars of ACNE lesions. The appearance of pockmarks can be improved by a variety of techniques, including dermabrasion, chemical peels etc.

poikiloderma Pigment changes of the skin, causing a dappled or mottled appearance with areas of both increased and decreased color.

poison ivy (*Toxicodendron radicans; Rhus toxicodendron*) Sensitivity to this plant's oil (urushiol) is the most common allergy in the country, affecting almost half of all Americans at one time or another. In a few cases, it can be quite serious; if symptoms such as swelling appear within 4 to 12 hours, patients should seek immediate medical treatment.

One of the most common poisonous plants in the United States, its leaves are glossy green, may be notched or smooth, and almost always grow in groups of three—two leaves opposite each other and one at the end of the stalk.

However, according to some experts there are exceptions, and leaves may sometimes appear in groups of five, seven or even nine. In early fall, the leaves sometimes turn bright red. While it usually grows as a long, hairy vine (often wrapping itself around trees), it can also be found as a low shrub growing along fences or stone walls. Poison ivy has waxy yellow-green flowers and greenish berries, which can help identify the plant in late fall, winter and early spring before the leaves

appear. Poison ivy is found throughout the United States, although it is most common in the eastern and central states.

Cause The itching and blistering is caused by the reaction of the body's blood vessels to the plant's urushiol oil, causing blisters and oozing sores. Sensitivity to this oil ranges from nonexistent to severe, and an allergy can spring up in previously immune people at any time. The urushiol oil that causes the rash is a colorless or slightly yellow resin, whose name comes from a Japanese word meaning lacquer. The entire plant contains this oil, and is therefore poisonous: leaves, berries, stalk and roots.

Urushiol is easily transferred from an object to a person, so anything that touches poison ivy (clothing, gardening tools, a pet's fur, athletic equipment) can be contaminated with urushiol and cause poison ivy in anyone who then touches the object. Urushiol remains active for up to one year, so any equipment that touches poison ivy must be washed. Even the smoke from burning poison ivy is toxic and can irritate the lungs, since urushiol can be carried in smoke. Therefore, individuals should never burn poison ivy plants as a way to get rid of them; the smoke given off by these burning plants is particularly dangerous and can enter the nasal passages, throat and lungs of anyone who breathes it.

As the leaves die in the fall, the plant draws certain nutrients and substances (including the oil) into the stem. But the oil remains active, so even in winter if broken stems are used as firewood kindling or as vines on a Christmas wreath they may cause a rash.

Symptoms: While not every person is allergic to poison ivy, about 7 out of 10 people are sensitive to urushiol and will develop contact dermatitis if exposed to a large enough dose.

Children rarely have allergic reactions to urushiol, primarily because it usually takes several exposures to develop a sensitivity to the resin. Symptoms vary from one person to the next; some people exhibit only mild itching while others experience severe reactions, which may include terrible burning and itching with watery blisters. The skin irritation, swelling, blisters and itching may appear within hours or days, usually developing within 24 to 48 hours in a sensitized person. The skin becomes reddened, followed by watery blisters, peaking about five days after contamination and gradually improving over a week or two, even without treatment. Eventually, the blisters break and the oozing sores crust over and then disappear.

Despite a common misconception, poison ivy is *not* spread by scratching open blisters or by skin-to-skin contact, but by the oil (urushiol) found in the plant. Anything that brushes against this oil is contaminated and can cause poison ivy if it contacts the skin. Poison ivy is not spread from person to person either, since only contact with the oil spreads the rash.

However, for this reason, doctors still recommend not scratching blisters, since any remaining urushiol that hasn't been washed off can be transmitted to another part of the body. In addition, scratching the blisters may cause a skin infection from bacteria present on the fingernails.

Animals can also transmit poison ivy from their fur to their owners' skin. Any animal suspected of coming in contact with poison ivy should be given a bath.

Allergy to poison ivy may also indicate that a person is allergic to related plants, including cashews, pistachios, mangos and Chinese or Japanese lacquer trees.

Prevention Most important is proper protection—gloves, long sleeves, heavy socks and pants tucked into boots. Before going out and working in a poison ivy–infested area, try spraying your deodorant or antiperspirant on arms, legs, clothes and pets. Deodorant sprays contain activated clay known as organoclay, and antiperspirants contain the clay and aluminum chlorohydrate, both of which have been found to neutralize urushiol oil. Antiperspirant contains both oil-fighting ingredients, but it is also irritating and should not be sprayed on the face or in body folds.

Short of avoiding the plant, the best method for preventing a rash from exposure to poison ivy before the allergic reaction takes hold is to *immediately* wash off the oil—first with alcohol, followed by water (soap is not necessary). Or, wash the affected area immediately after contact (within 10 minutes, if possible) with yellow laundry soap (such as Castile) and *cold* water, lathering several times and rinsing the area in running water after each sudsing. Do not scrub with a brush.

If you've come in contact with poison ivy out in the wild, wash in a cold running stream. If no water is available, there are a host of other possibilities, including rinsing with paint thinner, acetone, horse urine, ammonia and meat tenderizer. Organic solvents (paint thinner or acetone) work very well in washing off the urushiol oil, but they should not be used on a regular basis. (Regular skin contact with solvents can cause a rash). Solvents *are* recommended for eliminating the poison ivy oil on garden tools, car upholstery etc.

Other products designed to prevent poison ivy and poison oak are presently being investigated by the Food and Drug Administration.

Treatment If you aren't successful in washing off the oil before the allergic reaction begins, the best non-prescription treatment is generally considered to be CALAMINE LOTION, a soothing skin protector that cools the skin and absorbs the oozing, forming a protective crust that keeps the skin from sticking to clothes.

Because the cooling effect of calamine shrinks the blood vessels, this also helps stop the blister formation. Make sure to stop using calamine once the oozing stops, so as not to dry the skin too much and worsen itching again.

Itching also can be treated with compresses soaked in cold water. Products containing local anesthetics (such as benzocaine) should be avoided because they themselves cause a contact dermatitis. Some experts recommend cooling counterirritants such as phenol or menthol, which may be effective, although it may sting and may not be strong enough to stop the discomfort.

Nonprescription oral antihistamines (such as Chlor-Trimeton or Benadryl) may also be effective; systemic antihistamines do not work against the rash, although their sedative action may help the patient sleep. Nonprescription cortisone creams, however, are too weak to be very effective, although they may provide minor relief for minimal itching.

Colloidal oatmeal (such as Aveeno, available at drugstores) will dry up oozing blisters, and can be applied with a cloth or used in the bath.

Any clothing that might have come in contact with urushiol must be washed several times. If the urushiol is washed off, there is little or no further treatment of mild cases of the rash.

Widespread, severe poison ivy is treated by dermatologists with topical steroids; if quite severe, systemic steroids by mouth may be administered.

CAUTION A small percentage of sensitive individuals are seriously allergic, and will begin to develop a rash and swelling in only 4 to 12 hours after contact (as opposed to the normal 24 to 48). One of the few real emergencies in dermatology, such an extreme sensitivity should be immediately treated at the hospital as soon as possible; a shot of corticosteroids will lessen swelling.

Vaccines Extremely sensitive individuals may be desensitized to the effects of poison ivy with allergen extracts, although results have been disappointing sometimes and often don't last longer than one season. Vaccine is given by mouth or injection. The procedure requires a great deal of time (three to six months) and effort. Adverse reactions to the desensitization include swelling, dermatitis, gastroenteric disturbances, fever and inflammation at the injection site. Because of these problems, immunization is only recommended for those sensitive people who live or work near the ivy. Convulsions have occurred in children following oral administration of the plant's extract. No cream, lotion or spray has been proven effective as protection against the allergen, although studies are continuing.

Alternatively, recent research suggests a different vaccine may be available for millions of Americans tormented each summer with the itchy rash. Researchers at the University of Mississippi have developed an experimental vaccine that seems to prevent an allergic reaction and may lessen the painful symptoms after the rash appears. Researchers explain the vaccine works best as an injection, and probably would be most helpful for those who are highly sensitive to the plants. The agent has been tested on animals, but has not yet been tested on humans. Researchers at the university have been studying the oily compounds of the plants that make the skin blister and itch to create less-toxic forms of the oil, which allow the body to tolerate the plants in the laboratory.

polyarteritis nodosa See SYSTEMIC NECROTIZING VASCULITIDES.

polychondritis, relapsing See RELAPSING POLYCHONDRITIS.

polycystic ovary syndrome See STEIN-LEVENTHAL SYNDROME.

polymorphic light eruption An allergic reaction to certain wavelengths of the sun that affects 10 percent of the population, causing bumpy, scaling, blistering, itchy or red patches hours or days after exposure to the sun. More women than men are affected by this condition, which usually appears between adolescence and the 30s. See also SOLAR URTICARIA; PHOTOSENSITIZING DISORDERS.

Symptoms The eruption is characterized by red macules, papules, plaques and blisters, and begins anywhere between an hour and 24 to 36 hours after exposure to the sun, and lasts three to five days. The itch can be quite severe.

Treatment Avoid the sun and always use a sunscreen of at least SPF 15; patients tend to improve as the summer progresses. Slow exposure to the sun can increase tolerance. Nonprescription topical steroids or prescription steroids and antihistamines also may be effective.

polymyositis-dermatomyositis A rare systemic connective-tissue disease characterized by inflamed, weak muscles with or without rash. The disorder may affect children under age 10 and adults between ages 40 and 60. There have been reports of cases associated with cancer in up to 40 percent of adult cases.

The course of this disease varies and is unpredictable, lasting for many years or sometimes leading to death within 12 months.

Symptoms Reddish purple discolored swollen eyelids, scaly red flush over the cheeks and forehead, red papules over the surfaces of finger joints, and a dusky red rash on the arms and upper back, plus pigment changes of the skin (POIKILODERMA).

Treatment Corticosteroids may be given in the early stages; the disease may be chronic, requiring therapy for years. In those who fail to respond to steroids, immunosuppressive drugs (such as METHOTREXATE, cyclophosphamide, azathioprine and chlorambucil) may be effective. A combination of corticosteroids and methotrexate is probably most

effective, especially in childhood dermatomyositis.

polymyxins A group of antibiotics derived from the bacterium *Bacillus polymyxa* used to treat infections of the skin. These drugs, which include colistin and polymyxin B, are often given as drops or in ointment form and are often used in antibiotic eye drops or skin ointments. Taken orally, colistin is associated with pseudomembranous enterocolitis—a severe, life-threatening type of diarrhea sometimes caused by antibiotics.

pompholyx The appearance of VESICLES on the hands or feet without known cause. Once called dyshidrotic pompholyx, this term is no longer used since the sweat glands play no part in the disease's cause. *Pompholyx* means "bubble" in Greek and the words simply denote a blistering eczema of the palms and soles, respectively.

Symptoms In general the blisters are found on the sides of the fingers, spreading to the central palms and the soles of the feet. They often merge into large bullae (see BULLA). Itching is intense and secondary infection is common (especially on the feet). In some cases on the hands are initially affected and in other cases the reverse is true.

Treatment Low- or mid-potency steroids are often not very effective; high potency steroids are required. Soaking the hands in a potassium permanganate solution, normal saline or BUROW'S SOLUTION for 10 or 15 minutes followed by WET DRESSINGS (0.05 percent silver nitrate solution or shake lotions) gives rapid relief. However, the silver nitrate or potassium permanganate may stain the hands.

pore The tiny opening of the sebaceous (oil) or SWEAT GLANDS at the skin's surface, called the follicular orifice in the medical profession. The size of a pore is regulated by heredity, and contrary to popular opinion, it's not possible to shrink large pores. In addition, hot water doesn't open pores, and cold water doesn't close them.

You can make pores *appear* smaller by using an alcohol-base astringent that contains aluminum chloride or aluminum hydroxide. This will temporarily reduce oiliness and minimize light reflection, which can magnify pore size. In addition, RETIN-A and prescription strength GLYCOLIC ACID can refine the skin's texture, which may also help pores *look* smaller.

Women can also use a water-based foundation and powder to make pores look smoother and more even.

porokeratosis A disorder of keratinization that includes three separate autosomal dominant syndromes, all featuring a lesion with a raised border and central furrow or depression; the center may be scaly or atrophic.

In *porokeratosis of Mibelli,* the lesions—crater-like patches with a raised border that enlarge to form lesions—may appear anywhere on the body, either alone or in groups arranged in a line or in segments. This rare, chronic progressive skin disorder is seen usually in males and first appears in early childhood (usually before age 10). Lesions slowly enlarge as the child grows older.

Disseminated superficial actinic porokeratosis is an autosomal dominant skin disorder occurring on sun-exposed areas in fair-skinned individuals (usually women) over age 16. It is characterized by many brownish red macules with depressed centers and sharply-ridged borders. The palms and soles are spared. Unlike the Mibelli form, the border of the lesion is less distinct, the centers of the lesions are not as atrophied and they are often itchy. Number of lesions will increase with time.

The lesions of *porokeratosis plantaris, palmaris et disseminata* are most similar to those of disseminated superficial actinic porokeratosis, although they occur at an earlier age (in the second decade) and lesions first appear on palms and soles. The number of lesions will increase with time.

Treatment Because of the danger of the development of SQUAMOUS CELL CARCINOMA, albeit small (especially in the Mibelli type), physicians should follow this disease closely. FLUOROURACIL 2 percent or 5 percent cream applied twice daily for three weeks may be useful in some patients.

In the Mibelli form, surgical removal of small lesions (especially on arms and legs) may be effective.

Patients with the disseminated superficial actinic form should avoid sunlight and use sunscreens. Lesions (if not too numerous) may be treated with LIQUID NITROGEN.

porphyria A group of rare, inherited disorders that cause a rash or skin blistering that in some instances is brought on by sunlight, as a result of abnormalities of the metabolism of chemicals in the body called "porphyrins." The diseases result in the increased production and excretion of porphyrins; each type has distinct clinical, biochemical and genetic features.

Cause Porphyrins are involved in the manufacture of heme, a component of hemoglobin (the oxygen-carrying pigment in the blood). When blocks occur in the chemical process that produces heme, porphyrins build up.

Porphyria includes the more common types of acute intermittent porphyria, variegate porphyria and porphyria cutanea tarda, and rare varieties, including hereditary coproporphyria, protoporphyria and congenital erythropoietic porphyria.

Estimates of the combined prevalence of the disease in the United States is about 1 per 10,000 to 50,000.

Symptoms Porphyrias with skin symptoms include variegate porphyria and hereditary coproporphyria, both of which cause blistering of sun-exposed skin, together with abdominal pain, cramps in the arms and legs, muscle weakness, psychiatric disturbances etc. Attacks also may be brought on by a variety of drugs, including barbiturates, phenytoin, birth control pills and tetracyclines. Porphyria cutanea tarda causes blistering skin, but there are no abdominal or nervous system problems. In this variety, wounds are slow to heal and the urine may be pink or brown. Protoporphyria often causes mild skin symptoms after exposure to sunlight, such as burning and stinging without blister formation.

Treatment Specific treatment depends on the variety of porphyria. For prophyria cutanea tarda, avoiding causative agents such as alcohol and estrogen and treatment with phlebotomy and/or antimalerials such as hydroxychloroquine is recommended.

Portuguese man-of-war stings See JELLY-FISH STINGS.

port-wine stain The common name for nevus flammeus, a permanent large purple-red birthmark. Present at birth, port-wine stains are usually sharply outlined and flat, although the surface may sometimes have a pebbly feel. Most commonly appearing on the face, they can range in size from a few milimeters in diameter to half the body's surface. They do not grow as a child grows, but they become darker and raised over time.

Port-wine stains may appear by themselves as part of a multisystem disorder, such as STURGE-WEBER SYNDROME, which also features seizures and eye abnormalities such as glaucoma.

Treatment A simple port-wine stain, when it does not occur as part of another syndrome, is primarily a cosmetic problem. If treated early in childhood, the psychological burden on the family and the child may be relieved. Pulsed dye laser therapy to remove the stain is the most effective treatment.

Until the late 1980s, the argon laser was the treatment of choice for these birthmarks.

The laser works by emitting light that is absorbed by the hemoglobin in the dilated blood vessels that make up the birthmark. However, this therapy is limited because of its substantial rate of scarring—the continually delivered laser energy dissipates into the surrounding dermis, causing thermal damage. Less-than-optimum treatment can result in pale, immature port-wine stains. In addition, the extent of clearing and the rate of scarring is highly dependent on the skill and experience of the operator.

Choosing a wavelength that is more selectively absorbed by hemoglobin and delivering it in a pulse shorter than the cooling time of the abnormal vessel produces better results.

The most successful method of laser treatment employs the pulsed dye laser, popular because it has a low rate of scarring and its effectiveness is not as dependent on an operator's experience. In one study, 34 of 36 port-wine stains in children treated with the pulsed-dye laser cleared up completely without adverse effects after an average of 6.5 treatments, regardless of the age of the patient, the location of the lesion, or its color. Atrophic scarring developed in only two cases.

In larger studies of infants (6 to 30 weeks) and children, substantial but incomplete removal occurred in the majority of cases, without serious side effects.

Excision and grafting for smaller lesions, or tattooing for larger ones, are alternative treatments. CAMOUFLAGE COSMETICS also may be used to mask lesions.

postherpetic neuralgia Pain that occurs six weeks following an outbreak of SHINGLES. Because they are damaged after a shingles attack, nerves produce strong pain impulses even after the shingles blisters heal; this pain may last for months or years. The older the patient and more severe the shingles, the more likely postherpetic neuralgia will occur.

Zostrix (capsaicin) is a derivative of red pepper and may be effective in relieving the postherpetic neuralgia.

potassium iodide A simple chemical that has been used for a century to effectively treat lymphatic SPOROTRICHOSIS (chronic fungal skin infection). In saturated solution, it is prescribed on a slowly increasing dose until adverse effects appear, or until a response is noted. Potassium iodide is not effective against any other fungal infection.
Side effects Common side effects include acne-like lesions, nausea and vomiting, and hypothyroidism.

potassium para-aminobenzoate A chemical used to treat lichen sclerosis et atrophicus and SCLERODERMA. However, there is little scientific evidence that it works.

potassium permanganate An antiseptic drug with an astringent effect on the skin useful in treating inflammation (DERMATITIS). It is applied directly to the skin, as a dressing, or dissolved in water for a soak.

Once a popular remedy for dermatitis, its staining skin, nails and clothing purple has caused this drug to lose favor among physicians. Moreover, if not fully dissolved, potassium permanganate can cause a chemical burn on contact with skin.

poultice A warm pack made of a soft, moist substance such as kaolin (white clay) spread between layers of soft fabric as a way of providing moist heat to the skin. In the past, poultices were widely used to reduce pain or inflammation and improve circulation in a particular area, or to soften the skin to allow matter to be expressed from a boil. Poultices containing kaolin retain heat for a long period of time.

precancerous conditions Conditions in which cancer has a tendency to develop. Pre-cancerous conditions of the skin include AC-TINIC KERATOSES, DYSPLASTIC (or atypical) NEVI, LENTIGO MALIGNA, BOWEN'S DISEASE, and SQUAMOUS CELL CARCINOMA in-situ.

pregnancy and the skin A wide variety of skin changes can be brought about by pregnancy. While it is true that many women notice an improvement in the condition of their skin during pregnancy, some annoying skin problems also can occur. Changes during pregnancy may also be associated with pre-existing skin conditions such as ACNE, ATOPIC DERMATITIS and PSORIASIS.

Some of the many skin changes that arise during pregnancy include itchiness, stretch marks, blood vessel overgrowths and broken blood vessels, mole growth or darkening, and skin darkening in patches or all over.
Normal skin changes A certain number of physiological changes occur in the skin because of hormonal changes that take place during pregnancy. While they don't affect health, they may be psychologically distressing. About 90 percent of pregnant women experience an increase in pigmentation, usually a mild darkening of areas of the body that are already darkly pigmented (such as the underarms, the nipple and areolae, vulva, anus and inner thighs). A dark line often appears in the middle of the abdomen from the pubic bone to the belly button. (This line is already present on the skin, but doesn't really become visible until pregnancy).

Ordinary FRECKLES, some scars and many MOLES may also darken. These are harmless, but since malignant melanomas and premalignant DYSPLASTIC NEVI are sensitive to hormonal change, any suspicious-looking moles should be brought to the attention of a physician. Hyperpigmentation is usually most pronounced among dark-haired, dark-skinned women and usually begins in the first trimester, continuing throughout the nine months and usually fading after the birth. Generally, however, the sites that became darkened never return to their exact pre-pregnancy color.

Melasma Called the "mask of pregnancy," or chloasma, this is a special type of hyperpigmentation affecting the face that may appear in up to 75 percent of all pregnancies. It is more common in dark-skinned women, is often worsened by sun exposure, and also occurs in up to one-third of women on birth control pills. It has been suggested that this condition may be hereditary.

Pruritus gravidarum This common disorder is characterized by itching, which in some is mild and in others is generalized and severe. It occurs in the third trimester and disappears after the birth, but tends to recur with subsequent pregnancies or with the administration of birth control pills. Symptoms include itching over the entire body, loss of appetite, nausea and vomiting.

PUPPP Another common disorder is pruritic urticarial papules and plaques of pregnancy (PUPPP), which appears during the third trimester only in first pregnancies and is characterized by itching and red papules that resemble HIVES. They usually begin on the abdomen and later spread onto the thighs, buttocks and arms. There is no increase in fetal problems or death associated with this syndrome. Patients usually respond to antihistamines and topical corticosteroids, although some women need a brief course of oral corticosteroids to control the itching. The disease does not reappear after birth, nor is there a recurrence with birth control pills or subsequent pregnancies.

Papular dermatitis Spangler's dermatitis of pregnancy is a rare, severely itchy disorder that may begin at any time during the nine months. It is associated with a 30 percent chance of stillbirth or spontaneous abortion. The disorder, which can recur during subsequent pregnancies, may be characterized by red papules that become crusted and excoriated, followed by a darkening of skin after the lesions fade. The disorder is treated with oral corticosteroids.

Immune progesterone dermatitis of pregnancy This rare disorder of the first three months of pregnancy is characterized by papules and pustules on the arms, legs and buttocks that may resemble ACNE or PSORIASIS. The problem may recur with subsequent pregnancies. Administration of estrogens can suppress the lesions, which may be brought on by the administration of birth control pills with progesterone.

Herpes gestationis This unusual autoimmune blistering disorder is similar to bullous pemphigoid. It appears in one in 50,000 pregnancies, can occur at any time during pregnancy and is characterized by blistering and itching. It is treated with topical and sometimes systemic steroids. There is no conclusive proof that it is associated with an increased risk for fetal injury and death. There is a tendency for the condition to recur, with increased severity, in subsequent pregnancies.

Prurigo gestationis of Besnier This third-trimester disorder is characterized by small papules that are crusted and excoriated on the arms, backs of hands, tops of feet, thighs, legs and trunk. It is not associated with any fetal or maternal problems.

Impetigo herpetiformis This type of pustular PSORIASIS occurs primarily during the third trimester and may occur during subsequent pregnancies. It is thought to be associated with a significant increase in death rates for mother or child. Associated with hypoparathyroidism, it is characterized by symptoms such as fever, chills, prostration, vomiting, diarrhea, convulsions and weight loss. Skin symptoms include red macules followed by sterile pustules, especially in body folds and mucous membranes. The individual lesions may itch and burn. Treatment is the same as for pustular psoriasis, except for antimetabolites or ETRETINATE are avoided.

Jaundice This yellowing of the skin may appear during the last trimester, caused by obstruction of liver ducts. It is not usually a serious problem and resolves quickly after delivery.

Blood vessel lesions Vascular spider angiomas caused by circulating estrogens appear in the first or second trimester, but most (75 percent) have already faded seven weeks after the birth. Spider veins and varicose veins may also occur.

pressure sores See BEDSORES; PRESSURE INJURIES.

pressure injuries, chronic Continuous pressure on the skin can cause several different problems, including CORNS, calluses and DECUBITUS ULCERS (pressure sores). Trauma to the skin thickens the STRATUM CORNEUM. A corn appears when there is focal pressure over a bony prominence or a bone spur. Although they are most common on the foot, calluses, which are larger and less focal than corns, can form on any surface where there is recurrent pressure or friction (such as the soles of runners' feet, the fingers of guitar players, or the middle finger of people frequently holding a pencil or pen).

The initial thickening of the stratum corneum is an attempt by the skin to protect itself; pain and fissures may develop if the pressure continues. Eliminating this pressure or friction usually produces a permanent cure, but sometimes surgical removal may be necessary. Special inserts in shoes, wearing two pairs of sox, and wearing well-fit shoes may help to prevent the cause of sores.

Pressure sores form over any bony prominence (especially on the heels, base of the spine, and elbows) and are caused by continual pressure on the skin, which interferes with blood flow in patients who are unconscious, bedridden or who have abnormal sensations. The process is affected by a person's age, nutrition, and general physical shape.

Prevention Skilled, vigilant nursing care can prevent most of these ulcers from forming; any reddened area should receive special attention. Bedridden patients should be turned every two hours to distribute their weight, and the skin should be kept clean and dry. Urine and feces should be promptly removed before they irritate the skin; dusting powder may also help. Other preventive aids include sheepskins, water and air mattresses, and foam rings.

pretibial fever See LEPTOSPIROSIS.

prickle cell layer See STRATUM SPINOSUM.

prickly heat An irritating skin rash also known as heat rash, that is associated with obstruction of the SWEAT GLANDS and accompanied by aggravating prickly feelings. The medical term for prickly heat, miliaria rubra, or "red millet seeds," refers to the appearance of the rash. A milder form of the condition, miliaria crystallina, sometimes appears first as clear, shiny, fluid-filled blisters that dry up without treatment.

Symptoms Numerous tiny, red itchy spots occur, covering mildly inflamed parts of the skin where the sweat collects (especially the waist, upper trunk, armpits and insides of the elbows). With prickly heat it is comfortable to sleep only in cool surroundings, and lack of sleep and intense skin irritation can make the patient irritable.

Cause While physicians aren't completely sure of the mechanism behind the development of prickly heat, it is thought to be associated with sweat that is trapped in the skin.

Treatment Slow acclimation to hot weather will reduce the chance of prickly heat. Avoiding heavy activities in the heat will also help prevent the problem. Frequent cool showers and sponging the area will relieve the itching. Calamine lotion and dusting powder may also ease the discomfort. Clothing should be clean, dry, starch-free and loose to help sweat evaporate. Sweating from fever can be reduced with anti-pyretic drugs such as acetaminophen.

procarbazine (Matulane) A chemotherapy drug used to treat certain cancers of the skin, among other conditions. It inhibits grown of cancer cells by preventing cell division.
Adverse reactions In addition to typical anti-cancer drug side effects, which include nausea and vomiting, procarbazine may cause a sudden rise in blood pressure if taken with certain foods or drinks (such as cheese or red wine), which can be fatal.

progeria A rare autosomal recessive disorder characterized by premature old age, including excessive wrinkling of the skin. The condition is usually diagnosed at 6 to 12 months of age. The two forms of this disease are both very rare. In *Hutchinson-Gilford* syndrome, aging starts around age four; within eight years the affected child has all the external features of old age, including sagging skin on face and trunk, baldness, loss of fat, together with internal degenerative changes. Death usually occurs at puberty. *Werner's syndrome,* or adult progeria, begins in early adult life and follows the same rapid progression as the juvenile form. Most patients die during their adolescence.
Cause Unknown. Cells taken from affected patients show only a few generations of cell division before they stop reproducing, instead of the 50 generations that occur in cells from healthy youngsters.

progressive systemic sclerosis See SCLERO-DERMA.

prolidase deficiency A rare inherited disease in which the enzyme prolidase is absent. Skin symptoms include chronic recurrent ulcers of the lower legs, diffuse spider veins (TELANGIECTASIA) and shallow scarring with darkened skin color over face and buttocks.

Other skin symptoms include fragile skin; purple papules (PURPURA); gray hair; reddened fissures of hands and feet; papular lesions on face, arms and legs; and dry crusted areas on face and buttocks.

Other findings associated with this enzyme deficiency include nose abnormalities, jaw problems, multiple dental cavities, mental retardation, joint problems and recurrent ear and sinus infections. There is no treatment.

promethazine An antihistamine drug used to relieve itching in a variety of skin conditions, including HIVES and ECZEMA. The drug is also used to relieve nausea and vomiting, and as a premedication sedative.
Adverse effects Dry mouth, blurred vision and drowsiness.

Propionibacterium acnes A type of bacterium that is one of the more important factors in the development of ACNE. *P. acnes* is found deep in the sebaceous follicle. While it is important in the development of inflammatory acne, acne is not a bacterial infection; instead, inflammation probably stems from the effect of the byproducts of this bacterium within the cell.

propylene glycol A substance used to improve spreadability of a topical product that can worsen ACNE.

protozal infections Infection caused by single-celled animals account for a number of skin conditions, including LEISHMANIASIS, TRYPANOSOMIASIS, amebiasis, TRICHOMONIASIS and TOXOPLASMOSIS. See also PARASITIC INFECTIONS.

prurigo The general term for several itchy skin eruptions consisting of dome-shaped PAPULES and nodules. See also PRURIGO NODULARIS.

prurigo nodularis A skin condition characterized by intense itching. It is believed that the disease may represent some problem with skin sensory innervation. It primarily affects middle-aged women and drives affected individuals to pick and dig at their skin. Repeated picking produces nodular lesions. Lesions are found most often on the upper back, back of the neck, arms and shins. They are skin-colored with a warty, rounded surface topped by a crust.

Treatment There is no one specific treatment for this condition but picking must be stopped. Topical or intralesional steroids are often administered, while some patients respond slowly to a modified GOECKERMAN REGIMEN of tar ointments and daily exposure to ultraviolet-B light (UVB). CRYOTHERAPY also may be helpful in treating the lesions.

pruritic urticarial papules and plaques of pregnancy (PUPPP) A common disorder that appears during the third trimester of pregnancy characterized by itching and red papules that resemble HIVES. Lesions may first appear in the abdominal area, spreading to the thighs, buttocks and arms. The lesions usually fade away within one or two weeks after the birth. There is no evidence of death of either the fetus or the mother.

The disorder, which appears in one out of every 300 first-time pregnancies, does not occur in repeat pregnancies.

Treatment Antihistamines (for itching) and topical corticosteroids are effective, although initial control may require a brief course of oral corticosteroids. The disorder does not reappear after birth, nor does it recur with subsequent pregnancies or with the use of birth control pills.

See also PREGNANCY AND THE SKIN.

pruritis gravidarum This common itchy condition, also known as intrahepatic cholestasis of pregnancy, usually appears in up to 2.4 percent of pregnancies during the last tri-

mester and disappears after birth. This reversible condition, which appears to have a genetic component, causes itching without producing primary skin lesions. It tends to recur with subsequent pregnancies or with birth control pill use.

While the health of the mother is not affected by this condition, its effect on the fetus is more controversial. Some experts report premature births and intrauterine asphyxia among infants whose mothers have the condition, but most argue that there is no fetal risk.

Symptoms Itching that is localized at first and then spreads over the entire body may be associated with anorexia, nausea and vomiting and, rarely, jaundice. The liver may be enlarged and tender; stools are clay-colored and urine dark.

Cause Unknown, but lab studies reveal elevated bilirubin (a bile pigment); the itchiness is proportional to the concentration of bile acid in the skin (not the blood). Placental estrogens and progestins are believed to interfere with the liver's excretion of bile acids.

Treatment While the itching can be severe, it virtually always ceases after the birth. Oatmeal baths and antihistamines are effective, although in a few cases more aggressive treatment is necessary, involving the administration of cholestyramine and vitamin K. Phenobarbital has been effective in promoting bile excretion.

pruritus Itching.

pseudoacanthosis nigricans See ACANTHOSIS NIGRICANS.

pseudofolliculitis barbae (of the beard) A condition of ingrown hairs in the beard area very common among black patients but occurring in either sex on any part of the body that is shaved. Shaving increases the chances of this problem by sharpening the free hair end. Also, short, curly hairs are more likely to penetrate the skin than long straight ones.

Pseudofolliculitis may occur in any shaved location, but the beard area is the most common site of the problem. While early lesions include reddened papules with pustules, those who have suffered with the problem for a long time have firm, hyperpigmented papules.

Symptoms Numerous inflammatory papules and pustules (ranging from just a few to hundreds) in any hairy area (usually the beard) together with darker skin color. The disease disappears if the beard or other hair is allowed to grow.

Treatment The best treatment is to discontinue shaving, which will reduce the appearance of new lesions, ultimately allowing some of the embedded hairs to be released from the skin. As the beard grows, apply warm-water compresses for 10 minutes, three times daily to smooth lesions and remove crusts. The beard may be trimmed during this time, but to no shorter than half an inch. Release ingrown hairs each day with a clean toothpick or sterile needle; *do not pluck, since this may cause more irritation when the hair breaks through the hair follicle.* After releasing the hair, apply a topical corticosteroid lotion. If there is infection, systemic antibiotics may be prescribed.

If the beard must be shaved, avoid a close shave to stop the immediate penetration by sharpened hairs. Before shaving, first scrub your face with an abrasive soap and rough washcloth to loosen embedded hairs. Then, massage areas of ingrown hairs with a toothbrush. Rinse face after shaving with water, and apply warm-water compresses for several minutes. Next, apply shaving cream. Use a single-blade razor (not a double blade) and shave only with the grain, in one direction, using short, even strokes. Some people find relief with special razors designed to prevent a close shave, and some electric shavers are also designed to prevent close shaving. Don't

pull the skin tight, since the released skin falls on the stubble and causes more shaving bumps. Release any ingrown hairs after shaving, and then apply a nonirritating aftershave. If the lotion causes any itching or burning, try a prescribed topical corticosteroid lotion instead.

Alternatively, chemical hair-removers may be effective. For some people, topical RETIN-A (tretinoin) or glycolic acid is effective over the long term, although heightened irritation may occur at first. (See also PSEUDOFOLLICULITIS BARBAE PROJECT; BLACK SKIN.)

Pseudofolliculitis Barbae Project An association that seeks solutions for patients with PSEUDOFOLLICULITIS BARBAE (PFB), a skin disorder primarily of black men characterized by a bump-like rash on the face, aggravated by shaving. Because there is no cure for the problem, the best solution is to allow the beard to grow. The project believes that individuals who suffer from the disorder and are forced to shave by employers are victims of racial discrimination. Therefore, it provides legal assistance to those who may be discriminated against because of PFB. The project supports research on PFB and maintains a library. (See also BLACK SKIN; Appendix D.)

pseudoxanthoma elasticum A chronic hereditary disease involving abnormalities in connective tissue, resulting in fragmentation and calcification of elastic fibers. The condition is characterized by yellow-tan papules in areas of the skin that crease and are flexed in the presence of gastrointestinal hemorrhage. There are four different forms of pseudoxanthoma elasticum, two caused by autosomal recessive inheritance (the most common) and two caused by autosomal dominant inheritance. The condition is a genetic autosomal dominant trait, which means that only one defective gene (from one parent) is needed to cause the syndrome.

One of any of the four types of this condition can appear in one out of every 40,000 live births.

Symptoms Skin symptoms include thickened, yellow-tan skin that has lost its elastic capability appearing in mucous membranes of the mouth, cheek and inner lips, in the armpits, groin, the navel and the neck. Other general characteristics of the disorder include vision problems caused by hemorrhages in the retina, persistent high blood pressure, severe chest pain and dizzy spells. There are also visual and speech problems and transient ischemic attacks (brief, minor strokes), with abdominal pain and severe pain in the calf muscle. While intelligence is not affected, the lifespan is considerably shortened because of the complications of internal bleeding and arterial blocks.

Treatment There is no treatment for this disorder.

psoralens Organic compounds found in many plants such as limes, lemons, celery and parsnips that stimulate the formation of MELANIN in combination with ultraviolet light (UVA). Capable of inducing phototoxic reactions in the skin when exposed to sunlight, this substance, ironically, is now being studied for its therapeutic benefits.

Many years ago, a Cairo dermatologist found out that indigenous people along the Nile used plants containing oil of bergamot (contained in some fruits and vegetables) as a folk remedy to treat VITILIGO, a skin disorder in which the immune system attacks and destroys the skin's pigment. While researchers aren't sure why it works, they believe that psoralens, when combined with sunlight, may suppress the immune system and stop the attack on the skin's pigment while stimulating melanin production. Psoralens also stops cell from making DNA, eventually killing them, which may explain why it helps those with disorders characterized by rapid cell replication, such as PSORIASIS.

Psoralens, together with ultraviolet light-A (UVA), is the most commonly used form of photochemotherapy. Called psoralen-UVA (or PUVA), it became clinically available in the mid-1970s. PUVA therapy consists of oral or topical administration of a psoralen and irradiation of the skin with UVA light. The most widely used psoralen in the United States is 8–methoxypsoralen, administered orally and followed by a one-hour exposure to UVA. PUVA may interfere with the migration of inflammatory cells to the skin, and is highly effective in the management of psoriasis (it alleviates the problem in almost 90 percent of cases). It may also be used in the treatment of other forms of psoriasis, for cutaneous T-cell lymphomas, atopic dermatitis, LICHEN PLANUS and vitiligo.

Psoralen alone may produce itching and nausea in a small number of patients, and the risks of PUVA can be either acute or chronic. Sunburn-like redness may occur together with blisters. These effects can be prevented by carefully assessing dose. However, the chronic long-term toxicity is not yet determined. PUVA is known to be carcinogenic in experimental situations. Hyperpigmentation occurs in most patients, and some experience LENTIGINES and mottling of skin color. The risk of premature aging of the skin, ACTINIC KERATOSES, BOWEN'S DISEASE and SQUAMOUS CELL CARCINOMA is increased. Prior skin cancer, previous exposure to ionizing radiation, arsenic ingestion and (perhaps) the previous use of tar preparations may increase the chance of abnormal growths in those patients. The formation of cataracts is another risk, although there have been few reports of premature cataracts in those patients treated with PUVA without eye protection.

psoriasis A chronic skin disorder affecting more than 4 million men and women, producing silvery, scaly plaques on the skin. The most common type of psoriasis is called plaque psoriasis (or psoriasis vulgaris), characterized by raised, inflamed lesions covered with silver-white scales. Other, far less common forms include pustular, guttate, inverse and erythrodermic psoriasis. In erythrodermic psoriasis, red scaly involvement of the entire skin makes temperature and fluid control difficult, placing a signficiant strain on internal organs such as the heart and kidneys, that may require hospitalization.

Psoriasis usually starts in adolescence or after age 60, affecting 2 percent of the population.

The condition is considered mild if only 10 percent or less of the body is affected; 10 to 30 percent involvement indicates a moderate problem, and psoriasis over more than 30 percent of the body is considered severe. The *location* of the symptoms, more than the extent, influences how disabling the condition may be. Psoriasis only on the palms and soles of the feet can be physically disabling, while psoriasis on the face can be emotionally disabling.

Normally, a person with psoriasis experiences cycles of improvement and flare-ups; the disease can go into remission for a periods ranging from one to 60 years.

Cause The cause of psoriasis is unknown, although researchers believe that some type of biochemical stimulus triggers the abnormal cell growth in the epidermis. While normal skin cells take a month to mature, patients with psoriasis have skin cells that over-multiply, forcing the cells to move up to the top of the skin in only seven days. As the number of cells builds up, the epidermis thickens and the extra cells pile up in raised, red and scaly lesions. The white scale(s) covering the red lesion(s) is made up of dead cells that are continually shed; the inflammation is caused by the buildup of blood needed to feed the rapidly dividing cells.

Skin trauma, emotional stress and some kinds of infection may trigger the development of psoriasis. The condition sometimes forms at the site of a surgical incision or after a drug reaction. Psoriasis that appears after trauma is known as the "Koebner phenomenon." Alcohol abuse makes psoriasis more aggressive and more difficult to treat and control.

Symptoms The first lesions of plaque psoriasis appear as red, dotty spots that can be very small; these eruptions slowly get larger, producing a silvery white surface scale that is shed easily. When forcibly removed, the scales may leave tiny bleeding points known as the AUSPITZ'S SIGN. The plaques, which often appear in the same place on the right and left sides of the body, often cover large areas of skin, merging into one another. The most common sites are elbows, scalp, and genitals. Lesions vary in size and shape from one person to another.

While anyone can develop psoriasis, there appears to be a hereditary link and a family association in one out of three cases. It is not known whether just one gene or a collection predisposes a person to the condition, but it is believed that one gene modified by others in combination with certain environmental factors produces psoriasis. This may be why there is not one pattern of inheritance from one generation to another.

Both men and women can develop psoriasis at any age, but most patients develop lesions between ages 10 and 35 or after age 60, although a few people may contract the disease in early childhood or even infancy.

Certain races do seem more susceptible to developing psoriasis. Caucasians have the highest percentage, although East Africans are also at risk; African Americans have a low incidence of the disease, probably because their origins are primarily West African.

The most common places to find the scaly patches are on the scalp, elbow, knees and trunk, although they can be found anywhere on the body. Patches spread over wide expanses of skin can lead to intense itching, skin pain, dry or cracking skin and swelling;

body movement and flexibility may also be affected.

Potentially more disabling than the physical discomfort of psoriasis is the emotional impact of a potentially disfiguring disease. Psoriasis can be unsightly and erode self-confidence, inducing depression, guilt or anger.

Complications About 10 percent of patients develop psoriatic arthritis. Mild cases are milder than rheumatoid arthritis but in several cases can be very disabling. Psoriatic arthritis causes inflammation and stiffness, often affecting the fingers and toes.

Diagnosis Psoriasis is usually diagnosed by observation. There are no blood tests for the disease, although physicians sometimes examine a skin biopsy under the microscope to confirm the diagnosis. Sometimes small pits in the fingernails, yellow discoloration of the nail or collections of scaly skin under the nail can help to diagnose the condition.

Treatment There is no cure for psoriasis, but there are treatments that can clear plaques or significantly improve the skin's appearance. Treatment is aimed at slowing the excessive cell division, resulting in remissions lasting up to a year or more. Once the treatment is effective, it is discontinued until the psoriasis returns. Type of treatment depends on the type of psoriasis, its location and severity, patient age, and medical history.

Topical medications (EMOLLIENTS, steroids, Vitamin D derivatives, ANTHRALIN and COAL TAR preparations) are used for mild to moderate psoriasis. These may be used alone or in combination with each other or with ultraviolet light (UV-B). Regular sunbathing may help clear up a case of psoriasis for some patients because of the exposure to natural UV-B.

For more severe cases, the topical treatments above will be combined with psoralen plus UV-A, chemotherapy (methotrexate) and oral retinoid medications (Tegison). Treatments for severe psoriasis are toxic and must be weighed against their potential risks.

Dermatologists usually begin with the mildest therapy and work up to the one that is most effective in clearing up the skin problem. No single treatment works for everyone, and each patient reacts differently to the drugs.

For more information, contact the National Psoriasis Foundation, 6600 S.W. 92nd Avenue, Suite 300, Portland, OR 97223; request publications at (800) 248–0886.

Psoriasis Research Institute A professional group that creates projects for the study, diagnosis, treatment and eventual cure of PSORIASIS. The institute collects and disseminates information about psoriasis. It maintains a Psoriasis Medical Center, which offers advanced treatment programs and equipment to treat all aspects of the disease, counseling and biofeedback stress control. The institute compiles statistics, conducts epidemiological studies of patients, and sponsors monthly self-help workshops for patients using audiovisual presentations, written materials and discussions. It was formerly known as the International Psoriasis Research Foundation.

Founded in 1979, the group hosts the quadrennial International Psoriasis Symposium. It publishes the thrice yearly *Psoriasis Newsletter* that contains innovative treatment concepts, patient education tips and updates on basic science and clinical research programs. The institute also publishes the brochure *Psoriasis Medical Center*, research papers and pamphlets. For address, see Appendix D.

psoriasiform A medical term meaning "like PSORIASIS." It refers to any sharply-marginated plaque with thick scales.

psoriatic arthritis About 5 to 10 percent of patients develop psoriatic arthritis that is similar to, but milder than, rheumatoid arthritis. It may appear at any age, although it occurs most often during the 40s or 50s. There are five distinct forms of arthritis associated with PSORIASIS; the most common is a nonsymmetric type primarily affecting the hand joints.

As with psoriasis, the reason behind the development of arthritis is unknown but both genetic and environmental factors seem to play a role. It most commonly occurs in those with severe skin disease, especially with nail involvement. Usually, the skin symptoms of psoriasis occur before the arthritis.

Symptoms Psoriatic arthritis causes inflammation and stiffness often affecting a variety of joints from the low back to the hips, knees, ankles and wrists, to small joints of the hands and feet. The degree of arthritis doesn't correlate with the extent of skin involvement, but it usually improves as the psoriasis goes into remission.

Treatment Nonsteroidal anti-inflammatory agents (NSAIDs) are prescribed, although there may be a risk of worsening associated skin disease with these drugs. Steroid injections, oral gold, immunosuppressive therapy and surgery are used for difficult cases. Oral steroid therapy usually has no role in the management of this disorder. Methotrexate and PUVA may control the arthritis and the skin condition, which suggests the common role of inflammation in both diseases.

pulsed dye laser A type of laser that uses flashes of light that are only a few millionths of a second long, which is unlike the argon laser, which requires a continuous beam of light. Also unlike the argon laser, the pulsed dye laser emits light with a wavelength that is only absorbed by the target.

For instance, in use with blood vessels, only yellow light is used to target hemoglobin—the substance that gives blood its red color. As a result, when used to treat birth defects of blood vessels, only the abnormal blood vessels are destroyed; surrounding tissue is left undamaged by the laser light. In treating pigment disorders such as liver spots

and cafe au lait macules, green light is chosen to target the melanin.

This type of laser is particularly effective in removing birthmarks such as PORT WINE STAINS. The argon laser, once the preferred means of destroying the cluster of small blood vessels staining the skin, can cause heavy scarring, especially in children.

PUPPP See PRURITIC URTICARIAL PAPULES AND PLAQUES OF PREGNANCY.

purpura A group of disorders characterized by purplish or reddish brown areas of discoloration, visible through the skin and caused by bleeding within underlying tissue. "Purpura" also refers to the discolored purple areas themselves, which range from the size of a pinhead to an inch in diameter. Smaller bleeding points are called PETECHIAE; larger areas of discoloration are called BRUISES or ecchymoses.

Causes/Symptoms Common purpura (or senile purpura) is the most common of all bleeding disorders. It affects mostly middle-aged or elderly women, causing large discolored areas on the thighs but especially on backs of the hands and forearms, the result of thinning of the tissues supporting blood vessels beneath the skin. Bleeding may also be seen in the membrane lining the mouth.

Purpura caused by a lack of platelets in the blood, called thrombocytopenia, is usually the result of a disease of the bone marrow such as leukemia or aplastic anemia, or a side effect of drugs or excessive radiation.

Henoch-Schonlein purpura (or anaphylactoid purpura) is caused by inflammation of blood vessels in the skin, and is associated with inflammation of blood vessels in the gut, joints and kidney as well.

Other types of purpura can be found in SCURVY, resulting from a vitamin C deficiency, and in certain infections, autoimmune disorders, blood poisoning, or blood chemical disturbances.

Treatment Common purpura is difficult to treat. Avoidance of systemic and topical steroids are advised as they thin the skin even further. Avoiding trauma (even that as gentle as a slap on the wrist) is essential. Henoch-Schonlein purpura responds only to immunosuppressant drugs and systemic corticosteroids. In severe cases, plasmapheresis (removal of blood, replacement of plasma and retransfusion) can be effective. Platelet deficiency is treated by curing the underlying cause. Autoimmune thrombocytopenia purpura is usually treated with corticosteroid drugs or a splenectomy.

pus The product of inflammation, this is a pale yellow or green creamy fluid composed of millions of dead white blood cells, fluid, partly digested tissue, bacteria and other substances found at the site of a bacterial infection. A collection of pus in solid tissue is an ABSCESS.

The main organisms that form pus include staphylococci, streptococci, pneumococci and *Escherichia coli*. Some bacteria (*pseudomonas aeruginosa*) produce blue-tinged pus.

pustule A small pus-containing skin blister found on skin that may or may not be caused by infection. They are often found at the opening of hair follicles (folliculitis). *Staphylococcus aureus* is a frequent cause of bacterial folliculitis, while the pustules in ACNE are not infectious.

PUVA The combination of the oral or topical photosensitizing chemical PSORALEN (either trioxsalen or methoxsalen) plus long-wave ultraviolet light-A (UVA), the most commonly used form of photochemotherapy helpful in treating PSORIASIS, VITILIGO, MYCOSIS FUNGOIDES, and several other skin disorders. Only becoming clinically useful in the mid-1970s, PUVA therapy consists of oral or topical administration of a psoralen and irradiation of the skin with UVA light. Treatments (which last five to 10 minutes) are given two or three times a week until remission, when the therapy is reduced to one a week or every other week. The most widely used psoralen in the United States is 8–methoxysoralen, administered orally followed by a one-hour exposure to UVA.

The exact reason why PUVA works is not known, but it leads to a decrease in the rate of DNA synthesis, which may explain why it helps those with disorders characterized by rapid cell replication (such as psoriasis). PUVA may also interfere with the migration of inflammatory cells to the skin. PUVA is highly effective in the management of psoriasis (it clears the problem in almost 90 percent of the time). It may also be used in the treatment of other forms of psoriasis, for cutaneous T-cell lymphomas, atopic dermatitis, LICHEN PLANUS and vitiligo.

Adverse effects Patients who receive too much drug or ultraviolet light can develop severe sunburns. Psoralens alone may produce itching and nausea in a small number of patients, and the risks of PUVA can be either acute or chronic. Sunburn-like redness may occur together with blisters; these effects usually can be prevented by carefully assessing doses. However, the chronic long-term toxicity is not yet determined; PUVA is known to be carcinogenic in experimental situations. Hyperpigmentation occurs in most patients, and some experience LENTIGINES and mottling of skin color. The risk of premature aging of the skin, ACTINIC KERATOSES, BOWEN'S DISEASE AND SQUAMOUS CELL CARCINOMA is increased. Prior skin cancer, previous exposure to ionizing radiation, arsenic ingestion and (perhaps) the previous use of tar preparations may increase the chance of abnormal growths in those patients. The formation of cataracts is another risk, although there have been few reports of premature cataracts in those patients treated with PUVA without eye protection.

pyoderma   A purulent (containing or characterized by pus) condition of the skin.

pyoderma gangrenosum   A rare ulcerative condition characterized by ulcers that are surrounded by bluish gray discolored skin; it is found in about 5 percent of patients with ulcerative colitis. It may be associated with internal disorders involving the gastrointestinal, and musculoskeletal systems, or the bone marrow.

Symptoms Lesions begin as pustules that quickly progress to a necrotic (composed of dead tissue) ulcer; lesions often enlarge several centimeters each day. In about a third of cases, injury to the skin precedes the onset of the lesion. The blue-gray necrotic edge of the ulcer is characteristic of this disease.

Treatment Pyoderma gangrenosum can be very difficult to treat, and the underlying disease must be identified. Treatment of such underlying disease often helps to heal and prevent new ulcers. Treatment may involve topical and systemic corticosteroids, DAPSONE, SULFAPYRIDINE, anti-cancer drugs, MINOCYCLINE and CLOFAZIMINE. The lesions should be protected from injury and any underlying disease should be treated.

pyogenic granuloma   A capillary tumor, neither infectious nor composed of granular tissue, that may appear anywhere on the skin but is frequently seen on the lips, gums, digits, arms, legs or trunk (often after trauma). The solitary lesion usually begins as a small red papule that quickly grows; as it develops, it becomes friable and bleeds easily. The condition is common in pregnant women (granuloma gravidarum), especially in the gums.

Treatment Surgical excision by electrosurgery or CURETTAGE AND ELECTRODESICCATION, or laser (argon, CO_2 and dye lasers have all been successful.) Some pyogenic granulomas recur after surgery and may require treatment.

pyridoxine deficiency   See VITAMIN B_6 DEFICIENCY.

pyrilamine   An antihistamine drug used to treat HIVES (urticaria) that, unlike other antihistamines, rarely causes drowsiness.

Q

Quartz lamp A vacuum lamp of melted quartz glass used as a source of ULTRAVIOLET RADIATION.

Queensland tick typhus A disease in the spotted fever group caused by ticks infected with organisms (*Rickettsia australis*) that share a group antigen, also known as North Queensland tick typhus. The first sign of this disease is usually a local lesion at the site of the tick bite that becomes a necrotic (composed of dead tissue) ulcer up to 5 mm across with a red areola, also called the *tache noir* ("black spot").

Treatment Specific antibiotics and administration of fluids and electrolytes are recommended, as well as prompt treatment of the associated high fever. Tetracycline and chloramphenicol are effective, responding within 24 hours. Therapy should be continued for two weeks after the onset of fever. Treatment with corticosteroids has been effective for neurological complications of this infection.

quick-tanning lotions See SELF-TANNING PRODUCTS.

quintana fever See TRENCH FEVER.

R

racket nail One of the most common congenital nail deformities. It is caused by a problem with the thumb, which is shorter than normal, producing a nail that is very short and wide. This genetic trait is an autosomal dominant trait, which means that only one defective gene (from one parent) is needed to cause the syndrome. Each child of an affected person usually has a one in two chance of inheriting the defective gene and of being affected. The condition, which occurs most often in women, can affect either one or both thumbs.

radiation dermatitis See DERMATITIS, RADIATION.

radiation and the skin In the first half of this century, an X-ray machine was commonly found in every dermatologist's office. With the dawn of a host of other treatments, including antibacterials, antifungals, corticosteroids, chemotherapy and improved surgical treatment, and as the long-term consequences of radiation therapy became better known, radiotherapy became less frequently used. Today, it is confined largely to the treatment of skin tumors.

The penetration of X-ray radiation varies; the shorter the wavelength, the deeper it can penetrate tissue. X rays must be chosen to match tissue penetration. Superficial X-ray radiation is primarily used to treat BASAL CELL and SQUAMOUS CELL CARCINOMA of the face. While most of these cancers are treated by surgical excision, in some patients radiation is the treatment of choice (it is nontraumatic and better preserves cosmetic appearance). X-ray radiation is also used to treat eyelid cancers.

Other skin tumors (KAPOSI'S SARCOMA and MYCOSIS FUNGOIDES) may also be treated with superficial radiation.

Electromagnetic radiation includes a spectrum of wavelengths, beginning with the shortest (X rays and gamma rays), followed by ultraviolet (UV), visible light, infrared, microwave, and radio waves.

Ionizing radiation (as produced by X rays) produces FREE RADICALS in tissue, which lead to damage and structural changes in cells, delaying the growth and eventually killing the cells. See also DERMATITIS, RADIATION; RADIATION ERYTHEMA; BASAL CELL CARCINOMA; RADIATION THERAPY FOR SKIN CANCER; RADIATION ERYTHEMA; RADIODERMATITIS.

radiation erythema Also known as Roentgen erythema, this is a brief reddening of the skin with varying amounts of swelling following exposure to radiation of between 300–400 cGy. The transient redness lasts between 24 and 72 hours; a longer-lasting reddening follows in a week, and may last for another week. It appears to be an early response to injury to the EPIDERMIS and DERMIS (first and second layer of skin). Darkening of the skin caused by the excess production of MELANIN follows. There is usually no significant pain associated with this level of radiation exposure. See DERMATITIS, RADIATION; RADIATION AND THE SKIN; RADIATION THERAPY FOR SKIN CANCER; RADIODERMATITIS.

radiation therapy for skin cancer Treatment of BASAL CELL or SQUAMOUS CELL CARCINOMA by X rays that produce ionizing radiation. As the radiation passes through disease tissue, it destroys the abnormal cells. If the correct dosage of radiation is given, normal cells suffer little or no damage. Radiation, which is usually passed through diseased tissues by X rays (or electrons) produced by a linear accelerator, cures most skin cancers.

Side effects Radiation of skin cancer may produce fatigue, nausea and vomiting, and hair loss from the affected area. Early on, skin reddening and blistering after treatment are frequent and may be alleviated with corticosteroid drugs. Long-term side effects may include skin cancer in areas of chronic radiodermatitis (atrophy of the skin and loss of hair and/or sweat glands). Basal cell carcinoma is the most common cancer.

radioallergosorbent test See RAST TEST.

radiodermatitis A mottled increase and decrease in skin pigment caused by exposure to ionizing radiation. The area usually has no hair and is covered with dilated blood vessels over the thin surface of the patch. Radiodermatitis is considered to be a precancerous condition that may eventually progress to a malignant skin tumor.

The skin may have been exposed to ionizing radiation either by accident, or deliberately during radiation therapy; in either case, the radiation energy either injures or kills the individual cells, or causes a DNA mutation. The degree of radiation that reaches the cells depends on the type of radiation (X rays, gamma rays or neutrons); high-energy radiation used to treat deep tumors may actually cause less total energy to the skin than lower-energy radiation of X rays. Temporary hair loss may follow 300–400 cGy of superficial radiation to the skin; hair loss may be permanent following larger doses.

Radiation erythema causes a temporary reddening of the skin that lasts up to 72 hours, followed by a longer-lasting redness that appears in about a week and may take another week to fade. Hyperpigmentation due to excess MELANIN production follows. There is no

discomfort associated with this type of radiodermatitis.

Acute radiodermatitis can be expected following radiation therapy for cancer; it may also occur following accidental exposure to radiation. In this acute form, the skin reddening does not disappear after a week, but instead progresses to an inflammatory reaction by the second week, characterized by blistering, crusting and pain. As the inflammation begins to heal over the ensuing months, a nonpigmented scar and TELANGIECTASIAS appears; hair and sweat glands may be permanently destroyed.

Chronic radiodermatitis can appear years after large amounts of radiation exposure, characterized by atrophy of the skin, with telangiectasias and mottling. The skin becomes dry and easily injured, healing slowly. There is no hair on the exposed area, and sweat and sebaceous glands may be destroyed. There is an increased risk of skin cancer (most commonly BASAL CELL CARCINOMA). When SQUAMOUS CELL CARCINOMA develops, it is often more aggressive than this type of cancer induced by sun exposure.

Treatment Acute *radiodermatitis* should be treated with cool tap water and protective dressings; itching can be relieved with emollients, shake lotions or witch hazel. Mild analgesics may relieve pain; avoid rubbing the area. Treat secondary infection with antibiotics. Topical steroids are not effective with this type of skin condition. There is no treatment for *chronic radiodermatitis*, other than protecting the area from injury or exposure to the sun and watching carefully for early signs of skin cancer. See also RADIATION AND THE SKIN; RADIATION ERYTHEMA; RADIATION THERAPY FOR SKIN CANCER.

rash The popular term for a group of spots or red, inflamed skin that is usually temporary and is only rarely a sign of a serious underlying problem. It may be inflammatory, infectious, cancerous or it may represent an underlying disease.

RAST test The abbreviation for radioallergosorbent test, a type of radioimmunoassay used to detect antibodies to specific allergens. They are used to diagnose allergies. The principle behind these tests is that there is a specific antigen for every antibody. Any antibody will bind only to its own antigen.

rat-bite fever A condition following the bite of a rat that causes two similar type diseases—*sodoku,* caused by *Spirillum minus,* and *septicemia* caused by *Streptobacillus moniliformis. Spirillus minus* causes skin ulcers and recurrent fever; *Streptobacillus moniliformis* causes skin inflammation, muscular pain and vomiting. Following the rat bite, the wound heals but after one to three weeks, it becomes tender and swollen. Skin lesions appear, together with enlarged lymph nodes, general malaise, loss of appetite and joint pain.
Treatment Intravenous administration of penicillin G is effective in both cases.

Raynaud's phenomenon A disorder of blood vessels that causes the skin of the fingers to turn white in the cold; in rare cases, the blood flow is permanently decreased, leading to ulceration or gangrene at the tips of affected fingers and toes. Fingers of young women are most often affected.

On exposure to cold, the blood vessels of people with Raynaud's phenomenon suddenly contract, cutting off blood flow.

Possible causes of Reynaud's phenomenon include arterial diseases (Buerger's disease, atherosclerosis, embolism and thrombosis), connective tissue disease (rheumatoid arthritis, SCLERODERMA and systemic LUPUS ERYTHEMATOSUS) and drugs (ergotamine, methysergide and beta blockers).

Raynaud's phenomenon is also a recognized occupational disorder in some people who use pneumatic drills, chain saws or other vibrating machines; it is also sometimes seen in typists, pianists and those whose fingers suffer repeated trauma.
Symptoms During exposure to cold, the skin of the digits turns white. As blood flow returns, the skin turns blue; upon being reheated, the skin turns red. Feelings of tingling, numbness or burning may occur during an attack.
Treatment Hands and feet of affected individuals should be kept as warm as possible. Cigarette smoking further constricts the blood vessels and can worsen the condition and thus should be avoided. Vasodilator drugs may be administered to relax the blood vessel walls and help prevent vasoconstriction. In severe cases, sympathectomy (cutting of the nerves controlling the caliber of arteries) may be effective.

Patients with Raynaud's phenomenon should wear the proper clothes for the temperature. Keep in mind that perspiration is more responsible for cold hands and feet than cold temperatures, so it is important to wear fabrics that soak up excess sweat and keep it from contacting the body. Hands and feet are especially prone to getting cold because they are natural areas of perspiration, which is why woolen socks and fleece boots make you sweat and leave you chilly instead of warm.

This condition can occur in any season and is related to changes in termperature, so that grocery shopping or going to an air-conditioned theater in summer can provoke Raynaud's phenomenon.

razor bumps The common name for PSEUDOFOLLICULITIS BARBAE.

reactive perforating collagenosis A rare skin disease characterized by small papules with a central plug of oily material. They are caused by seeping of abnormal COLLAGEN through the overlying EPIDERMIS (top layer of skin). This hereditary condition usually appears in childhood. The lesions are usually found on the backs of the hands, forearms, elbows and knees.

Treatment No treatment is needed, since the lesions usually disappear on their own, but removing the lesions by freezing with LIQUID NITROGEN or ELECTRODESICCATION may be effective.

von Recklinghausen's disease See NEURO-FIBROMATOSIS.

reconstructive surgery See PLASTIC SURGERY.

reduction mammoplasty See MAMMOPLASTY.

Refsum's disease A rare genetic metabolic disease caused by a lack of the enzyme phytanic acid oxidase that causes mild scaling of the skin on the trunk, arms and legs similar to ICHTHYOSIS. This results in a buildup in many organs of phytanic acid, a compound chiefly of dietary origin.

The disorder is an autosomal recessive trait, which means that a defective gene must be inherited in a double dose to cause the abnormality. Generally, both parents of an affected person are unaffected carriers of the defective gene. Each of the children has a one in four chance of being affected, and a two in four chance of being a carrier.

Symptoms In addition to the skin symptoms, the disease is characterized by night blindness, cataracts and other eye problems, skeletal abnormalities, kidney or heart problems, and hearing problems.

Treatment Eating a low-phytanic acid diet is recommended. Some patients find relief with plasma exchange (a procedure that reduces the concentration of unwanted substances in the blood).

relapsing polychondritis A rare chronic autoimmune inflammatory disease in which cartilage in the ear, nose, joints, eyes, blood vessels, trachea and bronchial tubes may be destroyed.

About 30 percent of patients usually die within four years, usually as a result of obstruction or collapse of the airway. Even if heart and bronchial tube defects don't occur, the disorder can cause deformities of the ears and nose.

Symptoms Skin signs are characterized by abnormal cartilage in the outer ear, which is large, swollen, tender and red, lasting for one or two weeks before it fades and then recurs. Recurrent attacks will eventually destroy the cartilage, and result in "cauliflower ear." There are a number of other symptoms affecting other areas of the body; death can occur from aneurysms and cardiac valve disease.

Treatment Topical steroids do not work, but high doses of systemic corticosteroids can control or ease inflammation. Because of the frequent spontaneous remissions and recurrences, it is hard to evaluate response to therapy. DAPSONE, which may be safer than steroids, has been effective for some patients, but it also can cause serious side effects.

renal failure and skin symptoms See KIDNEY DISEASE AND SKIN SYMPTOMS.

reportable skin diseases Skin conditions (CHICKEN POX, MEASLES, syphilis, tuberculosis, and RUBELLA etc.) that must be reported to local health authorities by the physician responsible for care of the affected person. In turn, local health authorities must report some of these diseases to the national Centers for Disease Control.

Notification of certain potentially harmful infections is important because it enables public health officials to take the necessary steps to control the spread of infection. Reporting also provides valuable statistics on the incidence and prevalence of the disease, which can be used to formulate health policies such as immunization programs and improvements in sanitation.

resorcinol (trade name: Rezamid) An ointment that causes the skin to peel, used to treat ACNE, DERMATITIS and fungal infections, and contained in hair lotions for dandruff. Its mechanism of action is unknown.

It is available in concentrations of 2 percent or less. In preparations of 3 percent resorcinol and higher, local toxicity (swelling, dermatitis, itching and peeling) may occur. More seriously, there is also the possibility of systemic toxicity; if the drug is absorbed into the body, it can cause a decrease in activity of the thyroid gland and convulsions. For this reason, products containing resorcinol should not be applied to broken skin or to large areas of the body. In addition, resorcinol may discolor dark or black skin.

Resorcinol is usually added to sulfur as an acne treatment, although experts aren't sure why it works. Resorcinol by itself is not considered to be effective against acne, but it appears to enhance the action of sulfur. The Food and Drug Administration allows a combination of 8 percent sulfur with 2 percent resorcinol, or 8 percent sulfur with 3 percent resorcinol monacetate.

Resorcinol is considered to be a rather old-fashioned agent and is no longer used frequently.

Retin-A A synthetic form of vitamin A (see RETINOIC ACID) used as a prescription ACNE medication and wrinkle cream; it may also prevent skin and cervical cancer. The newest form of Retin-A is Retin-A(R)Micro (tretinoin gel) microsphere 0.1%, that uses a microsponge system designed to minimize irritation. Retin-A is used to treat acne and sun-damaged, wrinkled skin. While it has not been approved as an anti-aging ingredient, there is scientific evidence of beneficial results from its use in stimulating the basal layer of the epidermis where the cells are produced, boosting cell turnover and improving blood vessel growth and production of collagen and elastin that results in tightened skin and fewer wrinkles.

Although Retin-A is in the same family as vitamin A, the two are not the same. For many years, different compounds of vitamin A have been included in cosmetics (as retinol, retinyl, retinylacetate or retinyl palmitate) because these ingredients are not considered to be drugs by the U.S. Food an Drug Administration. Retin-A, the acid of vitamin A, has unique properties and because it is available by prescription only in this country, it is not included in any cosmetic skin-care product. It is available without a prescription in Mexico.

The first reports of Retin-A's ability to smooth out wrinkles appeared in the *Journal of the American Medical Association* in 1988, when researchers at the University of Michigan reported that subjects with sun-damaged skin showed significant improvement in number of wrinkles after applying Retin-A. Up to that time, dermatologists used Retin-A mostly for acne patients until Albert Kligman, M.D., a prominent dermatologist at the University of Pennsylvania, noted his acne patients' reports and began using Retin-A on sun-damaged skin.

In another recent study, University of Michigan dermatologists discovered that older patients who took Retin-A had 80 percent more of a protein that helps to form COLLAGEN (a substance that helps keep skin firm) than they had had before treatment.

Many studies have now shown that Retin-A is effective in removing facial wrinkles, smoothing coarse skin and improving lentigines. It is not effective for improving coarse wrinkles.

It is also extremely effective in the treatment of acne, although—as with the case of wrinkles—there is a lag time before it becomes effective. Some individuals even notice their skin becomes worse after the first two or three weeks. At the beginning, Retin-A can cause dryness and irritation.

How to apply The higher the concentration of Retin-A used, the faster and more significant the results. Retin-A is often irritating, however, and for this reason many doctors start patients with the milder forms available: 0.025 percent to 0.05 percent cream every other night, slowly increasing the strength and frequency of application. Higher concentrations of the product (0.1 percent) work best, but these are more irritating to the skin. Consumers should first wash the skin thoroughly with a gentle cleanser, pat dry and then wait 15 minutes; spread a tiny amount of cream over the entire face. Retin-A may be applied under the eyes, being careful to avoid the eye itself. Early on you will notice pinkness and flakiness. It takes three to six months before benefits are apparent. On less sensitive areas (such as the backs of the hands) it can be started more quickly and used every night relatively early on.

Side effects Retin-A is a powerful drug, and side effects can include burning eyes and peeling or reddening of the skin that lasts for weeks; this reaction is most common in women who sunburn easily and who normally have very sensitive skin. Benefits often don't appear until between 6 and 12 months. Newer forms of Retin-A have far milder side effects.

Users should always layer a high SPF block under makeup (even during winter) to protect the skin from harmful exposure. Wear protective hats and avoid the sun.

Dr. Kligman (the University of Pennsylvania dermatologist who developed the drug) recommends careful use under the supervision of a physician. Incorrect use of Retin-A can lead to extreme irritation (so can using the wrong strength), so consumers should see a dermatologist to obtain their own personal prescription.

Because of a lack of well-controlled studies of Retin-A and pregnancy, it may be advisable to avoid this drug if you are, or plan to become, pregnant.
See also ACNE; ACTINIC CONDITIONS; AGING AND SKIN; ALPHA HYDROXY ACIDS; BENZOYL PEROXIDE; CHLORACNE; COLLAGEN; EXFOLIANTS; ISOTRETINOIN; ISOTREX; PHOTOSENSITIVITY; STRETCH MARKS; VITAMIN A; WRINKLES.

retinoic acid See RETIN-A.

retinoids Synthetic or naturally occurring derivatives of vitamin A that have a range of effects on the skin, including wound repair, inhibiting tumor promotion, etc. Today, retinoids are widely used in the treatment of stubborn cases of ACNE, PSORIASIS, prevention of SKIN CANCER, reversal of aging, disorders of keratinization (the depositing of keratin within the cell).

Primary dietary sources of vitamin A are the beta-carotenes in the yellow and green leafy vegetables and also in some animal fats and fish oils. Vitamin A (retinol) is sent to the liver, where more than 90 percent of the body's stores are stockpiled.

They may be used topically (RETINOIC ACID) or systemically (ISOTRETINOIN, the generic form of Accutane, or ETRETINATE, the generic term for Tegison).

retinol The principal form of vitamin A found in the body. It is essential for growth, vision in dim light and maintenance of soft mucous tissue.

retinyl palmitate A form of vitamin A that some studies suggest may be transformed into the acid from RETIN-A in the skin. Retinyl palmitate is less irritating than RETINOIC ACID, but many experts believe that commercial skin care products do not contain enough of this substance to prevent or reduce aging. See also RETINOID.

rhinophyma Bulbous deformity and redness of the nose found almost exclusively in men, usually as a complication of severe ROSACEA (a skin disorder of the cheeks and nose). As nose tissue thickens, small blood vessels enlarge and the sebaceous glands become overactive, making the nose excessively oily.

Treatment Rhinophyma can be treated with a variety of surgical procedures; the swollen tissue is cut away until the nose is restored to a satisfactory shape. Skin grafting is not necessary, since the remaining tissue rapidly regenerates. It can be reshaped with a CO_2 laser electrosurgery or scalpel surgery.

rhinoplasty See NOSE REPAIR.

rhinoscleroma A bacterial infection caused by *Klebsiella rhinoscleromatis* that is chronic and common in rural areas with poor hygiene throughout the world.

Symptoms The disease begins with increased nasal secretion and crusting, followed by an enlargement of the nose, upper lip, palate or neighboring areas. If the infection spreads to the respiratory tract, breathing may become difficult and a tracheotomy may be necessary. The condition may be fatal due to breathing obstructions or continuing infection.

Treatment This progressive disease is difficult to treat; systemic antibiotics such as gentamicin and tobramycin have been effective. Alternatively, oral administration of ciprofloxacin may help, although this drug has not been widely studied as a therapy for this condition.

rhytidectomy See FACELIFT.

Richner-Hanhart syndrome The common name for tyrosinemia type II, this is a hereditary metabolic disease caused by the absence of the enzyme tyrosine aminotransferase.

The condition is inherited as an autosomal recessive trait, which means that a defective gene must be inherited from both parents to cause the abnormality. Generally, both parents of an affected person are unaffected carriers of the defective gene. Each child of parents who both carry the defective gene has a one in four chance of being affected, and a two in four chance of being a carrier.

Symptoms Skin signs include skin erosions on fingers, palms and soles of the feet that appear in symmetric lines that become crusted and wasted. The lesions may be so painful that they interfere with movement. Other systemic signs include mental retardation, excess tearing and eye problems.

Treatment Diets low in tyrosine and phenylalanine are advised. If diagnosed early enough, it's possible to prevent some of the systemic problems (including mental retardation) associated with the disease.

rickettsial infections Diseases caused by the bite or feces of intracellular parasites called rickettsiae. They can be grouped as the spotted fevers (ROCKY MOUNTAIN SPOTTED FEVER, RICKETTSIAL POX, other tickborne fevers); the TYPHUS group (epidemic or louseborne typhus, endemic or murine typhus and scrub typhus); Q fever; and trench fever.

Except for Q fever, all rickettsial infections are transmitted by arthropods (including ticks, mites and insects). All rickettsial diseases except Q fever are characterized by rash, fever and headache, although the skin manifestation differs from one disease to the next.

rickettsial pox An urban disease transmitted by mites on common house mice that has been reported in cities since 1946. The responsible microorganism is *Rickettsia akari*, which belongs to the spotted fever group of these parasites.

Symptoms A local lesion develops between one and three weeks after a mite bite, beginning as a red papule that breaks down into an area of dead crusted skin, at which time it may be associated with local swelling of lymph nodes. Within a week after the lesion appears, fever, chills, headache and myalgias occur, followed in a few more days by a rash over the body. This rash develops into an eruption similar to CHICKEN POX. The lesions may not be very severe, and the disease itself is mild and self-limiting.

Treatment Antibiotics (tetracyclines or chloramphenicol), fluid and electrolytes, and prompt treatment of complications.

Rickettsia rickettsii A type of intracellular parasitic microorganism that looks like a small bacterium but which can reproduce only by invading cells of another life form. These parasites live primarily off insects and insect-like animals such as lice, fleas, ticks and mites. In turn, these insects can transmit the parasite to rodents, dogs or humans through saliva or feces. Human diseases spread by different types of these microorganisms include ROCKY MOUNTAIN SPOTTED FEVER and various forms of TYPHUS.

rifampin An antibacterial drug used to treat LEPROSY that is usually prescribed with other antibacterials because some strains of bacteria quickly develop resistance to rifampin alone. It is also used to eradicate *staphylococcus aureus* from nasal cavities.

Side effects Harmless, orange-red discoloration of urine, saliva and other body secretions; muscle pain; nausea and vomiting; diarrhea; jaundice; flu-like symptoms; rash and itching.

ringworm The popular term for TINEA, a superficial fungal infection of the skin.

Ritter's disease The former name for staphlococcal SCALDED SKIN SYNDROME.

Rocky Mountain spotted fever A rare infectious disease caused by the parasite rickettsia (similar to a bacteria) characterized by a spotted rash. Transmitted to rabbits and other small mammals primarily by tick bites, it is found most often in wooded areas along the Atlantic coast, but it gets its name from its original occurrence in the Rocky Mountain states. The incidence of the disease has been rising steadily since 1980; there are more than 1,000 cases reported each year. Diagnosis may be difficult because the disease has symptoms resembling several other infections. Lab tests on blood and tissues are needed to confirm the diagnosis.

Symptoms Mild fever, loss of appetite and slight headache may develop slowly about a week after a tick bite. Sometimes, however, symptoms appear suddenly—high fever, prostration, aching, tender muscles, severe headache, nausea and vomiting. Two to six days after symptoms appear, small spots appear on wrists and ankles, spreading centrally over the rest of the body. The illness subsides after about two weeks. Untreated cases with very high fever may end in death from pneumonia or heart failure.

Treatment Antibiotic drugs tetracycline or chloramphenicol usually cure the disease.

Prevention People in tick-infested areas should use insect repellant and examine themselves daily for ticks.

rodent ulcer The popular term for BASAL CELL epithelioma (tumor of the covering of the internal and external surfaces of the body) that has become large and eroded.

Rogaine The brand name of the drug MINOXIDIL, used for treating hair loss.

rosacea A long-term disorder affecting facial skin of the nose, cheeks, chin or forehead that may include redness, pimples, pustules, solid raised lesions, dilated blood vessels (telangiectases) and, less commonly, disfigurement and enlargement of the nose.

While it is sometimes called "adult acne" because the pimples usually occur during the 30s and 40s, rosacea is actually a different condition than acne. The pimples are not usually associated with blackheads and whiteheads. While it tends to appear in those over 30, rosacea has been diagnosed in teenagers.

The condition affects fair-skinned patients more often than those with dark complexions, although it can affect all skin types. Most rosacea patients have a history of blushing more often and easily. Rosacea may also affect members of the same family because of similar skin conditions or genetic predisposition. Rosacea occurs at a particularly high rate among Irish Americans, although other nationalities—English, Scots or Eastern Europeans—are also likely to develop this conspicuous condition.

While women are more likely to develop rosacea, men are more likely to develop RHINOPHYMA (the large, bulbous nose associated with the condition). Rosacea is not associated with alcoholism, although alcohol may worsen the condition; teetotalers may also develop the condition.

Cause Unknown. Various theories suggest bacteria, mites, a fungus, a malfunction of the connective tissue under the skin, or psychological factors. While topical steroids may cause rosacea when applied to the face, after discontinuing use of the steroid, rosacea disappears. It seems likely there is no single cause, and that it develops in individuals who are susceptible due to a variety of factors, including skin color and skin structure.

Symptoms Rosacea develops slowly and usually gets worse unless treated. In most patients, the condition waxes and wanes repeatedly for no apparent reason. Earliest signs include a red face (especially on cheeks and nose) that may come and go. This redness is caused by enlarged blood vessels under the skin, and looks like a blush or sunburn. Gradually, the redness becomes permanent and more noticeable; facial skin also becomes very dry. As the redness gets worse, pimples may appear. Thin red lines (called TELANGIECTASES), which are really enlarged blood vessels, may appear on the surface of the skin. In the most advanced stages (especially in men) the nose may become lumpy and swollen from excess tissue.

Rosacea is aggravated by sun, hot liquids, spicy foods, alcohol, vigorous exercise, heat, cold and wind, fluorinated steroids, menopause, endocrine disturbances and emotional stress.

Treatment There is no cure for rosacea, but treatment can control the condition and improve the skin's appearance. Topical and oral medications can control redness and reduce papules and pustules; a combination of topical and oral forms of prescription drugs may be recommended. The most widely prescribed therapy for rosacea is topical metronidazole, which has been proven effective in clinical studies. Oral antibacterial medications such as TETRACYCLINE are also commonly used; they tend to produce better results and work more quickly than topical medications. Still, it usually takes several weeks for drugs to take effect, and they may have to be taken regularly to keep rosacea under control. Up to 80 percent of patients can expect significant improvement from oral or topical therapy, or a combination of both.

Prescription and nonprescription mild topical steroids are occasionally used on a short-term basis to help control redness; long-term use of topical steroids is not recommended.

Oral medications are usually taken twice a day; tetracycline should be taken on an empty stomach, since milk and certain foods may impair absorption.

Surgery may be used to correct the nose enlargement in rhinophyma. A fine electric needle or a laser may also be used to eliminate enlarged blood vessels, and also decrease the overall redness, thus improving appearance.

In addition, a dermatologist may recommend specific moisturizers, soaps, sunscreens or other products as needed to improve the condition of the skin. Use only very mild soaps or cleansers; avoid alcohol or irritating ingredients and excessive cleaning of the skin. Apply high quality moisturizers only after the topical medication has dried. Sunscreens of SPF 15 or higher are often recommended when prolonged sun exposure is expected.

*For more information, contact the National Rosacea Society, 220 South Cork Street, Suite 201, Barrington, IL 60010.

roseola infantum A common infectious disease of early childhood also known as *exanthema subitum* (Latin for "sudden rash") that can affect youngsters aged six months to six years. The disease, which is caused by the viruses human herpes virus 6 and 7, is characterized by the abrupt onset of irritability and a fever, which may climb as high as 105° F. By the fourth or fifth day, the fever breaks, suddenly returning to normal. At about the same time, a rash appears on the trunk, often spreading quickly to the face, neck and limbs, fading within hours and disappearing within two days. Other symptoms may include sore throat, enlarged lymph nodes and, occasionally, a febrile seizure. A single attack appears to confer permanent immunity.

Treatment There are no serious complications, and there is no specific treatment other than acetaminophen for the fever.

Rothmund-Thomson syndrome A recessive hereditary type of poikiloderma (pigmentary change causing a mottled or dappled appearance) also known as poikiloderma congenitale. It is characterized by skin changes, including the development of red patches and blisters on cheeks, forehead, arms, legs and buttocks, followed by dilation of blood vessels and skin lightening. One-third of patients are also extremely sensitive to light.

Other symptoms include short stature, small hands, photosensitivity and juvenile cataracts.

royal jelly A substance that is secreted from the digestive system of worker bees that is fed to male bees and workers for a few days after they are born. Because the queen bee eats royal jelly througout her life, royal jelly became associated with health and long life.

In humans, however, studies have shown that royal jelly does not prevent aging and is considered to be useless in humans.

rubella See GERMAN MEASLES.

rubber sensitivity See ALLERGIES OF THE SKIN; LATEX ALLERGY.

rubeola Another name for MEASLES.

rubor Redness.

Rud's syndrome A rare congenital syndrome characterized by mild to fairly severe ICHTHYOSIS (disease of rough, scaly skin), ACANTHOSIS NIGRICANS (dark, warty growths), excess sweating of palms and soles, epilepsy, hair loss, deformed teeth, mental retardation, seizures and hypogonadism.

S

St. Anthony's fire The common name for ERYSIPELAS, a potentially fatal streptococcal infection of the skin characterized by deep swellings on the face, with severe headache and blistering. Severe cases require hospitalization and intravenous antibiotics.

salicylic acid A drug used to treat a variety of skin disorders, including DERMATITIS, ECZEMA (topically), PSORIASIS, ICHTHYOSIS, ACNE and WARTS. The drug is also sometimes used for fungal infections.

For the treatment of warts, salicylic acid pads or solutions can be very effective. It is important to avoid treating normal surrounding skin to prevent its irritation. This can be avoided by coating the rim of the wart with zinc oxide paste or petroleum jelly.
Side effects This drug may cause inflammation and even skin ulceration if used for a long period of time or if applied to a large area of skin. It is poisonous and should never be ingested.

salmon patch See STORK BITE.

salve A healing, soothing (often medicated) ointment for the skin.

sarcoidosis A rare disease characterized by inflammation in the skin and other tissues throughout the body (especially the lungs) that occurs primarily in young adults. Often appearing abruptly, its incidence is highest among widely disparate ethnic groups—primarily blacks, but also Scandinavians, Irish and Puerto Ricans.

Despite decades of research, scientists still know very little about the disorder, and its cause remains unknown.

Sarcoidosis initially may be confused with tuberculosis or a deep fungal infection. The condition is often diagnosed by first ruling out these other problems. An unusual form of the disease, called Lofgren's disease, is characterized by a very rapid onset, with a HIVE-like skin rash and acute lung problems, enlarged lymph nodes and fever. This condition usually disappears as quickly as it came.
Symptoms The typical finding of the disease is the sarcoidal granuloma. Its most common symptom involves lung disease, but in the acute form of the disease ERYTHEMA NODOSUM (purplish swellings on the legs) may occur with fever, generalized aches and lymph node enlargement. Chronic sarcoidosis may cause a variety of symptoms, including a purple facial rash, painful joints, bloodshot eyes and numbness. However, about a third of affected people have no symptoms at all; in these people, X rays reveal enlarged lymph nodes in the center of the chest. In these symptom-free patients, the disorder will fade away with or without treatment in about two years.

In another third, the condition responds to drug therapy, but these patients may require treatment for many years.

Finally, about one patient in 20 will experience scarring and thickening of the lungs, abnormally high blood levels of calcium and kidney damage.
Treatment About 90 percent of patients recover completely within two years with or without treatment. However, the remainder develop a chronic form of the disease. Oral corticosteroid drugs (such as prednisone) may relieve erythema nodosum, fever and lung or eye problems. The steroids are given because their anti-inflammatory effects suppress the sarcoid granulomas often found in

the disease. This treatment usually produces a rapid reduction of symptoms within weeks, although it still takes about a year for the disease to disappear. Hydroxychloroquine is sometimes prescribed to treat skin abnormalities.

For the very seriously ill patient with life-threatening complications, more potent anti-inflammatory drugs (such as the anti-cancer drug METHOTREXATE) may be administered.

sarcoma Cancer of the connective tissue, blood vessels or the tissue surrounding and supporting organs. Examples of sarcoma include KAPOSI'S SARCOMA (mainly affecting the skin, common in AIDS patients), osteosarcoma and chondrosarcoma (both affecting bones).

Sarcoptes scabiei The mite responsible for the skin infestation of SCABIES.

scab A crust that forms on a healing superficial skin wound or infected area, composed of dried fibrin and serum leaked from the wound, along with PUS, skin scales and other skin debris. Another name for a scab associated with burns is ESCHAR.

scabicides Insecticides (such as LINDANE) designed to treat SCABIES by killing the mites that cause the infestation. These lotions usually kill the mites, but itching may continue for up to two weeks.

scabies A highly infectious skin infestation caused by the mite *Sarcoptes scabiei,* which burrows into the skin and lays its eggs. Mites are usually passed during close body contact.
Symptoms Tiny red scaly papules appear on the skin, between the fingers, on wrists and genitals and in armpits, that cause intense itching, especially at night. Reddish lumps may later appear on limbs and trunk.
Treatment Insecticide lotion (such as LIN-DANE, gamma benzene hexachloride or ele-

mite [permethrin]) should be applied to all skin below the patient's head, which kills the mites (although itching may continue for up to two weeks later). The insecticide is usually left on overnight for eight hours, and occasionally treatment is repeated the following night. Also, bedclothes and intimate apparel should be washed twice or the patient risks reinfection. All members of a family and close friends should be treated at the same time.

scald A burn on the skin caused by steam or hot liquid.

scalded skin syndrome, staphylococcal First recognized as a distinct condition in the mid-1800s, this disease has been incorrectly called by many different names, including Ritter's disease, TOXIC EPIDERMAL NECROLYSIS and pemphigus neonatorum. Only recently was its cause discovered to be a toxin-producing strain of *Staphylococcus aureus.*

This syndrome is primarily found in newborns and young children, where it carries a fatality rate of less than 4 percent. Epidemics have occurred in contaminated nurseries, and the strain of bacteria may be transmitted by a carrier who has no symptoms. The condition has also been reported among adults, most of whom had poorly-functioning immune systems.
Symptoms First symptoms usually include evidence of a primary staph infection, including IMPETIGO, conjunctivitis, ear infection or sore throat with fever, malaise or irritability. The center of the face becomes tender, and the skin around the mouth becomes reddened, weeping and crusting in a way that resembles potato chip scales. The trunk may also become involved. In some patients, the rash stabilizes, while in other cases flaccid blisters begin to develop all over the skin within 24 to 48 hours. Large areas of skin slough off, and hair or nails may be lost.

Treatment Prompt administration of anti-staphylococcal antibiotics, generally done in the hospital since patients often appear very ill with low fluid levels and risk of secondary infection. The skin is treated with wet dressings for crusted sites and antibiotic ointments such as bacitracin. Patients usually heal without scarring within a week.

scaling disorders of infancy It's completely normal for newborns to shed their skin, and it is particularly noticeable in babies that have gone beyond full term. However, excessive scaling may indicate one of the ichthyoses, a group of disorders featuring dry, rough and scaly skin caused by a defect in keratinization (the process by which skin cells become horny as they move upward toward the outer layer of skin).

There are four major types of ICHTHYOSIS, three of which occur during the neonatal period: X-linked ichthyosis, lamellar ichthyosis (nonbullous congenital ichthyosiform erythroderma) and epidermolytic hyperkeratosis. (The last type, ichthyosis vulgaris, rarely develops before age three months, and is most commonly found in older children). In addition, COLLODION BABY and HARLEQUIN FETUS describes the skin condition of some of these affected infants.
Symptoms In *X-linked ichthyosis,* up to a third of the affected male infants are born scaly, and the rest begin to show the signs by three months of age. This condition is characterized by dirty brown scales that usually cover the entire body, except for the face, palms and soles of the feet. Female carriers may have certain eye abnormalities, but they show no skin symptoms.

Babies with *nonbullous congenital ichthyosiform erythroderma* are born with red scaly skin over their body, including the palms, soles and flexible surfaces. As the babies age, the redness fades and yellow to brown thick scales appear over the body, especially in areas of the body that are flexed. These infants

may suffer with secondary infections due to the large areas of moist broken skin. The disorder is usually inherited in an autosomal recessive way, which means that a defective gene must be inherited in a double dose to cause the abnormality. Generally, both parents of an affected person are unaffected carriers of the defective gene. Each of the children has a one in four chance of being affected, and a two in four chance of being a carrier.

In *epidermolytic hyperkeratosis* (bullous congenital ichthyosiform erythroderma), affected infants develop crops of blisters over large areas of their body during the neonatal period. This causes dry, eroding, reddened skin, together with frequent secondary infection; sepsis (blood poisoning) may follow, especially in young infants. In this condition, the scales are wart-like and flake off easily in great numbers. Palms of the hands and soles of the feet are usually unaffected.

Other scaling conditions found in infancy include atopic eczema, seborrheic dermatitis (see DERMATITIS, SEBORRHEIC) and PSORIASIS.

scar An area of fibrous tissue left behind on the skin after damaged tissue has healed. When tissue is damaged, the body repairs the wound by increasing production of the tough protein COLLAGEN at the wound site. The collagen helps construct new connective tissue to free the defect. If the edges of the wound are brought together during healing (such as after the surgical excision of a MOLE), the scar is narrow and pale; if the edges remain wide apart (such as after a BURN), the scar is more extensive.

A KELOID is a large, irregular scar that outgrows the site of initial surgery. This type of scar is most common among blacks and Asians, and tends to run in families.

A HYPERTROPHIC SCAR is an overgrown scar that remains within the confines of the initial injury or cut. The tendency toward the development of hypertrophic scars may be inherited. Hypertrophic scars are usually present without symptoms, pink and relatively firm.

There is not always a clear-cut difference between keloids and hypertrophic scars, since both are characterized by the same type of fibrous connective tissue. Keloids tend to keep growing, whereas hypertrophic scars tend to reach a certain size, level off and spontaneously regress.

Treatment of both types of scars is generally not very effective; they tend to recur after surgical excision, and they can become larger and more unattractive than before the operation. New treatments, however, have improved the ability to deal with raised scars. Intralesional injections of corticosteroids, silicone gel dressings or pulsed dye laser therapy are each effective treatments for at least some scars. Prolonged application of pressure by special appliances after surgical removal may prevent recurrence, but it is frequently impractical.

Prevention Because wounds that heal quickly and neatly are less likely to scar, make sure all wounds are cleaned and slightly moist during healing. Refrain from picking scabs, which increases the likelihood of scarring.

To minimize scarring without stitching a wound, try using a butterfly bandage (available at most drugstores), which helps keep the wound closed. Eating a balanced diet, especially rich in the mineral ZINC, can help heal wounds quickly.

To help prevent keloids, earlobe puncturing and excision of nevi and other congenital lesions on keloid-prone areas should be done with caution in young people (especially those with dark skin). To help prevent hypertrophic scars, avoid injury to the skin (especially in early adulthood).

scarlet fever An infectious bacterial childhood disease characterized by a skin rash, sore throat and fever that is much less common and dangerous than it used to be. No longer a reportable disease, no one knows for sure how many cases occur today in the United States, although it is believed that the disease has been on the increase for the past several years.

Scarlet fever is caused by infection with group A streptococcus. Scarlet fever strains of group A strep produce toxins that are released in the skin, causing a bright red rash the consistency of sandpaper.

In the past, the disease was associated with poor living conditions. In 1737, a scarlet fever epidemic in Boston killed 900 people; another epidemic in New York City in the late 1800s killed 35 percent of children who contracted the disease; that same year, 19 percent of Chicago children who got the disease perished.

Inexplicably, by the 1920s the death rate of the disease dropped to 5 percent for reasons that are still not completely understood. It is believed that the scarlet fever bacteria underwent a natural mutation to make it less virulent. The introduction of penicillin reduced the death rate even more.

Today, most cases occur in middle-class suburbs, not in inner cities. Because it is possible to get streptococcal infection and scarlet fever more than once, and because the incidence of all strep infections is rising, prompt medical attention when streptococcus is suspected is important. A child with a sore throat or skin rash should be brought in for medical evaluation. Anyone can develop scarlet fever, but most cases are found among children aged four to eight.

Cause Scarlet fever bacteria are spread in droplets during coughing or breathing, or by sharing food and drink. When bacterial particles are released into the air, they can be picked up by others close by. For this reason, some experts advise children to avoid drinking fountains. The hallmark rash is caused by a toxin released by the bacteria.

Symptoms After an incubation period of two to four days, the first signs of illness is usually a fever of 103 to 104° F, accompanied by a severe sore throat. The face is flushed and the tongue develops a white coating with red spots, rather like a white strawberry. The patient may seem tired and flushed. Twelve to 18 hours after the fever, a rash appears as a mass of rapidly-spreading tiny red spots on the neck and upper trunk. The scarlet fever rash is unique in that it feels rough, like fine sandpaper, and is quite distinctive.

Other common symptoms include headache, chills and vomiting, and tiny white lines around the mouth, as well as fine red striations in the creases of the elbows and groin. After a few days, the tongue coating peels off, followed by a drop in fever and a fading rash. Skin on the hands and feet often peel.

Complications As with other types of sore throat caused by the streptococci bacteria, untreated infection carries the risk of rheumatic fever or glomerulonephritis (inflammation of the kidneys).

Treatment A 10–day course of antibiotics (usually penicillin or erythromycin), with rest, liquids and acetaminophen is usual. Children are contagious for a day or two after they begin treatment, but after that they can return to school. Alternative treatment is a shot of long-acting penicillin, which slowly releases the antibiotic over several weeks.

scarlatina Another name for SCARLET FEVER.

scarlatiniform Resembling SCARLATINA, the delicate red rash of SCARLET FEVER.

Schamberg's disease The common name for progressive pigmentary dermatosis, one of three subtypes of pigmented purpuric eruptions that share the symptom of rust-colored macules and papules (especially on the lower legs). The red pigment changes are caused by the leaking of blood into tissues.

In this subtype, there is no itching; the small macular spots and brown pinhead-sized macules are found on the lower part of the leg. The red color and tiny size give these lesions their name—CAYENNE PEPPER SPOT.

Treatment There is no really satisfactory treatment, but the condition is more of a cosmetic problem than a medical one, since internal organs are not involved and the lesions don't itch. Patients may find support stockings helpful. While systemic corticosteroids are usually effective, their risk is usually greater than any benefit that would accrue from their use. Topical corticosteroids (especially under wet dressings) may help.

schistosomiasis, visceral A parasitic disease (also called bilharziasis) that causes an itchy rash where flukes (flatworms) have penetrated the skin. The disease, found in most tropical countries, affects more than 200 million people around the world.

Symptoms While it also causes problems in other organs, the skin symptoms of this condition include dermatitis, hives and skin lesions, due to the deposits of eggs in the skin. The relatively minor skin symptoms of this form of schistosomiasis is quite different than the marked skin inflammation in SWIMMER'S ITCH (the second form of schistosomiasis).

About one to two months after the penetration of the skin, hives again appear. Skin lesions caused by the egg deposits may appear in the genital and perineal (the region of the body between the anus and the urethral opening) areas.

Cause The disease is caused by one of three types of flukes (schistosomes) acquired from bathing in infested lakes and rivers in the Far East, West Indies, Africa, South and Central America and the Middle East. The flukes penetrate the skin, where they develop within their host into adults. Their eggs provoke inflammatory reactions.

Treatment The new drug praziquantel has revolutionized the treatment of this form of schistosomiasis since the 1980s, since one dose can kill the flukes and prevent further damage. There is no vaccine to prevent the disease, and visitors to the tropics should assume that all lakes and rivers are unsafe for swimming. Alternative drugs are oxamniquine and metriphonate.

scleroderma A general term for several chronic autoimmune conditions (also called systemic sclerosis) that primarily affect the skin, arteries, kidneys, lungs, heart, gastrointestinal tract and joints. It is twice as common in women, especially between the ages of 40 and 60. Diseases include progressive systemic sclerosis, morphea, generalized morphea, linear scleroderma, morphea profunda, eosinophilic fasciitis and pansclerotic morphea.
Cause Unknown.
Symptoms While the symptoms vary widely, they include tight, shiny and thick skin on face and fingers, with puckering around the mouth, leading to a mask-like appearance. The taut skin often makes certain maneuvers (such as bending the fingers) very difficult.

There are wide variations among patients as to which body part may become affected. Other symptoms may include shortness of breath, swallowing problems, palpitations, high blood pressure, joint pain, stiffness and muscle weakness. Progression is often rapid in the first few years, and then slows down and even stops. In a small number of patients, however, degeneration is quite rapid, usually leading to death from heart, respiratory or renal failure.
Treatment There is no effective treatment. Symptoms may be controlled with antihypertensives, physical therapy, dialysis and corticosteroid drugs.

Scleroderma Federation A professional organization that promotes medical research to find a cure for SCLERODERMA; provides patients and the public with information and referrals to local organizations and medical specialists; offers encouragement and consultation services; and acts as a clearinghouse for information about the disease, its research, drugs and therapies. The federation maintains a speakers' bureau, compiles statistics and publishes a range of brochures and the quarterly *The Beacon*. Founded in 1983, the federation has 20,000 members and holds an annual seminar for patient education. For address, see Appendix D; see also SCLERODERMA INTERNATIONAL FOUNDATION; SCLERODERMA RESEARCH FOUNDATION; SCLERODERMA SUPPORT GROUP; UNITED SCLERODERMA FOUNDATION.

Scleroderma International Foundation International organization for individuals with SCLERODERMA, family and friends of patients, doctors and nurses that provides a supportive network and sponsors research into the cause, cure and control of the disease. The foundation provides information to patients, physicians and the public, and holds an annual meeting on the first Saturday of October in New Castle, Pennsylvania. Founded in 1971, there are 4,500 members in 11 countries. Publications include the quarterly newsletter *The Connector*, pamphlets and other brochures. For address, see Appendix D; see also SCLERODERMA FOUNDATION; SCLERODERMA RESEARCH FOUNDATION; SCLERODERMA SUPPORT GROUP; UNITED SCLERODERMA FOUNDATION.

scleroderma, localized One of several chronic types of scleroderma, a group of chronic autoimmune rheumatologic skin conditions of unknown cause. The localized skin forms of scleroderma include morphea, generalized morphea, linear scleroderma, morphea profunda, eosinophilic fasciitis and pansclerotic morphea. The various related disorders are all characterized by hardness of the skin, with thick, tightly-packed collagen fibers.

Morphea often improves on its own, but linear scleroderma that affects the scalp, face or extremities often involves progressive deterioration of underlying muscle and bone.

Symptoms In morphea, lesions first appear in purple to tan patches that are smooth; they then become white or porcelain-colored as they become shiny and firm. *Linear scleroderma* is associated with lines of hard, yellowish plaques that may be depressed into the skin, often found on the scalp, face, arms or legs; it affects all layers, including bone, and may lead to deep atrophy of the affected area. In *morphea profunda,* the collagen and inflammation are found in subcutaneous fat and even into fascia. *Eosinophilic fasciitis* is characterized by large, poorly-defined areas of hardened skin that impedes movement; deposits of thickened collagen are found as deep as the fascia.

Complications Morphea is usually uncomplicated. The greatest concern is usually the cosmetic appearance of the lesions and the concern that they might spread. In deeper forms of morphea, in linear schleroderma and in eosinophilic fasciitis, the primary complication is potential severe cosmetic deformities to the face and loss of movement in the arms and legs.

Treatment Plaques of morphea may fade by themselves. Administration of topical corticosteroids and emollients may be effective. Treatment of morphea profunda, pansclerotic morphea and linear scleroderma is difficult; the choice treatment is antimalarial drugs. Acute generalized morphea may respond to a brief course of systemic corticosteroids (such as prednisone) for a month.

Scleroderma Research Foundation A support and research group for interested individuals with firsthand experience of SCLERODERMA that supplements medical research on the cause, treatment and cure of the disease. The foundation also seeks to develop a national network of support centers for patients and their families; informs the medical community and public about symptoms; and encourages donations, bequests and memorials. The foundation holds meetings featuring speakers on various aspects of the disease and offers a slide/sound program. Founded in 1978, the foundation has 1,500 members and sponsors periodic meetings. It publishes a quarterly newsletter, the *Advance,* and the quarterly *Advance Research and Treatment: Informative Articles Pertaining to Scleroderma.* For address, see Appendix D; see also SCLERODERMA FOUNDATION; SCLERODERMA INTERNATIONAL FOUNDATION; SCLERODERMA SUPPORT GROUP; UNITED SCLERODERMA FOUNDATION.

Scleroderma Support Group A support group for patients with SCLERODERMA and interested individuals that provides information, raises funds for research and holds bimonthly medical meetings. Founded in 1989, the support group has 1,000 members. For address, see Appendix D; see also SCLERODERMA FOUNDATION; SCLERODERMA INTERNATIONAL FOUNDATION; SCLERODERMA RESEARCH FOUNDATION; UNITED SCLERODERMA FOUNDATION.

scorpion stings The bite of most species of scorpion cause pain similar to a bee sting, but the more dangerous varieties can cause sweating, restlessness, diarrhea and vomiting—and can be fatal to children.

Treatment Victims should seek immediate treatment, especially for children. Painkillers and cold compresses can alleviate pain; in severe cases, local anesthetics and powerful painkillers may be necessary. In addition, an antivenin to neutralize the poison may be given. (Antivenin against the venom of local, dangerous types of scorpions are available in most parts of the world where those species live).

Prevention In areas where scorpions live, clothing and shoes should be shaken out before dressing. Barriers (such as a porch at least 8 inches high) can discourage scorpions.

scratch A skin mark caused by the stroking of the skin with fingernails or a sharp instrument.

scrofuloderma Tuberculosis of the skin, where the skin breaks down over suppurating tuberculous glands, forming irregular-shaped ulcers.

Treatment Scrofuloderma responds better to anti-tubercular drugs than does LUPUS VULGARIS, another type of skin tuberculosis.

scurvy A disease caused by inadequate intake of vitamin C that results in skin hemorrhages, causing widespread bruising. It is rare today in developed countries because of widespread consumption of fresh fruit and vegetables; body stores of the vitamin can protect against scurvy for about three months. However, it is still seen in developed countries among the elderly who have poor diets. It has primarily been associated with sailors, who used to suffer from scurvy because of a lack of fresh fruit.

Cause The body's normal production of COLLAGEN is disrupted by inadequate supplies of vitamin C; as the collagen production becomes unstable, it weakens small blood vessels and slows wound healing. Hemorrhages and widespread bruising occur, together with bleeding gums and loosening of teeth. Pain results from bleeding into muscles and joints. Follicular purpura of the skin is classical.

The disease is especially serious in children, since bleeding into the membranes around the long bones may interfere with growth. Fatal hemorrhages in and around the brain may also occur.

Prevention The body can obtain enough vitamin C through modest consumption of fruit (especially citrus fruit) and vegetables; other sources of vitamin C include milk, liver, kidneys and fish.

Treatment Large doses of vitamin C will stop bleeding within 24 hours, quickly easing bone and muscle pain.

seabather's eruption A rash of red bumps that appear on the skin covered by a bathing suit and the skin creases after swimming in salt water. The symptoms usually become noticeable within several hours of swimming, and last for several days before clearing up. Apparently, some people are more susceptible to the condition than others, since in any group of swimmers only certain people will experience seabather's eruption. It is thought that seabather's eruption is a contact dermatitis from an unknown allergen in salt water.

Treatment Calamine lotion and, in severe cases, a course of systemic steroids. Antihistamines relieve itching and topical emollients may provide relief from symptoms.

sea urchins The spines of sea urchins can break off in or underneath the skin, causing an immediate burning, swelling or itching, and redness or a delayed reaction featuring a flesh-colored nodule appearing several months after being stung.

Treatment For the immediate reaction, put your foot in extremely hot water for at least a half hour to relieve pain; spines must be surgically removed in an emergency room to eliminate the risk of infection, but even if this is done, some species will remain lodged and will take several months to be ejected by the body's defenses.

seaweed A plant whose gelatin-like properties make up the main ingredient in peel-off masks that allow the skin to retain moisture. Seaweed is also used in face creams and lotions to help provide body to the products.

seaweed dermatitis See DERMATITIS, SEA-WEED.

sebaceous cyst A nonspecific term for a harmless large, smooth nodule under the skin, usually found on the face, ear, scalp, trunk or genitals (a cyst on the scalp is called a wen). These cysts may grow very large and may become red and inflamed either spontaneously or after trauma. The inflammation is usually the result of disruption of the cyst wall, causing the contents (usually a mixture of keratin) to leak out. These cysts are often wrongly thought to be infected because of their appearance, and antibiotics are incorrectly administered. The correct treatment is incision and drainage. Inflamed cysts should not be excised until the inflammation has subsided.

Treatment Large or bothersome cysts should be removed surgically under local anesthetic; if the entire cyst wall is removed, recurrence is rare.

sebaceous glands Tiny glands that secrete a lubricating substance called SEBUM either into hair follicles or directly onto the skin's surface. Most of these glands are located on the scalp, face and around the anus; none are found on the hands or soles of the feet. The production of sebum is partly controlled by male sex hormones. Problems with the sebaceous glands may lead to excessively oily skin (SEBORRHEA), ACNE, RHINOPHYMA or sebaceous hyperplasia.

seborrhea Excess SEBUM secretion causing increased facial oiliness and a greasy scalp. While the exact cause of this excess production is not understood, male sex hormones (androgen hormones) do play a role in the problem. Not surprisingly, therefore, the problem is most common in adolescent boys and men.

Tretment Seborrhea usually disappears by adulthood without treatment, but people

Cross section of Skin Revealing Sebaceous Gland

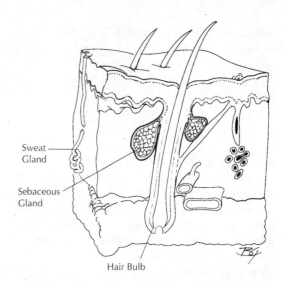

Sweat Gland

Sebaceous Gland

Hair Bulb

with seborrhea are also more likely to have other skin problems such as ACNE vulgaris and seborrheic DERMATITIS. Seborrhea is very difficult to treat. Washing the face frequently and the use of acne products reduce skin oiliness only temporarily. The only product known to reduce sebaceous gland activity is Accutane, which reduces the size of the glands during treatment and for several months afterwards. The side effects of Accutane usually preclude its use for seborrhea.

seborrheic dermatitis See DERMATITIS, SEBORRHEIC.

seborrheic keratoses See KERATOSES, SEBORRHEIC.

sebum An oily substance produced by the SEBACEOUS GLANDS in the skin. Composed of fat and wax, sebum lubricates the skin and protects it from becoming soggy when wet, or cracked when exposed to hot, dry temperatures. Sebum also helps protect the skin from bacteria and fungi. Oversecretion of sebum causes SEBORRHEA (oily skin and scalp) and may lead to seborrheic DERMATITIS or ACNE.

sebum-suppressive agents The only drug known to suppress sebum production is Accutane (ISOTRETINOIN), which works by suppressing the sebaceous glands. Topical agents may be used to defat the skin, but sebum activity is *not* affected and within minutes, the skin's oiliness returns.

self-tanning products A cosmetic product designed to produce an "artificial" tan without requiring exposure of the skin to the sun. The main ingredient in most topical products is DIHYDROXYACETONE (DHA), a chemical that acts only on the skin's superficial cell layers. When the DHA combines with certain amino acids and keratin in the skin's outer layer, it produces a natural golden color. However, as the skin sheds its dead cells, the tan fades—usually within a few days of application.

Some self-tanning products also include a sunscreen up to 15 SPF; others contain no sunscreens at all. Topical self-tanning products should be applied at least several hours before going out in the sun, and preferably the night before. Sunscreen should then be applied at least an hour before going outside.

For best results, users should exfoliate before application because the DHA may be absorbed unevenly in areas where there is a thick layer of dead cells—especially hands, elbows and knees. The depth of color is determined by how often the product is reapplied, not by how much is applied at one time. It can take between three to five hours for a self-tanner to develop fully.

Most self-tanning formulations have a short shelf-life once opened because DHA degrades quickly, and should be used up within three months of opening.

Tanning *pills* are another self-tanning product, but these drugs are available only outside the United States and are not recommended by dermatologists. There are two types; one type of drugs contain canthaxidine, a chemical that colors the skin but can damage the eyes and liver. The second contains psoralen, also available as a psoralen-containing cream. Neither is available in the United States, and both are considered dangerous by dermatologists because of the potential for severe sunburns.

The newest self-tanning product on the horizon is a synthetic hormone that colors the skin and also seems to protect against sun damage. This melanocyte-stimulating substance increases melanin, the pigment responsible for skin color.

Senear-Usher syndrome The common name for the blistering disease pemphigus erythematosus; it is usually limited to the face, where it appears as a butterfly rash over the nose and cheeks. Its severe scales and crusts may also appear on the scalp and the upper areas of the chest and back.
Treatment Topical medications including cleansing baths using Burow's solution or silver sulfadiazine cream, and application of topical corticosteroids may ease symptoms. Systemic corticosteroids are the primary method of treatment, beginning with doses high enough to completely stop the formation of new blisters. Immunosuppressive therapy together with corticosteroids improves control of the disease.
Side effects Most patients on long-term systemic corticosteroids develop side effects, such as high blood pressure, weight gain, infection, potassium loss, gastrointestinal bleeding, osteoporosis and cataracts.

senile keratoses See KERATOSES, SENILE.

sensitive skin Some people appear to have skin that is extraordinarily sensitive, easily itching, burning, chafing, stinging. This type of skin is also called problem-sensitive skin. Individuals with sensitive skin often develop difficulties while using cosmetics. While popular myth holds that fair or thin-skinned women have the most sensitive skin, in fact any type of skin in men or women can be highly reactive to a variety of irritants.

Some of the most common irritants are cold air, dry air, water and ultraviolet light. Other nonenvironmental irritants that can induce contact dermatitis include primary and secondary irritants. Primary irritants can cause the skin to react the very first time they contact the epidermis. (This group includes strong acids or alkalies that burn the skin). Secondary irritants are milder, and produce an irritation only after the skin has become sensitized to the substance over time. For example, these could include soaps, detergents, moisturizers, sunscreens, etc.

"Hypoallergenic" cosmetics and products are designed for the consumer with sensitive skin. This may indicate that a product has no added fragrance or that the manufacturer has avoided certain compounds known to be irritating. Unfortunately, when a person has become sensitive to a range of ingredients, it can become harder and harder to find products that don't trigger an allergic response. This group of patients is not necessarily allergic to agents, but they may more easily develop irritant reactions. See also DERMATITIS, IRRITANT; DERMATITIS, CONTACT; DERMATITIS, ALLERGIC.

serum sickness A brief illness featuring a skin rash that develops about 10 days after an injection with an antiserum derived from animals (such as anti-rabies serum equine obtained from horses). Antiserums can be obtained from either human or animal blood that contains specific antibodies (substances that play a role in immunity), and may be given to protect against dangerous infections.

When an antiserum is prepared from animal blood, a protein in the serum may be identified by the body's immune system as a potentially harmful foreign substance (called an antigen). In serum sickness, the person's immune system produces antibodies that combine with the antigen to form particles called immune complexes. They are deposited in various tissues, stimulate more immune reactions and lead to inflammation and other symptoms. Serum sickness is different from anaphylactic shock, another type of hypersensitivity reaction in response to antiserums.

Anyone who has ever had serum sickness should note the injection to which they are sensitive and warn medical personnel against future use of the antiserum.

Symptoms About a week after exposure to the antiserum, an itchy rash may appear, followed by enlarged lymph nodes, painful joints and fever. In severe cases, a state similar to shock develops. Symptoms usually fade within a few days.

Treatment Soothing lotions may help with the itching; nonsteroidal anti-inflammatory drugs may relieve joint pain and an antihistamine may curtail the illness period. In severe cases, systemic corticosteroids may be prescribed.

Sezary syndrome A rare T-cell lymphoma causing total body redness (with scaling), because of an abnormal overgrowth of lymphoid cells in the skin, liver, spleen and lymph nodes. Sezary syndrome primarily affects middle-aged and elderly patients.

Symptoms The patchy redness appears first, followed by hair loss, thickening of the palms and soles and distorted nail growth. Malignant T-cells also accumulate in the bloodstream.

Treatment Treatments include topical and systemic anticancer drugs, electron beam radiation and PUVA therapy. Low doses of METHOTREXATE also has been reported to help a group of patients, and does not cause secondary leukemia. Also beneficial may be photopheresis—giving the PSORALEN methoxsalen followed by irradiation of the blood with UVA.

shagreen patch A sign of TUBEROUS SCLERO-SIS, this is a large area of protruding skin usually found on the lower back.

shake lotion A suspension of powder in a liquid, such as water or oil.

shampoo Liquid cleaner designed to wash hair of dirt and oil. All shampoos clean hair by removing oil (produced from the oil glands in the scalp) and debris the oil attracts to the hair shaft. Inexpensive shampoos may be about 90 percent water with added detergent cleansing agents—usually either sodium laureth sulphate, sodium lauryl sulphate, ammonium laureth sulfate and ammonium lauryl sulfate. More expensive products vary from 30 to 50 percent solids. Other shampoo ingredients include slip agents or oils such as dimethicone, lecithin, cyclomethicone and mineral oil, with thickeners and ingredients to add lubrication and texture, such as stearyl alcohol, cetyl alcohol or protein; detangling agents such as tricetylmonium chloride, benzalkonium chloride or quaternium 1 through 80; foaming agents (linoleic DEAL or cocamide DEAL); preservatives, coloring agents and/or fragrances. Many manufacturers add other ingredients, including aloe vera, amino acids, collagen, vitamins, herb or fruit extracts and a variety of unusual oils.

The formulation of shampoos for various types of hair is very complex; even the addition of .1 percent of an active ingredient can change the formula. Therefore, it is difficult to judge any product's performance based on the label ingredients alone, since performance is determined by the *concentration* of ingredients and how they function when mixed with other ingredients. Even expert cosmetic chemists cannot judge the performance of a product based on reading label ingredients alone.

Some manufacturers have begun to add sunscreens in shampoo, but they are not given an SPF rating, because rating is based on the ability of a sunscreen to allow greater sun exposure to an individual without producing a sunburn. Since a sunburn is evaluated by skin redness, the test is impossible to do on hair. Instead, manufacturers have proposed establishing measures of "hair protective factors" as a way of measuring a product's ability to protect hair. Hair is very susceptible to damage from ultraviolet light, especially if it has been colored or permed. Sunscreen for hair is most effective when included in conditioners or finishing sprays.

How to use Shampoo should be applied to the scalp, especially if you have long or chemically treated hair. Hair near the scalp will be oilier, and look flat and sticky with oil buildup; hair at the ends doesn't get nearly the lubrication. Those with seriously damaged or dry hair should never apply shampoo to the ends of the hair shaft; enough shampoo will reach this area as the hair is rinsed.

Shampoo *must* be thoroughly rinsed out of the hair, or it will make the shafts look dull and flaky with residue.

Anyone with coarse, permed, color-treated or damaged hair should not use a combination shampoo and conditioner. A shampoo and conditioner's uses are actually opposite; the shampoo is designed to clean oil off the hair, while the conditioner coats the hair.

Those with oily hair should not use conditioner unless the hair is colored or permed, since conditioners add lubricants and coatings to the hair, which is already struggling with excess oil. For those with chemically treated hair, use conditioners designed for oily hair (these products use little or no oils and lighter weight lubricants), and apply it only to the ends of the hair, avoiding the scalp.

Don't scrub your hair dry with a rough towel; dry gently by a blotting or gentle squeezing motion. Rough treatment on wet hair can damage the cuticle.

shaving and the skin It may be possible that men's skin stays younger looking than women's because daily shaving exfoliates the skin.

The best way to get a non-damaging shave is to first soften the hair with warm, not hot, water, because hot water can inflame the skin. Use shaving soap or cream to help hold moisture, softening and lifting the hairs. Gel and cream-containing moisturizing shaving creams help individuals with dry or easily irritated skin. Avoid shaving creams that contain OIL OF BERGAMOT (found in some lime scents), which can cause a photosensitivity reaction when you go out in the sun. Also avoid shaving creams with benzocaine, since some people are allergic to these products.

Change blades after three to six shaves, and don't stretch the skin as you shave; a light touch with smooth, even, long strokes along the grain produces the closest, least-irritating shave. In the case of nicks, use a styptic pencil (aluminum chloride).

After shaving, apply cool water or a mild after-shave lotion to tighten pores and smooth skin. If alcohol is irritating to your skin, choose a product that is low in this ingredient. Talcum powder after shaving doesn't really provide much benefit. Applying a mild moisturizer after shaving may be helpful, however.

shingles Caused by the VARICELLA-ZOSTER VIRUS, a virus of the herpes family, this is a painful, red blistering viral infection of the nerves that supply certain areas of the skin. The problem begins during a CHICKEN POX attack (usually in childhood); after the spots fade, the virus lies dormant in sensory nerves for many years. For reasons that aren't entirely clear, the virus may reemerge and cause an eipsode of shingles. This is found most often in those over age 50.

Although rarely fatal, shingles has been the scourge of the elderly and the immunocompromised because it causes such terrible pain; each year, the condition affects several hundred patients per 100,000 in the United States. Researchers believe that current population trends will bring more cases of shingles as the numbers of elderly and those with failing immune systems increases.

Symptoms The first sign of shingles is an excessive sensitivity in an area of skin, followed by pain. After about five days a rash appears, turning first into tense blisters, and then yellow lesions within three more days. The blisters then dry out and crust over, gradually dropping off, leaving small pitted scars behind. Because the nerves have been damaged after the shingles attack, once the blisters heal the nerves constantly produce strong pain impulses that may last for months or years. The older the patient and more severe the rash, the more likely the pain (called POST-HERPETIC NEURALGIA) will persist.

Shingles often affects a belt of skin over the ribs on one side, which is where herpes zoster gets its name (*zoster* is the Greek word for belt). Sometimes the disease affects the lower part of the body or the upper half of the face on one side. The common name for the disease—shingles—comes from the Latin word for belt—*cingulus*.

Treatment Although there is no cure, several new drugs are currently being studied, and a newly-approved chicken pox vaccine also may offer hope to those at risk for shingles. Prompt use of antiviral drugs—such as ACYCLOVIR (Zovirax) or the newly approved famciclovir (Famvir) can shorten the rash and lessen the chance of pain later. Both are most effective if used within 72 hours after the rash appears; patients should seek medical help at the first sign of shingles. Both drugs slow reproduction of the virus and shorten the course of the infection. There is some evidence that the drugs may also decrease the chances for nerve pain following an attack.

Another recently approved drug is Valtrex, the Glaxo-Wellcome trade name for valacyclovir, which is converted to acyclovir in the body. Because acyclovir is itself not well absorbed, the new drug may provide better relief at lower doses.

BV-araU, under development by Bristol-Myers Squibb, is now undergoing clinical trials around the world. If it is found to be safe it could be even more effective than other drugs now on the market.

No agents have been demonstrated to routinely prevent post-herpetic neuralgia. Some experts maintain that steroid drugs such as prednisone can prevent this pain; other combine steroids with vitamins B or C complex, a multivitamin and a mineral tablet. Antidepressive drugs may also be effective, not by fighting depression, but by interfering with chemicals that transmit pain signals.

For do-it-yourself relief, you can try applying a cold, wet compress to the blisters and avoiding direct heat on the lesions. The mediction Zostrix (active ingredient: CAPSAICIN, a red pepper derivative) may help relieve the post-herpetic neuralgia, once all the blisters have disappeared. A counterirritant, it works by fighting fire with fire, but some patients may find it is too irritating. Experts believe the capsaicin blocks the production of a chemical necessary for pain impulse transmission between nerve cells. It should not be applied to active shingles blisters; as a counterirritant, Zostrix is designed to be used on unbroken, healed skin that hurts, not for open, oozing infections.

For severe pain from shingles, some experts recommend injecting a sympathetic nerve block in the appropriate place to block the nerves supplying the area of pain. This block typically relieves pain in up to 80 percent of patients. In some cases, it can permanently end shingles pain. Prompt intervention by a pain specialist can sometimes head off post-herpetic neuralgia.

shock, electrical See ELECTRICAL BURN; ELECTRICAL INJURY.

Shwartzman phenomenon A severe reaction involving tissue death caused by the injection of endotoxin into the skin 24 hours after an intravenous injection of the same or another endotoxin at a site other than the original site.

sickle cell ulcers Skin symptoms that occur in about half of patients with sickle cell anemia, a hereditary disease that affects blacks characterized by the production of an abnormal type of hemoglobin. The skin ulcers associated with this condition usually appear between ages 10 and 20 and appear on the lower legs, with recurrent attacks of fever and pain in the anus, legs and abdomen. They are caused by partial obstruction in the blood vessels and decreased oxygen in certain areas caused by abnormal hemoglobin.
Symptoms The sickle cell lesions look like well-defined punched-out skin defects that are painful and heal slowly; they may be complicated by infection.
Treatment Affected limbs should be elevated and immobilized. Clean the ulcers with hydrogen peroxide or antibacterial solutions; the wounds should also be debrided in order to promote healing. Blood transfusions may be necessary.

silica A mineral included in face and body powders and paste-type masks. Silica is soothing and forms a moisture-retaining film on the skin.

silicone implant A synthetic implant once widely used in cosmetic surgery because it was resistant to body fluids, permeable to oxygen and not rejected by the body. The implants have been used in breast reconstruction or breast enlargement for several million American women. Medical-grade silicone is included in more than 500 products, including a range of over-the-counter medications, and in hair spray, processed foods, skin creams and cosmetics.

Of the more than 2 million women who have had breast implants containing a soft polymer called polydimethylsiloxane (PDMS), reported illnesses from reactions to the implants include autoimmune disorders such as LUPUS ERYTHEMATOSUS, rheumatoid arthritis and chronic fatigue. In some cases, silicone invades the surrounding tissue or implant capsule.

In recent research, scientists at the Armed Forces Institute of Pathology in Washington, D.C. found that of three types of implants (those filled with PDMS gel, saline implants and those with PDMS gel covered with polyurethane), only the saline implants leached no silicone into breast tissue.

History Silicone gel–filled breast implants have been available since 1963 and were originally made out of a thick, smooth envelope of silicone rubber filled with a silicone gel. In the early 1980s, the shell was reformulated to minimize the amount of certain types of silicone that "bled" through the envelope.

In 1992, based on complaints that the implants ruptured or caused systemic disease, the FDA called for a voluntary moratorium on the use and distribution of silicone gel–filled breast implants. This call followed a 1991 advisory panel ruling that found "no evidence that these implants are unsafe" but noted that "there is also insufficient evidence to prove safety."

Today, while the FDA has not formally approved silicone gel–filled breast implants, they have allowed their continued use under certain guidelines. The FDA also concluded that the implants were of significant benefit for reconstructive patients, and ruled that the implants should be available to those who want them. However, only a small number of women who want the gel-filled implants for cosmetic augmentation are allowed to have them; these women must be part of a research study and their names must be re-corded in a registry. The FDA also requires manufacturers to conduct more studies to prove the device's safety and effectiveness.

Women who have an "urgent need" for an implant will have immediate access to the device; these include women who have expanders, whose implants have ruptured, or who are facing mastectomy and who want reconstruction with silicone.

Procedure Surgical insertion of the device can be performed under local or general anesthesia, and is usually an outpatient procedure. It can be placed either directly beneath the breast tissue or under the muscles. For reconstructive surgery after mastectomy, the existing surgical incision is usually used, and the implant can be placed at the time of mastectomy or at a later date.

Side effects There have been a variety of different problems that women have experienced, which has led the FDA to crack down on silicone implants.

Hardening of the implant The most common side effect is called "capsular contraction." Normally a surgical pocket is created for the implant that is larger than the device itself. A membrane called a capsule forms around the implant, and under the best circumstances, it maintains its original dimensions, allowing the implant to rest inside it. However, for reasons that seem to be related to a person's individual characteristics, the scar capsule shrinks in some women and squeezes the implant, causing the implant to become hard. These levels of contracture are measured on a scale of one to four (one so soft as to be undetectable, and four to be as hard as a grapefruit). The contraction may occur right after surgery, or only many years later, in one or both breasts. Some researchers believe that a low-grade bacterial contamination may trigger this process.

This hardening is not hazardous to the health, but it can interfere with the cosmetic result and cause discomfort or pain. If it becomes troublesome, a physician may recommend surgically scoring the tight capsule of scar tissue or surgically removing it. However, hardening can recur.

For some women who have developed hardened implants, a "closed capsulotomy" can provide dramatic immediate relief. In this procedure, a forceful squeeze of the breast can tear the scar capsule, allowing additional space for the implant and restoring softness. This simple procedure causes very little pain and—when it works—the relief is immediate, eliminating the necessity for surgery.

However, in some women excessive force is required to tear the capsule, which can be painful and sometimes ruptures the implant. The FDA states that a closed capsulotomy should not be performed, although some physicians feel the procedure is appropriate for some patients. If the implant does break, a closed capsulotomy can push the loose gel into nearby tissues.

Rupture Sometimes the implants break on their own. This could happen in the wake of a car accident or normal breast movement and compression. This type of "silent rupture" may be detected on a mammography or by physical examination, although neither method is 100 percent successful. If this should happen, the free gel will usually be kept within the scar-tissue capsule around the implant.

You should suspect a rupture if the breast changes in appearance or texture. Rarely, an accident can tear the scar envelope itself, and push the gel into subcutaneous areas such as the chest wall, down into the abdomen, the arm or the breast tissue.

Within two to six weeks, gel that has escaped is surrounded by new scar tissue and can form granulomas, which can either mask or mimic a tumor. This is one reason why direct injection of silicone into the breast is not recommended.

Cancer An FDA advisory panel in 1991 concluded that the potential risk from cancer from polyurethane-coated implants is probably less than one in 1 million. Studies of women who have had implants for 10 or 20 years have found no higher incidence of breast cancer in this group than in those women without implants.

Other experts are concerned that the implants may block the detection of breast tumors via mammography. The American College of Radiology, the American Cancer Society and the American Society of Plastic and Reconstructive Surgeons agree that a woman with breast implants should have routine mammography at the same rate as a woman without implants, but that she should be referred to mammographic facilities accredited by the American College of Radiology who are familiar with the special "Eklund" views required for adequate evaluation of the breast. If possible, these women should return to the same place for all future mammograms. This type of mammography is more expensive, since a minimum of four X rays is required to adequately evaluate the breast; thus, the amount of radiation is also higher.

Rheumatic disorders Some experts have speculated that there may be an association between silicone and autoimmune or rheumatic disorders, especially SCLERODERMA and LUPUS ERYTHEMATOSUS. Since scleroderma, lupus and similar diseases aren't commonly found in the population, it is difficult to research and compare the link between them and implants.

Silvadene   See SILVER SULFADIAZINE.

silver nitrate   A salt of silver that is applied in creams or solutions to destroy warts and treat wounds and burns. It is also used as eyedrops to prevent a serious form of conjunctivitis in all newborns.

Side effects Silver nitrate may cause irritation or pain and if used for a long time, it may cause permanent blue-black skin discoloration. It is extremely poisonous when ingested.

silver sulfadiazine An antibacterial cream used to prevent infections in skin grafts or second- and third-degree burns. It is especially helpful in keeping burn sites sterile, thereby reducing the chance of secondary infection.

Adverse effects Possible side effects include allergic reactions (with rash, itching or burning). Although rare, long-term use may produce serious blood disorders or kidney damage. It is not recommended for patients who are sensitive to sulfonamide drugs, nor should it be used for newborns or premature infants.

Sjogren's Syndrome Foundation A foundation for individuals with Sjogren's Syndrome, specialists, internists, immunologists, rheumatologists, otolaryngologists, ophthalmologists, gynecologists, gastroenterologists, pulmonologists, dermatologists, pharmaceutical companies and dentists. The foundation hopes to increase public awareness and medical knowledge about the syndrome, educate patients and their families and allow patients to share coping tips. See Appendix D for address.

skin The outermost covering of body tissue that weighs twice as much as the brain—about 6 to 9 pounds, stretching over 18 square feet. It is also a sensory organ, and contains many cells sensitive to touch, temperature, pain, pressure and itching. The skin protects the internal organs and keeps the body at the correct temperature—not too warm and not too cold.

When the body is hot, the sweat glands in the skin perspire, cooling the body and helping the blood vessels in the dermis to dilate, dissipating the heat. If the body gets cold, the blood vessels in the skin constrict, conserving

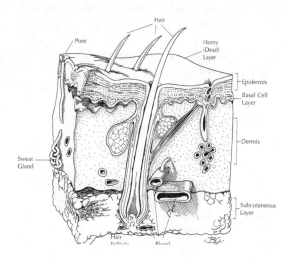

Cross section of Skin

the body's heat. The skin also takes in oxygen and secretes waste, and manufactures hair, nails and vitamin D.

The skin completely renews itself every 30 days; as older cells are sloughed off on the surface, new cells are produced in lower layers of skin. After these new cells have grown and divided, they begin to migrate over a two-week period up to the surface, where they replace older cells.

The hair and nails are extensions of the skin and are primarily made up of KERATIN, the main constituent of the top layer of the skin.

There are two layers of skin—the EPIDERMIS and DERMIS. The *epidermis* is the top skin layer, whose thickness varies from about a 1/2 inch on soles of feet and palms to 1/25 inch over the eyelids; most of the epidermis is no thicker than a page in this book, made up of about 20 overlapping layers near the skin surface. The epidermis is good at holding water, which helps make the skin elastic and maintains the body's balance of fluid and electrolytes.

A small proportion of epidermal cells are called Langerhans cells, and are located in the mid-zone of the stratum spinosum, the middle layer of the epidermis. They are also found in the dermis, lymph nodes and thymus, and they are important in recognizing and presenting antigens to keratinocytes and to lymphocytes. They serve as the early warning system of the body's immune system, picking up antigens in the skin and circulating to the draining lymph areas via the dermal lymphatics in order to elicit an immune reaction.

The epidermis is also divided into three layers—the basal layer (named because its cells form the *base* of the epidermis)—is also referred to as the *Stratum germinativum* because this layer of cells is always producing—or germinating—new cells. The second subdivision of epidermis is called the prickle cell layer (or *Stratum spinosum*), composed of squamous cells. The topmost layer is called the "horny layer" (*Stratum corneum*). The basal layer is also home to the class of cells called MELANOCYTES, the pigment-producing cells that give birth to MELANIN (responsible for giving color to the skin). One out of every six cells in the basal layer is a melanocyte. Production of the melanin is under the control of a hormone secreted from the hypothalamus of the brain called melanocyte-stimulating hormone (MSH). It is believed that melanin is capable of absorbing ultraviolet light and thus protecting against the harmful effects of the ultraviolet rays that occur with suntanning.

Differences in skin color are due to genetically determined differences in how much melanin there is, and where it is found in the body. In general, the darker the skin the more melanin in the epidermal cells, and the more densely arranged. Sunlight stimulates this melanin production, and a suntan simply means that more melanin has been produced as a way of protecting the skin against the harmful effects of the sun. While our culture may consider a suntan to be a characteristic of attractiveness, to the body it means a protective response to injury.

The epidermis is modified in different areas of the body; it is thick over the palms of the hands and soles of the feet, and contains more keratin. This contrasts with the thin epidermis over most of the rest of the body. The epidermis can get even thicker with use, and can result in a callus on hands or feet.

The junction where epidermis and dermis meet is an area of many furrows called rete ridges, which anchors the epidermis with the dermis and allows the exchange of nutrients between the two.

The *dermis* is the second layer of skin, made up of connective tissue and various specialized structures like HAIR FOLLICLES, SWEAT GLANDS and SEBACEOUS GLANDS that produce oily SEBUM. It is the sebum that makes the skin waterproof, allowing a person to sit in a tub without soaking up water like a sponge. Blood vessels, lymph vessels, and nerves are also found throughout the dermis. Hair and sweat glands are actually epidermal appendages that migrate into the dermis during fetal development.

skin biopsy The most common procedure in dermatology, this technique involves cutting a small piece of skin for analysis and requires only a local anesthetic. It is used to establish a diagnosis by providing specific, reliable information about the problem. The biopsy will include all of the skin and some subcutaneous tissue that is large enough to contain hair complexes and sweat glands.

Most commonly, the sample will be taken for histopathologic examination by routine light microscopy, but special studies (immunofluorescence microscopy or electron microscopy) may be performed. It may also be processed for a bacterial, fungal or viral culture.

Dermatologists commonly use four different techniques—punch, shave, excisional or wedge (incisional) biopsy. The punch (trephine) biopsy is most commonly used by dermatologists for a routine diagnostic biopsy. It is used to remove a portion of a larger lesion, to remove small lesions completely or to sample a representative area involved in widespread disease.

Shave biopsy is a simple technique used to remove lesions (or parts of them) protruding above the skin's surface. This technique is quick and easy and provides good cosmetic results afterward. However, it does not allow for the sampling of the dermis underlying the lesion. This type of biopsy is often used to rule out cancer in seborrheic keratoses and cutaneous horns. It is rarely used to diagnose an inflammatory skin disease.

Excisional biopsy is occasionally used to excise an entire lesion, especially in the case of malignant melanoma (see MELANOMA, MALIGNANT) and DYSPLASTIC NEVI, since the appearance of the cells may differ widely within one lesion in these conditions. Excision also allows for a much bigger chunk of tissue than a punch biopsy. However, this type of biopsy carries greater risk of significant scars, bleeding and infection.

The *wedge (incisional) biopsy* involves a narrow incision that extends deep into a nodule or subcutaneous tissue that is used when it is important to assess the subcutis. This type of biopsy may be used to diagnose panniculitis, large vessel vasculitis or a deep fungal infection. While the technique is similar to an excisional biopsy, the incision is usually narrower and extends more deeply.

skin cancer Skin cancer is the most common of all cancers, affecting more than 600,000 Americans each year—a number that is rising rapidly. But it is also the easiest cancer to cure if diagnosed and treated early. Prolonged exposure or intermittent overexposure to sunlight is the primary cause of skin cancers. In fact, about 90 percent of all skin cancer is related to sun exposure, and most skin cancers are found on parts of the body exposed to sunlight.

Because ultraviolet light can damage DNA, exposing the skin to sunlight increases the risk that an individual will develop skin cancer.

Skin type is also a very important factor in the development of skin cancer, since fair-skinned individuals who tend to burn easily and tan poorly are at greatest risk and dark skinned people are at a reduced risk.

Recently, French scientists have discovered they can determine a person's skin cancer risk by measuring a specific mutation in a tumor-suppressor gene called p53. They found specific changes in the building blocks for this gene in three-quarters of samples taken from sun-exposed skin of cancer patients, according to scientists at the International Agency for Research on Cancer in Lyon. Almost no DNA from nonexposed skin of these patients—or the skin of those who spend less time outdoors—had this mutation.

There are three basic types of skin cancer: Basal cell, squamous cell and melanoma. BASAL CELL CARCINOMA usually appears as a small, shiny bump on sun-exposed areas, such as the face, neck, chest, upper back and hands, primarily in fair-skinned people (especially those who burn easily). The lesions gradually grow and may crust, bleed or ulcerate, although they usually don't spread. Local destruction of the skin and underlying tissues may be considerable if this type of cancer is left untreated.

SQUAMOUS CELL CARCINOMA usually appears as a red, scaly patch. It grows slowly, occasionally becoming a nodule and frequently becoming crusted and eroded. Bleeding is common. Basal cell and squamous cell cancers are almost certainly related to cumulative sun exposure, occurring mostly on exposed places. Unlike basal cell carcinoma, squamous cell cancers grow and may spread (metastasize).

Basal and squamous cell cancers account for about 500,000 new cases each year; cure rates are excellent if these lesions are discovered and effectively treated early.

MALIGNANT MELANOMA is the third type of cancer, the most deadly of the three. Melanomas are usually small brown, black or multicolored patches, plaques, or nodules with an irregular outline. They may crust on the surface or bleed, and many of them appear in preexisting MOLES. Melanoma is much more dangerous than other forms of skin cancer because of its tendency to spread rapidly to vital internal organs as the lungs, liver and brain.

Diagnosis Because the skin is so easily visualized, skin cancer can be easier to spot than internal malignancies. To make sure that skin cancer is recognized early, dermatologists recommend that everyone examine his or her skin twice yearly, using a full length and a hand-held mirror. When doing a self-exam, look for the early warning signs (see box) but also look for any *changes* in the skin. Coupled with yearly skin exams by a physician, self-exams are the best way to ensure early detection and treatment of skin cancer. (For a free brochure illustrating how to do the skin surface exam step-by-step, send a stamped self-addressed business-sized envelope to the Skin Cancer Foundation, Box 561, Department SE, New York, NY 10156.)

Treatment Most skin cancers—even malignant melanoma—can be cured if discovered early enough, which is why attention to symptoms and regular self-examination is highly recommended. When cancers of the skin are discovered early, there are a variety of treatment possibilities, depending on the type of tumor, size, location and other factors affecting the patient's general health. A biopsy is often studied before a definitive therapy is selected.

Prevention Use sunscreens and avoid excess sun exposure, scientists have found that some foods and nutrients *may* counteract the development of melanoma: best choices are fish with omega-3 fat, and antioxidants (including vitamin E, vitamin C and beta carotene). Avoid tanning beds.

SKIN CANCER WARNING SIGNS

Any spot that:

· changes color
· increases in size or thickness
· changes in texture
· is irregular in outline
· is bigger than 6mm (the size of a pencil eraser)
· appears after age 21
· A spot or sore that continually itches, hurts, crusts, scabs, erodes or bleeds
· Any sore that does not heal
· A skin growth that increases in size and appears pearl-colored, translucent, tan, brown, black or multicolored

---

Skin Cancer Foundation, The The only international organization concerned solely with the world's most prevalent malignancy—skin cancer. A nonprofit foundation, it conducts public and medical education programs and provides support for medical training and research to help reduce the incidence, morbidity and mortality of skin cancer.

More than 6,000 medical specialists from a wide variety of specialties, including dermatology, plastic and reconstructive surgery, oncology, surgery, radiology, pathology, photobiology, immunology, general and family practice, internal medicine, otolaryngology, ophthalmology and psychiatry, are affiliated with the foundation through its honorary fellows program.

The major goals of the foundation are to increase public awareness of the importance of taking preventive measures against the damaging rays of the sun, and to teach people how to recognize and act on the first warning signs of skin cancer. It distributes brochures, posters, books, newsletters and audiovisual materials to the general public, the media and to physicians offices, screening clinics, health fairs and corporate and community wellness programs.

The foundation has created teaching materials for distribution to schools, community education seminars and consumer awareness programs in pharmacies and department stores.

The Children's Sun Protection Program includes a book for five- to nine-year-olds, *Play It Safe in the Sun*, illustrated by a 10–year-old artist; an educational poster distributed to 60,000 elementary schools; and brochures, *Sunproofing Your Baby* and *For Every Child Under the Sun*, giving advice on sun protection from infancy onward.

The foundation offers audiovisual materials for use in physician's offices and waiting rooms, schools, communities, and corporate education programs. The foundation publishes an annual journal (the *Skin Cancer Foundation Journal*) and a quarterly newsletter (*Sun & Skin News*). It also grants its Seal of Recommendation to sunscreens of SPF15 or higher that meet its stringent criteria developed by an independent committee of photobiologists.

The foundation provides funding for basic research and clinical studies in the diagnosis, treatment and prevention of skin cancer. A vaccine to treat malignant melanoma has been developed under the foundation's sponsorship and has shown promising results in clinical testing on patients with the disease.

For address, see Appendix D.

skin, cleansing Skin should be cleansed daily to remove dirt and grease, bacteria and odor. Soaps are the products used for these purposes. There are differences in the types of soaps that may be used on the skin, and they differ in outward appearance, fragrance, cost and composition.

For example, superfatted soaps, which are designed to improve mildness, contain excess fatty material and leave an oily residue on the skin. Transparent soaps contain glycerin and varied amounts of vegetable fats. Other soaps may be produced for specific purposes, such as oatmeal soap for skin that tends to break out. The choice of a proper soap depends on a person's age, skin texture, skin problems and personal needs. All soaps are good at cleansing, but because of age, heredity, climate and skin texture, there are many different methods of proper skin cleansing.

Infancy In infancy, the skin's oil glands are not very active, although the SWEAT GLANDS are quite active. Tepid water is recommended for bathing, and a mild soap may be used sparingly to remove skin oil. The diaper area requires special attention: Soiled diapers should be changed frequently to avoid the harsh irritant potential of urine and feces. Removal of fecal material may require gentle rubbing with a cotton ball soaked in warm water. Avoid using soap if an irritating rash appears—in fact, a great deal of soap is not required at this early age. It is not necessary to wash the skin after removing a diaper soaked in urine only, since an infant's urine is sterile.

Childhood As the child gets older, the need for soap increases, but if a rash appears, then the soap should be discontinued. It may be particularly difficult to use soap on a child who has atopic dermatitis, an inherited dry, scaly condition of the skin. Preteens have a greater need for daily soap and bathing, as the sweat and oil glands are now functioning with more efficiency and can withstand repeated use of soap.

Teenagers During puberty (13 to 19 years) the oil glands function at peak capacity—especially on the scalp, forehead, face and upper chest. Some degree of acne and an oily complexion are quite common, and routine showering or bathing should become a habit. While frequent washing may appear to decrease oiliness, it will not alleviate acne by itself.

Adulthood As the skin continues to age, the oil glands secrete much less oil, and soap may begin to cause drying. While some people may continue to cleanse with soap for a long time without any adverse effects, others will experience excess dryness. Seasonal variations affect the skin, too, and must be taken into consideration. Cold, wind, sunlight and other environmental factors play a role in skin dryness.

If soap is used too often in later life, skin disease may develop; it may be better to cut down on the use of soap, especially on the lower extremities—especially during the colder months. Cleansing creams or lotions may be good substitutes, although certain areas of the body may continue to require soap. It's especially important to cleanse the body folds with soap.

skin care for infants When babies are born, their pigment production is not complete; even children who will go on to have dark eyes and hair are fairly light at birth. Slowly, as the child gets older the skin color changes and begins to correspond more closely to that of the parents. While young skin heals faster than older skin, it is also less able to protect itself from injury (including injury from the sun).

Examine your child's skin regularly, while diapering, bathing and dressing. Any change (mole, growth, spot or sore) should be pointed out to your baby's doctor or dermatologist. While it is normal for toddlers to develop new moles and other brown spots, ones that continue to change should be checked by a doctor.

Some medications make skin ultra-sensitive—when prescribed, ask the physician if the sun should be avoided.

Preventing sunburn in infants It may take several years until an infant's melanin pro-

duction is fully developed; until then, the skin is especially vulnerable to the sun—even darker skin.

Because a baby's skin constitutes a larger percentage of total body mass than an adult's, they are especially vulnerable to anything affecting the skin. A bad sunburn can cause serious fluid and electrolyte loss, fever, faintness, delirium, shock, low blood pressure and irregular heart beat.

Under six months As sunscreens have not been approved for their age group, infants under six months of age should be kept out of the sun entirely. Use carriage hoods, canopies and tightly woven umbrellas, and make sure baby wears a lightweight but tightly woven hat. Try to limit time in the sun to short trips, and keep to the shade as much as possible. Since sand, concrete, snow and water reflect ultraviolet radiation, it's better to park a baby carriage on grass instead of a patio; if you're at the beach, stay away from the water and put an old blanket under the carriage. Be aware that even on overcast days, as much as 80 percent of the sun's harmful radiation can still penetrate the clouds.

Over six months For babies over age six months, avoid the hours from 10 A.M. to 3 P.M. when the sun is most intense. Cover up with tightly woven hats and clothes (a broad-brimmed hat will shade ears, nose and lips, and may reduce your baby's chance of cataracts in later life.) Be aware that the sun can penetrate some fabric (even cotton undershirts, which only have an SPF of about 8)—so don't rely on clothes alone for protection. Limit time spent in the sun, regardless of hour or season.

After a baby reaches six months of age, experts agree on the importance of using sunscreen. Unscented sunscreens are a better choice because they don't attract insects. The sun protection factor (SPF) should be at least 15, manufactured by a major drug company and purchased at a store with a large turnover. Look for an expiration date (lack of one probably indicates there are no ingredients that won't deteriorate). Some sunscreens are available without PABA, which can cause skin irritation in some people.

No matter how safe and effective the product seems, it's a good idea to test it on your child's skin before regular use. Place a small amount on arm or abdomen; if redness or irritation appear, select another product. Normally, creamy products work best on youngsters because they don't dry the skin and can be easily seen.

Apply the sunscreen on all exposed areas, and under thin clothing, 15 to 30 minutes before exposure (it takes that long for the ingredients to penetrate the skin).

For a baby under one year, sunburn should be treated as a medical emergency. If the child is over age one, call the doctor if there is pain, blistering, decreased urine output, lethargy or fever over 101° F.

Treatment Give water or juice to replace fluids, especially if the child is not urinating. Give acetaminophen for fever over 101° F. Soak the skin in tepid, clear water, followed by a light moisturizing lotion. If touching the skin is painful, do not apply lotion. Dabbing plain calamine lotion may help, but don't use one that includes antihistamines.

DO NOT apply alcohol, which may cool the skin too much, and don't use any medicated cream (such as hydrocortisone or benzocaine) unless your baby's doctor prescribes it. Keep the child completely out of the sun until the burn is healed, and make sure your infant never gets another sunburn.

Sunscreen Look for a sunscreen with an SPF of 15 or higher, and look for a SPF 15 lip balm for face and hands—the waxy form stays on and doesn't sting or taste bad. Toddlers can even apply it themselves. Do a patch test by applying a small amount of sunscreen on the inside of baby's wrist the day before you plan to use it all over. If irritation or rash develops, ask your physician to recommend a nonirritating alternative.

Coat the child's skin well, rubbing in the lotion; don't forget hands, ears, nose, lips and areas around the eyes. Avoid contact with eyes or eyelids. It may help to apply sunscreen to your hands first, and then rub on baby.

Apply before going into the sun, and every two hours thereafter. Apply more often if the child plays in water or is perspiring. Teach children to use sunscreen early and they will be more likely to use it regularly as adults, according to recent studies.

Zinc oxide on the nose and lips may give more protection. Never put baby oil on the child before going outdoors—it makes the skin translucent, letting the sun's rays pass through more easily.

skin care product, allergy Allergic reactions to skin care products are rare (only 210 for every 1 million applications), but they can develop after years of trouble-free use. The perfuming agents in creams, soaps and cosmetics are often the cause (even some products called "unscented" contain tiny amounts of fragrance to hide chemical odors). See also COSMETIC ALLERGY.

skin characteristics A description of a person's skin—oily, dry or in-between—often referred to as "skin type" among consumers and cosmetician.

Oily skin People with this type of skin usually have enlarged pores, a shiny nose and a tendency to have breakouts, acne or blackheads. People with an oil problem should keep their skin especially clean, while not scrubbing too hard, which can stimulate the overproduction of oil.

Buy only products formulated for oily skin. In the oiliest areas, use an astringent or toner with a high alcohol content. Oil-free moisturizers may be used, and women with oily skin should only use water-based makeup.

On the positive side, people with oily skin are less likely to experience premature aging lines, although eventually even the oiliest skin becomes drier, causing wrinkles and lines.

Dry skin People with this type of skin usually have invisible pores and a tendency to itch, flake, get chapped and develop tiny premature wrinkle lines around mouth or eyes.

This type of skin should be cleaned with soaps that moisturize; transparent soaps are a good choice, but their added alcohol may leave skin dry, so be sure to follow with a moisturizer. Lips may need special protection against chapping in winter. One suggestion is to use a humidifier or pan of water indoors during winter to keep indoor air moisturized.

Combination skin The majority of people with this type of skin have basically trouble-free complexions with a supple, flexible smooth texture. Some areas of the skin may be dry (such as forehead and eyes) and other parts may be oily (such as the nose). It's a good idea to use products designed for normal skin, but use specially designed products on spots that are oily or dry.

skin color There are three pigments that give skin its color—MELANIN, which provides brown tones, carotene, which produces yellow tones, and hemoglobin, the red pigment in blood that provides red and pink color. A person's skin is actually a blend of the various pigmentations, and the healthy "rosy glow" comes primarily from hemoglobin. In some people, lack of this healthy rosy color is caused by low hemoglobin levels or impaired circulation of the blood in the skin. See also BLEACHING CREAMS; PIGMENT CELLS; PIGMENTATION; PIGMENTATION, DISORDERS OF; PIGMENTING AGENTS.

skin, congenital absence of See APLASIA CUTIS.

skin cream Lotions designed to retain moisture and keep skin smooth and soft. These products usually include at least one of the following: LANOLIN, petrolatum, collagen, mineral oil and squalane.

Many products also include preservatives that keep the product stable and fresh. The most common preservatives include parabens (ethyl-, methyl- and butyl-), quaternium-15 and imidazolidinyl urea. In addition, because many fragrances can cause allergies, many skin creams and other products also offer fragrance-free products.

skin disorders Despite its surprising resiliency, any number of things can go wrong with the skin: it can become irritated and inflamed; it can be burned. The skin is also prey to production problems—too little or too much oil, melanin or skin cells.

In fact, skin-related complaints account for up to 10 percent of all ambulatory patient visits in this country. Since the skin mirrors the general condition of the patient, many systemic conditions may be accompanied by dermatologic manifestations. And because disorders of the skin are so readily visible, dermatologic complaints are often the primary reason for patient visits.

Congenital skin conditions Birthmarks are pigmented skin blemishes present at birth that include MOLES, MONGOLIAN SPOTS and HEMANGIOMAS.

Infection/infestations The skin can be infected with either viruses, bacteria or fungi. Viral infections include CHICKEN POX, WARTS, HERPES SIMPLEX, MOLLUSCUM CONTAGIOSUM and HERPES ZOSTER. Bacterial infections include BOILS, CELLULITIS, ERYSIPELAS and IMPETIGO. Fungal infections include ATHLETE'S FOOT, JOCK ITCH and RINGWORM. Parasites include scabies, worms, fleas, ticks and lice.

Tumors (neoplastic disorders) Noncancerous tumors are very common skin problems, and include seborrheic keratoses and most types of NEVI. Types of skin cancer are BASAL CELL

CARCINOMA, SQUAMOUS CELL CARCINOMA, MALIGNANT MELANOMA, PAGET'S DISEASE OF THE NIPPLE, MYCOSIS FUNGOIDES and KAPOSI'S SARCOMA.

Autoimmune disorders Caused when the body attacks its own tissues, these skin disorders include LUPUS ERYTHEMATOSUS, VITILIGO, DERMATOMYOSITIS, MORPHEA, SCLERODERMA, PEMPHIGOID and PEMPHIGUS.

Disorders of hypersensitivity A wide range of skin symptoms can occur because of hypersensitivity. These include contact dermatitis, hives and anaphylaxis, reactive erythemas, drug reactions, vasculitis and photosensitivity diseases.

Scaling and bullous disorders Although uncommon, the bullous diseases are a dramatic and serious group of skin diseases. They include PEMPHIGUS, BULLOUS PEMPHIGOID, HERPES GESTATIONIS, EPIDERMOLYSIS BULLOSA ACQUISA, DERMATITIS HERPETIFORMIS and HAILEY-HAILEY DISEASE.

Trauma The skin's role as protector of vital underlying organs means that it is vulnerable to injury itself. Injuries may be due to cold (CHILBLAINS, IMMERSION FOOT or FROSTBITE), to heat (BURNS or erythromelalgia), or to pressure (CALLUSES, CORNS or BEDSORES).

Occupational skin conditions Injuries excluded, dermatoses account for nearly half of all remaining occupational illnesses. They can include systemic disease due to skin absorption; contact dermatitis (see DERMATITIS, CONTACT); PHOTOSENSITIVITY DISORDERS; ACNE; PIGMENT DISORDERS; tumors; connective tissue disease; granulomatous reactions; and disorders of the hair or nails.

Disorders of structure/function These can include inherited skin diseases; disorders of keratinization (ICHTHYOSIS, REFSUM'S DISEASE, FOLLICULAR HYPERKERATOSES, ACANTHOSIS NIGRICANS etc.); disorders of pigmentation (LENTIGO SIMPLEX, NEVUS SPILUS, NEUROFIBROMATOSIS, FRECKLES, MELASMA etc.); diseases of the dermis (CUTIS LAXA or PROGERIA); disorders of the subcutaneous tissue (such as POLYARTERITIS NODOSA); ACNE or ROSACEA; disorders of hair (such as ALOPECIA); disorders of the nails (such as PACHYONYCHIA CONGENITA); MAST CELL DISEASES (such as URTICARIA PIGMENTOSA); and diseases of nutrition and metabolism (such as VITAMIN A DEFICIENCY or PHENYLKETONURIA).

skin graft A technique used by both dermatologists and plastic surgeons to repair areas of lost or damaged skin in which the healthy skin is removed from one part of the body and reattached to the damaged area. If successful, new cells grow from the graft and cover the damaged area with fresh, new skin.

Skin used for a graft may be removed from another part of the patient's body, or taken from an identical twin; otherwise, skin from anyone else is rejected as foreign by the recipient's body. (Skin from an unrelated donor may provide temporary cover, however). Although all skin grafts leave scars, a skin graft is performed when the damaged area is too large to be stitched together or because an ungrafted area would result in unsightly or restrictive scarring.

There are two types of skin grafts—split thickness and full thickness grafts. A *split-thickness graft* is used when large areas (such as burns) must be covered; the area that has been "harvested" will regenerate in a few days to weeks and can provide more donor skin. *Full-thickness grafts* include a deeper, thicker section of the skin, and are often used for facial grafts because the transferred skin looks more normal. They have a more natural color and texture, and contrast less than split-thickness grafts. However, full-thickness grafts are less likely to successfully attach themselves. In addition, donor sites cannot be reharvested, and must be stitched closed after the graft section has been removed. Split-thickness grafts are usually cut from the abdomen or thigh; full-thickness grafts are often taken from behind or in the crease in front of the ear.

Pinch grafts may be used in an attempt to treat leg ulcers when there is good granulation tissue. In this procedure, grafts are taken from anesthetized skin (usually the upper thigh) by pinching a small amount of skin with a needle and slicing it with a scalpel or razor blade. The grafts are transferred to the ulcer bed with a small space between grafts, sprayed with an adhesive and covered with a semipermeable dressing with edges extending beyond the margin of the ulcer. Gauze and an elastic dressing cover the wound, which is left in place for three or four days. Strict bed rest is required. The physician can examine the pinch graft through the semipermeable dressing, draining accumulated fluid when necessary. Dressings may be removed in five or six days, or left in place if there is no infection. Cleansing with alcohol helps the wound to form a firm crust that will fall off in two or three weeks. The grafts will extend to the skin of the adjacent graft and fill up the ulcer.

skin infections Because the skin represents the outer barrier to the world, it is responsible for defending the interior of the body against a wide range of attackers, including bacteria, viruses, insect venom and fungi. Skin infections can range from a local superficial problem (such as IMPETIGO) to a widespread and possibly fatal infection.

Examples of bacterial skin infections include IMPETIGO, ECTHYMA, FOLLICULITIS, BOILS, CARBUNCLES, ERYSIPELAS, SCARLET FEVER, CELLULITIS etc. Viral infections with skin symptoms include HERPES SIMPLEX, CHICKEN POX and SHINGLES, WARTS, MEASLES, GERMAN MEASLES, RUBEOLA, FIFTH DISEASE, AIDS etc.

Fungal infections can be noninvasive, invasive and systemic. They include RINGWORM (tinea), CANDIDA infection, CHROMOMYCOSIS, CRYPTOCOCCOSIS etc.

Rickettsial infections are conveniently groups as the spotted fevers (ROCKY MOUNTAIN SPOTTED FEVER, RICKETTSIALPOX etc.), the typhus group (TYPHUS), Q FEVER and TRENCH FEVER.

Parasitic infections are endemic in many developing countries, where poverty, poor hygiene and inadequate sanitary facilities create favorable conditions for infection. The infections enter the United States with the immigration of foreign students, diplomats and immigrants. Protozoal infections include LEISHMANIASIS and AMEBIASIS; helminthic infections (worms) include PINWORMS, HOOKWORMS, STRONGYLOIDIASIS, CUTANEOUS LARVA MIGRANS, FILARIASIS etc. Ectoparasite (a parasite that lives on the outside of the host) infections include SCABIES and LICE. See also SKIN DISORDERS.

skin, nerves of The skin is filled with a vast web of nerves that have considerable functional overlap, producing sensitivity to temperature, touch, pressure, itch and pain. The nerve endings are found within the papillary and reticular dermis—some extend into the lower portion of the EPIDERMIS (outer layer of the skin). Great collections of sensory nerves also surround hair follicles and hair bulbs which enable fine body hairs to act as a sort of sensing antenna.

There are three types of special nerve endings found in the skin—MEISSNER'S TOUCH CORPUSCLES, pacinian corpuscles and hederiform endings. Meissner's touch corpuscles are composed of oval coils of terminal axons within collagen fibers, found mostly on the palms and soles of the feet and thought to be associated with touch. Pacinian corpuscles are composed of an axon core inside a capsule found in the deep protein of the feet and palms; they may be especially tuned to detect vibration.

Hederiform ("ivy-shaped") endings include the Merkel cells, found alone or in groups in the basal epidermis, which may function as touch receptors, although their exact function is not clear.

skin, newborn At birth, the skin of an infant may be covered by a soft, cheesy white material called vernix that serves to protect young skin; in the past this was almost always immediately removed, but lately more physicians assume it may have a protective benefit.

Many babies are born with skin marks, splotches or rashes that are quite normal and temporary. Some newborns have ACNE, as a result of the mother's hormones still in the baby's system; these fade away in a few months. There may be scratch marks, superficial bruises or a purplish mottling of the skin due to a temporary instability of the blood vessels. Sucking blisters on the lips, feet or hands are normal, and will fade away.

More than half of all babies and up to 80 percent of premature infants experience jaundice, a yellow discoloration of the skin due to a buildup of bilirubin (a product released normally when blood cells are broken down). It may be that an infant's liver is not ready to handle the job, but there is not usually cause for concern. Bilirubin levels may normalize on their own, or the baby may need to rest under special blue lights for a few days or refrain from nursing until the levels drop.

Birthmarks are often apparent, and in most cases should be left alone. However, some experts believe that a mole (or congenital nevus) present at birth should be removed to forestall the potential later transmutation into a malignant melanoma. A STORK BITE nevus (a type of HEMANGIOMA) is a harmless small flat pin skin blemish found in up to half of all infants, usually around the eyes, that disappears within the first year of life. Those around the nape of the neck may persist indefinitely. See NEVUS, CONGENITAL.

skin patch Also called a transdermal patch, this is a multilayered disk that ranges in size from that of a small coin to several square inches. It introduces a controlled release of a drug into the system through the skin. The patches are painless and usually do not irritate the skin. The patch works by maintaining a reservoir of the drug and releasing it through the skin via an adhesive-coated polymer membrane. Effective drug levels can be maintained this way for several days.

To offset motion sickness, patches have been used to deliver scopolamine; nitroglycerin and other nitrates to treat heart disease; and nicotine to people trying to stop smoking. Researchers are studying ways to introduce estradiol to postmenopausal women who need estrogen replacement, and to administer timolol and clonidine hydrochloride to treat high blood pressure, among other things.

Questions remain about long-term use of the patch. Critics worry about the levels of drugs that are administered, whether drug tolerance will develop, or whether the variability of skin permeability may affect the level of medication that is absorbed by the patient. There have also been concerns raised about contact dermatitis, especially with transdermal introduction of nitroglycerin and clonidine.

skin scams Many beauty products promise to *reverse the tracks of time* by removing wrinkles. Unfortunately, this is something no skin cream can do. Terms like "anti-aging," "rejuvenation" and "cellular renewal" sound wonderful, but they do not permanently alter the characteristics of aging skin. In truth, these skin products simply moisturize the skin, plumping it up so lines and creases are less noticeable. Experts say the special wrinkle-fighting ingredients in the supercream formulas are of limited value.

COLLAGEN, for example, is commercially manufactured from animal protein with the idea that, applied topically, it will enhance the production of a person's own collagen. But collagen molecules are just too large to be absorbed into the skin. Other anti-aging skin formulas include RNA and DNA, superoxide dismutase and glycosphingolipid, which some claim can "rejuvenate" cells. None of them has been shown to have any effect on internal body chemistry, experts say.

According to the Food and Drug Administration, if skin products alter the structure or function of the skin, they are regarded as drugs, not cosmetics. Manufacturers would have to submit data to demonstrate that these products were safe and performed their intended function—something not now required of cosmetics.

Other products with little value include quail egg omelettes for the face, seaweed cleansers, moisturizers with bee jelly and oils squeezed from turtles, sharks and minks.

skin tags Known medically as "acrochordons," these common lesions are small brown or flesh-colored flaps of skin that usually occur spontaneously and tend to run in families.

They are found most often in middle-aged women, on the neck, under the arm, under the breasts and on the eyelids.

Skin tags don't usually cause problems, although they may be irritated by rubbing clothing or jewelry. Anal tags often occur as a complication of anal fissures or hemorrhoids. Skin tags appear to be more common in overweight individuals.
Treatment Not normally necessary, skin tags can usually be removed with electrosurgery or by cryosurgery. Larger lesions may be removed with scissors or a scalpel, followed by electrodesiccation or cauterization.

skin tuberculosis See TUBERCULOSIS, SKIN.

skin tumor, benign A group of skin tumors that are not cancerous. For example, these include CUTANEOUS SKIN TAGS, SEBORRHEIC KERATOSES, ACTINIC KERATOSES, BIRTHMARKS, LIVER SPOTS, MOLES, KELOIDS and WARTS.

skin tumor, malignant See SKIN CANCER.

skin type While the phrase "skin type" has come to mean the skin's *characteristics* (whether the skin is oily, dry or in-between), dermatologists use the term "skin type" to indicate a person's relative sensitivity to sun exposure. Because a person's skin characteristics can vary from one part to another, dermatologists prefer to treat specific areas and conditions of each area of the skin. Skin characteristics tend to become more oily in summer, under stress, during adolescence and in hot, humid climates.

Skin type, according to dermatologists, is classified into six groups, according to its tendency to sunburn.

SUNBURN TYPE
TYPE 1: Always burns, never tans. Very fair with red or blond hair and freckles.
TYPE 2: Burns easily, tans minimally. Usually fair skinned
TYPE 3: Sometimes burns, gradually tans
TYPE 4: Minimum burning, always tans. Usually white with medium pigmentation
TYPE 5: Very seldom burns, always tans. Medium to heavy pigmentation
TYPE 6: Never burns but tans darkly. Blacks as well as others with heavy pigmentation

SLE See SYSTEMIC LUPUS ERYTHEMATOSUS.

smallpox A highly infectious viral disease causing skin rash and flu-like symptoms that has been totally eradicated since 1980. A medical scourge of the 19th century, smallpox was characterized by a rash that spread over the body, turning into pus-filled blisters that crusted and sometimes left deeply pitted scars. Complications included blindness, pneumonia and kidney damage, and there was no effective treatment for the disease, which killed up to 40 percent of affected individuals.

Smallpox was eradicated through a cooperative international vaccination program that was successful because the disease affected only humans. Victims were easily recognized and infectious only for a short time. As a result of the eradication program, smallpox vaccination certificates are no longer required for international travel. Most countries have stopped vaccinating because the vaccine itself is now more dangerous than the disease, since the vaccine can cause encephalitis and there is now no chance of contracting smallpox.

The virus responsible for smallpox is still maintained at laboratories at the Centers for Disease Control in Atlanta and at a research institute in Moscow. A recent suggestion to destroy the virus was met by such criticism among the scientific community, who value the virus for scientific purposes, that any attempt to do so has been postponed.

soap and the skin Soap is an emulsifier that attaches to water molecules and to oil and dirt molecules, pulling them together. This is why soap is better at washing away oily dirt than water alone.

Many people choose to clean their skin with soap (in fact, Americans take nearly 60 billion showers and baths each year) and the choices of soap are almost limitless—from 100 percent pure, hard-milled and scented to translucent bars or liquids. Soap has been around for quite some time (scented bars of soap were excavated from Pompeii and Phoenicians were milling soap 700 years before that), and the majority of Americans still turn to a bar of soap to clean their skin.

The downside of soap is that some skins are irritated by heavily perfumed products, and deodorant soaps may be troublesome to others. Moreover, some people with very dry skin or with ECZEMA may find that soap's fatty acids are too irritating; for them, a soapless cleanser or detergent (acid rather than alkaline) is a good choice. (Soaps are made from natural animal fat, while detergents are synthetic).

Antibacterial soap Dermatologists note that there is a place for the antibacterial cleanser such as Dial, Safeguard or Liquid Lever 2000, a mild new product that contains moisturizer in addition to deodorant and antibacterial agents and safe for children over age 18 months. Antibacterial soap is ideal for cleaning the fingers before inserting contact lenses, after handling suspicious things or after being around people with coughs and colds. These cleansers should be used on hands, or all over the body if skin is oily, or after exercise in hot weather.

Old-fashioned soap In grandmother's day, soap was made by combining an alkali with fat (such as vegetable oil) and water. Soaps like Ivory come under this heading, but many other products that seem like soap are really detergents.

Detergent soap While many consumers assume that "detergent" is synonymous with "household cleaner" and is therefore too harsh for the skin, in fact many companies add extra emollients to detergent formulas to make their products milder. Still, detergents do tend to be harsher than soap. Dove is an example of a soap that is really a detergent.

Superfatted soap A cleansing product with extra oils or fats (such as coconut or mineral oil, lanolin, or cold cream) included in the formula. In addition, excess fatty acids are added to ensure that the pH is not too alkaline. These products tend to leave an oily film.

Glycerin soap Usually transparent, these soaps contain the humectant GLYCERIN as an ingredient. Examples include Basis and Neutrogena.

Castile soap Often advertised as being especially pure, the real difference between castile and other soaps is that castile products are made with olive oil instead of other fats.

Medicated soap This cleansing product, which includes antibacterial ingredients, is considered to be a drug and is therefore subject to drug regulations. In fact, some medicated soaps, such as soaps containing salicylic acid or benzoyl peroxide, are sold only by prescription.

Deodorant soap These cleansing products (such as Dial) contain ingredients that fight body odor by killing bacteria. They are not recommended as facial cleansers.

Whatever kind of soap is used, it must be completely rinsed off the skin or the resulting residue can dry the skin and attract dirt.

Old beauty advice held that any type of soap was bad for the skin. The reasoning was that no matter how mild or pure, soap was still too drying. Formerly, people were advised to use a nonsoapy cosmetic cleanser containing no alcohol or grains, followed by a toner or astringent.

But today, many skin care experts note that there are plenty of mild, non-drying soaps available that are fine for everyone, such as glycerin or superfatted soaps. In fact, more than 50 new soaps were introduced in 1993 alone. A consumer should select the mildest product that is effective, according to dermatologists.

Despite the plethora of fancy "beauty bars," featuring milk and honey, essence of eucalyptus, pear nectar and freesia, for example, all soaps still contain sodium or potassium salts. It may not be glamorous, but soap works by emulsifying surface oils, carrying dirt away in the foam.

All soaps (by definition) are alkaline, made by the action of alkali on animal and vegetable fats, and strip the skin of its outside oily layer. Some soaps have a neutral or slightly acid pH, until they come in contact with water, whereupon they become alkaline. Therefore, no matter what a particular company may claim, a soap cannot truly be pH-balanced.

How to use soap It is important not to *overclean* the skin; even those with oily or problem skin should wash with soap just twice a day (or once in the evening if skin is very dry). Experts recommend 10 rinses to ensure that the skin is free of residue. If the skin has a tight, drawn feeling after washing, most likely the skin has been overcleansed or too strong a soap has been used.

Skin condition may change drastically with the seasons. In cold, harsh weather the skin is prone to dryness and chapping. Hot, humid weather may lead to more washings, which could irritate the skin. (See also SKIN CARE; CLEANSING AGENTS).

Society of Clinical and Medical Electrologists
A professional society of electrologists (those who remove superfluous hair for cosmetic or medical reasons). The society conducts continuing education and leadership development seminars. Founded in 1985, the society has 1,000 members and sponsors an annual convention. For address, see Appendix D; see also COUNCIL ON ELECTROLYSIS EDUCATION; INTERNATIONAL GUILD OF PROFESSIONAL ELECTROLOGISTS; NATIONAL COMMISSION FOR ELECTROLOGIST CERTIFICATION.

Society for Investigative Dermatology
A professional society promoting research in dermatology and allied subjects. Founded in 1937, the society has 2300 members and hosts an annual conference. It also publishes the monthly *Journal of Investigative Dermatology*. For address, see Appendix F.

Society for Pediatric Dermatology
A professional organization of pediatricians, dermatologists, pediatric or dermatologic house

officers, manufacturers of children's skin products and researchers in biomedicine whose concentration is in pediatric dermatology. Founded in 1975, the group has 450 members, conducts research programs and bestows awards.

Publications include the quarterly *Society for Pediatric Dermatology*, a newsletter that reviews current publications in the field of pediatric dermatology, including reviews in allergy and immunology, genetics and syndromes, infectious diseases, diagnosis and treatment. For address, see Appendix E.

sodium lauryl sulfate A detergent cleanser and emulsifier in creams and lotions that may cause allergic reactions in some people.

soft tissue augmentation Treatment that gets rid of serious wrinkles such as smile lines, furrows in the forehead, and vertical lines between the eyebrows with a bit of collagen, FIBREL (a gelatin extracted from the patient's own plasma) or fat suctioned from other places in the body (microliposuction).

Dermatologists use collagen to fill out scars, frown lines and wrinkles around the lips and on the forehead. Fibrel works better for acne scars and skin defects. Using your own fat to fill in deep wrinkles or restore youthful facial contours is more complex, however, because it requires two procedures: One to remove the fat and another to inject it into the lines that need to be removed.

The cost for soft-tissue augmentation ranges from several hundred to several thousand dollars, depending on how much work is being done, and the procedure will need to be repeated within two years because eventually the filler gets absorbed into the body.

solar keratoses See ACTINIC KERATOSES.

solar lentigo This condition is an acquired hyperpigmentation (skin darkening) due to an excess of MELANOCYTES (melanin-produc-ing cells). Solar lentigo appears in patients with fair skin who have a history of chronic sun exposure, developing the lesions usually after age 40.

Symptoms Moderately dark brown, large spots (called "age spots" or "liver spots") with irregular borders. The epidermis (outer skin layer) is atrophied with fine, paperlike wrinkles. Like LENTIGO SIMPLEX, solar lentigo does not fade in the winter or darken in the summer.

Treatment The most important part of treatment is to avoid any further hyperpigmentation by avoiding the sun, and applying sunscreens or sunblocks before going outside. Bleaching creams applied every day for up to a year may be effective. More aggressive treatment includes LIQUID NITROGEN cryotherapy, and short pulsed laser treatment such as Q-switched RUBY LASERS.

solar urticaria The medical term for sun-induced hives, this is an allergic reaction to certain wavelengths of the sun that appears immediately after exposure to the sun. See also POLYMORPHIC LIGHT ERUPTION.

Treatment The treatment of choice is a nonsedating antihistamine such as terfenadine.

solar warning index A new daily warning index forecasting the ultraviolet light radiation exposure for 58 cities in the United States designed to help people avoid skin cancer. The index is issued daily to forecast the amount of dangerous ultraviolet light that will reach the Earth's surface at noon the next day. The scale is generally from 1 to 10 in most areas, rising to 1 to 15 in regions that receive stronger solar radiation. The higher the number, the greater the level of radiation from the sun.

The goal of the warnings, issued by the National Weather Service, is to remind people of the danger of the sun to their skin so they will use sunscreens, sunglasses and reduce exposure to themselves and their children. Damage from sun exposure accumulates over time, and much of the injury is done when people are youngsters.

THE GENERAL CATEGORIES OF HAZARD ARE:

Minimal (index of 0–2): Fair-skinned people may burn in 30 minutes; those with darker skin may be safe up to two hours.

Low (3–4) Fair-skinned people may burn in 15 to 20 minutes; mothers may be safe from 75 to 90 minutes.

Moderate (5–6) Fair people may burn in 10 to 12 minutes; others may be safe for 50 to 60 minutes.

High (7–9): Fair people may burn in 7 to 8 1/2 minutes; others may be safe for 33 to 40 minutes.

Very high (10 and up): Fair people may burn in 4 to 6 minutes; others may be safe for 20 to 30 minutes.

The Environmental Protection Agency worked on the index with the National Oceanic and Atmospheric Administration and the Centers for Disease Control and Prevention.

sore The common term for a skin lesion.

SPF See SKIN PROTECTION FACTOR.

spider angioma A type of vascular lesion with a central pulsating body and radiating legs, often associated with pregnancy (between the second and fifth months) or cirrhosis. Believed to be caused by circulating estrogens, up to 75 percent of the pregnancy lesions fade by the seventh week after birth. The lesions may also appear in children and healthy adults, and then disappear or last for a long period. They tend to appear on the face, neck, upper throat and arms.

Treatment The central feeder vessel can many times be destroyed by electrosurgery using a very fine wire electrode that is threaded down into the vessel before cauterizing. Laser destruction has also been effective, using either the pulsed dye laser or a variety of continuous wave and quasi continuous wave lasers, such as the argon, krypton or copper lasers.

spider bite Two species of spider are responsible for most of the serious spider bites in the United States; widow spiders (*Latrodectus*) (see BLACK WIDOW SPIDER BITES) and band-spinning spiders, or BROWN RECLUSE SPIDERS (*Loxosceles*).

spongiform pustule An accumulation of white blood cells between epidermal cells that may lead to a spongy appearance and the appearance of fluid between the cells. It is characteristic of PSORIASIS.

spongiosis Swelling between the epidermal cells. It is a hallmark of ECZEMA.

sporotrichosis A chronic fungal infection of the skin that often follows trauma caused by the fungus *Sporothrix schenckii*, characterized by the formation of painful abscesses and ulcers. The fungus affects both men and women around the world, who come in contact with the fungus through soil, vegetation, untreated plants, or decaying vegetable.

There are several forms of the disorder; most patients (80 percent) develop the acute chancriform or lympho-cutaneous form of sporotrichosis. In this form of sporotrichosis, numerous scaly papules that erode and form chronic ulcers usually form in a line starting at the initial site of injury, spreading up the limb along the course of the lymphatics. There is also a disseminated systemic form, which invades the eye, nervous system or other organs in a true systemic fungal infection. The skin lesions that may accompany this type of musculoskeletal sporotrichosis are more chronic, and their outlook may not be so positive.

Treatment Specific treatment depends on the form of sporotrichosis. In the cutaneous form, iodides (given as an oral solution of potassium iodide) are the preferred method of treatment for up to six weeks. Amphotericin B and flucytosine have also been used to treat the chancriform sporotrichosis. Itraconazole has also been found to be effective.

Systemic sporotrichosis does not respond well to iodide treatment. For this form of sporotrichosis, amphotericin B is usually necessary. Systemic sporotrichosis in particular may be fatal.

spun-glass hair See UNCOMBABLE-HAIR SYNDROME.

squamous cell Keratinocytes (keratin-producing cells) that make up most of the EPIDERMIS, lying above the BASAL CELL layer. See also SQUAMOUS CELL CARCINOMA.

squamous cell carcinoma The second most common SKIN CANCER (after BASAL CELL CARCINOMA), squamous cell cancer affects more than 100,000 Americans each year. Arising from the EPIDERMIS layer of the skin, this type of cancer begins in the squamous cells that comprise most of the upper layer of skin. Squamous cell cancers may be found on all areas of the body, including the mucous membranes, but they are most often found on areas exposed to the sun.

While squamous cell carcinomas start in the epidermis, they can eventually spread to underlying tissues if untreated. Rarely, they spread to distant tissues and organs; this spread (metastasis) can be fatal. Squamous cell carcinomas that metastasize most often begin from chronic inflammatory skin conditions or on the mucous membranes, lips or ears.

Causes Chronic exposure to sunlight causes most cases of squamous cell cancer, which is why tumors are usually found on areas of the body that are exposed to sunlight. The rim of the ear and the lower lip are particularly prone to this type of cancer.

Squamous cell cancers may also appear on skin that has been injured by burns, scars, long-standing sores, sites previously exposed to X rays or chemicals (such as arsenic and petroleum byproducts). In addition, chronic skin inflammation or medical conditions that suppress the immune system for long periods of time may encourage squamous cell carcinoma.

Sometimes squamous cell carcinoma begins spontaneously on what seems to be normal, healthy skin. Some researchers believe this type of cancer may be hereditary.

Anyone with a long history of sun exposure can develop squamous cell cancer, but those with fair skin, light hair and blue, green or gray eyes are at highest risk. Dark-skinned individuals are far less likely to develop any form of skin cancer, but more than two-thirds of all skin cancers in blacks are squamous cell carcinomas found most often on sites of preexisting inflammatory skin conditions or burn injuries.

There are some skin conditions that are associated with eventual development of squamous cell carcinoma. These conditions include ACTINIC KERATOSIS, actinic cheilitis, LEUKOPLAKIA and BOWEN'S DISEASE. These "precursor" conditions, if properly treated, can be prevented from developing into a squamous cell carcinoma.

Symptoms Symptoms include a persistent, scaly red patch with irregular borders that sometimes crust or bleed; an elevated growth with a central depression that sometimes bleeds; a wart-like crusting growth that may bleed; an open persistent sore that bleeds and crusts. The lesions usually look like rough, thick scaly patches that bleed if bumped. They often look like warts, and sometimes an open sore will develop with a raised border and a crusty surface.

Treatment A diagnosis is made after physical exam and biopsy (removal and examination of a piece of tissue). If tumor cells are found, the physician will outline possible treatment. The treatment is based on type, size and location of the tumor and on the patient's age and health. It is usually performed on an outpatient basis. Local anesthetics are used to prevent pain during the procedure.

A physician may use electrosurgery (curettage and electrodesiccation) in which cancerous tissue is scraped from the skin with a curette (sharp ring-shaped device) while an electric needle burns a safety margin of normal skin around the tumor at the base of the scraped area. This technique is repeated several times to make sure the tumor has been completely removed.

With CRYOSURGERY, the physician does not cut the growth but instead freezes the lesion by applying LIQUID NITROGEN with a special spray or a cotton-tipped applicator; this method doesn't require anesthesia and produces no bleeding. It is easy to administer and is the treatment of choice for those who have bleeding disorders or are intolerant to anesthesia. Patients experience redness, swelling or blistering, and crusting after this treatment.

LASER SURGERY is used to focus a beam of light onto the lesion either to excise it or destroy it by vaporization. The major advantage of this technique is that it seals blood vessels as it cuts.

The most frequently used treatment is excision of the entire growth and an additional border of normal skin as a safety margin (excisional surgery). The site is then stitched closed and the tissue is sent to the lab to determine if all malignant cells have been removed.

In radiation therapy, X rays are directed at the malignant cells. It usually takes several treatments several times a week for a few weeks to totally destroy a tumor. Radiation therapy is most often used with older patients or with those in poor health. Radiation may be less traumatic for the elderly.

Mohs surgery (microscopically controlled surgery) involves the removal of very thin layers of the malignant tumor, checking each layer thoroughly under a microscope. This is repeated as often as necessary until the tissue is free of tumor. This method saves the most healthy tissue and has the highest cure rate. It is often used for tumors that recur, for large tumors, or for areas where recurrences are most common (nose, ears and around the eyes).

Outlook When removed early, squamous cell carcinomas are easily treated, but the larger the growth the more extensive the treatment. While squamous cell carcinoma does not spread to vital organs very often, if it does it can be fatal. Since removal of a tumor scars the skin, large tumors may require reconstructive surgery and skin grafts.

If a patient is diagnosed with one squamous cell carcinoma, there is a greater chance of developing other squamous cell carcinomas in the future. And having had a BASAL CELL CARCINOMA also makes it more likely that a squamous cell cancer will develop. No matter how carefully a tumor is removed, another can develop in the same place (or nearby), usually within the first two years after surgery. If the cancer recurs, the physician may recommend a different type of treatment the second time. It is therefore important to examine the surgical site periodically. (See also BASAL CELL CARCINOMA; MALIGNANT MELANOMA; SKIN CANCER.)

staphylococcal infections A group of infections caused by staphylococci bacteria that are a common source of skin conditions. Staphylococcal bacteria are normally found on the skin of most people, but if the bacteria accumulate within the skin, they can cause a wide variety of skin infections (PUSTULES,

BOILS, ABSCESS, STY or CARBUNCLE). One strain of the bacteria produces a toxin that can cause a severe blistering rash in newborn babies called staphylococcal SCALDED SKIN SYNDROME. Another produces the toxin responsible for TOXIC SHOCK SYNDROME.

staphylococcal scalded skin syndrome See SCALDED SKIN SYNDROME.

Stein-Leventhal syndrome A form of hirsutism (excess hairiness) also known as polycystic ovary syndrome. In this disorder, the ovaries increase testosterone production, increasing blood levels of the male hormone. About 20 percent of women with this problem have ACNE. This disorder is characterized by incomplete development of follicles in the ovary due to inadequate secretion of luteinizing hormone; the follicles fail to ovulate and remain as multiple cysts, distending the ovary. Hormone imbalance results in obesity and HIRSUITISM, and the sufferer becomes infertile due to the lack of ovulation.
Treatment Administration of antiandrogens such as spironolactone, cimetidine or cyproterone acetate and the oral contraceptive pill to suppress gonadotropic hormones. A wedge resection of the ovaries may help some women.

Stevens-Johnson syndrome A rare, acute condition involving the skin and mucous membranes (ERYTHEMA MULTIFORME MAJOR) characterized by fever and a variety of skin lesions, including red papules, erosions and blisters. When the condition affects only the skin, it is called erythema multiforme minor, or simply erythema multiforme. The condition is most often caused by drug reactions, and while it may occur at any age, it is most common in children and young adults. A fever and malaise may precede by several days the appearance of skin lesions, and there may be extensive involvement of the skin, lips, oral areas and mucous membranes.

Treatment Painkillers and sedatives may relieve the pain; while Stevens-Johnson patients usually respond to treatment, they may become seriously ill if shock or infection set in. Patients usually survive iwth some scarring, eye problems and nail dystrophy. Controversy exists over whether systemic steroids are indicated in this condition. See ERYTHEMA MULTIFORME.

Stewart-Treves tumor A type of tumor that is closely related to angiosarcoma that often appears in the upper extremities after radical mastectomy for breast cancer. The tumor, which is unrelated to the breast cancer, usually appears about 10 years after the original surgery and after long-standing swelling in the lymph nodes in the upper extremity.

Onset of this tumor is usually fairly quick, with the appearance of a blue-purple patch on the upper arm followed by red-blue or purple nodules or blisters. Larger lesions may spread quickly, through the lymph system and blood vessels, to the lungs, pleura and thoracic wall.
Treatment There is no truly effective treatment; the tumors and lesions usually recur even after radical surgery.

sting An injury caused by a plant or animal toxin introduced into the skin.

stork bite nevus A type of vascular malformation, this is a harmless small flat pink skin blemish found around the nape of the neck in up to 50 percent of newborn babies that may persist indefinitely.

Salmon patches are similar blemishes found around the eyes in a similar percentage of newborns. These blemishes usually disappear within the first year.

stratum corneum Latin for the "horny layer," the top layer of EPIDERMIS that consists of dead cells. Because the surface of this layer is acidic, it is sometimes also referred to as the acid mantle. The *Stratum corneum* gets its name from the fact that when tightly compacted, its cells toughen, like an animal's horn (and mammal horns *are* made of the same protein material that makes up the stratum corneum).

The cells of this SKIN layer are constantly sloughed from the skin's surface and are completely replaced about every two weeks by cells migrating upwards from below. If for some reason horny cells accumulate on the skin surface, the result will be flaky skin. This is a particular problem for those with dark skin because of the sharp contrast between the gray flakes and the surrounding skin.

This layer of the skin provides the major physical barrier of the body, and also serves as a shield to the sun's harmful ultraviolet rays. It also blocks the penetration of most substances that touch the skin. Normally only substances smaller than a water molecule can easily penetrate the horny layer, which means that your skin can't drink up vitamins, nutrients, collagen or elastin because their molecular structure is larger than water.

stratum germinativum The base of the EPIDERMIS also known as the basal layer where SKIN cells are constantly germinated anew. New cells are constantly produced in the basal layer, eventually migrating upward through the epidermis to the surface of the skin. The basal layer is composed not only of basal cells, but also of MELANOCYTES, the pigment-forming cells of the skin that produce MELANIN, responsible for giving skin its color.

stratum granulosum A part of the EPIDERMIS, the stratum granulosum consists of two or three rows of cells lying directly below the STRATUM LUCIDUM, which lies below the STRATUM CORNEUM.

stratum lucidum The epidermal cell layer between the STRATUM CORNEUM and the STRATUM GRANULOSUM.

stratum malpighii The major layer of the EPIDERMIS, consisting of six to 10 layers of keratinocytes.

stratum spinosum The middle layer of the EPIDERMIS also known as the skin's "prickle cell layer," because of its spiny, hairlike prickly projections linking the cells in this area. The cells within this thickest part of the epidermis are called SQUAMOUS CELLS (basal cells that have matured and migrated upward through the epidermis). See also SKIN.

strawberry birthmark Also called strawberry nevus, strawberry hemangioma or superficial hemangioma, this is a bright red BIRTHMARK. Hemangiomas are proliferative lesions of blood vessels in which the number of vessels is greater than normal. The marks usually appear shortly after birth, when they enter a rapid growth phase during the first several months of life. Growth then gradually slows down and stops, usually beginning to regress by age one. All superficial hemangiomas regress by age seven, although residual fatty tissue is frequent.

Treatment Because these birthmarks eventually disappear on their own, treatment is not always recommended. Despite preliminary data that shows a good response to the pulsed dye laser, many believe that routine treatment of these benign lesions is questionable. The pulsed dye laser is effective at slowing growth during the proliferative phase, and may help to speed resolution of an already-regressing hemangioma.

Instead, many dermatologists recommend a cautious approach, unless the hemangioma grows rapidly or interferes with function of vital organs.

streptocerciasis A type of tissue round-worm (*Dipetalonema streptocerca*) found only in the tropical rain forests of western and central Africa, where it causes a chronic DER-MATITIS similar to onchocerciasis (a tropical skin disease caused by a parasitic worm).

streptococcal infections A group of infections caused by bacteria of the streptococcus family, among the most common bacteria that affect humans. These infections are responsible for a wide range of health problems, including such skin conditions as ERYSIPELAS, CELLULITIS, ECHTHYMA, SCARLET FEVER or wound infections. Some types of strepococcal bacteria exist harmlessly in people's throats; if the bacteria gets in the bloodstream, it is usually destroyed—unless the patient has a heart condition, which may lead to bacterial endocarditis. Other types of streptococcal bacteria can lead to sore throats, tonsillitis, middle ear infections or pneumonia.

stress and the skin Your skin is the "window to the mind," and to an astonishing degree your skin can reveal your emotional state—you blush when you're embarrassed; you blanch when you're afraid. When you're angry, your skin turns bright red. It's not surprising that stress, which can have a profound impact on the emotions and the physical health of the body, can also cause profound effects on your skin. In fact, experts believe a wide range of skin problems (ACNE, ECZEMA, ROSACEA, HERPES, PSORIASIS and HIVES) can be worsened or even triggered by stress.

Stress can make new skin lesions appear, or make already existing skin problems worse. In fact, people who are most at risk for developing stress-related skin problems are those who have problem skin to start with. This is most likely due to the fact that when people are under stress, they may work long hours, eat unhealthy meals, neglect their exercise or sleep needs.

Abusing alcohol can also damage the skin, since alcohol increases the flow of blood to the skin. Alcohol use is particularly troubling to skin conditions such as rosacea, hives, flushing and psoriasis. Nicotine, on the other hand, constricts blood vessels, which reduces the supply of blood to the skin. This is one reason why the skin of chronic smokers looks pale and deeply lined, leading to the "smoker's mask."

Treatment If you think stress is worsening the condition of your skin, try these general tips:

· Avoid picking or scratching your skin
· Use a noncomedogenic moisturizer; it won't clog pores but will combat dryness.
· Avoid exotic ingredients that could cause an allergic reaction.
· Drink more water; it will affect the skin's tone and texture
· Learn how to minimize or eliminate your stress through relaxation techniques, biofeedback, etc.

stretch marks Also known medically as "striae," these are lines on the skin caused by thinning and loss of elasticity in the underlying skin area (DERMIS). Stretch marks first appear as red, raised lines that turn purple, flatten and fade to form shiny streaks between a quarter-inch and a half-inch wide. These marks may strike during adolescence, appearing on thighs and hips of young girls during their growth spurt. They are also common in pregnancy; about 75 percent of pregnant women experience the marks on breasts, thighs and lower abdomen. In addition, purple stretch marks may occur in patients with Cushing's syndrome and in those using excess corticosteroid hormones, which suppress the formation of collagen (skin fiber), causing COLLAGEN to waste away.

Treatment Tretinoin (RETIN-A) has been found to help fade stretch marks significantly, and in some cases even make them disappear, as long as the marks are new and still pink. Retin-A does not work on stretch marks that have turned white. *Pregnant women and nursing mothers should not use Retin-A, because it crosses the placenta and is also found in breast milk and may harm the baby.*

Most recently, studies suggest striae may improve with treatment by pulsed dye lasers.

striae See STRETCH MARKS.

strongyloidiasis An intestinal infestation of tiny parasitic roundworms that cause itching and raised red patches where the worms enter the skin. The disease, caused by *Strongyloides stercoralis,* is found throughout the tropics, especially in the Far East. The worms are picked up by walking barefoot on soil contaminated with feces. The larvae enter the skin of the feet and migrate to the small intestines where they develop into adulthood, burrowing into the intestinal walls and producing larvae.

Symptoms After infestation, the worms cause redness, swelling, itching or hives, fading within two days. If the larvae penetrate the perianal area, skin lesions begin to radiate from the anus down the thigh or across the buttocks or abdomen as itchy bands. While the individual lesion may fade away within a few days, an infestation may continue in the host for many years and cause recurrent problems.

Complications Death may occur from blood poisoning or meningitis many years after the worms are picked up, but it is rare. Pneumonia may occur because of immune system damage.

Treatment Ivermectin administered in a single dose is the newest treatment of choice.

Sturge-Weber   Foundation A   support group for patients with STURGE-WEBER SYN-DROME and their families that serves as an information clearinghouse on the syndrome, PORT-WINE STAINS and Klippel-Trenaunay Weber syndrome. (Sturge-Weber syndrome is a congenital disorder characterized by facial port-wine stains, seizures, glaucoma and loss of motor control). The group, founded in 1986 with 750 members, provides information, offers support, maintains a speakers' bureau, compiles statistics and funds research. The foundation publishes a quarterly *Branching Out Newsletter* and sponsors an annual conference. For address, see Appendix D.

Sturge-Weber syndrome A rare congenital condition (also called trigeminal angiomatosis) that affects the skin and brain, characterized by a large purple PORT-WINE STAIN (birthmark caused by abnormal size and distribution of blood vessels) usually over one side of the face. Abnormal formation of blood vessels in the brain may cause some weakness on the opposite side of the body, progressive mental retardation, seizures, eye problems and epilepsy. Glaucoma may develop in the affected eye, causing partial or total blindness.

Treatment Visible light lasers (argon, dye and heavy metal lasers) are the treatments of choice, although lesions respond variably according to their color, thickness, size and site. The birthmark can be hidden with specially designed masking makeup, and seizures can be controlled with anticonvulsant drugs. In severe cases, surgery on the affected part of the brain may be performed.

See CAMOUFLAGE COSMETICS.

sty A small pus-filled ABSCESS (also called a hordeolum) near the eyelashes caused by an infection with *Staphylococcus aureus.*

Treatment Warm compresses administered for 20 minutes, four times daily, may help eliminate the pus, reduce swelling and decrease pain. An antibiotic ointment designed for the eyes can help prevent a recurrence.

subcutaneous A medical term referring to the area beneath the skin.

subcutaneous fat, atrophy of See FAT ATROPHY.

subcutaneous fatty tissue Also known as subcutis, this is the bottommost layer of skin, found under the DERMIS. This layer serves as a cushion for internal organs and also as a storage site for reserve energy. The amount and distribution of this fatty tissue throughout the body is believed to be governed largely by heredity and by how much you eat.

subcutis See SUBCUTANEOUS FATTY TISSUE.

subungual hematoma A blood-filled bruise under the fingernail caused by direct trauma, such as slamming the finger in a door. The pain can be eased by puncturing the nail plate with a drill or fine scalpel blade; otherwise, the nail may be shed. If the injury affects the matrix of the nail, it may form permanent deformity of the nail, with ridging or a split.

Sulfamylon See MAFENIDE ACETATE.

sulfapyridine A long-acting sulfa drug used to treat blistering diseases such as DERMATITIS HERPETIFORMIS.
Side effects This drug can cause severe allergic reactions, anemia and a decrease in the number of white cells in the body. To prevent kidney problems, patients should drink plenty of liquids.

sulfonamide drugs The first available antibacterial drugs, these are used to treat skin infections, among other things (such as uri-

nary tract infections, some types of pneumonia and middle ear infections). Before the development of penicillin drugs, the sulfonamides were widely used to treat other infections.

The sulfa drugs are usually given by mouth, and most are quickly absorbed from the stomach and small intestines.
Side effects A variety of side effects may occur, including nausea, vomiting, headache and appetite loss. More severe side effects include blood disorders, skin rashes and fever. Patients taking sulfa drugs should avoid sun exposure.

sulfones One of a group of drugs closely related to the sulfa drugs in their structure and the way they act. Sulfones are powerful agents in the fight against bacteria that cause LEPROSY. The two sulfones most often used in dermatologic practices are DAPSONE and SULFAPYRIDINE. Other diseases in which sulfones are used include subcorneal pustular dermatosis, acne conglobata, PYODERMA GANGRENOSUM, BULLOUS PEMPHIGOID, cicatricial pemphigoid, chronic bullous dermatosis of childhood, erythema elevatum diutinum, relapsing POLYCHONDRITIS, GRANULOMA ANNULARE, granuloma faciale, bullous eruption of systemic lupus erythematosus, leukocytoclastic vasculitis, actinomycotic mycetoma, alopecia mucinosa, pustular psoriasis, HERPES GESTATIONNIS, PEMPHIGUS, Weber-Christian PANNICULITIS, BROWN RECLUSE SPIDER BITES and HAILEY-HAILEY DISEASE.

Patients who take these drugs require frequent evaluation, including complete blood counts with differential white counts, a chemistry profile (including liver and kidney tests), urine tests and methemoglobin level.

sulfur An important mineral component of vitamin B1 and of several essential amino acids (protein building blocks). Sulfur is particularly necessary for the body's production of COLLAGEN, which helps to form connective tissue. Sulfur is also a component of KERATIN, the chief ingredient in hair, skin and nails.

In addition, sulfur is one of the oldest of the modern drugs and a popular acne treatment, although its action is still not well understood. Researchers believe that it is effective by controlling bacteria and exfoliating the skin.

Many studies suggest that a combination of benzoyl peroxide and sulfur is more effective than sulfur used alone. Sulfur is thought to dissolve the top layer of dry dead cells and slow down oil-gland activity, which is why it is used in acne soaps, lotions and dandruff shampoos.

The highest concentration of sulfur in over-the-counter medication is 10 percent. Sulfur may cause a mild sensitivity and allergic reactions, and can irritate the eyes. Discontinue use if skin sensitivity occurs.

While most experts consider benzoyl peroxide and sulfur safe when used as single ingredients, products that combine the two increase the possibility of sensitivity to benzoyl peroxide. Therefore, combination products are not available without prescription.

In addition, sulfur is sometimes added to RESORCINOL (a drug that causes skin to peel) as an acne treatment, although experts aren't sure why this combination works. Resorcinol by itself is not considered to be effective against acne, but it appears to enhance the action of sulfur. Because resorcinol in concentrations above 3 percent appear to be toxic, products with this ingredient are only available over the counter in concentrations of 2 percent and less. Products containing resorcinol should not be applied to broken skin or to large areas of the body. In addition, resorcinol may discolor dark or black skin.

Sulfur is not the same as "sulfa," an abbreviation for a group of antibacterial agents including sulfadiazole and sulfathiazole.

sun blocks See SUNSCREEN.

sunburn Inflammation of the skin as a result of overexposure to the sun. Sunburn occurs when the ultraviolet rays of the sun destroy skin cells in the outer layer of the skin, damaging tiny blood vessels underneath. Sunburn is a particular problem in light-skinned individuals whose skin does not produce much MELANIN, the protective pigment that can guard against damage from the sun.

Symptoms Sun-exposed skin turns red, becomes very painful and may develop blisters; if the burn is severe, the individual may also experience symptoms of sunstroke, including vomiting, fever and collapse. Several days after the skin has burned, the skin may shed its dead cells by peeling. Repeated exposure to sunlight over the years may result in prematurely aged skin and SKIN CANCER; blistering sunburns before age 20 increase the risk of melanoma.

Treatment The best idea is to avoid getting sunburned in the first place, because once the skin is burned it has become damaged. While there are many so-called sunburn "remedies," none are highly effective. Compresses may help, using a variety of ingredients such as skim milk and water, aluminum acetate baths (as contained in Buro-Sol antiseptic powder or Domeboro's powder), oatmeal or witch hazel.

Cool (not cold) baths may also be soothing, especially if you add one cup of white vinegar, Aveeno powder (made from oatmeal) or baking soda. Don't use soap or bubble baths on sunburned skin (they can irritate tender flesh). After a compress or a soaking bath, be sure to apply moisturizer immediately afterward; pat skin dry, apply bath oil followed by a moisturizing cream or lotion (such as Eucerin).

You can also try a cornstarch paste, or apply raw cucumber or potato slices, yogurt or tea bags soaked in cool water. Aloe (the oil from the aloe plant) may be applied directly to the skin for sunburn relief—but first test your skin to be sure you're not allergic to it.

Prevention Limit exposure to strong sunlight to 15 minutes on the first day, especially in those with fair skin, increasing exposure slowly each day. Until the skin has tanned, it should be protected with a high-protection SUNSCREEN of at least 15 SPF. Fair individuals and those who are photosensitive should use a sunscreen with an SPF of 29 or higher. Avoid going out into the sun between the hours of 10 A.M. and 3 P.M. Aspirin and nonsteroidal anti-inflammatory drugs (NSAIDs) can prevent sunburn only if taken before exposure to the sun; once burned, they are not effective. New types of protective clothing are now available that are equivalent to an SPF of 30; typical clothing is only about as effective as SPF 6.

sun poisoning A lay term for a temporary condition of red, itchy bumps caused by a variety of causes of sun sensitivity. Some of these causes include POLYMORPHIC LIGHT ERUPTION, photocontact dermatitis involving an agent applied to the skin (such as PABA or oxybenzone in SUNSCREENS), photosensitivity to a systemic drug (such as tetracycline). If you stay out of the sun, the bumps should disappear within a week. Patients should see a doctor if weeping, oozing blisters develop, since this may indicate a possible infection. (See also SOLAR WARNING INDEX; SUNBURN; SUNSCREEN; SKIN CANCER.)
Treatment Cool compresses and over-the-counter hydrocortisone cream or oral antihistamines.

sun protection factor (SPF) A rating system for sunscreen products that measures how effectively the sunscreen works; the higher the SPF, the greater the amount of protection from the sun. For example, an SPF of 15 means that an individual using the sunscreen could spend up to 15 times longer in the sun without burning than if he or she weren't wearing it. However, the SPF applies only to UVB; no rating for UVA currently exists.

Experts suggest that sunscreen should have a minimum SPF of 15 to avoid the burning, drying and wrinkling that results from overexposure to the harmful rays, which are the single most damaging element to the skin. On the other hand, experts at the Food and Drug Administration criticize sunscreens with SPFs up to 50, charging that consumers may have a false sense of security by using products with very high SPF values.

An SPF of 50 implies that a person can tolerate 50 times the amount of sun that it would normally take to burn, which isn't necessarily true. And even a sunscreen with an SPF of 50 lets *some* UVB rays through, so using it doesn't allow a person to bake for hours in the sun without any risk of cancer or wrinkling, according to some dermatologists.

In addition, the higher the SPF number, the faster the proportional increase in protection diminishes. For example, the difference between an SPF of 45 and one of 30 is only a few percentage points. As a result of these concerns, the FDA recently proposed legislation that would limit SPF labelling to 30.

There are still some physicians and sunscreen manufacturers who believe that higher SPFs should be available for those who choose to use them. Rather than cut off protection at 30, these physicians suggest the FDA ask manufacturers to explain the percentage of ultraviolet rays blocked by each of the different SPF numbers.

For overseas travelers, it is important to realize that not all SPFs are the same. In Europe, the SPF is called DIN (Deutsches Institut fur Normung, the company that developed the system). The DIN uses lower numbers than the American SPF system for equivalent sun protection. For example, an SPF 12 is equal to DIN 9; SPF 19 is DIN 15.

sunscreens Products that protect the skin from the harmful effects of sunlight's harmful radiation; all sunscreen products protect against ultraviolet-B (UVB); some products protect against both ultraviolet-A (UVA) and UVB. Sunscreens are used primarily to avoid SUNBURN and suntanning, although they can also be used to prevent the rash in patients' PHOTOSENSITIVITY. They also prevent skin cancer and the aging effects of the sun on the skin.

While some skin exposure to sunlight is necessary for the body to produce VITAMIN D, overexposure can have a range of harmful effects, especially in fair-skinned people. Most sunscreens, including those preparations containing PARA-AMINOBENZOIC ACID (PABA) or benzophenone, work by absorbing ultraviolet rays of the sun. Products containing other substances (such as TITANIUM DIOXIDE, an uncolored relative of ZINC OXIDE) *reflect* the sun's rays.

Sunscreens are designed to protect against UVB light, the type of radiation that causes sunburn. Most common sunscreens aren't designed to protect against UVA, another kind of ultraviolet light produced by the sun that used to be considered less dangerous because it didn't directly damage skin. However, new research suggests that UVA can damage the skin and may play a role in malignant melanoma simply because sunlight contains so much of it. (Think UVA-*aging,* UVB-*burn* plus *aging*).

Only a few sunscreens offer significant protection from UVA rays; those that do list the ingredient "Parsol 1789" (avobenzone), the only ingredient approved by the FDA specifically for blocking the UVA rays.

Many more products contain certain other ingredients are also allowed to claim UVA protection, but none can say how much. Since each of these chemicals block only part of the UVA spectrum, it's a good idea to choose a product with more than one of them. Check the label for some of these names: dioxybenzone, oxybenzone, sulisobenzone, methyl anthranilate, octocrylene and octyl methoxycinnamate (also called ethylhexyl p-methoxycinnamate).

The best sunscreens offer a broad spectrum of protection, and include such ingredients as oxybenzone, titanium dioxide, zinc oxide or Parsol 1789. But while sunscreens aren't perfect, they do prevent sunburn, future freckling and brown spots, ACTINIC KERATOSES (precancerous lesions) and SKIN CANCER.

But you can still develop sun-induced aging and skin cancer even if you don't get a sunburn. The only way to completely protect yourself against aging skin cancer is to avoid the sun.

SPF Sunscreen products are labeled with a SUN PROTECTION FACTOR (SPF), which is a measure of how effectively the sunscreen works; the highest factor indicates the greatest amount of protection. Use sunscreen with a minimum SPF of 15 to avoid burning, drying and wrinkling that results from chronic overexposure. An SPF of 15 means that individuals using the sunscreen could spend up to 15 times longer in the sun without burning than if they weren't wearing it. However, the SPF applies only to UVB; no effective rating for UVA currently exists.

An SPF 15 blocks 94 percent of UVB rays and an SPF 30 blocks 98 percent. However, since some people skimp when applying sunscreen or apply it unevenly, experts rationalize that if you skimp when applying SPF 15 you might end up with the equivalent of an SP6, whereas if you skimp using an SPF of 30 or higher, you'll still get adequate protection.

The U.S. Food and Drug Administration (FDA) established guidelines for safety of sunscreens in 1978; they are currently revising its sunscreen labeling to include a maximum SPF 30 on all sunscreens, the use of the terms "water-resistant" and "very water resistant" instead of "waterproof," charts to match skin types with the appropriate SPF numbers, and stricter guidelines on anti-aging claims.

How to apply Experts suggest that adults should use an ounce of sunscreen (about a shot glass full) to properly protect an average-sized person. Sunscreens should be reapplied every two hours, and again after swimming; waterproof or water-resistant sunscreens can be applied less often, but experts recommend an extra application after swimming if there is any uncertainty about the need for more.

Apply sunscreen before you go outside (even in cloudy weather, since 80 percent of the sun's rays break through the clouds).

Sunscreen allergies Some people are allergic to the chemicals contained in sunscreens and can develop a skin rash. The most common ingredients to cause an allergic reaction are PABA and oxybenzone. If you break out when wearing a sunscreen, you should consult a dermatologist, who may perform a patch test to determine what ingredient is to blame for the rash.

Fortunately, new chemical-free sunscreens are now being developed that contain physical sunblocks (such as titanium dioxide and talc) broken down into tiny particles that can be formulated into clear, invisible lotions instead of the white zinc-oxide creams. The nonchemical sunscreens block both UVA and UVB rays far better than most chemical sunscreens.

Other protective factors A more controversial approach to sunscreen developments is the addition of other protective factors, such as vitamins E and C (antioxidants that neutralize free radicals, which are unstable oxygen molecules that damage skin). The goal is to prevent or delay damage to skin cells by screening out some of the premature-aging effects of sunlight while allowing the triggering of vitamin D, but many dermatologists are skeptical.

Because the wavelength of light that stimulates vitamin D production in the skin is UVB, some have voiced concern regarding the overuse of UVB sunscreens. However, since it takes only 15 minutes two or three times a week to spur vitamin D synthesis in the skin, very few people have to worry about not getting enough sun exposure.

Rating sunscreens The Skin Cancer Foundation rates sunscreens; consumers should look for their seal of approval on all sunscreen products. Sunscreens that have the Foundation's "SEAL" on the label have met stringent criteria that exceed those of the FDA; in order to rate the foundation's approval, the product must prove that it helps prevent sun-induced damage to the skin. The product must have an SPF of 15 or higher and include substantiation for any claims that a sunscreen is waterproof, water- or sweat-resistant. The *Seal* is also granted to SELF-TANNING PRODUCTS that include a sunscreen; this sunscreen must meet the same requirements as regular sunscreen. Clothing is still considered to be the best protection against sun-induced skin aging and SKIN CANCER of all types. See also SUN POISONING; SOLAR WARNING INDEX.

SAFE EXPOSURE TIMES USING SUNSCREENS			
PROTECTION FACTOR	**4**	**8**	**15**
SKIN TYPE		SAFE EXPOSURE TIME	
Fair	10 minutes	40-80 minutes	1.5-2 hours
Medium	50-80 minutes	2-2.5 hours	5-5.5 hours
Dark	1.5-2 hours	3.5-4 hours	all day
Black	4 hours	all day	all day

Protective clothing Finally, it's a good idea to wear some type of sun-protective clothing specially designed to block the harmful rays of the sun, such as Frogwear or Solumbra.

sunstroke Also called heatstroke, this condition is caused by excess exposure to heat and the sun, and is characterized by feelings of dizziness and nausea. However, in some people (especially the elderly) it can involve a very high body temperature and lack of sweating followed by loss of consciousness. For these individuals, this condition is potentially fatal unless treated quickly.
First aid Quick cooling is the most important aspect of treatment for sunstroke. Apply an ice bag or crushed ice, or wrap a wet sheet and hose it down with cold water until emergency medical help arrives.

suntan The result of the body's attempt at protecting itself from the damage of the sun's ultraviolet rays. During exposure to the sun, the skin begins to produce more of the dark pigment called MELANIN to absorb the damaging rays. The result is a darkened skin tone.

While a suntan is widely considered to be desirable, it is in fact a sign that the skin has been damaged. Melanin provides some protection from skin damage and is the reason why dark-skinned individuals usually get fewer wrinkles than fair-skinned individuals given the same amount of sun exposure.

Even with frequent applications of SUN-SCREEN, sunbathers may be at risk for developing skin cancer, including melanoma (the most serious form of skin cancer). Newest findings have found that not only ultraviolet-B (UV-B) light (rays that cause sunburn, between 280 and 320 nanometers) but also light with longer wavelengths—including ultraviolet-A (UV-A) light—can fuel a series of changes in skin cells.

In the past, scientists had linked melanoma to damaged DNA because those who inherit a defect in their DNA-repairability are more than 1,000 times more likely than others to get this type of cancer. Because DNA absorbs only UV-B energy, many researchers believed that only this type of light caused the damage. Others *suspected* UV-A light, but lacked hard evidence of a link between the light and cancer.

But while studying light exposure with fish susceptible to the development of melanoma, scientists at Brookhaven National Laboratory in Upton, N.Y., found that exposure to a wavelength of 365 nanometers (UV-A used in black lights) resulted in tumors in 38 of 85 fish tested. Of the 61 fish treated with violet light (405 nanometers), 18 developed melanoma; only one of 20 control fish kept in subdued yellow light got cancer. It is believed that melanin absorbs light, setting off a chemical reaction that produces compounds damaging to DNA.

The sun's rays don't just stay on the surface of the skin; they also penetrate deep beneath the skin, where they can damage the COLLAGEN network, the springy web of fibers that support and strengthen skin. This damage actually can be reversed in part by staying out of the sun and by long-term use of RETIN-A. See also MELANOMA, MALIGNANT; SUN BLOCKS; SUNBURN; SUN PROTECTION FACTOR; TANNING BEDS.

suppuration The formation of PUS at the site of bacterial infection. The pus may also accumulate, forming an ABSCESS (in solid tissue) or a BOIL or PUSTULE on the skin. Open sores often weep pus like this, especially when they don't heal well, because the exposed tissue gets reinfected with bacteria again and again.

surfer's nodules Lesions caused by repeated friction of the tops of the feet and the knees against a surfboard. This condition will disappear if you stop surfing; otherwise, local injections of a low-dose cortisone will help.

sweat and the skin Sweating is the body's way of keeping its internal temperature at a constant 98.6°. When the body's temperature rises, the body's SWEAT GLANDS are stimulated to start producing water to cool off the body. When this happens, sweating is heaviest on the forehead, upper lips, neck and chest.

Sweat is made primarily of water and some tiny amounts of other substances (such as salt). Perspiration itself, regardless of the type of sweat gland from which it originates, is odorless—the smell occurs when sweat mixes with bacteria (especially in the armpits).

Sweating is an involuntary process, a response to the environment, or to psychological factors such as embarrassment or stress. People who experience constant sweating (hyperhidrosis) need to be referred to a physician, since such sweating may be a sign of hormonal imbalance.

sweat glands Sweat glands are spread out all across the body in varying concentrations that are designed to produce perspiration. Each gland has a tube for secreting sweat, and a narrow passage that carries sweat to the skin's surface. Most people have about 3 million sweat glands in two types—apocrine and eccrine glands.

Apocrine glands lie heavily coiled in mostly hairy areas (the armpits, the nipples, genital and anal areas, and around the navel), located deep within the fatty tissue (subcutis). This is the gland that secretes the type of sweat associated with body odor, mostly under the armpits. Apocrine glands secrete a milky sweat into the upper portion of the HAIR FOLLICLE, and from there to the skin surface. This sweat is broken down by bacteria on the skin, causing body odor. While it is believed that the apocrine glands in other mammals serve as a sexual stimulant, their function in humans is not known. Like SEBA-

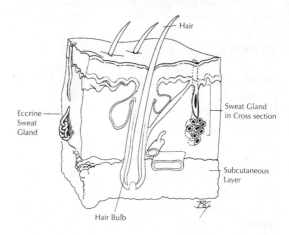

Cross section of Skin Showing Sweat Glands

CEOUS GLANDS, the apocrine glands do not mature and begin secreting until puberty.

Eccrine glands are the most common (especially on hands and feet), and like apocrine glands they are heavily coiled in the fatty tissue layer. Eccrine glands secrete clear, watery sweat through their own pores, not along hair follicles. Exercise, hot weather, fever and emotional stress can stimulate eccrine sweating over the entire surface of the body (but concentrated on the soles of the feet, forehead palms and armpits). They appear to be more strongly linked to stimulation by emotional stress than by heat. Eccrine glands are mostly water and do not cause body odor; they serve to regulate body temperature and to help eliminate waste salts. See also HYPER-HIDROSIS; SWEAT GLANDS, DISORDERS OF.

sweat glands, disorders of There are a number of disorders that can affect the sweat glands (eccrine and apocrine). The most common is PRICKLY HEAT, an intense, irritating skin rash caused by blocked glands. Less commonly, the sweat glands may be affected by HYPERHIDROSIS, a type of profuse sweating that often requires medical treatment and can cause highly embarrassing social problems. HYPOHIDROSIS (reduced sweating), a less frequent problem, occurs in ectodermal dysplasia syndrome.

swimmer's ear See OTITIS EXTERNA.

swimmer's itch The common name for cutaneous SCHISTOSOMIASIS, or cercarial dermatitis, this is an itchy skin inflammation caused by schistosome bites (bites from flatworms). This disorder features a distinctive papular eruption after swimming in or having contact with fresh water populated by ducks and snails.

This type of dermatitis is a potential risk whenever people use an aquatic area with animals and mollusks who harbor the schistosomes. In the United States, the worst outbreaks occur in the lake regions of Michigan, Wisconsin and Minnesota. A more serious tropial disease is visceral schistosomiasis.
Symptoms After exposure to water affected by the schistosomes, a prickling or itchy feeling begins that can last up to an hour while the flukes enter the skin. Small red macules form, but there may be swelling or wheals among sensitive people. As these lesions begin to disappear, they are replaced after 10 or 15 hours by discrete, very itchy papules surrounded by a red area. Vesicles and pustules form one or two days later; the lesions fade away within a week, leaving small pigmented spots. Different symptoms depend on how sensitive the patient is to the schistosome. Each reexposure causes a more severe reaction.
Prevention The best way to alleviate the problem is to destroy the snails by treating the water with copper sulfate and carbonate, or with sodium pentachlorophenate. A thick coating of grease or tightly woven clothes can protect against infestation. Bathing with a hexachlorophene soap before swimming may help to some degree. Briskly rubbing the skin with a towel after swimming may help remove some organisms.

Treatment Calamine lotion or oral antihistamines may help control the itch until the lesions begin to disappear on their own.

swimming pool granuloma A disorder of the skin caused by a mycobacterium characterized by abscesses usually seen on the hands over the fingers, or on the knees in people who clean swimming pools. The problem is also found in those who own tropical fish tanks; if a person cleans the tank and scratches a hand against objects in the tank, the organism can penetrate the abrasion; weeks later, an abrasion may form.
Treatment Treatment includes local heat therapy and minocycline.

sycosis vulgaris See BARBER'S ITCH.

syphilis A sexually transmitted infection found around the world that causes (among other symptoms) a skin sore and rash. Also present as a congenital (at birth) infection, syphilis was first recorded as a major epidemic in Europe during the 15th century, after Columbus returned from his trip to America.

Today, the infection is transmitted almost exclusively by sexual contact. Since the 1970s and early 1980s, the incidence of syphilis in the United States has been on the rise.
Cause Syphilis is caused by a spirochete *Treponema pallidum* that enters broken skin or mucous membranes during sexual intercourse, by kissing or by intimate bodily contact with an infected person. The rate of infection during a single contact with an infected person is about 30 percent.
Symptoms During the first (or primary) stage, a sore (chancre) appears between three to four weeks after contact; the sore has a hard, wet painless base that heals in about a month. In males, the sore appears on the shaft of the penis. In women it can be found on the labia, although it is often hidden so well that the diagnosis is missed. In both

sexes, the sore may be seen on the lips or tongue.

Six to 12 weeks after infection, the patient enters the *secondary stage,* which features a skin rash that may last for months. The rash has crops of pink or pale red, round spots, but in black patients the rash is pigmented and appears darker than normal skin. The eruption can be mistaken for PITYRIASIS RO-SEA. In addition, the lymph nodes may be enlarged, and there may be backache, headache, bone pain, appetite loss, fever, fatigue and sometimes meningitis. The hair may fall out and the skin may exhibit gray or pink patches (condylomata) that are highly infectious. The secondary stage may last up to a year.

The *latent stage* may last for a few years or until the end of a person's life. During this time, the infected person appears normal; about 30 percent of these patients will develop tertiary syphilis.

Tertiary syphilis (end stage) usually begins about 10 years after the initial infection, although it may appear after only about three years or as late as 25 years later. The person's tissues may begin to deteriorate (a process called "gumma formation"), involving the bones, palate, nasal septum, tongue, skin or any organ of the body. The most serious complications in this stage include heart problems, brain damage (neurosyphilis) leading to insanity, and paralysis.

Treatment Penicillin is the drug of choice for all forms of the disease; early syphilis can often be cured by a single large injection; later forms of the disease may require a longer course of the drug. More than half of syphilis patients treated with penicillin develop a severe reaction within six to 12 hours caused by the body's response to the sudden killing of large numbers of spirochetes.

Prevention Infection can be avoided by maintaining monogamous relationships; condoms offer some protection, but they are not absolutely safe. People with syphilis are in-fectious during the primary and secondary stages, but not in the late latent and tertiary stages.

systemic disease, skin symptoms of In many ways, the skin can be a window into the health of the body, mirroring internal disease. Changes can appear in thickness, color, texture or sensation. Problems with immune function or with blood flow can trigger the appearance of HIVES, PURPURA (purple skin patches), blisters or deadened areas of skin.

Skin findings may be important in diagnosing cancer and a host of systemic diseases affecting any of the body's organ system, such as the gastrointestinal tract, eye, kidneys, lungs, heart, blood vessels, cardiovascular system, musculoskeletal or endocrine system.

Generalized itching is one skin symptom that may be associated with systemic disease. If there are no other skin diseases to explain it, itching of unknown origin (or "idiopathic" itching) may be associated with Hodgkin's disease, polycythemia rubra vera, liver or kidney disease, thyroid disease, hypoparathyroidism, infections or drug reactions.

systemic lupus erythematosus (SLE) The more serious and potentially fatal form of the chronic circulatory disease LUPUS ERYTHEMATOSUS that affects many systems of the body. (The milder form is DISCOID LUPUS ERYTHEMATOSUS, or DLE). SLE is probably not one, but several, conditions; while many systems of the body may be affected, it's also possible that the disease may affect just the skin. Although typically a disease of young women, it can affect either sex and all age groups without regard to race. The disease commonly waxes and wanes, and its etiology is affected by heredity, autoimmunity, certain drugs, sex hormones, ultraviolet light and viruses.

The relationship between DLE and SLE is controversial. Between 2 and 20 percent of patients who are first diagnosed with DLE go on to develop SLE. It is not uncommon for typical SLE to go into remission, leaving lesions of chronic DLE. On the other hand, DLE may spontaneously subside, remain constant, worsen or progress to active SLE after some stress.

The prognosis for patients with SLE depends on which organs are involved; kidney or central nervous system involvement implies a poor prognosis. In most patients the disease is chronic; more than 90 percent of patients survive for at least 10 years.

Symptoms Typically there is a red scaly rash on the face, affecting the nose and cheeks, arthritis and progressive kidney damage; the heart, lungs and brain may also be affected by progressive attacks of inflammation followed by the formation of scar tissue. In the milder form (DLE) only the skin is affected.

Treatment Local corticosteroid creams and ointments, or a therapeutic trial of salicylate. Immunosuppressive agents are sometimes used, especially among those who have experienced side effects from corticosteroids.

systemic necrotizing vasculitides A group of inflammatory diseases of the small and medium-size arteries causing palpable nodules, ulcers, purple patches (purpura) or plaques. This group of diseases includes polyarteritis nodosa and WEGENER'S GRANULOMATOSIS.

The survival rate for untreated polyarteritis nodosa is 13 percent; corticosteroid treatment improves the survival rate to 48 percent and a combination approach using corticosteroids and immunosuppressive agents hikes the rate to 80 percent.

In a variety of polyarteritis nodosa, cutaneous polyarteritis nodosa, patients don't usually develop systemic signs and their prognosis is quite good.

Symptoms Skin symptoms include palpable purpura (see LEUCOCYTOELASTIC VASCULITIS), tender nodules, purple patches, LIVEDO RETICULARIS and ulceration. There are a wide variety of non-skin symptoms, including fever, malaise, weight loss, joint or muscle problems, kidney problems, nausea and vomiting, abdominal pain, congestive heart failure, high blood pressure, strokes and neuropathy.

Symptoms of Wegener's granulomatosis include ulcers, papules and plaques on legs, with ulcers in the mouth. "Saddle nose" may appear as a result of destruction of the cartilage in the nose.

Treatment A combination of corticosteroids (prednisone) and cyclophosphamide is the treatment of choice for both diseases, together with a careful control of high blood pressure. In addition, additional treatment with aspirin, sulfapyridine and DAPSONE may be considered.

systemic sclerosis See SCLERODERMA.

T

tachyphylaxis The rapid decrease of response to an anti-inflammatory and antimitotic effects of topical steroids. Patients treated with topical corticosteroids after only one or two weeks but usually after several weeks may find that the product seems to have stopped working. After a week-long rest of that specific corticosteroid, however, the drug usually begins working again.

Substituting one corticosteroid for another type with a slightly different chemical structure may eliminate this problem.

tan See SUNTAN.

tanning booths/beds A special booth or bed that emits ultraviolet (UV-A) rays that cause the skin to tan. While an estimated 2 million Americans still aim for a rich golden tan from a bed or booth, experts have concluded that the practice is neither safe nor foolproof.

These devices were once billed as a way to get a "safe" tan because the artificial ultraviolet light they emit is made up of primarily UVA rays, not UVB rays (the main component of sunlight). However, new research suggests that in fact, both types of ultraviolet light may be dangerous.

New research also suggests that tanning beds may promote aging of the skin and skin cancer. Many consumers don't realize that just 30 minutes in a tanning bed is equal to six to eight hours of nonstop sunning on the beach.

Experts also caution that there is no such thing as a "safe" tan that so many desire from a tanning bed, and such a tan is just as damaging as a tan acquired at the beach.

Only 24 states have laws regulating indoor tanning, and there are no government standards for how much exposure time is safe for different skin types. Furthermore, many salons are staffed by part-time attendants who are poorly trained in safe tanning-bed procedures.

Finally, many prescription drugs are photosensitizing, including some antibiotics (such as tetracycline) and thiazides (blood pressure pills). If you are taking a medication that is photosensitizing, using a tanning parlor can have severe consequences.

tanning pills Sometimes called "French bronzing pills," these are drugs designed to provide an artificial tan. They are sold outside the United States (and occasionally by mail order or through health food stores in this country). The drugs contain beta-carotene and/or canthaxidine canthaxanthin), chemicals that color the skin but also can damage the eyes and possibly the liver. They are not recommended by dermatologists.

Some tanning pills are advertised as a safe method of tanning, while others are designed to bolster resistance to sun damage. Regardless of the reason they are used, they should only be used with close medical supervision.

The Food and Drug Administration (FDA) does not approve the sale of pills that contain beta-carotene and/or canthaxanthin, both relatives of vitamin A (although beta-carotene is available by prescription). According to both the FDA and the Skin Cancer Foundation, some of the ingredients in these pills can have toxic side effects.

Beta-carotene is a natural component of many fruits and vegetables (such as oranges, carrots and tomatoes), and is sometimes used as a food additive in butter or cheese to add color. However, the pills may do the same thing to human skin, turning it yellow or orange instead of a handsome tan. In combination with the canthaxanthin, beta-carotene accumulates in the skin and colors it. At the same time, it forms deposits in the blood, fatty tissue, liver and other organs, sometimes becoming toxic.

Another kind of tanning pill contains 5- or 8-methoxypsoralen, a form of PSORALEN that is used to treat PSORIASIS, ALOPECIA AREATA and VITILIGO. Physicians have sometimes prescribed this chemical for those with sensitive skin as a way to resist sun damage on the theory that the chemical may thicken the skin and accelerate melanin production. It has been prescribed for those who are allergic to sunblocks, but can't avoid the sun.

It is recommended that it be used only under close medical supervision. It is available in other countries, and it does produce a deep, protective tan—but the risk of bleeding is significant.

tar compounds Crude and refined tars are an effective treatment for PSORIASIS, and are used either alone or in combination with ultraviolet light therapy. Tar decreases the turnover of the top-most layer of skin, and helps to reduce scaling and flakiness. However, the color and smell of these products don't make them popular choices. Tar is usually applied to the skin a few hours before light therapy.

Tar is a mixture of hundreds of compounds; a more cosmetically acceptable tar compound is liquor carbonis detergens (LCD) usually mixed with cold cream in a 5 to 10 percent concentration. LCD is a distillate of crude coal tar not dissimilar to road tar. Other tar preparations are available as soaps, gels or shampoos. There are lots of newer cosmetically acceptable preparations, such as LCD tar-gel or fragranced clear shampoo.

Tar shampoos are one of the treatments of choice for scaly scalp conditions such as seb-

orrheic dematitis (see DERMATITIS, SEBORRHEIC) DANDRUFF or PSORIASIS.

tattooing The process of instilling permanent colors into the skin, usually to create words or a design. Practiced for thousands of years as a form of identification or tribal marking, today tattoos are almost always used just for decoration. Even when performed by professionals, however, tattooing can be dangerous, leading to AIDS or hepatitis if the tattoo artist does not follow strict sterile procedures to clean needles that inject the dyes.

There are no state or federal regulations regarding tattooing. Neither the procedures nor the pigments used in the tattooing process are regulated.

Tattoos can be removed using short pulsed lasers including the Q-switched ruby, Ng:YAG, Alexandrite and 510 nanometer pulsed dye laser. Amateur tattoos can usually be entirely removed, as can black professional tattoos. Multicolored professional tattoos are more difficult to remove and require several different wavelengths for the different colors.

Tegison The trade name for ETRETINATE.

telogen The resting stage of the hair growth cycle.

telogen effluvium Generalized hair shedding, often after an acute illness or pregnancy. Normally, healthy adults lose between 75 and 100 hairs daily, but certain events can prompt an increase in hair loss by inducing the hair follicles to enter the telogen (resting) phase of hair growth.

About 95 percent of women develop some degree of hair loss after giving birth, or after stopping birth control pills. Other causes may include high fever, surgery and psychiatric stress, bulimia, dieting, malnutrition, blood loss, shock. See also ALOPECIA AREATA.

Treatment No treatment is needed, since new hairs replace those falling out. If hair loss persists for longer than three months you should consult a dermatologist.

terfenadine (trade name: Seldane) An oral antihistamine used to treat allergic skin problems such as HIVES, terfenadine does not induce sleepiness and is used by people who wish to avoid drowsiness.
Adverse reactions Possible problems include nausea, appetite loss or rash. Interaction with certain drugs, including erythromycin and ketoconozole, may result in irregular heartbeat.

tetracyclines A group of antibiotic drugs used to treat a range of conditions including ACNE, SYPHILIS, and ROCKY MOUNTAIN SPOTTED FEVER. (It is also used to treat bronchitis, gonorrhea, nonspecific urethritis, pneumonia, cholera, and brucellosis.)
Adverse effects Possible problems include nausea and vomiting, diarrhea, photosensitivity rash and itching. Tetracyclines may increase the overgrowth of yeasts in the vagina and interfere with the absorption of over-the-counter drugs taken concurrently. They may also discolor developing bones and teeth, and are not prescribed for youngsters under age 12 or for pregnant women. Tetracyclines may also worsen kidney disease in patients with kidney problems.

thalidomide The infamous anti-nausea drug never approved for use in the United States that caused widespread birth defects in other parts of the world when given to pregnant women. Thalidomide is currently being studied for use in treating certain types of LEPROSY, aphthous ulcers, LUPUS ERYTHEMATOSUS, and GRAFT VS. HOST DISEASE.

theque An island of MELANIN-producing cells situated at the junction of the DERMIS and EPIDERMIS, or within the dermis.

thrush The common name for candidiasis, a superficial fungal infection of the mucous membranes of the mouth. See CANDIDA INFECTION.

thymol An antiseptic that is derived from PHENOL that used to be used to treat ECZEMA, PSORIASIS and ACNE. It is an effective drying agent for the treatment of PARONYCHIA.

thyroid disorders, skin symptoms of There are a range of skin symptoms that accompany thyroid disorders. Hyperthyroidism is characterized by fine, thin hair, red palms, increased sweating, onycholysis, diffuse darkening of skin and itching. Hypothyroidism includes dry, lax skin; thick lips and tongue; cool skin; thinning hair; carotenemia; itching; xerosis; brittle nails. Hashimoto's thyroiditis is associated with several other auto-immune conditions such as VITILIGO, ALOPECIA AREATA (hair loss), DERMATITIS HERPETIFORMIS, PEMPHIGOID, LUPUS ERYTHEMATOSUS, and SCLERODERMA.

ticks and disease Ticks aren't so much a primary cause of skin disease as carriers of infectious agents that produce disease. They can transmit ROCKY MOUNTAIN SPOTTED FEVER, LYME DISEASE, TULAREMIA and other diseases.

Ticks bury their heads into the skin to feed, become engorged with their host's blood and swell to many times their size. Sometimes generalized HIVES associated with toxic symptoms may develop. While a tick bite itself does not usually cause problems, it may result in persistent nodules or papules after forced removal of the tick. Other skin reactions to tick bites include papular hive-like lesions, patchy scalp hair loss, painful local swelling, ulceration and erythema chronicum migrans in Lyme disease.
Treatment Ticks can be removed by touching the parasite with a lighted match or cigarette, or by applying gasoline, kerosene, phenol, or

soft paraffin. This should make the tick withdraw its head. Gently pulling the tick parallel to its axis can often remove it competely as well. Inflammatory papules and nodules caused by a tick bite can be treated with a potent topical corticosteroid cream. Excision of nodules may be necessary, although persistent reactions have occurred in spite of excision.

Prevention Apply tick repellents. Low concentrations of routine bug repellants such as DEET don't work very well at repelling ticks.

Tinactin See TOLNAFTATE.

tinea The medical term for ringworm, a group of common fungus infections of the skin, hair or nails caused by various species of the fungi *Microsporum, Trichophyton* and *Epidermophyton.* It affects humans as well as animals. Ringworm is highly contagious and can be spread either by direct contact or via infected material. Infections can be contracted from other people, and from animals, soil or an object (such as a shower stall).

The term "tinea" is often followed by the part of the body affected by the fungus, such as tinea pedis (ATHLETE'S FOOT).

Symptoms Symptoms vary according to the part of the body affected by the infection. The most common affected area is the foot (ATHLETE'S FOOT), with cracking, itchy skin between the toes. Tinea cruris (JOCK ITCH) is more common in males, and produces a red, itchy area from the genitals outward over the inside of the thighs. TINEA CORPORIS (ringworm of the body) is characterized by itchy circular skin patches with a raised edge. TINEA CAPITIS (ringworm of the scalp) causes round, itchy circles of hair loss found most commonly in children living in large cites or in overcrowded conditions. Tinea unguium (ringworm of the nails, or ONYCHOMYCOSIS) is characterized by thick, white or yellow nails. Ringworm can also affect the skin under a beard (TINEA BARBAE) or the facial skin.

Treatment Antifungal drugs as creams, lotions or ointments can successfully treat most types of tinea. For widespread infection (or those affecting hair or nails), systemic treatment is usually required. Treatment should continue after symptoms have faded to ensure the fungi have been destroyed. Mild infections on the surface of the skin may be treated for four to six weeks. Toenail infections may require treatment with griseofulvin for up to two years, but with the new drugs three-month treatment may be sufficient. Until recently, the standard treatment was griseofulvin. It is relatively effective for skin and hair fungal infections but of limited use in the treatment of nail infections. Three new antifungals that are better at killing fungi are presently in the process of being approved by the FDA for fungal infections of the skin.

tinea barbae Ringworm infection of the skin under the beard, caused primarily by *Tinea mentagrophytes* or *T. verrucosum.* See TINEA.

tinea capitis The medical term for ringworm of the scalp, this fungal infection causes several round, itchy patches of hair loss on the scalp. It is most commonly found in children who live in cities or who are subject to crowded conditions where the fungi spread more easily.

Treatment Antifungal drugs, usually taken by mouth for four to six weeks, are administered.

tinea corporis The medical term for ringworm of the body, this fungal infection is characterized by itchy round patches with raised edges.

Treatment Treatment consists of antifungal drugs in cream, lotion, ointment or oral form administered for four to six weeks.

tinea cruris See JOCK ITCH.

tinea manuum Ringworm infection most often caused by *Tinea rubrum*, often found together with a foot infection. The condition is characterized by thickened scaly skin of palms and fingers, especially in the creases of the skin.

Treatment Topical antifungal preparations such as imidazole or allylamine antifungals are preferred. Topical agents may not be enough to cure this problem; therefore, an oral antifungal drug (such as GRISEOFULVIN or KETOCONAZOLE) is usually required and should be taken for two to three months.

tinea nigra palmaris A superficial ringworm infection of the palms, although the soles of the feet may also be affected. While the condition is found throughout the world in both men and women of all ages, it is uncommon in North America. Compared to other types of fungal infections, the incidence of tinea nigra palmaris is low, even in South America where it is most often found.

Symptoms The condition is characterized by the appearance on the palm or sole of a single brown-black macule with sharply defined margins that tends to spread in a circular pattern. It may mimic malignant melanoma (see MELANOMA, MALIGNANT).

Treatment Most infections respond to topical antifungals such as Whitfield's ointment, topical imidazoles or allylamines, Keralyt gel or 40 percent urea. Removal by scraping with an emery pad is helpful. Recurrence is rare. There are no established oral medications.

tinea pedis See ATHLETE'S FOOT.

tinea unguium See ONYCHOMYCOSIS.

tinea versicolor A common skin condition (also known as pityriasis versicolor) characterized by patches of white, brown or salmon-colored flaky skin on the trunk and neck. It primarily affects young and middle-aged adult men, and is not contagious.

Cause A yeast (living on most people's skin) causes the condition when it colonizes the dead outer layer of skin.

Treatment Thorough application of antifungal cream or lotion from ears to knees for several consecutive nights after shampooing with an anti-yeast shampoo, such as one containing selenium sulfide or ketoconazole, will eradicate the fungus, provided not one spot is missed. It is also important to wash underwear and night clothes and sheets thoroughly. The treatment will cure the condition, but it may take many months for the skin patches to return to a normal color. Relapses are frequent. A simpler approach requires taking an anti-yeast pill, ketoconazole, for just two doses.

tissue expansion A technique of plastic surgery that uses neighboring skin to cover birth defects, injuries or cosmetically displeasing areas by slowly stretching the skin.

This procedure began to gain popularity in the early 1980s and was first practiced to reconstruct breasts after mastectomy. Today it is used to cover birth defects, areas of skin after tumor removal, skin damaged by trauma, as well as for breast enlargement and creation of new, hair-bearing scalp for bald men.

In the past, the only way to replace skin marred by defects or injuries was to cut a flap of healthy flesh from elsewhere on the body, and transplant it over the problem area. Unfortunately, this caused scarring in both the donor and recipient area of the skin, as well as a mismatch between skin type. For example, the skin from the abdomen or back looks very different from the flesh on the breast or face in the color, thickness, and texture and ability to grow hair.

With the tissue expansion technique, a small silicone balloon is implanted beneath the skin, usually next to the area to be covered or enlarged. After the incisions have healed, the balloon is gradually filled by injection with saline solution until the skin has expanded enough to cover the desired area. This expansion process takes from six weeks to four months depending on the location and size of the defect. When the skin has been expanded enough, the balloon is withdrawn, any deformed tissue is removed and the newly stretched skin is positioned and sutured into place. Studies have shown that during expansion, the outer layer of skin (the EPIDERMIS) actually thickens as the cells multiply in reaction to the pressure.

In contrast, the underlying connective tissue, which is squeezed between the epidermis and the expanding balloon, becomes thinner. The body also forms a membrane of scar tissue around the expander, adding to the look of fullness. These changes, however, disappear about five months after the expander is removed.

toad skin See PHRYNODERMA.

tobramycin (trade names: Nebcin, Tobrex) An antibiotic drug used to treat severe skin infections, usually given by injection in combination with penicillin.
Adverse effects Possible side effects when giving tobramycin in high doses may include kidney damage, nausea and vomiting, inner ear deafness, headache and itchy rash.

toe web infection Disorders of the spaces between the toes are usually called ATHLETE'S FOOT, and most are caused by fungal infections. Although the fungus is the primary cause of tissue destruction, subsequent bacterial infiltration can contribute to the problem and interfere with treatment success. Independent bacterial infection also produces toe web infection.
Symptoms Maceration, cracking, discomfort, foul smell and oozing in the spaces between toes.
Treatment Because so many different types of organisms are involved in toe web infec-

tions, several different types of treatment must be used in order to be effective. If the lesions are dry and scaly, topical antifungal agents (such as imidazoles or allylamines) are effective. For soft, wet lesions, treatment must include removal of excess moisture, daily compresses with saline or albumin subacetate (Burow's solution), broad-spectrum topical antimicrobial agents, long-term use of antifungals, and oral GRISEOFULVIN.

tolnaftate (trade names: Aftate, Tinactin) An antifungal treatment for some types of TINEA (including ATHLETE'S FOOT). It is available without a prescription as a cream, powder or aerosol.
Adverse effects In rare cases, it may cause skin irritation or rash.

topical medications Drugs that are applied to the skin surface (instead of being injected or swallowed). Topical drugs also refer to suppositories inserted into the vagina or rectum, and drugs administered to the ear canal or surface of the eye.

toxic epidermal necrolysis See NECROLYSIS, TOXIC EPIDERMAL.

toxic shock syndrome An uncommon condition characterized by a distinctive skin rash resembling sunburn on the palms and soles of the feet that peels within one or two weeks. The condition, first recognized in the 1970s, is associated with the use of certain brands of highly absorbent tampons (now taken off the market). About 70 percent of cases occur in women who are using tampons when symptoms begin. Most recent cases have been related to staphylococcal infections unrelated to tampon use, however.
Symptoms In addition to the skin rash, symptoms include sudden high fever, vomiting and diarrhea, headache, muscular aches and pains, dizziness and disorientation. Blood pressure may drop rapidly and shock

may develop. Death occurs in about 3 percent of cases, usually due to a prolonged drop in blood pressure or lung problems.

Cause The condition is caused by a toxin produced by *Staphylococcus aureus.*

Treatment Antibiotic drugs and IV infusion (to prevent shock), plus treatment for any complications as they occur. Recurrence is common: women who have had toxic shock syndrome should not use tampons, cervical caps, diaphragms or vaginal contraceptive sponges.

transforming growth factor (TGF) beta A biological compound produced by the body that is essential for the normal production of COLLAGEN and elastin, which lies beneath the skin and make it supple. One of the newest compounds currently being studied, TGF may one day be available as a daily beauty treatment to slow down the physical signs of aging and keep skin young.

tretinoin See RETIN-A.

triamcinolone (trade names: Aristocort, Aristospan, Kenalog, Triacet, Triamolone) A corticosteroid hormone used to treat skin inflammations, with uses similar to cortisone. It reduces inflammation but doesn't cause water retention.

Side effects Dizziness, headache, muscle weakness, low blood pressure may be evident.

trichauxis An increase in the size and number of hairs.

trichiasis Ingrown eyelashes that grow toward the eyeball instead of outward as they normally would. If the lashes grow to the point where they touch the eyeball, they can cause severe pain and may damage the cornea.

Treatment Temporary treatment consists of removing the eyelashes that are growing the wrong way, but the lashes will regrow. Permanent treatment requires the destruction of the growth follicles of the wayward eyelashes via ELECTROLYSIS.

trichosporosis Also known as piedra, this is a fungal condition in which the hair shafts are coated with hard masses of white (*Trichosporon cutaneum* or *T. beigelii*) or black (*Piedraia hortai*) fungus. The black fungus appears as small dark nodules along the hair shaft, visible to the naked eye and under the microscope. It is found primarily in the tropics. The white variety is found around the world, and is characterized by soft nodules on primarily facial and pubic hair.

Treatment Removal of the affected hairs by clipping or shaving.

trichotillomania The habit of pulling out one's hair, often associated with psychological stress and sometimes mental illness or psychotic illness (such as schizophrenia). Hair-pulling may also take place among children who are anxious and frustrated. Typically, the patient pulls, twists or breaks off chunks of hair, leaving bald spots. Children sometimes eat the removed hair, which may cause a hairball in the stomach.

Treatment Psychotherapy and/or antipsychotic drugs are sometimes used.

tuberculin test A skin test used to determine whether or not a person has been infected with tuberculosis. The test is used to diagnose suspected cases of tuberculosis prior to vaccination against the disease.

During the test, the skin is first disinfected, usually with an alcohol swab, and a small dose of tuberculin (a protein extract of the tuberculosis bacilli) is introduced into the skin in one of a variety of ways. In the Mantoux test, the extract is injected into the skin with a needle—in the Sterneedle test, the extract is dropped on the forearm as a spring-loaded instrument circled with a sharp prong that forces the tuberculin into the skin.

After two days, the skin is inspected at the site; if the skin is unchanged, the reaction is negative, indicating the person has never been exposed to tuberculosis and has no immunity. Skin that becomes red, firm and raised after the injection indicates that the person has been exposed to tuberculosis, either through vaccination or infection. See also TUBERCULOSIS, SKIN.

tuberculosis, skin Tuberculosis of the skin is characterized by breakdown of the skin over pus-filled tuberculous glands, forming irregular-shaped ulcers tinged with blue. TB was uncommon and decreasing in prevalence in developed countries until the past few years. Recently, there has been a resurgence in TB cases, especially in the inner city. There are two basic forms of this type of TB: localized and disseminated.

The *localized* form may develop after the introduction of the tubercle bacilli into a wound in patients who have never been exposed to TB. It begins as an inflammatory nodule (called the "tuberculous chancre") and is followed by swelling of the lymph nodes. In those who are immune or partially immune, two types of lesions may appear: tuberculosis verrucosa and lupus vulgaris. In tuberculosis verrucosa, the bacilli leads to localized granulomatous solid elevated lesions or verrucose nodules. Lupus vulgaris begins in early life, with patchy lesions studded with what look like soft yellowish brown "apple jelly" nodules, when compressed with a glass slide. This is followed by swelling, ulcers and hypertrophy. In temperate climates, the majority of lupus lesions are on the face, while those of tuberculosis verrucosa are on the hands; the distribution may be different in tropical areas.

Scrofuloderma is another form of localized skin TB, in which tuberculosis of the lymph nodes extends into the skin, resulting in the development of ulcers. There may be many fistulas beneath ridges of bluish skin.

In the *disseminated* form, bacteria spread by patients with fulminating TB result in miliary tuberculosis of the skin. Papulonecrotic lesions that resemble acne appear on the face and arms and legs; these lesions end in chicken pox–like scars.

Treatment Treatment usually combines isoniazid, rifampin ethambutal. See also TUBERCULIN TEST.

tuberous sclerosis An inherited (autosomal dominant) disorder of pigmentation that affects the skin, characterized by an acne-like condition of the face called "adenoma sebaceum." In addition, patients often experience nervous system problems, benign tumors, epilepsy and mental retardation (although intelligence may be normal in mild cases). Seriously affected patients may not live beyond age 30. The gene for tuberous sclerosis can now be detected at an early stage of pregnancy.

Symptoms Other symptoms include ash leaf macules, which are white or light-colored and shaped like an ash leaf, anywhere on the skin; confetti spots (white, tiny macules scattered on the skin), SHAGREEN PATCH (an area of yellowish thickened skin usually on the lower back) and subungual fibromas (small overgrowths of fibrous tissue on the sides of the nails).

Treatment There is no cure; treatment is aimed at relieving symptoms. The adenoma sebaceum lesions can be removed with laser surgery, dermabrasion or electrosurgery.

tularemia An infectious disease of wild animals occasionally transmitted to humans, characterized by a red spot at the skin site of infection that eventually forms an ulcer.

Humans may contract the disease through direct contact with an infected animal (such as rabbits, squirrels or muskrats). The bacteria enters the body through a cut or scratch in the skin. It may also be acquired following a bite from a tick, flea, fly or louse or (rarely) by eating infected meat.

The disease is found only in North America (a few hundred cases yearly), some parts of Europe, and Asia.

Prevention A vaccine is available for those at high risk, such as hunters, trappers, game wardens or lab workers.

Symptoms In addition to the skin lesion, symptoms include enlarged lymph nodes, fever, headache, muscle pains and malaise. Sometimes the eyes, throat, digestive tract and lungs are affected.

Treatment Antibiotics (such as streptomycin, tetracyclines or intravenous gentamicin) treat the disease with a less than 1 percent fatality rate. Untreated, tularemia can be fatal in 5 percent of cases. The disease confers permanent immunity.

tumefaction A swelling.

tumbu fly bites These fly bites cause MYIA-SIS (skin infestation with fly larvae), most commonly in South Africa.

tunable dye laser Dye lasers use colored solids dissolved in organic solvents to produce laser light. The color of the laser light emitted is dependent on the color of solid material chosen. By changing the dye, the wavelength (or color) can be altered. Dye lasers are used for the treatment of blood vessel abnormalities (yellow light), and pigmented disorders (green light). See also PULSED DYE LASER.

Tunga penetrans A species of fleas found in tropical and subtropical America, commonly referred to as jiggers, sand flies or chigoes.

turban tumor Multiple benign growths called cylindramas, which cover the scalp, giving the sufferer the appearance of a person wearing a turban.

turtle oil One of the oldest products used in skin care because of its alleged benefits, its effectiveness was discredited as early as 1934. Extracted from the genitals and muscles of the giant sea turtle, the oil does have some vitamins and—like all oils—forms a film on the skin that helps retain moisture. It has no other value in skin-care products.

tylosis Callus formation.

tyrosine An amino acid that is used to produce MELANIN (skin pigment). Tyrosine is also used in some tan accelerators.

Tyndall light phenomenon The reflection of light by particles suspended in a gas or liquid that imparts a blue tinge to objects. In skin, melanin particles found at levels of the dermis give the skin varying degrees of a bluish tinge. This is the same process as the scattering of particles in the atmosphere that makes the sky appear blue.

typhus Any of a group of infectious diseases with similar symptoms, characterized by a measles-like rash, severe headache, back and limb pain, high fever, confusion, prostration, weak heartbeat and delirium. Untreated, a patient may die from blood poisoning, heart or kidney failure, or pneumonia.

In the past, epidemic typhus, spread by body lice, was the most significant type of this disease. Epidemics of this type swept across the world, killing hundreds of thousands of people during war, famine and natural disaster. It is rare today, except in some areas of Africa and South America.

Cause Typhus is caused by rickettsiae (microorganisms much like bacteria); in epidemic typhus, they are ingested by lice from the blood of infected patients. The lice deposit feces containing the rickettsiae on other people's skin. When they scratch their skin, the microorganisms enter the bloodstream.

Endemic (or murine) typhus is found in rats; it is spread to humans through flea bites. Scrub typhus is spread by mites in India and Southeast Asia.

Prevention Epidemic typhus may be prevented by vaccination and control of infestations via insecticides. Other types of typhus may be prevented by wearing protective clothes to prevent tick, mite and flea bites.

Treatment Antibiotic drugs (tetracyclines) treat typhus fever; other treatment is aimed at relieving symptoms. It may take a long time to recover from the disease. In the past, epidemic typhus was prevalent in crowded, unsanitary places and had a mortality rate of close to 100 percent.

tyrosine An amino acid used to produce MELANIN (skin pigment).

tyrosinemia type II See RICHNER-HANHART SYNDROME.

Tzanck smear Examination of cells from the floor of a VESICLE (blister). It is used to diagnose herpes virus infections and some blistering disorders such as PEMPHIGUS. A dermatologist removes the top of the blister and scrapes the jelly-like material from the base of the blister onto a microscope slide. The yield of this type of smear is better than in a culture of the virus in varicella-zoster virus infections, but lower than that of a culture in herpes simplex. However, the test is inexpensive and very reliable.

U

ulcer An open sore on the skin caused by the destruction of surface tissue. Skin ulcers, typically caused by inadequate blood flow, may be found anywhere on the body; the site is often helpful in a diagnosis. Leg ulcers are mainly caused by inadequate blood flow or poor blood return to the heart. Skin cancer can ulcerate, as can trauma or burns. More rarely, ulcers may be caused by BASAL CELL CARCINOMA. Genital ulcers may be caused by sexually transmitted diseases, including syphilis, gonorrhea, chancroid and herpes simplex.

ulerythema A skin disease causing atrophy and scarring, usually of the face. Typically, a portion of the eyebrow is affected and is lost.

ultraviolet light warning badge A self-adhesive waterproof badge that can be worn on clothing or on the skin that changes color with accumulated UV exposure. Watching the color changes on the badge helps even a child understand when excess exposure has occurred. See also ULTRAVIOLET LIGHT.

ultraviolet radiation The energy that comes to the earth from the sun is emitted as radiation of various wavelengths, called the electromagnetic spectrum. Included in this spectrum are radio waves, X rays, infrared rays, visible light and ultraviolet radiation.

Infrared radiation is experienced as heat, representing 45 percent of the sun's total energy. Another 49 percent of the total energy reaching the earth makes up the *visible light* spectrum, which we perceive as color.

Ultraviolet radiation makes up the rest of the total energy from the sun reaching the earth—radiation strong enough to cause pho-

tochemical reactions and penetrate the skin.

It is ultraviolet radiation that is responsible for both immediate and long-term damage to the skin. This radiation can cause anything from a beautiful tan to a painful sunburn. It causes skin to sag and wrinkle, brings out "sun spots" and ultimately can lead to skin cancer. Ultraviolet radiation stimulates melanocytes to produce brown pigment called MELANIN, which acts as a natural defense mechanism against ultraviolet radiation and gives skin a tanned look.

The amount of ultraviolet radiation people receive depends on how close they are to the equator, what time of day it is, what season it is, how high they are and the type of surrounding terrain. The potential for damage is greater at high altitudes because less atmospheric filtration occurs.

The closer to midday and the equator, the more damage from the sun because of the position of the sun in the sky: when the sun is directly overhead, its rays reach us vertically instead of at an angle, lessening the distance they must travel through the earth's protective atmosphere.

Seasonal changes also affect the ozone layer; the ozone layer is thinner and more dangerous, allowing more of the sun's rays to penetrate the atmosphere. Snow can be very hazardous because it reflects the sun more effectively even than sand and water. While clouds and pollution obstruct some ultraviolet radiation, they don't entirely eliminate it.

The ozone layer in Earth's stratosphere filters out most of this harmful radiation, but scientists warn that UV levels will climb as chemicals break down the ozone layer. Because the ozone layer is being depleted, higher concentrations of both UV-A and UV-B are now reaching the earth, which has significantly increased the risk of skin cancer among all people.

In the last several years, instruments have detected significant thinning of stratospheric ozone over much of the world, but it is not clear how UV levels at the earth's surface have changed, because no worldwide measurement network exists.

Interestingly, polluted air has been found to protect citizens from the ultraviolet radiation streaming through the earth's damaged ozone layer. Studies found that levels of UV light were nearly twice as high in the relatively clean air of New Zealand as they were in the more polluted area of Germany. Similarly, measurements in the Alps show a strengthening of UV intensity; those in the United States show a weakening.

There are three types of ultraviolet radiation emitted from the sun: UV-A, UV-B and UV-C. UV-C is toxic to human, plant and animal life but it is absorbed by the earth's atmosphere before it reaches the earth. UV-B (0.5 percent of the total energy reaching earth) is responsible for inducing skin redness and burning by penetrating the top two layers of the skin. UV-B has been considered to be more dangerous than UV-A, and is believed to be the direct cause of a range of major skin and eye problems.

Until recently, UV-A radiation was believed to be fairly harmless because it has a much lower intensity than UV-B. But this type of ultraviolet radiation can penetrate the dermis (the third layer of the skin), and since UV-A represents 5.5 percent of the total energy reaching the earth, it has grave potential for damage.

uncombable hair syndrome There have been about 50 cases of this problem, characterized by coarse, curly, tangled hair. It is also known as spun-glass hair, mostly affecting children aged 3 to 12. In the only case where the problem occurred in an adult with previously healthy hair, a 39-year old woman with thick, light-brown hair began taking the diuretic drug spironolactone for hair loss. After taking the drug the shedding decreased, but the hair that grew back was coarse, curly and so tangled that she could not comb it even with liberal use of conditioners. Under an electron microscope the hair shafts were found to be kidney bean or triangular shaped instead of round as normal hair shafts would be.

ungual Relating to the nail.

United Scleroderma Foundation Support group for SCLERODERMA patients, their families, physicians, nurses, allied health professionals and others interested in the disease. The foundation maintains support networks and encourages medical research. Established in 1975, the group was formerly known as the Monterey Bay Scleroderma Foundation; it currently has 5,000 members and sponsors an annual meeting. The foundation publishes a quarterly newsletter, brochures and a handbook. For address, see Appendix D; see also SCLERODERMA FOUNDATION; SCLERODERMA INTERNATIONAL FOUNDATION; SCLERODERMA RESEARCH FOUNDATION; SCLERODERMA SUPPORT GROUP.

Unna's boot A dressing of gelatin and ZINC OXIDE paste applied to the foot and leg to help to heal leg ulcers and other inflammatory skin conditions.

Urbach-Wiethe disease A rare hereditary metabolic disease involving the skin as well as other tissues and organs. The condition is an autosomal recessive trait, which means that a defective gene must be inherited from both parents in order to cause the abnormality. Generally, both parents of an affected person are unaffected carriers of the defective gene. Each of their children has a one in four chance of being affected, and a two in four chance of being a carrier.

Symptoms In the first two years of life, skin symptoms include pustules or blisters on the face and exposed areas of the arms and legs that heal, leaving behind white scars. Subsequent skin lesions include nodules, waxy yellow papules on the face, back of the neck, hands and fingers. Another characteristic sign is a line of lesions along the eyelids resembling a string of beads. In addition, there may be red warty plaques on elbows, knees, fingers, buttocks and face. Some patients develop a general yellow thickened skin and lose hair on the scalp, beard area, eyebrows and eyelashes.

Treatment There is no known treatment. Tracheostomy may be required for patients whose trachea becomes blocked with cartilage.

urticaria See HIVES.

urticaria, contact An acute localized allergic reaction characterized by a wheal-and-flare response (HIVES) after direct contact with an allergen, usually occurring within minutes after contact. It can be triggered by contact with a variety of antigens in food (especially fish or meat), drugs, cosmetics and textiles, and can also be set off by other mechanisms, such as jellyfish, nettles and chemicals. See also URTICARIA; URTICARIA, SOLAR.

Treatment Avoiding a known irritant is the only prevention. Antihistamines and anticholinergic drugs may sometimes provide relief in treatment.

urticaria pigmentosa Groups of mast cells (a large cell in connective tissue) that form brown MACULES or plaques that become itchy, red and swollen when irritated. See also MASTOCYTOSIS.

urticaria, solar A rare allergic response to the sun characterized by the appearance of HIVES within minutes of exposure. The lesions last from a few minutes to an hour, depending on the intensity of the exposure as well as the sensitivity of the individual. This condition may be chronic. Remissions are common and may be permanent.

Prevention Susceptible patients should avoid exposure to the sun by wearing protective clothes and opaque sunblocks. SUNSCREENS are not of much help. Gradual daily exposure to more and more of the sun will control the disease in many people, but this type of therapy is very difficult to carry out because of recurrent hives or even anaphylaxis; PUVA therapy is helpful in some patients. Recent studies have found that the more sedating antihistamine terfenadine is effective.

urushiol oil The active ingredient in POISON IVY that is one of the most potent external toxins known. The amount necessary to cause a rash in a sensitive person is measured in nanograms (a nanogram is one billionth of a gram). This means that 500 people could start itching from the amount of urushiol oil equal to the size of the period at the end of this sentence. Urushiol oil also boasts an incredible shelf life — specimens of poison ivy several centuries old have been known to trigger a reaction in sensitive individuals.

UV light See ULTRAVIOLET LIGHT.

V

vaccinia A viral cattle disease (cowpox) inoculated in humans to produce an antibody against SMALLPOX.

vaginal warts See WARTS.

van Lohuizen's disease See CUTIS MARMORATA TELANGIECTATICA CONGENITA.

varicella-zoster virus A member of the family of HERPES viruses named after the two illnesses it causes—varicella (CHICKEN POX) and zoster (SHINGLES). The virus first enters the upper respiratory tract of a nonimmune host in childhood and produces the skin lesions of chicken pox. About 90 percent of Americans get chicken pox, usually in childhood. The virus then becomes dormant in the nerve cells that transmit messages from the central nervous system to the skin, where it establishes a latent infection.

A person's immune system usually can successfully keep the virus from reactivating until later in life, when the patient's immunity to VZV may deteriorate. At that time, the virus replicates within the ganglia and results in shingles. Why and how the virus replicates is not well understood. In younger people shingles often may appear during periods of stress. It is much more likely, however, to affect people over age 50.

varicose veins Twisted, swollen veins just below the skin's surface, most often found in the legs. When valves in the leg veins become defective, they cause blood to pool in the superficial veins of the legs, which become swollen and distorted. Obesity, hormones during pregnancy or menopause, deep vein thrombosis, phlebitis, or pelvic vein pressure can all accelerate the formation of varicose veins. About 15 percent of adults suffer from varicose veins, which are more common among women and run in some families.

If backflow of blood from varicose veins is severe enough to cut off oxygen and nourishment to tissue, the skin over the veins may become thin, tight, dry, scaly and discolored, which can lead to ulcers. Bumping a large varicose vein may cause severe bleeding, which can be stopped by tying a clean handkerchief around the leg to apply moderate pressure and raising the affected leg.

Treatment In many cases, wearing elastic support stockings, exercising regularly, elevating the legs and standing still as little as possible will alleviate the problem. In severe cases, SCLEROTHERAPY (injecting an irritant solution into the veins to scar and block them, forcing other healthy veins to take over) is effective.

If they are very painful or if the overlying skin ulcerates, the veins may be removed using a surgical technique known as stripping. The patient must then keep the affected area bandaged for several weeks to help heal the wound.

variola Another name for SMALLPOX.

Varivax Brand name for the new CHICKEN POX vaccine developed by Merck and Co., which was approved by the U.S. Food and Drug Administration in April 1995. Its use has been recommended by the American Academy of Pediatrics for all children, teens and young adults who haven't had the disease.

Approval of the vaccine, which has been used in Japan for some time, has been controversial in this country, but most pediatricians recommend the vaccine for their patients.

Varivax vaccine is made from a live, weakened virus that works by creating a mild infection similar to natural chicken pox, but without related problems. The mild infection spurs the body to develop an immune response to the disease. These defenses are then ready when the body encounters the natural virus.

The vaccine is considered to be safe, although questions remain about how long the vaccine confers immunity and whether it may be linked with flareups of SHINGLES. Although there has been no evidence of impaired immunity, if the vaccine should wear off later in life adults could then be vulnerable to infection at an age when chicken pox can be more serious.

And since the virus belongs to the herpes virus group, there are some concerns that the vaccine might cause periodic reactivation of the varicella-zoster virus and resultant cases of shingles. However, research indicates that the vaccine causes fewer (or no more) cases of shingles than naturally contracted chicken pox.

The vaccine is recommended by doctors for all children, teenagers and young adults who haven't had chicken pox. One dose is needed for children up to age 12 (ideally given between 12 and 18 months of age); teenagers and adults need two shots, four to eight weeks apart. High-risk, susceptible patients may also obtain passive immunization with VZV immune globulin, which can abort or modify infection if administered within three days of exposure.

vascular tumors Tumors related to or supplied with blood from blood vessels. They include HEMANGIOMAS (including superficial strawberry hemangioma, deep (cavernous) hemangioma, cherry angioma, pyogenic granuloma); ANGIOKERATOMAS, spider nevus, lymphangioma, GLOMUS TUMOR, ANGIOSARCOMA and STEWART-TREVES TUMOR and PORT WINE STAINS.

vasculitis Inflammation of blood vessels. This is the underlying basic disease process in a number of diseases such as PERIARTERITIS NODOSA, ERYTHEMA NODOSUM, SCHONLEIN-HENOCH PURPURA, SERUM SICKNESS, temporal arthritis and Buerger's disease. The inflammation usually leads to narrowed, blocked blood vessels, which eventually destroy the surrounding tissues supplied by those damaged vessels. Symptoms depend on the size of vessel involved and their body location.

Vasculitis is caused in some cases by immune complexes in circulating blood. While these immune complexes would normally be destroyed by white blood cells, in certain disease states they settle in the blood vessel walls where they cause severe inflammation.

venereal warts See WARTS.

vernix The pale cheesy substance covering newborn skin consisting of fatty secretions and dead cells. It is thought to protect and insulate the baby's skin before birth.

verruca The medical term for WART.

vesicle A small skin BLISTER (usually filled with clear fluid).

viral diseases with skin symptoms Viral diseases are a common cause of skin disease. Some of these eruptions (such as WARTS) are exclusively infections of the skin, whereas others (such as MEASLES and CHICKEN POX) are the symptoms of systemic disease.

Viral diseases with skin symptoms include measles, dengue, erythema infectiosum (HHV-6), EXANTHEM SUBITUM, HERPES simplex (HSV-1 and HSV-2), SHINGLES, MILKER'S NODULE, ORF, PAPULAR ACRODERMATITIS, RUBELLA, chicken pox, COXSACKIE (hand, foot and mouth disease) and WARTS.

Other viral infections with only passing skin symptoms include Epstein-Barr virus (infectious mononucleosis), hepatitis and retroviruses (such as HIV).

vitamin A The vitamin necessary for healthy skin. Many foods contain this vitamin, but particularly good sources include liver, fish-liver oils, egg yolk, milk and other dairy products, margarine, and a wide range of fruits and vegetables.

Deficiency of this vitamin is rare in developed countries but a serious lack or excess intake can both cause dry, rough skin, among other problems.

Contrary to popular belief, ingesting too much carotene (by eating huge amounts of carrots) does *not* cause excess levels of vitamin A; however, it can produce carotenemia (high blood levels of carotene), which colors the skin deep yellow.

Synthetic vitamin A-like compounds called retinoids, such as tretinoin, applied directly to the skin have been used to treat acne and skin wrinkling and mottled pigmentation caused by chronic sun exposure. Used systemically, retinoids such as isotretinoin (ACCUTANE) and ETRETINATE treat acne and help to prevent skin cancer in those at very high risk.

vitamin A acid See RETINOIC ACID.

vitamin A deficiency The earliest signs of vitamin A deficiency appear in the eyes. These include night blindness, dry eyes and corneal ulcers. Skin symptoms of vitamin A deficiency include dryness, fine scaling and FOLLICULAR HYPERKERATOSIS.

vitamin B₂ (riboflavin) deficiency Deficiency of this vitamin may cause chapped lips and a sore tongue or sores in the mouth corners. While a balanced diet usually provides adequate amounts of riboflavin, some people are susceptible to a deficiency. These people include those taking phenothiazine antipsychotic drugs, tricyclic antidepressants, oral contraceptives and those with malabsorption disorders or severe alcohol dependence. Deficiency may also result from serious illness or injury, or surgery.

vitamin B₆ (pyridoxine) deficiency Deficiency of this vitamin causes a variety of skin conditions, inflammation of mouth and tongue and cracked lips. This vitamin plays a vital role in the activities of various enzymes and hormones involved in keeping skin healthy. Good dietary sources of vitamin B₆ are found in liver, chicken, pork, fish, whole grains, wheat germ, bananas, potatoes and dried beans. A balanced diet will provide sufficient amounts of this vitamin, which is also produced in small amounts by intestinal bacteria.

People who are at risk for developing a vitamin B₆ deficiency include breast-fed infants, people with poor diets and those with malabsorption disorders, severe alcoholics, and patients taking certain drugs (including penicillamine, hydralazine or birth control pills).

vitamin C Also known by its chemical name (ascorbic acid), this vitamin plays an important role in healing wounds in the skin (among other duties) and in preventing SCURVY. The primary dietary source of this vitamin is fresh fruits and vegetables, especially citrus fruits, tomatoes, green leafy vegetables, potatoes, green peppers, strawberries and cantaloupe.

A balanced diet usually provides enough vitamin C, but slight deficiencies may occur after surgery, fever, constant inhalation of carbon monoxide in tobacco smoke and traffic fumes, serious injury, or use of oral contraceptives.

vitamin D A naturally occurring substance produced by the interaction of sunlight with chemicals in the skin that helps the body absorb calcium from the intestinal tract and provides for the healthy development and growth of bones. About 15 minutes outdoors a day is enough to meet the body's requirements for the vitamin, although it is also found in many foods. A deficiency of vitamin D, either through a poor diet or lack of sunlight, can lead to rickets. Vitamin D has been added to milk since the 1930s as a way to reduce the incidence of rickets.

Many other foods are fortified with vitamin D, and supplements are also available. Other good dietary sources of vitamin D include oily fish, liver, dairy products and egg yolks. However, sunlight's interaction with the skin can provide enough vitamin D unless children drink no milk at all. Elderly people who don't drink milk and don't get out into the sunshine do have a potential risk for vitamin D deficiency.

Vitamin D is considered to be an antioxidant (see ANTIOXIDANT BEAUTY PRODUCT) and anticarcinogen, and may play a role in skin pigmentation. Since it can be absorbed by the skin, applying this vitamin topically can have an effect on the skin's health.

Vitamin D is toxic in very large amounts (between 5,000 and 10,000 IU daily for several months for D3 or D4), and megadoses should be avoided. Sunbathing, however, will not result in an overdose.

vitamin E (tocopherol) This vitamin has a long history of use for those with skin problems. Many people today use vitamin E for bruises, cuts skin irritations and to help heal wrinkles. Scientifically, it has never been shown to be effective when used topically as anything other than a moisturizer, since vitamin E cannot penetrate the outer skin's layers. Some studies have found that this vitamin can actually irritate the skin of the face, especially when it is used with an ACNE product that has a peeling effect. When spray-on vitamin E is forced through the layers of the skin it can lead to severe allergic reactions.

Vitamin E *is* an antioxidant. It can help prevent FREE RADICAL damage. Based on the observation that skin damage caused by the sun and by other environmental agents are induced by free radicals, there is the possibility that vitamin E may be effective in preventing skin damage. It is being used more and more in skin preparations as a way to fend off this damage.

Although topical use of vitamin E has few negative consequences other than the potential for allergic reaction, oral vitamin E overdoses can block the absorption of other fat-soluble vitamins such as A and D.

Vitamin E deficiency is extremely rare, and when it occurs it is usually caused by a disease that blocks its absorption from the gastrointestinal tract. This vitamin is found naturally in vegetable oils, including wheat germ oil; most people get an adequate supply by eating a typical American diet.

vitamins and the skin Experts have known for some time that vitamins affect the skin. Lack of vitamins can make skin lifeless, blotchy, dry or oily. Healthy skin requires a variety of vitamins to keep it resilient; specifically, vitamins A (found in carrots, broccoli, leafy green vegetables, asparagus, cantaloupe, apricots, peaches and sweet potatoes) and vitamin E (in whole-grain breads, wheat germ, oatmeal and eggs).

Furthermore, vitamins E and C (found in citrus fruits and vegetables) are the simplest forms of antioxidant. Antioxidants may help prevent skin damage from free radicals, a dangerously mutant form of oxygen that in large doses (from pollution, sunlight, etc.) can break through the membrane that protects the skin's cells and cause inflammation, visible lines and wrinkles, among other damage.

Vitamin A may help prevent sun damage and vitamin C may accelerate skin healing. There is also some evidence that vitamin C may pass through the layers of skin and help heal tissue damaged by burn or injury, although some experts dispute this. Vitamin D, absorbed through the skin's outer layers, may help heal the skin when applied topically, especially when combined with vitamin A.

vitiligo A common skin pigmentation disease characterized by irregular patches of various size totally lacking pigment. The unpigmented areas are extremely sensitive to ultraviolet radiation. The depigmented areas are particularly obvious in dark-skinned people, and are found most often on the face, hands, armpits and groin. In fair-skinned individuals, they are often only noticeable if the person tans.

While the condition may appear at any age, it usually develops in early adulthood and affects about one in every 200 people. Spontaneous repigmentation occurs in about 30 percent of patients.

Cause Vitiligo is believed to be an autoimmune disorder that leads to an absence of MELANOCYTES (specialized cells that secrete skin pigment MELANIN).

Treatment Makeup can disguise the disease, and in mild cases no further treatment is necessary. PHOTOTHERAPY using PUVA may induce repigmentation in more than half the cases, but many treatments are needed. Corticosteroid creams may also help. If the skin depigmentation is extensive, topical chemicals may be used to remove pigment from remaining areas of involved skin.

See also CAMOUFLAGE COSMETICS.

Voigt's line(s) Also known as Futcher's lines, these normal color patterns are seen in dark-skinned people (especially blacks and dark Japanese) in which the border between the darker segment of skin (usually on the upper arms) and the lighter area of skin is marked by a line.

voiles A new type of spray-on fragrance that is non-drying because of a lack of alcohol. The voiles (French for veils) are based on a water-in-oil emulsion and are helpful for consumers with dry skin who find alcohol-based fragrance to be too drying. The voiles are nondrying, and the oil in the formulation helps skin retain moisture.

volar melanotic macules A condition primarily affecting black skin characterized by darker macules on palms and soles resulting from local accumulation of MELANIN. The discoloration lasts throughout life and requires no treatment.

W

Waardenburg's syndrome A hereditary disorder of pigmentation and hearing loss that was first described in 1951. Symptoms include a white forelock of hair with a triangular white area of skin on the forehead (60 percent); piebald spots on extremities or trunk (five to 10 percent); medial folds of the eyes associated with flattening of the root of the nose (66 percent) and possibly two different colored eyes. About 50 percent of patients may have a nonprogressive sensorineural hearing loss ranging from mild to severe in one or both ears.

The disorder is genetically transmitted to offspring in a dominant manner, and carries a 50 percent risk that siblings may be born with a variation of the syndrome. Still, only a few people who have the abnormal form of the gene show all the features of the syndrome. Researchers believe there may be a connection between the development of pigmentation and hearing during pregnancy.
Treatment Therapy for the depigmentation of the skin is the same as for those with PIEBALDISM. Attempts to repigment the white areas of the skin with conventional methods (such as ultraviolet light and psoralens) have generally been unsuccessful. It is possible to surgically correct the problem with punch autografts, epidermal suction grafts and thin split-thickness grafts. Repigmentation does occur, and the appearance is often satisfactory. Opaque cosmetics can be used to conceal the more obvious depigmented areas.

wart removal preparations Substances that remove WARTS from the skin. Liquid nitrogen is used to freeze a wart and form a blister that lifts off the growth. Sometimes a blister-producing liquid (cantharidin) or a corroding acid liquid or plaster is used. The last two product groups usually contain salicylic acid, lactic acid or trichloracetic acid.

warts Harmless, contagious growths on the skin or mucous membranes caused by any of more than 50 varieties of PAPILLOMAVIRUS. Warts appear only on the very top layer of skin, without roots or branches. Occasionally, warts contain small black spots, which are capillaries that have become clotted due to the rapid skin growth caused by the virus. While all warts are basically the same type of growth, they may look different depending on where on the body they appear.

COMMON WARTS are firm, well-defined growths up to a quarter-inch wide, often with a rough surface. They usually appear in areas that are frequently injured, such as the hands, fingers, feet, toes, knees, and face, especially in young children. They often appear in crops, and can disappear spontaneously.

FLAT WARTS are flat-topped, sometimes itchy PAPULES found mainly on the wrists, backs of hands, legs and face. *Digitate warts* are dark-colored growths with finger-like projections. *Filiform warts* are long, slender growths found on the armpits, eyelids, or neck in middle-aged or overweight people.

PLANTAR WARTS are found on the soles of the feet, flattened by the pressure of the body on the bottom of the feet, forcing them to grow inward.

GENITAL WARTS are transmitted through sexual contact, and are characterized by pink or brown, flat or raised cauliflower-like groups of growths on the genitals. This type of wart needs prompt diagnosis and treatment, since there is evidence that some of these warts infecting a woman's cervix may predispose her to cervical cancer. *It is important that both partners be checked and re-*

checked, since the infection can be passed back and forth between them. Condoms can prevent the transfer of warts. Warts present around the genitals of young children may be a sign of sexual abuse.

Treatment About half of all warts disappear on their own between six months to a year after they appear. In many cases they can be left untreated to spontaneously resolve.

Common, flat and plantar warts may be removed with liquid nitrogen or a blister-producing agent, corroding acids or plasters. Surgical removal with a scalpel, electric needle or laser also may be used.

Genital warts may be removed by surgery or by the application of podophyllin. Recurrence rates with this type wart are very high and there is no specific treatment available. All treatments are destructive and not that effective.

Researchers at Children's Memorial Hospital in Chicago and New York University have found that the ulcer drug cimetidine may be an effective treatment of multiple warts in children. Multiple warts can be troublesome because they often resist common treatment such as topical medications, freezing, burning or laser surgery. Multiple warts also may reappear after successful treatment. But this new research found that young patients whose warts had not responded to other treatment showed signs of improvement after three daily doses of cimetidine. Within six to seven weeks, many of the warts had become flatter and less visible. Two months into the study, warts in almost 80 percent of the children had disappeared. Researchers report that cimetidine is safe for children, and does not appear to cause any side effects.

See also WART REMOVAL PREPARATIONS.

waxing A technique used to remove unwanted hairs (usually from the legs, bikini area and upper lip) by stripping them from their root. In the procedure, solid wax and resin mixtures are heated until they melt, and are applied to the hairy areas. As the wax cools, it traps the hair; when the wax is pulled off, the hair comes off with it.

Alternatively, tacky material on strips of cloth or paper may be used to remove hair on the body or face. Waxing is most often performed in beauty salons. When performed on the upper lip or legs around the hair follicle it may cause FOLLICULITIS, an inflammatory reaction.

webbing A flap of skin present at birth, located between toes or fingers that may affect two or more digits. Although mild webbing is harmless, surgery may be performed for cosmetic reasons. In severe cases, adjacent digits may be completely fused (called syndactyly). Webbing may have a genetic origin.

weeping Oozing of clear fluid from a superficial inflammation of the EPIDERMIS. When the ooze dries, it forms a crust.

Wegener's granulomatosis See SYSTEMIC NECROTIZING VASCULITIDES (VASCULITIS).

Weil's disease See LEPTOSPIROSIS.

Werner's syndrome A rare connective tissue disorder in men and women associated with premature aging and hardening of the skin, mottled skin color and spidery veins in the skin. Other symptoms include a distinctive appearance with short stature, beaked nose, premature gray hair, diabetes mellitus, hypogonadism, and leg ulcers.

The disease usually starts in the 20s and 30s and is transmitted as an autosomal recessive trait, which means that a defective gene must be inherited from both parents to cause the abnormality. Generally, both parents of an affected person are unaffected carriers of the defective gene. Each of their children has a one in four chance of being affected, and a two in four chance of being a carrier.

This syndrome usually is associated with an increased risk of cancer, for which there is no known treatment. Death usually occurs as a result of accelerated hardening of the arteries (atherosclerosis), generally when the patient is in his 40s.

wheal A hive—a smooth, raised area of skin that is usually itchy.

Whipple's disease A rare disorder found most often among middle-aged men that causes (among other things) abnormal skin pigmentation. Other symptoms include malabsorption, diarrhea, abdominal pain, progressive weight loss, joint pain, swollen lymph nodes, anemia and fever.
Cause Unknown, but probably due to an unidentified bacterial infection.
Treatment Antibiotics for at least one year.

whitehead Also known as an open comedone, this is a very common superficial dilated closed pore filled with debris and some white cells seen typically in patients with acne. Left untreated, some whiteheads progress to inflammatory pustules, which often clear spontaneously. See MILIA.

Whitmore's disease The common name for melioidosis, a bacterial infection of rodents caused by *Pseudomonas pseudomallei,* which is endemic in Southeast Asia and Australia. The disease, which is also found in pigs, cattle, sheep and horses, can be acquired by humans by breathing in the bacteria or by the bacteria's coming in contact with broken skin. The bacteria is also found in soil and water (especially rice paddies).

In humans, the disease takes three forms— an acute septicemic (blood poisoning) with diarrhea, a typhoidal form with local abscess formation and severe HIVES; and a chronic variety. The disease may be milder and more common than had been thought.

Treatment Abcesses must be surgically drained; antibiotics (tetracycline with chloramphenicol, piperacillin, gentamicin or doxycycline) are administered.

Wickham's striae Pale network of whitish lines on the surface of the PAPULES of LICHEN PLANUS. The lines are also highly visible in the mouth.

Wilson's disease An inborn defect of copper metabolism characterized by excess amounts of copper deposits in the liver (causing jaundice and cirrhosis) or the brain (causing mental retardation and parkinsonism). Known medically as hepatolenticular degeneration, skin symptoms include skin darkening (hyperpigmentation) along the front portion of the legs; blue-colored nails', spider ANGIOMAS and JAUNDICE. Other symptoms include tremor, psychiatric problems, hepatitis or cirrhosis, discolored corneal membrane, bony abnormalities, etc.

Scientists recently have discovered the gene that causes Wilson's disease. The gene prevents the liver from removing the excess copper ingested in food; eventually, the copper accumulates in the body, damages the liver and leaks into the brain. The discovery could lead to a screening test and more effective treatment.
Treatment Administration of D-penicillamine for life. For those who cannot tolerate this drug, trientine is a safe alternative. If treated early, patients can expect to live a normal lifespan. Untreated patients eventually develop a fatal failure of many organs.

winter itch Itchy, dry skin related to the cold winter season.

Wiskott-Aldrich syndrome This hereditary disease is characterized by a DERMATITIS that resembles atopic dermatitis (see DERMATITIS, ATOPIC), recurrent infections and a reduced number of platelets in the blood (thrombocytopenia).

The disease is an X-linked recessive trait, which means that it is caused by a defect on the X chromosome, usually leading to problems in males only. Women can be carriers of the defect, and half of their sons may be affected.

Symptoms The first sign of this disease is usually a hemorrhagic eczematous dermatitis, and by the end of the year other infections appear, often followed by lymphoreticular cancers. Death from bleeding or cancer usually occurs early.

Treatment Infections are treated by replacement of immunoglobulins and blood platelets; bone marrow transplants have helped some patients.

witch hazel An extract of the leaves and bark of the *Hamamelis virginniana* plant used as an effective astringent. It can dry out spots, reduce oil on the skin, and soothe bruises and sprains. Puffy eyes can be refreshed with refrigerated witch hazel–soaked pads.

wound Damage to the skin and/or underlying tissue resulting from an accident or surgery. Wounds in which the skin is broken are called *open* wounds; wounds associated with unbroken skin are called *closed* wounds.

Incised wounds involve skin that is cleanly cut or surgically incised; an *abrasion* is a graze in which the surface skin is scraped away; a *laceration* involves torn skin. A *penetrating wound*, which penetrates all skin layers, would include a stab or gunshot wound, and a *contusion* is a bruise caused by a blunt instrument that damages underlying tissue.

Treatment Many minor wounds may be treated with first aid, but deeper wounds require professional care. Any foreign material or dead tissue must be removed. The wound should be cleaned with an antiseptic solution to decrease the chance of infection.

Clean, freshly incised wounds may be stitched closed, and usually heal with little scarring. The jagged edges of a laceration may need to be removed before stitching. Contaminated wounds are not usually stitched shut. Instead, they are usually filled with layers of sterile gauze and covered with a bandage. After four or five days, if there is no sign of infection, the wound can then be closed. Otherwise, the wound will be left open to heal on its own. It may be necessary to draw off blood from a severe bruise through a needle to aid healing.

wound healing Research has shown that cuts and scrapes heal best with a broad-spectrum antibacterial ointment and a proper bandage. Some individuals, however, may be allergic to some compounds in these ointments, especially those that contain neomycin or preservatives.

It's best to keep cuts and scrapes clean and moist and not exposed to the air, which forms scabs that cut down on cell growth. Bandages that keep the wound moist (such as those impregnated with petroleum jelly) enable cells to regenerate rapidly.

Woronoff ring A skin symptom of PSORIASIS in which a white halo forms at the periphery of skin lesions. It is thought to be related to vasoconstriction of vessels surrounding psoriatic plaques caused by the elaboration of prostaglandins.

wrinkles A crease or furrow in the skin caused by the natural process of aging or by excessive exposure to the sun's damaging rays. Wrinkles are caused by reduced COLLAGEN production and subsequent loss of elasticity in the skin. While wrinkles are most obvious on exposed areas, they occur all over the body. "Expression lines" may be caused by the contraction of facial muscles during smiling or frowning; when these muscles contract, they pull the skin in, causing a line. And the muscles controlling frown lines between the brows may contract even when the muscle is resting, causing deep lines.

Treatment Treatments aimed at reducing wrinkles do not permanently restore skin elasticity. These treatments include adding things to the skin to fill the wrinkles (such as collagen, silicone, fat or gortex) and removing tissue to smooth the surface (DERMABRASION, CHEMICAL PEELS, LASER RESURFACING and FACE-LIFTS). While all of these treatments are considered permanent solutions, they work best on fine, shallow wrinkles.

Laser resurfacing with a pulsed CO_2 laser is one of the newest techniques for the treatment of medium-to-fine wrinkles, emitting a very brief pulse of high-intensity light that's fast enough to limit heat damage in the skin, yet strong enough to vaporize tissue cleanly. Since the heat penetrates the skin no deeper than half the thickness of a human hair, it can remove the wrinkled skin layer by layer without scarring. The procedure can be done on an outpatient basis, and takes on average about *30 minutes to an hour.*

Less expensive than a face-lift, laser resurfacing doesn't cause bleeding and doesn't require general anesthesia. While face-lifts are good for sagging skin, they aren't ideal for too much sagging skin. While laser resurfacing cannot *replace* a face-lift, it can improve the appearance after a face-lift has been performed by removing the fine lines that may remain.

Unlike other cosmetic techniques, most patients report little or no pain *during* the pulsed CO_2 laser treatment. Areas of the skin that can be completely anesthetized, such as the skin around the mouth, are usually pain free. After the technique, the skin may ooze and become puffy, crusting and red. The skin remains reddened for about six weeks, but can be covered completely by makeup after the first few days. Full healing takes place within about three months.

Many dermatologists today believe the pulsed CO_2 laser is a better way to treat wrinkles than either dermabrasion and chemical peels because it allows for better control and safety.

Dermabrasion is the surgical removal of the top layer of skin by high-speed sanding; it can leave the skin smooth and soft, but it also carries a risk of scarring and pigment changes. In an age of blood-borne infections such as AIDS, dermabrasion can be risky to health care workers since the technique tends to spray a great deal of blood.

Deep *chemical peels* also are more risky than laser treatment since the extent of the burn can be difficult to control and the final appearance of the skin may appear artificial. A chemical peel causes a deep, controlled second-degree burn using caustic chemicals; at least one of the chemicals (phenol) may adversely affect someone with poor liver, heart or kidney function.

Collagen injections, although temporary, is one of the less painful, and more conservative methods to temporarily reduce the appearance of facial wrinkles. The procedure involves the injection of tiny drops of collagen (derived from cowhide) into the skin to minimize lines, filling in deep vertical wrinkles between the eyebrows, deep wrinkles running from mouth to nose, and forehead wrinkles. Results last only between three and 18 months. The entire treatment may take up to only about 10 minutes, and patients recover in two to three hours. Afterward, there may be some redness lasting up to 10 days. A few patients experience bruising, temporary stinging or burning, faint redness, swelling or excessive fullness. Others may have no reaction. Risks include allergic reaction, contour irregularities, infection or local abscesses. Those who have a history of immunologtical disorders (such as LUPUS ERYTHROMATOSUS or rheumatoid arthritis) are not suitable candidates. Like all cosmetic procedures, its success depends on the skill of the physician:

ill-placed collagen can leave a bumpy surface.

A face-lift can smooth out wrinkles by stretching the skin, but the effects only last for five to 10 years. In facelifts and brow lifts, excess skin is removed at the edge of the face, leaving stretched, tighter skin behind.

One of the newest techniques to remove wrinkles is BOTOX (*Botulinum* toxin), a purified form of the toxin that causes botulism. Injected into the face, the substance temporarily and partially paralyzes the muscles underneath frown lines, giving the face a smoother, less furrowed look. While experts report up to a 90 percent reduction in wrinkling, the cost is high (between $500 and $1,000 per treatment) and critics point out that the treatment may give patients a lifeless look.

Wrinkles in men Wrinkle-reducing products recently have begun to be marketed for male consumers because a man's skin tends to be thicker and oilier than a woman's and therefore needs unique skin care products. Men's products tend to be more oil-free and concentrated. On the market today are a range of products just for men.

X

xanthelasma Yellowish patches that tend to occur on the eyelids as a result of cholesterol deposits. Common in elderly patients, they are usually no more serious than a cosmetic problem. However, they should be assessed by a physician since 50 percent of patients with this problem have abnormal cholesterol levels.

Treatment High cholesterol levels are treated by controlled diet and medication. The eyelid patches may be treated with a laser or excisional surgery.

xanthogranuloma, juvenile A benign disorder of infancy characterized by red-yellow nodules that gradually grow larger and then fade away. They first appear in the first six months of life, but they can occur in older children and adults.

Treatment These lesions usually require no treatment.

xanthoma A yellow deposit of fatty material in the skin, they may indicate a disorder of triglycerides or cholesterol.

There are several types of xanthomas, depending on the lipid abnormality. XANTHELASMAS are yellowish plaques on the eyelids that are related to lipid abnormality in 50 percent of patients.

Xanthomas may appear over joints such as elbows or knees (tuberous xanthomas) or scattered in showers over the trunk (eruptive xanthomas).

Treatment Dietary changes and agents that lower blood lipid levels can be effective for tuberous and especially eruptive xanthomas. Eruptive xanthomas usually disappear as triglyceride levels return to normal.

xanthomatosis A condition in which yellowish fatty deposits are found in various parts of the body (including the skin). When they occur in the eyelids only, the condition is known as XANTHELASMA. Xanthomatosis is often associated with a variety of disorders that cause higher levels of fats and cholesterol in the blood.

Treatment The best treatment is to lower levels of fat and cholesterol in the blood by means of a diet low in cholesterol and high in polyunsaturated fat. Drug therapy may also be effective in lowering cholesterol levels.

xenograft See HETEROGRAFT.

xeroderma pigmentosum This rare inherited skin disease causes an extreme sensitivity to light, so that the skin (normal at birth) becomes dry, wrinkled, freckled and prematurely old by age 5, with various types of benign and malignant skin tumors. Inherited as an autosomal recessive trait, it is often accompanied by eye disorders such as photophobia and conjunctivitis.

The condition is caused by the lack of an enzyme present in normal individuals that corrects light-induced DNA damage. In affected patients, the lack of this enzyme causes cells to reproduce abnormally, leading to vast numbers of skin cancers. BASAL CELL CARCINOMA, SQUAMOUS CELL CARCINOMA, KERATOACANTHOMAS and malignant melanoma (see MELANOMA, MALIGNANT) are common at an early age and may be fatal.

Symptoms Infants or young children exposed to sunlight develop a prolonged skin redness, freckles and TELANGIECTASIA. Skin hardening causes distortions of eyes, nose and mouth, and eye problems from damage caused by the sun. In some forms of the disease, there also may be microcephaly, mental retardation and testicular hypoplasia.

Treatment Patients must avoid exposure to sunlight by wearing protective clothing and using SUNSCREENS with an SPF of at least 15. Skin cancer is treated by surgical removal or with anticancer drugs.
See also MELANOMA, MALIGNANT.

xerosis Abnormal dryness of the skin.

Y

yaws One of the world's most prevalent infections, this is a childhood skin disease found throughout the poorer subtropical and tropical areas of the world, caused by a spirochete similar to the one responsible for SYPHILIS. Yaws, also known as frambesia, pian or bouba, is not a sexually transmitted disease. It is found between the Tropics of Cancer and Capricorn, where more than 50 million people have been treated with penicillin in an effort to eradicate the disease. As a result, its incidence has been reduced in many areas, although it still occurs in many communities. It is transmitted by direct contact with infected persons, their clothing, and possibly by a type of fly. The spirochetes enter through skin abrasions.

About a month after infection, a highly contagious, itchy tumor with yellow crusts appears on hands, face, legs and feet. Scratching spreads the infection, leading to development of more growths on other parts of the skin that may deteriorate into deep ulcers.

Treatment A single dose of penicillin will cure this disease. Without treatment, growths heal slowly over about six months, but recurrence is common. About 10 percent of untreated patients experience widespread tissue loss leading to destruction of skin, bones and joints of the legs, nose, palate and upper jaw.

yeast infections Skin infections caused by types of yeast, the most important of which is *Candida albicans,* which causes candidiasis. *Candida* can normally be found in the mouth, vagina and large intestine, but for unknown reasons it can cause infection in its host—most commonly in those who take antibiot-

ics, oral steroids or birth control pills, or in diabetics and the overweight. Age or sex has no effect on these infections. This type of yeast causes THRUSH (white patches on the inside of the cheeks), cheesy vaginal discharge, monilial intertrigo (damp red eruptions under the breasts, the foreskin and under-body folds in the obese). It also causes CANDIDA PARONYCHIA (redness and swelling around the nails).

Treatment Yeast infections respond to specific systemic agents designed to fight yeasts (such as nystatin or ketoconazole).

yellow fever A short-acting infectious disease that gets its name from the jaundiced yellow skin that is its most striking symptom.

Cause The yellow fever virus is transmitted by mosquitoes who spread the disease from monkeys to humans. Today it can be contracted only in Central America and a large part of Africa. In urban areas in those places, the disease is transmitted between humans by *Aëdes aegypti* mosquitoes.

Prevention Vaccination confers long-lasting immunity and should always be obtained before travelling through affected areas. A vaccination certificate is required for entry to many countries. A single injection of the vaccine gives protection for up to 10 years, but children under age one should not be vaccinated. In addition, eradication of the mosquito from populated areas has greatly reduced the incidence of the disease.

Symptoms Between three and six days after infection there is a sudden fever and headache accompanied by nausea and nosebleeds. Sometimes the patient recovers within three days, but often in more serious cases there is severe headache and neck, back and leg pain, followed by liver and kidney damage, jaundice, and kidney failure. This may be followed by agitation, delirium, coma and, in 10 percent of cases, death.

Treatment No drug is effective against the yellow fever virus, so treatment is aimed at maintaining blood volume via transfusion of fluids. In mild or moderate cases the prognosis is excellent. Relapses do not occur and one attack confers lifelong immunity.

Yersinia (Pasteurella) pestis A small gram-negative bacterium that causes PLAGUE and is transmitted from rodents to humans. Streptomycin is the antibiotic of choice in combatting the bacterium.

Z

Z-plasty A plastic surgical technique used to change the direction of a scar so it can be hidden in natural skin creases or to relieve skin tension caused by a skin CONTRACTURE. It is especially helpful in reducing unsightly scars on the face, and for releasing scarring across joints (such as on the fingers or armpits) that restrict movement.

In the operation, a Z-shaped incision is made with the central arm of the Z along the scar; two V-shaped flaps are created by cutting the skin away from underlying tissue. The flaps are then transposed and stitched.

zinc For many years, zinc has been used as an astringent, an antiseptic and a skin protectant. However, a recent advisory panel of the U.S. Food and Drug Administration has determined that zinc salts (ZINC OXIDE, zinc stearate and zinc sulfide) have no established effectiveness in the treatment of ACNE. Some dermatologists, however, recommend zinc to their patients for its anti-inflammatory effect, theorizing that zinc releases vitamin A which may normalize cells, and suggesting patients add zinc-rich food to their diet (lean beef, cheese and chicken). Zinc oxide also is an effective sunblock. See also DIET AND THE SKIN.

zinc deficiency Deficiency of this vitamin may cause skin inflammation and hair loss, diarrhea and low zinc blood levels. Skin symptoms are very similar to those of ACRODERMATITIS ENTEROPATHICA. Zinc is a trace element essential for normal wound healing. Small amounts are found in a wide variety of foods, including lean meat, whole-grain breads and cereals, dried beans and seafood.

A common cause of zinc deficiency is tube feeding without adequate zinc replacement,

usually after the second or third month of tube feeding.

Treatment Zinc supplements rapidly reverses the deficienty.

zinc oxide An ingredient in many skin preparations that has a mild astringent action and soothing effect. It can be used to treat painful, itchy or moist skin conditions (such as ECZEMA, DIAPER RASH and BEDSORES) and is an ingredient in diaper rash ointment. It can also ease the pain and itch of insect bites and stings and hemorrhoids, and will block the ultraviolet rays of the sun. An inert ingredient, it is often used to thicken lotions and creams.

Zostrix An ointment whose active ingredient is capsaicin, a red pepper derivative used to make chili powder, used to ease the pain of SHINGLES. *Zostrix should only be used once all the shingles blisters have disappeared,* and *never* applied on an active blister.

Experts believe that capsaicin blocks the production of a chemical (substance P) necessary for pain impulse transmission between nerve cells. As a counterirritant, Zostrix is designed to be used on unbroken, healed skin with a pain sensation, not for open, oozing infections. Zostrix does cause a burning sensation, and won't be effective unless used often and continuously for three weeks. The burning decreases or vanishes altogether if treatments of Zostrix are continued.

Zostrix has also been tested for treatment of PSORIASIS; however, it has been approved so far by the U.S. Food and Drug Administration only for use against shingles.

Zyderm The brand name for liquid collagen, it is available as a soft white gel that is injected into the skin to replace tissue lost as the result of age or trauma. Approved by the U.S. Food and Drug Administration in 1981, Zyderm works below the outer surface to re-create a firm dermis, replacing lost tissue and becoming a part of the individual's own tissue.

Zyderm injections can correct small de-pressions such as scars and wrinkles (espe-cially around the forehead and lines around the mouth). Only three out of 100 people are allergic to collagen. Treatments are usually given in a series of from two to six half-hour visits, usually with a two-week rest in be-tween. The physician uses a very thin needle to make multiple injections along the line of the wrinkle, which feels like a light scratch; this is followed by a slight temporary swell-ing and blanching, but with very little dis-comfort. Retreatment is needed in six months to a year because Zyderm becomes part of the skin and will age as normal skin. After several months, it is impossible to tell the dif-ference between Zyderm and the natural tissue.

Zyderm II is a recently introduced im-provement that has more collagen and less saline in each injection; this is better than Zyderm I for very deep aging lines and some scars; Zyderm I is better for fine lines.

Zyplast is used to correct deeper defects than Zyderm I and II, and must be injected deeper into the skin for longer-lasting re-sults.

GLOSSARY

abdominoplasty A tummy tuck.

abrasion A slight loss of epithelium (usually caused by a scrape) that causes oozing and crusting.

abscess A clearly defined walled-off inflammatory area (usually caused by infection) that contains pus.

acantholysis Loss of cohesion between skin cells caused by dysfunction in the formation of intercellular bridges, loss of an intercellular binding substance, or an autoimmune reaction against the intercellular bridges.

actininc Relating to sunshine.

actinic keratosis Rough slightly raised, pink or red papules that appear singly or in groups on sun-damaged skin.

acute condition A condition that appears suddenly.

adnexa Term that refers to hair, nails, sweat and oil glands.

allergen Substance that causes allergic reactions.

alopecia Hair loss.

aluminum sulfate A common aluminum salt used in astringents (very similar to alum).

ammonium thioglycolate A chemical relaxer used in products designed for hair waving and straightening that break the chemical bonds of the proteins giving the hair its shape.

anagen Growth phase of hair.

anaphylactic shock A severe life-threatening hypersensitivity reaction that occurs in people with an extreme sensitivity to a particular substance that causes the release of massive amounts of histamines and other inflammatory chemicals that affect body tissues. The dilation of blood vessels cause a drop in blood pressure; other symptoms include hives, constriction of the airway, leading to breathing problems, abdominal pain, and swelling of the tongue.

androgen Male hormone.

angioedema A soft tissue swelling of skin caused by excess fluid.

angioma A tumor comprised of blood or lymph vessels.

anhidrosis Absence of the ability to sweat.

aniline dyes Chemicals derived from coal tars used primarily in hair dyes. These dyes are found in almost all permanent hair-coloring products.

annular Ring-shaped.

antifungal A substance that destroys or suppresses the growth/reproduction of fungi.

antigen Any substance foreign to the body's system that causes an immune response.

antihistamine A drug that counteracts the action of histamine.

aplasia Lack of development of a tissue or organ.

apocrine A gland that releases cellular material and fluid. It usually applies to the type of sweat gland found only in hairy areas of the body and that develop after puberty.

arcels Substances used as emulsifiers in creams, lotions and sunscreens that keep the product's oil and water molecules together in order to maintain a non-separating solution. Arcels do not affect the skin itself, but are designed to refine the skin care product.

atrophy Wasting away.

Auspitz's sign Pinpoint bleeding when the scale of a psoriatic lesion is removed.

axillary Referring to the armpit area of the body.

basal cells Germinative cells found along the basal layer of the epidermis (topmost layer of the skin).

benign   Not malignant.

blackhead   A darkened plug of sebum and keratin blocking the outlet of a sebaceous (oil-forming) gland in the skin. (Another name for open comedo.)

blue nevus   A group of nevus cells that produce a bluish or blue-black papule or nodule.

bromhidrosis   Foul-smelling sweat produced by the apocrine sweat glands, caused by bacterial decomposition.

bubo   Enlarged, inflamed lymph node (especially under the arm or in the groin) caused by infections (such as plague, tuberculosis or syphilis).

bulla   A fluid-filled blister.

cafe au lait macules   Medium brown-colored patches that may appear without an underlying disorder or in patients with neurofibromatosis.

calcinosis cutis   Abnormal deposits of calcium in the skin.

callus   Thickening of the stratum corneum in certain areas (especially on the hands and feet), often caused by friction.

Candida   A genus of fungi characterized by yeast cells, mycelia and blastospores.

canker sore   A small painful ulcer usually found in the mouth or on the lips.

capillary hemangioma   A benign tumor made up of a proliferation of small blood vessels.

carbuncle   A staphylococcal infection of skin and skin tissue made up of a cluster of furuncles.

carcinoma   A malignant growth of cells.

carcinoma in situ   Limitation of cancer to its place of origin.

carotenemia   Yellowed skin (similar to jaundice) caused by too much carotene in the skin. It is most often caused by eating too many carrots.

cavernous hemangioma   A vascular tumor of large blood vessels found in the deep dermis (middle layer of the skin), extending into the subcutaneous fat.

cayenne pepper spots   Tiny red spots seen in pigmented purpuric disorders.

cellulitis   Inflammation of tissues of the skin usually caused by bacterial infection.

chancre   A papule or ulcer at the site of infection in the skin caused by diseases such as syphilis or tuberculosis.

cold sore   The common term for a herpes simplex infection (usually on the lips).

collagen   The primary supportive protein of the skin.

comedo   Another name for blackhead or whitehead (also called "comedone").

compound nevus   A collection of benign nevus cells both at the dermal epidermal junction and in the dermis (melanin-producing cells).

corn   A tender, horny thickened growth produced by friction or pressure, resulting in a cone-shaped mass pointing into the dermis (middle layer of skin).

corticosteroid   A group of drugs based on the structure of cortisone (a hormone produced by the adrenal glands) with anti-inflammatory properties.

crust   Outer layer of solid material caused by drying of a secretion by the body.

curet   An instrument with a tip shaped like a spoon or loop used to remove abnormal tissue or growths.

curettage   The removal of skin tissue with a curet.

cutis   The skin.

cyst   A sac containing either a liquid or semisolid.

depigmentation   Loss of pigment (usually melanin).

dermabrasion   Surgical removal by mechanical methods of the epidermis (outermost layer of skin) and as much of the dermis (middle skin layer) as necessary.

dermatitis   Skin inflammation.

dermatofibroma   A benign skin nodule found most often on the extremities, composed of a proliferation of fibroblasts and collagen.

dermis Part of the skin lying directly under the epidermis, made up primarily of connective tissue.

diaphoretic A substance that produces or increases perspiration.

ecchymosis Bruise.

eccrine The name for the common sweat gland and its related structures.

ecthyima A shallow infection caused by bacteria that often causes scarring.

eczema Dermatitis.

edema Collection of excess fluid in the skin leading to swelling.

elastosis Degeneration of elastic tissue.

electrodesiccation Dehydration and destruction of skin tissue using a high-frequency electric current.

emollient A substance used to moisten, soften or smooth the skin.

emulsifier A substance that binds two dissimilar substances together (such as the mixture of an egg, oil and vinegar to make mayonnaise).

emulsion One liquid broken down into globules and distributed throughout a second liquid.

ephelis Freckle (plural: ephelides).

epidermis The very thin outer layer of the skin that covers the dermis; it contains the stratum basal, stratum spinosum, stratum granulosum, stratum lucidum and stratum corneum.

epidermolysis A condition of the epidermis (topmost skin layer) characterized by blisters forming either spontaneously or after trauma.

erosion A superficial ulcer, resulting in loss of epidermis (outer skin layer) that heals without scars.

eruption Visible rash or production of lesions.

erythema Blanchable red skin color.

erythroderma Generalized redness of the skin.

eschar Crusted dead skin produced by burns, corrosive agents or gangrene.

exfoliative Diffuse scaling.

factitial Produced artificially.

fibroma A tumor of fibrous or mature connective tissue.

fissure Crack or split in the skin.

flush Redness and warmth (usually of the face and neck).

follicle A sac, cavity or depression

fungus Simple parasitic life forms that make up a plant phylum (including yeasts, rusts, molds, smuts, mushrooms, mildews etc.).

furuncle Another name for a boil that usually involves a hair follicle.

genodermatosis A genetic skin disorder.

granular The presence of granules or grains.

granuloma A chronic, proliferative lesion of cells often associated with chronic inflammation anywhere in the body.

hemangioma A benign tumor composed of blood vessels.

hematoma A localized accumulation of blood (usually clotted) in skin caused by a rupture of a blood vessel wall.

hidradenitis Inflammation of a sweat gland (usually an apocrine gland).

histamine A chemical found in cells all over the body that is released during an allergic reaction; it is one of the substances responsible for inflammation.

hives An eruption of itchy wheals (raised white lumps surrounded by red areas) on the skin (also called urticaria).

hyperhidrosis Excessive sweating.

hyperpigmentation An abnormal excess of pigmentation (or darkening) of the skin.

hyperplasia An increase in the number of keratocytes that cause a thickened epidermis (topmost layer of the skin).

hypersensitivity A condition of heightened reactivity in that the body responds with an exaggerated reaction to a foreign substance.

hypertrichosis Excess hair growth.

hypertrophic scar Enlarged or thickened scar.

hypertrophy Thickened epidermis (topmost skin layer) caused by the increase in keratinocyte size.

hypopigmentation A reduction of pigment resulting in a lightening of skin.

ichthyosis Several generalized skin disorders characterized by rough, dry, scaling skin caused by excess production or retention of keratinocytes.

integument The skin.

intertrigo Inflammation found on opposite and touching sides of the skin, such as the creases of the neck, under the arms, in the folds of the groin, underneath the breasts.

keloid A sometimes-tender scar that is sharply elevated and larger than the original wound.

keratin The principal protein constituent of epidermis, hair and nails.

keratinization The process by which the epidermal cells (outer layer of the skin) turn into keratin.

kerion A deep fungal infection of hair-bearing skin that produces a nodular swelling covered with pustules.

laceration Torn, ragged skin wound.

lanugo The fine hair covering the fetus.

lentigo Pigmented macule on the skin (liver spot).

lichenification Thickened epidermis with exaggerated normal markings.

liniment Oily liquid preparation.

lipoma A benign tumor composed of mature fat cells.

lotion A liquid preparation in suspension or dispersion for external application to the body.

macerate Soften by wetting or soaking.

macule Nonpalpable area of skin that has a different color or texture from surrounding skin, less than 1–2 cm. in diameter.

malignant Cancerous.

melanocyte Melanin-producing cells found in the basal cell of the epidermis (topmost skin layer) and the hair matrix.

mesoderm The middle layer of the three primary germ layers of the embryo.

milia Small white cysts.

mole A nevocellular nevus.

morbilliform Eruption resembling measles.

mycosis Any disease caused by a fungus.

myxedema A condition of dry, waxy swellings with abnormal mucin deposits in the skin seen in conjunction with thyroid disease.

necrosis Death of cells.

neurodermatitis Skin irritation caused by scratching.

ointment A greasy semisolid preparation applied to the skin.

papule Raised pimple that is smaller than a pea.

petechia A tiny non-blanchable red spot caused by a capillary hemorrhage.

pilar Pertaining to the hair.

poikiloderma Dappled, mottled with areas of hypo- and hyperpigmentation and atrophy.

porphyria A group of diseases caused by dysfunction in porphyrin metabolism, characterized by increased production and excretion of porphyrins.

poultice A moist hot pack applied to the skin.

prickly heat The common term for milia rubra, an itchy rash caused by obstructed sweat glands.

prurigo An itchy area of skin.

pruritus Itching.

psychocutaneous The psychological aspects of skin function and disease.

purpura The generic term for hemorrhage into tissue. It may appear as pinpoint bleeding (petechiae) or larger areas (bruise).

pus A liquid caused by inflammation consisting of leukocytes, dead tissue and fluid.

pustule A raised skin lesion (papule), usually less than 1 cm, containing pus.

pyoderma A condition of the skin involving pus-filled lesions.

rash Skin eruption.

Raynaud's phenomenon Intermittent episodes of vasoconstriction of digital blood vessels leading to blanching of the fingers or toes caused by exposure to the cold, followed by blue and red discoloration.

scale The thin cells of the epidermis (outer layer of the skin) that is shed from the skin.

sclerosis Hardening.

seborrhea Excess secretion of sebum.

sebum The oily secretion produced by the oil (sebaceous) glands, consisting of fats and waxes designed to lubricate the skin and keep it supple.

shake lotion A suspension of a powder in a lotion.

squamous cell Flat cell between the basal and granular cell layers of the epidermis (topmost skin layer).

systemic Refers to the internal administration of medications and the combined organs of the body; the term may also refer to a disease that affects many or all of the organs or systems of the body.

telangiectasia Dilation of small group of blood vessels.

tinea Superficial fungal skin infection.

topical medication Drugs that are applied directly to the surface of the skin.

tumefaction Swelling.

ulcer An erosion or loss of skin layers from the surface of the skin downward.

urticaria The medical term for hives or wheals.

verruca A wart.

vesicle A small blister less than 1 cm. in diameter.

xerosis Skin dryness.

APPENDIX A: COSMETIC INGREDIENTS

For the latest information about dozens of topics concerning cosmetics ingredients and color additives call the FDA hotline at (800) 270-8869.

ABRASIVE AGENT
pumice

ACNE TREATMENT
benzoyl peroxide
biotin
birch
ergocalciferol

ANTI-BACTERIAL
methylbenzethonium chloride

ANTI-INFLAMMATORY AGENT
coltsfoot
elder
hypericum
juniper
restharrow

ANTIOXIDANT
ascorbyl palmitate
BHA
BHT
hydrogen peroxide
propyl gallate
salicyclic
sodium ascorbate
sodium bisulfate
tricosan

ANTIPERSPIRANT
aluminum chlorohydrate
sage

ANTISEPTIC
balsam
benzalkonium chloride
benzoin
boric acid
chamomile
colloidal sulfur

eucalyptus
geranium
horsetail
juniper
lemon
menthol
myrrh
phenol (carbolic acid)
pine needle
propylene glycol
resorcinol
thyme
zinc phenolsulfonate

ANTI-WRINKLE
orange
rose
royal jelly
tocopherol
turtle oil

ASTRINGENT
ammonium alum
apricot
bentonite
birch
boric acid
coltsfoot
hectorite
horse chestnut
kaolin
lemon
nettle
potassium alum
quercus
rose
sage
salicylic acid
thyme
zinc sulfate

362

BLEACHING AGENT
ascorbic acid
fennel
hayflower
hydrogen peroxide
hydroquinone
lemon
linden
orange
parsley
phosphoric acid
wild lettuce

CLEANSER
acetone
ether
isopropyl alcohol
mineral oil
petrolatum
SD alcohol
sodium laureth sulfate
yarrow

CONDITIONING AGENTS
alanine
amino acid
amniotic liquid
aspartic acid
benzoin
carrageenan
chondroitin sulfate
collagen
cysteine
cystine
elastine
glutamic acidglutathione
hydrolized animal proteins
lysine
menthionine
P.E.G. 2 stearyl quaternium 4
proteins
tyrosine

DEPILATORY
glyceryl thioglycolate

DETERGENT
benzalkonium chloride
sodium laureth sulfate

DISINFECTANT
benzoyl peroxide

DRAWS SKIN IMPURITIES TO THE SURFACE
almond bitter oil
bentonite
hectorite
kaolin
magnesium aluminum silicate
titanium dioxide
silica
zinc oxide

DRYING AGENT
benzoyl peroxide
kelp

EMOLLIENTS
acetamide
almond sweet oil
althea
apricot kernel oil
avocado oil
beeswax
benzoin
butyl stearate
caprylic/capric triglyceride
carnauba
carrot
castor oil
ceresin
cetearyl alcohol
cetearyl octanoate
cetyl alcohol
cocoa butter
cocoanut acid
cocoanut oil
coltsfoot
diisopropyl adipate
glycerin
glyceryl monostearate
hexyl alcohol
hexylene glycol

isocetyl stearate
isopropyl isostearate
isopropyl myristate
isopropyl palmitate
isostearic acid
laneth
lanolin
lanolin alcohol
lanolin hydrogenated
lard
lauryl alcohol
lauryl lactate
lecithin
magnesium lanolate
microcrystalline wax
mineral oil
mink oil
myristyl alcohol
myristyl lactate
oleic acid
oleyl alcohol
olive oil
palm oil
petrolatum
polyethylene
polyethylene glycols
polyoxethylene lauryl ether
poilyoxypropylene 15 stearyl ether
P.P.G. (followed by a number)
propylene glycol stearate
purceline
sesame oil
silicone
spermaceti
squalane
stearic acid
steryl alcohol
vegetable oils
wheat germ

EMULSIFIER
octoxynol
stearic acid
acetamide M.E.A.
ammonium laureth sulfate
ceteareth

ceteth
choleth
disodium monolauryl sulfosuccinate
disodium phosphate
glyceryl stearate
isopropyl (lanolate, linoleate, myristate, ole-
    ate, palmitate or stearate)
isosteareth 20
lanolinamide DEA
lauramide DEA
laureth
lauroyl sarcosine
linoleamide
magnesium lauryl sulfate
nonoxynol
octoxy glyceryl palmitate
oleamide DEA
oleth
pareth
poloxamer
polysorbate
quaternium
sodium borate
sodium cocoyl isethionate
sodium isostearoyl 2 lactylate
sorbeth (followed by a number)
sorbitan
steareth
stearoyl sarcosine
sucrose

HEALING, SOOTHING AGENT
allantoin
allantoin acetyl methionine
aloe
apricot
arnica
azulene
balm mint
biotin
birch
boric acid
calendula
coltsfoot
cucumber
elder

honey
hops
horsetail
hypericum
mallow
menthol
peach
peppermint
restharrow
riboflavin
spearmint
thyme
tocopherol
witch hazel

HUMECTANTS
amniotic liquid
butylene glycol
cholesterol
diethylene glycol
glycerin
glycol (usually followed by another name)
lactic acid
laneth
lavender
lecithin
lime
P.P.G. (followed by a number)
propylene glycol
royal jelly
sorbitol solution
stearic acid
urea

MISCELLANEOUS
chlorhexidine (skin activity booster)
dimethicone (silicone)
folic acid (essential for cell growth)
ginseng (promotes cell growth)
papaya (natural exfolient)
pyridine (helps synthesize vitamins)
pyridoxine (helps metabolize fat)
resorcinol (peels dead cells)
retinol (improves dry skin)
rosemary (tonic, antispasmodic)
salicylic acid (peels dead skin cells)

sodium bicarbonate (increases pH of a cosmetic)
sodium xexameta phosphate (water softener)
titanium dioxide (whitens powders)
tocopherol (slows formation of dark spots)

PIGMENTS
bismuth oxycholoride
chromium oxide green
D&C and FD&C
erric ammonium ferrocyanide
ferric ferrocyanide
iron oxides
manganese violet
mica
titanium dioxide (white pigment)
ultramarine blue

PRESERVATIVES, ANTIOXIDANTS AND CHEMICAL STABILIZERS
benzylparaben
benzoin
boric acid
butylparaben
disodium EDTA
ethylparaben
fructose
imidazolidinyl
lactic acid
methylparaben
parabens (ethyl-, methyl- and butyl-)
potassium sorbate
propylparaben
quaternium-15
sodium chloride
sodium dehydroacetate
sorbic acid

SEBACEOUS GLAND REGULATOR
camphor
eucalyptus
hops
lime
linoleic acid
menthol
methionine

myrrh
rosemary
royal jelly
thyme

SOLVENTS

acetone
ascetic acid
alcohol
ether
ethoxydiglycol
isopropyl alcohol
toluene

STABILIZERS/VISCOSITY BUILDERS

amphoteric
cholesterol
glycol
lecithin
phosphoric acid (stabilizer)
sodium laureth sulfate

STIMULANT

anise
apricot kernel oil
chamomile
dandelion
gentian
juniper
matricaria
myrrh
parsley
thyme

SUNSCREEN

cetyl dimethyl paba (escalol)
cucumber
dihydroxyacetone
homosalate
matricaria
myrrh
para-aminobenzoic acid (PABA)

THICKENING/STIFFENING/ SUSPENDING AGENTS

acacia
acrylate/acrylamide copolymer
agaraluminum stearate
carbomer
cellulose
dextrin
gelatin
glutam gum
hydrated silica
potassium alginate
potassium carrageenan
rosin
xanthan

TONER

althea
balsam
hops
horse chestnut
hydrolized animal proteins
lavender
matricaria
mint
pine needle
quercus
rose
spearmint
thiamine H.C.I.
turtle oil
witch hazel

VASO-CONSTRICTOR

camphor
elder
geranium
horsetail
lime
menthol
mint
pine needle
witch hazel

APPENDIX B: COSMETIC INGREDIENTS TO AVOID

CONDITIONERS
Irritants: Quaternium 15, Benzalkonium chloride, stearalkonium chloride
Carcinogens: DEA

DEODORANTS
Irritants: Fragrance, lanolin, parabens, propylene glycol, triclosan
Carcinogens: Cocamide DEA

LIPSTICKS
Allergens/irritants: Synthetic colors
Carcinogens: Some synthetic colors, octyl dimethyl PABA

LOTIONS
Irritants: Lanolin, beeswax, propylene glycol, parabens, some preservatives
Carcinogens: TEA

MOISTURIZERS
Irritants: Beeswax, cocao butter, PABA, propylene glycol, parabens, preservatives

Carcinogens: Polyethylene glycol, TEA, octyle dimethyl PABA

SHAMPOO
Allergens/irritants: Sodium lauryl sulfate, preservatives
Carcinogens: Cocamide DEA

SHAVING CREAMS
Allergens/irritants: Lanolin
Carcinogens: Cocamide DEA, TEA

SOAPS
Allergens/irritants: Almond, coconut, lavender, oak moss, potassium hydroxide
Carcinogens: DEA

SUNSCREENS
Irritants: PABA, octyl methoxycinnamate, lanolin, cocoa butter, cocoanut oil
Carcinogens: TEA; padimate-0 or octyl-dimethyl PABA *may* be carcinogenic

APPENDIX C: TYPES OF LESIONS

ABNORMAL KERATIN FORMATION
Acanthosis nigricans
Actinic keratosis
Ichthyosis
Keratosis of soles and palms
Keratosis follicularis
Warts

BLISTERS
Burns
Chemical warfare
Dermatitis herpetiformis
Drug eruption
Epidermolysis bullosa
Erythema multiforme
Frostbite
Herpes gestationis
Impetigo
Pemphigoid
Pemphigus
Phototoxicity
Plant allergies
Porphyria
Toxic epidermal necrolysis
Toxic dermatitis

DEPOSITS
Amyloid: systemic amyloidosis
Calcinosis: scleroderma, dermatomyositis
Cholesterol: xanthoma and xanthelasma
Mucus: mucinosis, diffuse myxedema, pretibial myxedema

ERYTHRODERMA
Allergic contact dermatitis
Atopic dermatitis
Congenital ichthyosiform erythroderma
Dermatoleukemia
Lymphoma
Psoriasis

MACULES
Drug eruptions
Infectious exanthemas

HIVES
Cold, warmth or irradiation
Food or drug allergies
Insect bites

PAPULES
Atopic dermatitis
Leishmaniasis
Leprosy
Lichen planus
Localized neurodermatitis
Lymphocytoma
Metabolic disorders
Molluscum contagiosum
Rosacea
Sarcoidosis
Secondary syphilis
Tuberculosis
Warts

NODULES
Erythema nodosum
Granuloma annulare
Leishmaniasis
Leprosy
Lymphomas
Nodular vasculitis
Sarcoidosis
Tumors

PUSTULES
Acne
Folliculitis barbae
Fungal infections
Mercury dermatitis
Pustular psoriasis
Pyodermas
Reiter's disease

VESICLES
Allergies
Contact dermatitis
Dermatitis herpetiformis
Duhring's disease
Fungal infections
Herpes simplex
Miliaria
Mycosis
Nummular eczema
Shingles

APPENDIX D: ORGANIZATIONS

ALBINISM

National Foundation for Vitiligo and Pigment
  Disorders
9032 South Normandy Drive
Centerville, OH 45459
(513) 885-5739

National Organization for Albinism and Hypopigmentation (NOAH)
1530 Locust Street
Box 29
Philadelphia, PA 19102
(215) 545-2322; (800) 473-2310
E-mail: noah@albinism.org

ALLERGIES

American Allergy Association
PO Box 7273
Menlo Park, CA 94026
(415) 322-1663

ALOPECIA AREATA

National Alopecia Areata Foundation
710 C Street, Suite 11
PO Box 150760
San Rafael, CA 94915
(415) 456-4644

BEHCET'S SYNDROME

American Behcet's Association
PO Box 54063
Minneapolis, MN 55454
(800) BEHCETS 723-4238

BIRTHMARKS

Klippel-Trenaunay Support Group
4610 Wooddale Avenue
Minneapolis, MN 55424
(612) 925-2596
E-mail: vesse001@maroon.tc.umn.edu

National Congenital Port Wine Stain Foundation
125 E. 63rd Street
New York, NY 10021
(516) 867-5137

BURNS

Burns United Support Groups
441 Colonial Court
Grosse Pointe Farms, MI 48236
(313) 881-5577

National Burn Victim Foundation
32-34 Scotland Road
Orange, NJ 07050
(201) 676-7700

Phoenix Society for Burn Survivors
11 Rust Hill Road
Levittown, PA 19056
(215) 946-BURN
(800) 888-BURN

CANCER

American Cancer Society
1599 Clifton Road, NE
Atlanta, GA 30329
(404) 320-3333; (800) 227-2345

National Cancer Care Foundation
1180 Avenue of the Americas
New York, NY 10036
(212) 221-3300

Nevoid Basal Cell Carcinoma Syndrome Support Network
162 Clover Hill Street
Marlboro, MA 01752
(508) 485-4873; (800) 815-4447
E-mail: Souldansur@aol.com

Skin Cancer Foundation
245 Fifth Avenue, Suite 2402
New York, NY 10156
(212) 725-5176

CHICKEN POX/SHINGLES

VZV Research Foundation
36 E. 72nd Street
New York, NY 10021
(212) 472-3181

COSMETOLOGY

American Electrology Association
106 Oak Ridge Road
Trumbull, CT 06611
(203) 374-6667; FAX (203) 372-7134

Council on Electrolysis Education
46 S. Holmes Street
Memphis, TN 38111
(901) 458-1431

International Guild of Professional Electrologists
202 Boulevard, Suite B
High Point, NC 27262
(919) 841-6631

DERMATITIS HERPETIFORMIS

American Celiac Society
58 Musano Court
West Orange, NJ 07052
(201) 325-8837

ECTODERMAL DYSPLASIA

National Foundation for Ectodermal Dysplasias
219 E. Main Street
PO Box 114
Mascoutah, IL 62258
(618) 566-2020
http://www.nfed.org

ECZEMA

Eczema Association for Science and Education
1221 S. W. Yamhill, Suite 303
Portland, OR 97205
(503) 228-4430

EHLERS-DANLOS SYNDROME

6399 Wilshire Boulevard, Suite 510
Los Angeles, CA 90048

(213) 651-3038
E-mail: LooseJoint@aol.com

EPIDERMOLYSIS BULLOSA

Dystrophic Epidermolysis Bullosa Research Association of America
40 Rector Street, 8th Floor
New York, NY 10006
(212) 995-2220

HAIR

American Hair Loss Council
100 Independence Place, Suite 207
Tyler, TX 75703
(903) 561-1107; (800) 274-8717; FAX: (903) 561-8603

National Alopecia Areata Foundation
710 "C" Street, Suite 11
PO Box 150760
San Rafael, CA 94915
(415) 456-4644

HERPES

Herpes Resource Center
American Social Health Association
PO Box 13827
Research Triangle Park, NC 27709
(919) 361-8488

ICHTHYOSIS

Foundation for Ichthyosis and Related Skin Types
PO Box 669
Ardmore, PA 19003
(610) 789-3995; (800) 545-3286
E-mail: ichthyosis@aol.com

INCONTINENTIA PIGMENTI

National Incontinentia Pigmenti Foundation
41 E. 57th Street, 5th Floor
New York, NY 10022
(212) 207-4636
E-mail: nipf@pipeline.com

KLIPPEL-TRENAUNAY SYNDROME

Klippel-Trenaunay Support Group
4610 Wooddale Avenue
Edina, MN 55424
(612) 925-2596
E-mail: vesseool@maroon.tc.umn.edu

LEPROSY

American Leprosy Missions
1 ALM Way
Greenville, SC 29601
(800) 543-3131; (803) 271-7040

Damien Dutton Society for Leprosy Aid
616 Bedford Avenue
Bellmore, NY 11710
(516) 221-5929

International Christian Leprosy Mission
PO Box 23353
Portland, OR 97281
(503) 244-5935

American Leprosy Foundation
11600 Nebel Street, Suite 210
Rockville, MD 20852
(301) 984-1336

LICE

National Pediculosis Association
PO Box 149
Newton, MA 02161
(800) 446-4NPA; (617) 449-6487

LUPUS ERYTHEMATOSUS

American Lupus Society
3914 Del Amo Boulevard, Suite 922
Torrance, CA 90503
(310) 542-8891; (800) 331-1802

Lupus Foundation of America
1300 Picard Drive, Suite 200
Rockville, MD 20850
(301) 670-9292; (800) 558-0121

Lupus Network
230 Ranch Drive
Bridgeport, CT 06606
(203) 372-5795

MELANOMA

American Melanoma Foundation
USC/Norris Cancer Center
2025 Zonal Avenue
GH-10-442
Los Angeles, CA 90033
(213) 226-6352

NATIONAL NEUROFIBROMATOSIS FOUNDATION

95 Pine Street, 16th Floor
New York, NY 10005
(212) 344-6633 or (800) 323-7938

NEVI

Nevus Network
Congenital Nevus Support Group
1400 South Joyce Street
Number C-1201
Arlington, VA 22202
(703) 920-3249; (405) 377-3403

OSLER-WEBER-RENDU SYNDROME

HHT Foundation International
PO Box 8087
New Haven, CT 06530
(313) 561-2537; (800) 448-6389

PLASTIC/RECONSTRUCTIVE SURGERY

National Foundation for Facial Reconstruction
317 E. 34th Street, Suite 901
New York, NY 10016
(800) 422-FACE; (212) 263-6656

Children's Craniofacial Association
10210 N. Central Expressway, Suite 230
Lockbox 37
Dallas, TX 75231
(214) 368-3590; (800) 535-3643

PORPHYRIA

American Porphyria Foundation
PO Box 22712
Houston, TX 77227
(713) 266-9617
http://www.enterprise.net/apf/

PORT WINE STAIN

National Congenital Port Wine Stain Foundation
123 E. 63rd Street
New York, NY 10021
(516) 867-5137

PSEUDOFOLLICULITIS BARBAE

PFB Project
1875 Connecticut Avenue
Suite 1140
Washington, DC 20009-5728
(202) 588-5300

PSEUDOXANTHOMA ELASTICUM

National Association for Pseudoxanthoma Elasticum, Inc. (NAPE)
1420 Ogden Street
Denver, CO 80218
(303) 832-5055
E-mail: derkhn@ttuhsc.edu

PXE International, Inc.
23 Mountain Street
Sharon, MA 02067
(617) 784-3817
E-mail: PXEInter@aol.com

PSORIASIS

Canadian Psoriasis Foundation
1565 Carling Avenue
1306 Wellington Street, Suite 500 F
Ottawa, ONT
CANADA K1Y-3B2
(613) 728-4000; in Canada, call (800) 265-0926

National Psoriasis Foundation
6600 S.W. 92nd Avenue, Suite 300
Portland, OR 97223
(503) 244-7404; Fax: 503/245-0626
Publications request line: (800) 723-9166
E-mail: 76135.2746@compuserve.com

Problem Psoriasis Clinic
909 Ridgeway Loop Road
Memphis, TN 38120
(901) 767-3612

Psoriasis Research Association
107 Vista del Grande
San Carlos, CA 94070
(415) 593-1392

Psoriasis Research Institute
600 Town and Country Village
Palo Alto, CA 94301
(415) 326-1848; FAX: (415) 326-1262

Psoriasis Society of Canada
PO Box 25015
Halifax, NS B3M 4H4
CANADA
(902) 443-8680

ROSACEA

National Rosacea Society
800 S. Northwest Highway, Suite 200
Barrington, IL 60010
(847) 382-8971
E-mail: rosacea@aol.com

SCLERODERMA

Scleroderma Federation, Inc.
Peabody Office Building
1 Newbury Street
Peabody, MA 01960
(508) 535-6600; (800) 422-1113

Scleroderma Info Exchange, Inc.
150 Hines Farm Road
Cranston, RI 02921
(401) 943-3909

Scleroderma International Foundation
704 Gardner Center Road
New Castle, PA 16101
(412) 652-3109

Scleroderma Research Foundation
2320 Bath Street, Suite 307
Santa Barbara, CA 93105
(805) 563-9133

Scleroderma Society
1725 York Avenue, Suite 29-F
New York, NY 10128
(212) 427-7040

Scleroderma Support Group
8852 Enloe Avenue
Garden Grove, CA 92644
(714) 892-5297

United Scleroderma Foundation
PO Box 399
Watsonville, CA 95077
(408) 728-2202; (800) 722-HOPE
E-mail: outreach@scleroderma.com

SJOGREN'S SYNDROME

National Sjogren's Syndrome Association
21630 N. 19th Avenue
Phoenix, AZ 85023
(800) 395-NSSA; (602) 516-0787

Sjogren's Syndrome Foundation
333 N. Broadway, Suite 2000
Jericho, NY 11753
(516) 933-6365; (800) 4-sjogren

SKIN DISEASE RESEARCH

American Skin Association
150 E. 58th Street, 32nd Floor
New York, NY 10155
(212) 753-8260

Dermatology Foundation
1560 Sherman Avenue
Evanston, IL 60201
(708) 328-2256

SKIN DISORDERS

National Institute of Arthritis and Musculoskeletal and Skin Diseases
9000 Rockville Pike
Building 31, Rm 9A04
Bethesda, MD 20892
(301) 496-8188

STEVENS-JOHNSON SYNDROME

The Stevens-Johnson Syndrome Foundation
9285 N. Utica Street
Westminster, CO 80030
(303) 430-9559

STURGE-WEBER SYNDROME

Sturge-Weber Foundation
PO Box 418
Mt. Freedom, NJ 07970
(201) 895-4445

TUBEROUS SCLEROSIS

National Tuberous Sclerosis Association
8181 Professional Place, Suite 110
Landover, MD 20785
(301) 459-9888; (800) 225-6872
http://www.ntsa.org/

VITILIGO

Frontier's International Vitiligo Foundation
4 Rozina Court
Owings Mills, MD 21117

National Vitiligo Foundation, Inc.
PO Box 6337
Tyler, TX 75711
(903) 534-2925; FAX: (903) 534-8075
E-mail: 73071.33@compuserve.com

XERODERMA PIGMENTOSUM

Xeroderma Pigmentosum Society
57 Sleight Plass Road
Poughkeepsie, NY 12603
(914) 473-4735
E-mail: xps@mhv.net

APPENDIX E: WEB SITES

ALBINISM

The National Organization for Albinism and
Hypopigmentation
http://www.albinism.org/

ALOPECIA AREATA

National Alopecia Areata Foundation
http://weber.u.washington.edu/~dvictor/
natl.html

ATAXIA

The A-T Children's Project
http://www.med.jhu.edu/ataxia/

BEHCET'S SYNDROME

American Behcet's Association
http://www.w2.com/behcets.html

CANCER (SKIN)

Nevoid Basal Cell Carcinoma Syndrome
http://www.kumc.edu/GEC/support/
nevbasal.html

ECTODERMAL DYSPLASIA

National Foundation for Ectodermal Dysplasia
http://www.nfed.org

EHLERS-DANLOS SYNDROME

http://www.edf.org/

HERPES

American Social Health Association
http://sunsite.unc.edu/ASHA/

INCONTINENTIA PIGMENTI

National Incontinentia Pigmenti Association
http://www.medhlp.netusa.net/www/
nipf.htm

KLIPPEL-TRENAUNAY

Klippel-Trenaunay Support Group
http://www.tc.umn.edu/nlhome/m474/
vesse001/k-t.html

LEPROSY

World Health Organization Action Pro-
gramme for the Elimination of Leprosy
http://www.WHO.CH/programmes/lep/
lep__home.htm

LUPUS

Lupus Foundation of America, Inc.
http://www.lupus.org/lupus/

MASTOCYTOSIS

The Mastocytosis Society
http://www.gil.com.au/comm/mast/

PORPHYRIA

American Porphyria Foundation
http://www.enterprise.net/apf/

PSEUDOXANTHOMA ELASTICUM

PXE International, Inc.
http://www.med.Harvard.edu/programs/
PXE

PSORIASIS

National Psoriasis Foundation
http://www.psoriasis.org/npf.shtml

ROSACEA

National Rosacea Society
http://www.rosacea.org/

SCLERODERMA

United Scleroderma Foundation
http://www.scleroderma.com/

SJOGREN'S SYNDROME

Sjogren's Syndrome Foundation, Inc.
http://www.sjogrens.com/

SKIN CANCER

Oncolink–University of Pennsylvania Cancer
   Center
http://www.cancer.med.upenn.edu/disease/
   skin1

STEVENS-JOHNSON SYNDROME

The Stevens-Johnson Syndrome Foundation
http://members.aol.com/sjsupport/

TUBEROUS SCLEROSIS

National Tuberous Sclerosis Association
http://www.ntsa.org/

VITILIGO

National Vitiligo Foundation, Inc.
http://www.nvfi.org

XERODERMA PIGMENTOSUM

Xeroderma Pigmentosum Society, Inc.
http://www.xps.org/

APPENDIX F: PUBLICATIONS

American Osteopathic College of Dermatology Newsletter
American Osteopathic College of Dermatology
800 W. Jefferson Street
PO Box 7525
Kirksville, MO 63501
(800) 449-2623

Cutis
North American Clinical Dermatologic Society
Mayo Clinic
4500 San Pablo Road
Jacksonville, FL 32082
(908) 223-2000

Dermatoloqy Focus
Progress in Dermatology
Stewardship Report
Dermatology Foundation
1560 Sherman Avenue, Suite 302
Evanston, IL 60201
(708) 328-2250

Epidermolysis Bullosa Currents
EB Reporter
Dystrophic Epidermolysis Bullosa Research Association of America
40 Rector Street, 8th Floor
New York, NY 10006
(212) 995-2220

Ichthyosis Focus
Foundation for Ichthyosis and Related Skin Types
PO Box 669
Ardmore, PA 19003
(610) 789-3995
(800) 545-3286

International Journal of Dermatology
International Society of Dermatology: Tropical, Geographic and Ecologic
200 1st Street SW
Rochester, MN 55905
(507) 284-3736

Journal of the American Academy of Dermatology
American Academy of Dermatology Bulletin
American Academy of Dermatology
930 N. Meacham Road
Schaumburg, IL 60173
(847) 330-0230

Journal of Cutaneous Pathology
American Society of Dermatopathology
550 Building
550 N. Broadway, Suite 408
Baltimore, MD 21205
(410) 955-2332
FAX: (410) 955-2445

Journal of Dermatologic Surgery and Oncology
International Society for Dermatologic Surgery
930 N. Meacham Road
Schaumburg, IL 60173
(847) 330-0230
FAX: (708) 689-4382

Journal of Investigative Dermatology
Society for Investigative Dermatology
Department of Dermatology
2074 Abington Road
University Hospitals of Cleveland
Cleveland, OH 44106
(216) 844-3682
FAX: (216) 844-8993

Hair Loss Journal
American Hair Loss Council
100 Independence Place, Suite 207

Tyler, TX 75703
(903) 561-1107
(800) 274-8717
FAX: (903) 561-8603

National Neurofibromatosis Foundation Newsletter
National Neurofibromatosis Foundation
95 Pine Street, 16th Floor
New York, NY 10005
(212) 344-6633; 800-323-7938

National Psoriasis Foundation Bulletin
National Psoriasis Foundation—Pharmacy News
National Psoriasis Foundation
6600 S.W. 92nd Avenue, Suite 300
Portland, OR 97223
(503) 244-7404
FAX: 503/245-0626
Publications request line: (800) 723-9166 (Brochures: *A Guide to Understanding Psoriasis; Psoriasis: How It Makes You Feel; Things to Consider: In Talking with Your Physician; Making Treatment Decisions; Knowing your Rights as a Patient*

National Vitiligo Foundation Newsletter
National Vitiligo Foundation, Inc.
PO Box 6337
Tyler, TX 75711
(903) 534-2925
FAX: (903) 534-8075

Perspective Newsletter
National Tuberous Sclerosis Association
8000 Corporate Drive, Suite 120
Landover, MD 20785
(301) 459-9888
(800) 225-6872

Psoriasis Newsletter
Psoriasis Research Institute
600 Town and Country Village
Palo Alto, CA 94301
(415) 326-1848
FAX: (415) 326-1262

Rosacea Review
National Rosacea Society
800 S. Northwest Highway, Suite 200
Barrington, IL 60010
(847) 382-8971

Sjogren's Digest
Patients' Education Series
National Sjogren's Syndrome Association
21630 N. 19th Avenue
Phoenix, AZ 85023
(800) 395-NSSA; (602) 516-0787

Society for Pediatric Dermatology—Newsletter
Society for Pediatric Dermatology
University of Michigan Hospitals
1910 Taubman Health Care Center
Ann Arbor, MI 48109
(313) 936-4086
FAX: (313) 936-6395

APPENDIX G: HOTLINES

Rosacea Hotline
708-382-8971
(general information about rosacea)

Look Good, Feel Better Hotline
800-395-LOOK
(for name of local programs that offer free classes in makeup, hair and nails for cancer patients)

National Psoriasis Foundation
800-248-0886
(publication request line)

National Pediculosis Association
(800) 446-4NPA
(brochures, publicity materials)

BIBLIOGRAPHY

Abel, Elizabeth, Rigel, Darrell and Seigler, Hilliard. "Reversing the melanoma surge," *Patient Care,* 25 (June 15, 1991):122–134.

Abel, Elizabeth, Bercovitch, Lionel and Stoll, Howard L., Jr. "When actinic keratoses are a problem," *Patient Care* 26 (July 15, 1992):115–128.

Adler, Tina. "Sunscreen can't give blanket protection," *Science News* 145 (1/22/94):54–55.

Alexander, Paul. "Is it a mole or a melanoma?" *Cosmopolitan* 213 (September 1992):152–53.

Anastasi, Joyce and Rivera, Julie. "Identifying the skin manifestations of HIV," *Nursing* 22 (Nov. 1992):58–61.

Armstrong, B. "Epidemiology of a malignant melanoma: Intermittent or total accumulated exposure to the sun?" *Journal Dermatology Surgical Oncology* 14 (1988):835–849.

Armstrong, B. K. and Kricker, A. "How much melanoma is caused by sun exposure?" *Melanoma Research* 3(6)(December 1993):395–401.

Armstrong, Robert. "Clinical panel assessment of photodamaged skin treated with isotretinoin using photographs," *JAMA, The Journal of the American Medical Association* 268 (Aug. 12, 1992):720.

Arnott, Nancy. "Your baby head to toe," *American Baby,* 54 (June 1992):48–51.

"Artificial fat aids skin replacement," *USA Today* 121 (June 1993):3.

Associated Press. "Retin-A May Prevent Skin, Cervix Cancer," *New York Newsday,* May 25, 1993.

Atkins, Andrea. "Skin care: news to help you look and feel better," *Better Homes and Gardens* 68 (March 1990):26.

Beardsley, Tim. "A gentler therapy? Retinoic acid turns off a form of leukemia," *Scientific American* 264 (April 1991):20.

———, "Shear bliss: a bioreactor grows cells that resemble real tissue," *Scientific American* 266 (Feb. 1992):27.

Belcove, Julie, Cara Kagan and Soren Larson. "Beauty companies ride acid wave," *Women's Wear Daily* 167 (March 18, 1994):S4–5.

Berkley Wellness Letter. "Cosmeceuticals: the latest wrinkles," *University of California, Berkeley Wellness Letter* (March 1994):3.

Bikowski, Joseph. "Effectively treating acne vulgaris," *The Physician and Sportsmedicine* 20 (August 1992):100–106.

Bleicher, P. A., Dover, J. S. and Arndt K. A. "Lichenoid dermatoses and related diseases, Part I" *Journal of American Academy of Dermatology* 22 (Feb. 1990):288–92.

———. "Lichenoid dermatoses and related diseases, Part II" *Journal of American Academy of Dermatology* 22 (April 1990):671–5.

Bondeson, J. and Rausing, A. "Reversible scleroderma, fasciitis and perimyositis," *Clinical and Experimental Rheumatology* 12(1)(Jan./Feb. 1994):71–73.

Bonifas, J. M., Rothman, A. L. and Epstein, E. H., Jr. "Epidermolysis bullosa simplex: evidence in two families for keratin gene abnormalities," *Science* 254 (Nov. 22, 1991):1202–1206.

Bourguignon, Jean-Pierre, Pierard, Gerald, Ernould, Christian, Heinrichs, Claudine, Graen, Margarita, Rochiccioli, Pierre, Arrese, Jorge, and Franchimont, Claudine. "Effects of human growth hormone therapy on melanocytic naevi," *The Lancet* 341 (June 12, 1993):1505–1507.

Boyer, Pamela. "The perfect tan: Save-your-skin tans without the dangers of sun exposure," *Prevention* (May 1993):116–121.

———. "Moisturizers for the 21st century," *Prevention* 44 (Dec. 1992):81–85.

Brazzelli, V. *et al.* "Effects of fluid volume changes during hemodialysis on the biophysical parameters of skin," *Dermatology* 188 (2) 1994:113–116.

Bronaugh, R.L. "Dose response relationship in skin sensitization," *Food and Chemical Toxics* 32 (February 1994) 113–117.

Brumberg, Elaine. "What Price Beauty?" *Modern Maturity* (Aug./Sept. 1993):74.

Bulengo-Ransby, Stella, Griffiths, Christopher, Kimbrough-Green, Candace, Finkel, Lawrence, Hamilton, Ted, Ellis, Charles and Voorhees, John. "Topical tretinoin therapy for hyperpigmented lesions caused by inflammation of the skin in black patients," *The New England Journal of Medicine* 328 (May 20, 1993):1438–1443.

Caldwell-Brown, Dorothea, Stern, Robert S., *et al.* "Lack of efficacy of phenytoin in recessive dystrophic epidermolysis bullosa," *JAMA* 327 (July 16, 1992):163–168.

Campbell, Laurel. "Assessing pediatric rashes," *RN* 56 (April 1993):58–65.

Cardinal, David. "20 ways to wipe away 10 years; age erasers," *Men's Health* 5 (June 1990):62–66.

Champsi, Jamila and Deresinski, Stanley. "Cutaneous tuberculosis," *JAMA* 268 (Sept. 9, 1992):1339.

Chase, Deborah. *The New Medically Based No-Nonsense Beauty Book.* New York: Henry Holt and Co., 1989.

Collier, Elizabeth. "When it comes to skincare products and makeup with sunscreen, can there be too much of a good thing?" *Vogue* 180 (May 1990):152.

Colwell, Shelley. "Treatment cosmetics: more than just a pretty face," *Soap-Cosmetics-Chemical Specialties* 70 (March 1994):22–26.

Consumer Reports. "It won't kill you to dye," *Consumer Reports On Health* (June 1994):69.

Coopman, Serge, Johnson, Richard, *et al.* "Cutaneous disease and drug reactions in HIV infection," *The New England Journal of Medicine* 328 (June 10, 1993):1670–1675.

Costikyan, Barbara. "Cosmo talks to Norman Orentreich, M.D., dermatologist," *Cosmopolitan* 208 (Feb. 1990):122–123.

Cowen, Ron. "Dermatophagy: Waste Not, Want Not?" *Science News* (June 19, 1993):397.

Current Health editors. "Birthmarks: lifelong companions," *Current Health* 18 (April 1992):30–32.

Darmstadt, G. I. and Karizler, M. H. "Subcutaneous fat necrosis of newborn," *Archives of Pediatrics and Adolescent Medicine* 148 (Jan. 1994):61–62.

Davis, Donald. "Boggy ground," *Drug & Cosmetic Industry* 154 (March 1994):22.

DeCoste, Susan and Stern, Robert. "Diagnosis and treatment of nevomelanocytic lesions of the skin: a community-based study," *JAMA* 269 (March 24, 1993):1554.

van Deuren, Marcel. "Rapid diagnosis of acute meningococcal infections by needle aspiration or biopsy of skin lesions," *JAMA* 270 (July 21, 1993):326.

Discover. "Skin deep," *Discover* 12 (August 1991):16.

Dover, Jeffrey S. and Arndt, Kenneth. "Dermatology," *JAMA* 265 (June 19, 1991):3111–3114.

Dover, Jeffrey S. and Johnson, R. A. "Basal cell carcinoma," *New England Journal of Medicine* 329 (Aug. 1993):545.

———. "Cutaneous manifestation of HIV-infected patients, Part II" *Archives of Dermatology* 127 (Oct. 1991):1549–1558.

———. "Cutaneous manifestation of HIV-infected patients, Part I" *Archives of Dermatology* 127 (Sept. 1991):1383–1391.

Dover, Jeffrey S., Kilmer, S. I. and Anderson, R. R. "What's new in cutaneous laser surgery," *Journal of Dermatologic Surgery and Oncology* 19 (April 1993):295–298.

Edelson, Sharon. "Color treats skin right," *Women's Wear Daily* 162 (Aug. 9, 1991):C8.

Eden, Alvin. "A sensitive subject—diaper rash," *American Baby* 54 (Dec. 1992):10–11.

———. "Getting to the bottom of diaper rash," *American Baby* 54 (Nov. 1991):16–17.

Edwards, Libby. "Treatment of cutaneous squamous cell carcinomas by intralesional interferon alfa-2b therapy," *JAMA* 269 (Feb. 3, 1993):578.

Elias, S., Emerson, D. S., et al. "Ultrasound-guided fetal skin sampling for prenatal diagnosis of genodermatoses," *Obstetrics and Gynecology* 83 (March 1994):337–341.

Eller, Daryn. "Danger: Rays. How safe are we from UVAs?" *Health* 23 (May 1991): 74–80.

Elston, Dirk and Bergfeld, Wilma. "Skin diseases of the hands and feet," *The Physician and Sportsmedicine* 22 (March 1994): 40–48.

Epstein, Ervin. "Molecular genetics of epidermolysis bullosa," *Science* 256 (May 8, 1992):799–805.

Esgleyes-Ribot, T., Chandraratna, R. A. et al. "Response of psoriasis to a new topical retinoid," *Journal of the American Academy of Dermatology* 30 (April 1994):58l–590.

Evans, R. D., Kopf, A. W., Lew , R. A., et al. "Risk factors for the development of malignant melanoma I: Review of case-control studies," *Journal of Dermatology Surgical Oncology* 14 (1988):393–408.

Ezzell, Carol. "Skin genes underlie blistering disorder," *Science News* 140 (Sept. 28, 1991):197.

Fackelmann, Kathy A. "Vitamin A-like drug may ward off cancers," *Science News* 141 (May 30, 1992)):358.

Fairley, Janet. "Tretinoin revisited," *The New England Journal of Medicine* 328 (May 20, 1993):1436–1437.

Farndon, P. A., Del Mastro, R. G., Evans, D. and Kilpatrick, M. "Location of gene for Gorlin syndrome," *The Lancet* 339 (March 7, 1992):581–582.

Fears, Linda. "How to look younger; some of the new nonsurgical techniques offer truly amazing results," *Ladies Home Journal* (April 1994):80–84.

Fernandez, D. F., Wolff, A. H., and Bagley, M. P. "Acute cutaneous toxoplasmosis presenting as erythroderma," *International Journal of Dermatology* 33 (February 1994):129–130.

Flory, Christy. "Skin assessment," *RN* 55 (June 1992):22–27.

Freundlich, Naomi. "Homing in on the genetic flaw that causes skin cancer," *Business Week* (November 23, 1992):87.

Frey, Nadine. "Skin outlook," *Harper's Bazaar* 124 (Jan. 1991):15–16.

Gage, Diane. "Fighting back: the side effects of Retin-A," *American Health* 9 (June 1990):18–19.

Gannon, Kathi. "Glycolic acid found helpful in treating problems of the skin," *Drug Topics* 135 (May 6, 1991):43–44.

Ganske, Mary Garner. "Nine skin signals that can save your life," *Family Circle* 105 (Nov. 3, 1992):52–54.

Garrett, Anne Wolven. "Dermal irritation continued," *Drug & Cosmetic Industry* 152 (June 1993):16–17.

———. "IPD—immediate pigment darkening," *Drug & Cosmetic Industry* 149 (August 1991):12.

Gavenas, Mary Lisa. "New cure for wrinkles?" *Glamour* 91 (February 1993):54.

Geronemus, Roy, Grimes, Pearl, Nordlund, James and Wiley, M. Denise. "What to look for in hyperpigmentation," *Patient Care* 25 (October 30, 1991):47–64.

Gibran, N. S., Isik, F. F. et al. "Basic fibroblast growth factor in the early human burn wound," *Journal of Surgical Research* 56 (March 1994):226–234.

Gillespie, Sheila, Carter, Matthew, Asch, Steven, Rokos, James, Gary, William, Tsou, Cecelia, Hall, David, Anderson, Larry and Hurwitz, Eugene. "Occupational risk of human parvovirus B19 infection for school and daycare personnel during an outbreak of erythema infectiosum," *JAMA* 263 (April 18, 1990):2061–2064.

Glaser-Sommer, Marjorie. "Taking a shot at wrinkles," *American Health* 11 (May 1992):28.

Gleason, Suzanne Gleckman. "Facing the bar," *Vogue* 184 (January 1994):80.

Godfrey, Jean. "Can you really get beautiful skin in eight weeks?" *Glamour* 92 (March 1994):222–225.

Goldstein, Randi. "Making things right for Morgan," *Good Housekeeping* 21 (June 1993):54–57.

Gorman, Christine. "Does sunscreen save your skin?" *Time* 141 (May 24, 1993):69.

Green, Howard. "Cultured cells for the treatment of disease," *Scientific American* 265 (Nov. 1991) 96–102.

Greene, Eva-Lynne. "Old wine in new bottles," *American Health* 11 (Sept. 1992):45.

Gregory, Richard, Roenig, Randall, and Wheeland, Ronald. "When and when not to use cutaneous laser therapy," *Patient Care* 25 (Nov. 30, 1991):67–84.

Griffiths, Christopher, Russman, Andrew, *et al.* "Restoration of collagen formation in photodamaged human skin by tretinoin," *The New England Journal of Medicine* 329 (Aug. 19, 1993):530–536.

Grossbart, Ted and Sherman, Carl. *Skin Deep: A Mind/Body Program for Healthy Skin.* New York: William Morrow Co., 1986.

Grosse, G. "Cutaneous histoplasmosis as opportunistic initial infection in AIDS," *JAMA* 271 (Jan. 19, 1994):186H.

Gutfield, Greg. "Sun downer: tretinoin smooths damaged skin," *Prevention* 43 (December 1991):18.

Gutfield, Greg, Meyers, Melissa and Sangiorgio, Maureen. "Tumor doomer: vitamin A drug may help shrug off head and neck cancer," *Prevention* 43 (Feb. 1991):18.

Hall, E. G. *et al.* "Acyclovir-resistant varicella-zoster and HIV infection," *Archives of Diseases in Childhood* 70 (February 1994):133–135.

Hamilton, Joan. "Sun Protection? There's a rub." *Business Week* 11 (June 1991):12–13.

Henriksen, Ole. *Seven-Day Skin-Care Program: The Scandinavian Method for a Radiant Complexion.* New York: Macmillan Publishing Co., 1984.

Henry, Linda. "Marked for death," *Muscle & Fitness* 53 (April 1992):140–144.

Hittner, Patricia. "Wintertime skin care," *Better Homes and Gardens* (February 1994):62–64.

Hoffman, Michelle. "A layer by layer look at the skin blister diseases," *Science* 254 (Nov. 22, 1991):1111–1112.

Hom, D.B. "The wound healing response to grafted tissue," *Otolaryngologic Clinics of North America* 27 (February 1994):13–24.

Hong, Waun Ki, Lippman, Scott M., Itri, Loretta, Karp, Daniel, Lee, Jin, Byers, Robert, Schantz, Stimson, Kramer, Alan, Lotan, Reuben, Peters, Lester, Dimery, Isaiah, Brown, Barry and Goepfert, Helmuth. "Prevention of second primary tumors with isotretinoin in squamous-cell carcinoma of the head and neck," *The New England Journal of Medicine* 323 (Sept. 20, 1990):795–802.

Horowitz, H. W., Sanghera, K., *et al.* "Dermatomyositis associated with Lyme disease:case report and review of Lyme myositis," *Clinical Infectious Diseases* 18 (February 1994):166–171.

Hruza, G. J., Geronemus, R. G. and Dover, J. S. "Lasers in dermatology," *Archives of Dermatology* 129 (Aug. 1993):1026–1035.

Hruza, G. J., Dover, J. S., *et al.* "Q-switched ruby laser irradiation of normal human skin," *Archives of Dermatology* 127 (December 1991):1799–1805

Hughes, B. R. and Cunliffe, W. J. "A prospective study of the effects of isotretinoin on the follicular reservoir and sustainable sebum excretion in patients with acne," *Archives of Dermatology* 130 (March 1994):31–38.

Hutter, Sarah. "Changing baby: here's the bottom line on diapering," *Working Mother* 16 (Feb. 1993):60–62.

Iglesias, M. E., Espana, A. *et al.* "Generalized skin reaction following tinea pedis," *Jour-*

nal of Dermatology 211 (January 1994):31–34.

Imai, S. "Reactions of uninvolved psoriatic skin and normal skin to ultraviolet radiation," Journal of the American Academy of Dermatology 30 (April 1994):657–660.

Jaroff, Leon. "Giant step for gene therapy: an experiment on a young girl opens a new era in the fight against hereditary diseases," Time 136 (Sept. 24, 1990):74–77.

Jick, Susan, Terris, Barbara and Jick, Hershel. " First trimester topical tretinoin and congenital disorders," The Lancet 341 (May 8, 1993):1181–1182.

Jimenez, Sherry. "Measles, mumps and pregnancy: here's how to protect yourself and your unborn baby from the effects of these childhood illnesses," American Baby 52 (November 1990):64–66.

Journal of the American Medical Association, the, "Anogenital warts in children: clinical and virologic evaluation for sexual abuse," JAMA 265 (April 17, 1991):1934.

Kahn, Henry, Nelson, Dorothy, Klag, Michael, Whelton, Paul, Coresh, Josef, Grim, Clarence and Kuller, Lewis. "Blood pressure and skin color," JAMA 265 (June 12, 1991):2957–2958.

Kalter, D.C. "Laboratory tests for diagnosing and evaluating of leishmaniasis," Dermatologic Clinics 12 (January 1994):37–50.

Kang, S. and Dover, J. S. "Successful treatment of eruptive pyoderma gangrenosum with IV vancomycin and mezlocillin," British Journal of Dermatology 121 (3)(September 1990):389–393.

Karagas, Margaret, Stukel, Therese, Greenberg, E. Robert, Baron, John, Mott, Leila, and Stern, Robert. "Risk of subsequent basal cell carcinoma and squamous cell carcinoma of the skin among patients with prior skin cancer," JAMA 267 (June 24, 1992):3305–3310.

Karlsrud, Katherine and Dodi Schultz. "What to do about birthmarks," Parents 68 (Septpmber 1993):70–72.

Klein, Nancy. "Face off against wrinkles," Muscle & Fitness 53 (May 1992):36–37.

Klinger, Georgette and Rowes, Barbara. Skincare. New York: William Morrow and Co., Inc. 1979.

Koh, Howard. "Cutaneous melanoma," The New England Journal of Medicine 325 (July 18, 1991):171–183.

Koike, Tadashi, et al. "Severe symptoms of hyperhistaminemia after treatment of acute promyelocytic leukemia with tretinoin," The New England Journal of Medicine 327 (Aug. 6, 1992):385–387.

Kraemer, K. H., et al. "Risk of cutaneous melanoma in dysplastic nevus syndrome types A and B," New England Journal of Medicine 315 (1986):1615–1616.

Kurimoto, Il, Arana, M. and Streilein, J. W. "Role of dermal cells from normal and ultraviolet B-damaged skin in induction of contact hypersensitivity and tolerance," Journal of Immunology 152 (7)(April 1, 1994):3317–3323.

Laman, S. D. and Provost, T. T. "Cutaneous manifestations of lupus erythematosus," Rheumatic Disease Clinics of North America 20 (February 1994):195–212.

Larson, Connie and Dennis West. "Photoreactions and photoprotection," Drug Topics 135 (April 8, 1991):77–83.

Laskin, J. D. "Cellular and molecular mechanisms in photochemical sensitization studies on the mechanism of action of psoralens," Food and Chemicals Toxics 32 (February 1994):119–127.

Lazarus, G. S., Cooper, D. M. et al. "Definitions and guidelines for assessment of wounds and evaluation of healing," Archives of Dermatology 130 (April 1994):489–493.

Lebowitz, Lisa. "Pollution solutions," Harper's Bazaar 124 (October 1991):147–148.

Lebowitz, Lisa and Cardozo, Constance. "Beauty blooms," Harper's Bazaar 124 (Jan. 1992):84–89.

Lee, M. N., Gellis, S., and Dover, J. S. "Eczematous plaques in a patient with liver failure," *Archives of Dermatology* 128 (February 1992):257, 260.

Leffell, David. "Aggressive-growth basal cell carcinoma in young adults," *JAMA* 267 (March 18, 1992):1456.

Lesher, Jack; Levine, Norman and Treadwell, Patricia. "Fungal skin infections: common but stubborn," *Patient Care* 28 (Jan. 30, 1994):16–31.

———. "Antifungals in office dermatology," *Patient Care* 28 (March 15, 1994):59–69.

Levine, Norman, Sheftel, Scott, Eytan, Ted, Dorr, Robert, Hadley, Mac, Weinrach, Jonathan, Ertl, Gregory, Toth, Katalin, McGee, Daniel and Hruby, Victor. "Induction of skin tanning by subcutaneous administration of a potent synthetic melanotropin," *JAMA* 266 (Nov. 28, 1991):2730–2737.

Lewin, A. H., *et al.* "Evaluation of retinoids as therapeutic agents in disease," *Pharmacology Research* 11 (February 1994):192–200.

Lister, Pamela. "Skin spots: not every blemish is cause for concern," *New Choices for the Best Years* 30 (August 1990):34–36.

Littlefield, Robin Wiest. "Are they safe? (sunscreens)," *American Health* 9 (May 1990):20.

———. "Long-distance dermatology; computer technology expert diagnosis," *American Health* 10 (Jan.–Feb. 1991):20.

Longley, B., Jack Morganroth, Greg, *et al.* "Altered metabolism of mast-cell growth factor in cutaneous mastocytosis," *The New England Journal of Medicine* 328 (May 6, 1993):1302–1305.

Lord, Shirley. "Green beauty: more and more companies are relying on plants for skin care," *Vogue* 180 (May 1990):129–130.

———. "The seven ages of skin," *Vogue.* 180 (Jan. 1990):208–213.

———. "Skin solutions: the New Year brings hope for ageless-looking skin, as a race for youth cream picks up speed," *Vogue* 184 (January 1994):78–79.

Mademoiselle editors. "A little hair science," *Mademoiselle* 96 (April 1990):230–233.

Maheux, R. "A randomized, double-blind, placebo-controlled study of the effects of conjugated estrogens on skin thickness," *American Journal of Obstetrics and Gynecology* 170 (February 1994):642–649.

Martin, Paul. "Skin cancer: scourge of the sun," *Safety & Health* 143 (May 1991):82–85.

Marwick, Charles. "Additional steps proposed to ensure antiacne drug used only in appropriate patient population," *JAMA* 263 (June 20, 1990):3125–3126.

Mayo Clinic editors. "Melanoma: what's your risk of developing this type of skin cancer?" *Mayo Clinic Health Letter* 9 (August 1991):1–3.

———. "Skin cancer: tried-and-true ways for dealing with the diagnosis," *Mayo Clinic Health Letter* 12 (March 1994):1–3.

Maytin, E. V. Horan, R. F. and Dover, J. S. "Tumorous nodules on the lower extremitiy in systemic mastocytosis," *Archives of Dermatology* 127 (March 1991):406–410.

McCann, Jean. "FDA set to classify all sunscreen products as drugs," *Drug Topics* 137 (Jan. 25, 1993):67–68.

McCarthy, Laura Flynn. "Research shows hair loss occurs among women for many reasons," *Vogue* 181 (Jan. 1991):88.

———. "Today's skin-care products give increasingly scientific explanations of their various benefits," *Vogue* 180 (July 1990):86.

———. "Overdoing cleansing or using the wrong products can irritate skin, but the marriage of medicine and cosmetics is helping to better educate consumers," *Vogue* 180 (April 1990):216.

Megahed, H. and Scharffetter-Kochanek, K. "Epidermolysis bullosa acquisita: successful treatment with colchicine," *Archives of Dermatological Research* 286 (1)1994:35–46.

Men's Health editors. "Just a trim, please. Leave some character," *Men's Health* 6 (October 1991):20.

Menter, Marcia. "Winning the wrinkle wars," *Redbook* 177 (October 1991):62–66.

Miller, C. C., *et al.* "Ultraviolet B injury increases prostaglandin synthesis through a tyrosine kinase-dependent pathway," *Journal of Biological Chemistry* 269 (5)(Feb. 4, 1994):3529–3533.

Miller, Laura. "Feeling the heat: sun protection for professionals," *Working Woman* 16 (July 1991):74–77.

Miles, R. H., Paxton, T. P., *et al.* "Systemic administration of interferon-gamma impairs wound healing," *Journal of Surgical Research* 56 (March 1994):288–294.

Mitchnick, Mark. "Microfine zinc oxide: a transparent total sunblock," *Drug & Cosmetic Industry* 153 (August 1993):38–43.

Nish, W. A. "The effects of immunotherapy on cutaneous late phase response to antigen," *Journal of Allergy and Clinical Immunology* 93 (February 1994):484–493.

Novick, Nelson Lee. *Super Skin.* New York: Crown Publishers, 1988.

O'Donnell, Brian Patrick. "Suramin-induced skin reactions," *JAMA* 267 (April 15, 1992):2022.

Ohtake, N., *et al.* "Brown papules and leukoderma in Darier's Disease," *Dermatology* 188 (2)1994:157–159.

Olbricht, Suzanne, Bigby, Michael and Arndt, Kenneth (eds.). *Manual of Clinical Problems in Dermatology.* Boston: Little, Brown and Co., 1992.

Orkin, Milton, Maibach, Howard and Dahl, Mark. *Dermatology.* Norwalk, Conn.: Appleton & Lange, 1991.

Osborne, R. and Perkins, M. A. "An approach for development of alternative test method based on mechanics of skin irritations," *Food and Chemical Toxics* 32 (February 1994):133–142.

Paller, A. S. "Laboratory tests for ichthyosis," *Dermatologic Clinics* 12 (January 1994):99–107.

Patient Care editors. "Melanoma detection: a new, improved method," *Patient Care* 26 (May 30, 1992):13–23.

Pavllichko, Joseph and Band, Phil. "The sci-

ence of minimizing wrinkles," *Soap-Cosmetics-Chemical Specialties* 68 (February 1992):33–37.

Peters, Sue. "A new light on birthmarks," *Health* 7 (Jan.–Feb. 1993):26–27.

Phillips, Tania and Dover, Jeffrey S. "Recent advances in dermatology," *The New England Journal of Medicine* 326 (Jan. 16, 1992):167–179.

Pope, Deborah. "Benign pigmented nevi in children: prevalence and associated factor," *JAMA* 268 (Nov. 18, 1992):2641.

Preston, Diana and Stern, Robert S. "Nonmelanoma cancers of the skin," *The New England Journal of Medicine* 327 (Dec. 3, 1992):1649–1662.

Prevention editors. "Fake and Bake: Indoor tanning is no day at the beach," *Prevention* (May 16, 1993).

———. "Warning spots: mole location may indicate melanoma risk," *Prevention* 42 (July 1990):11–12.

———. "Smoking's new wrinkle," *Prevention* 43 (October 1991):12.

———. "Skin cancer preventive: study shows potential for vitamin A derivative," *Prevention* 42 (Feb. 1990):19–20.

Probert, Christina. *Vogue Beauty and Health Encyclopedia.* London: Octopus Books, 1986.

Rae, Stephen. "Retin-A: acne remedy or wrinkle reducer?" *Modern Maturity* 34 (Dec.–Jan. 1991):76.

Rafal, Elyse, Griffiths, Christopher, Ditre, Cherie, Finkel, Lawrence, Hamilton, Ted, Ellis, Charles and Voorhees, John. "Topical tretinoin treatment for liver spots associated with photodamage," *The New England Journal of Medicine* 326 (February 6, 1992):368–374.

Ralston, Jennie. "The news may still be unpalatable, but the only tan that isn't damaging comes out of a bottle," *Vogue* 180 (March 1990):242–244.

Reali, V. M. "Sonographic evaluation of dermis and subcutaneous tissues during and after skin expansion," *Plastic and Reconstructive Surgery* 93 (5)(April 1994):1050–1055.

Reid, Ken and Vikhanski, Luba. "The sun's ominous side: skin cancer," *Medical World News* 33 (Feb. 1992):18–25.

Roddi, R. "Progressive hemifacial atrophy in patient with lupus erythematosus," *Plastic and Reconstructive Surgery* 93 (5)(April 1994):1067–1072.

Rose, Jeanne. *Kitchen Cosmetics.* Berkeley: North Atlantic Books, 1990.

Rudolf, Patricia. "Is your back fit to bare?" *Redbook* 175 (June 1990):128–129.

Rubenstein, Hal. "Dying of thirst: reviving your skin," *The New York Times Magazine* (March 27, 1994):S18.

Rundle, Rhonda. "Cells 'tricked' to make skin for burn cases," *The Wall Street Journal,* March 17, 1994, B1, E.

Rustad, O. J. "Outdoors and active: relieving summer's siege on skin," *The Physician and Sportsmedicine* 20 (May 1992):162–176.

Ryval, Michael. "The facts about fifth disease: how the virus affects children and pregnant women," *Chatelaine* 66 (Feb. 1993): 32.

Sangiorgio, Maureen, Gutfeld, Greg and Rao, Linda."Helping bad cells age," *Prevention* 44 (February 1992):18–19.

Sangiorgio, Maureen, Meyers, Melissa and Gutfeld, Greg. "So long stretch marks: Vitamin A offshoot may erase unwanted scars," *Prevention* 42 (December 1990):22.

Schempp, Christoph. "Further evidence of Borrelia burgdorferi infection in morphea and lichen schlerosus et atrophicus confirmed by DNA amplification," *JAMA* 270 (Oct. 20, 1993):1801.

Schneider Phyllis. "Skin caring," *Redbook* 174 (Feb. 1990):92–93.

Schneiderman, Henry. "What's your diagnosis: pearly penile papules," *Consultant* 31 (July 1991):39–40.

Schorr, Lia. *Skin Care for Men.* Englewood Cliffs, N.J.: Prentice-Hall, 1985.

———. *Seasonal Skin Care.* Englewood Cliffs, N.J.: Prentice-Hall, 1988.

Science News editors. "Hot answers to some 'bad hair' problems," *Science News* 144 (Dec. 11, 1993):391.

———. "Mutation reveals skin's exposure to sun," *Science News* 145 (Jan. 22, 1994):60.

Scuderi, N. and Onesti, M. G. "Anti-tumor agents," *Annals of Plastic Surgery* 32 (Jan. 1994):39–44.

Shapin, Alice Rindler. "Best faces forward," *Family Circle* 105 (April 21, 1992):15.

Sheehan, M. P. "Oral psoralen photochemotherapy in severe childhood atopic eczema: an update," *JAMA* 270 (Dec. 1, 1993):2550.

Shorell, Irma. *A Lifetime of Skin Beauty.* New York: Simon and Schuster, 1982.

Shum, D. T. "Usefulness of the dissecting microscope in surgical management of skin cancers," *Journal of Dermatologic Surgery and Oncology* 20 (April 1994):266–271.

Siegel, Mary-Ellen. *Safe in the Sun.* New York: Walker and Company, 1990.

Sioutos, N., *et al.* "Primary Cutaneous Hodgkin's Disease," *American Journal of Dermatopathology* 16 (1)(February 1994):2–8.

Smith, Mark. "Saving your skin," *Saturday Evening Post,* April 1994, 32–33.

Smith, Walter P. "Hydroxy acids and skin aging," *Soap-Cosmetics-Chemical Specialties* 69 (September 1993):54–58.

Sommi, Roger W. "Drugs that go on top," *Current Health II* 17 (April 1991):14–15.

Stambler, Irwin. "Tissue R&D produces skin replacements," *R&D* 35 (July 1993):18.

Stehlin, Dori. "Beyond measles and chickenpox: other childhood diseases cause rashes," *FDA Consumer* 26 (April 1992):32–35.

Steigleder, Gerd Klaus and Maibach, Howard. *Pocket Atlas of Dermatology.* New York: Thieme Medical Publishers, 1993.

Sumitra, S., and Yesudian, P. "Friction amyloidosis: a variant or etiologic factor in amyloidosis cuta," *International Journal of*

Dermatology 33 (January 1994):74.

Szentgyorgyi, Tom. "Artificial skin goes on trial," *Popular Science* 238 (April 1991):24.

Tardio, Amy. "The black man's guide to skin care," *Gentleman's Quarterly* 64 (March 1994):174–175.

Teot, L. and Bosse, J. P. "The use of scapular skin island flaps in the treatment of axillary postburn scar contractures," *British Journal of Plastic Surgery* 47 (2)(March 1994):108–111.

Toufexis, Anastasia. "Fountain of youth in a jar," *Time* 138 (Oct. 14, 1991):83–84.

Tran, L. P. *et al.* "Familial multiple glomus tumors," *Annals of Plastic Surgery* 32 (January 1994):89–91.

Ujihara, M., Hamanaka, S., *et al.* "Pemphigus vulgaris associated with autoimmune hemolytic anemia and elevated TNF alpha," *Journal of Dermatology,* 21 (1)(January 1994):56–58.

Valmy, Christine. *Skin Care and Makeup Book.* New York: Crown Publishers, 1982.

Walker, S. L., Morris, J., Chu, A. C. and Yong, A. R. "Relationship between the ability of sunscreens containing 2-ethylhexyl-4-methoxycinnamate to protect against UVA-induced inflammation, depletion of epidermal Langerhans cells and suppression of alloactivating capacity of murine skin in vivo," *Journal of Photochemistry and Photobiology* 22 (January 1994):29–36.

Walzer, Richard. *Healthy Skin: A Guide to Lifelong Skin Care.* Mount Vernon, NY: Consumers' Report Books, 1989.

"Want a shot of sunshine?" *Time* 138 (Dec. 2, 1991):85.

Ward, Debra. "The fresh face: new improved cleansers," *McCall's* 118 (July 1991):42.

Wasco, James. "What your hands say about your health,"*Woman's Day* 53 (Feb. 6, 1990):26.

Weis, Rick. "Melanoma shrinks from human monoclonals,"*Science News* 137 (May 26, 1990):324.

Widmer, J., Elsner, P. and Burg, G. "Skin irritant reactivity following experimental cumulative irritant contact dermatitis," *Contact Dermatitis* 30 (January 1994):35–39.

Wilson, Roberta. "Assaying UVA protection in sunscreen products," *Drug & Cosmetic Industry* 149 (Aug. 1991):24–27.

Winthrop, Anne. "New hope for port-wine stains," *American Baby* 53 (March 1991):12.

Woodley, David, Zelickson, Alvin, Briggaman, Robert, Hamilton, Ted, Weiss, Jonathan, Ellis, Charles, Voorhees, John. "Treatment of photoaged skin with topical tretinoin increases epidermal-dermal anchlring fibrils:a preliminary report," *JAMA* 263 (June 13, 1990):3057–3059.

Wooldridge, Wilfred. "Skin conditions that require further investigation," *Consultant* 32 (Feb. 1992):31–38.

INDEX

Boldface numbers indicate extensive discussion.